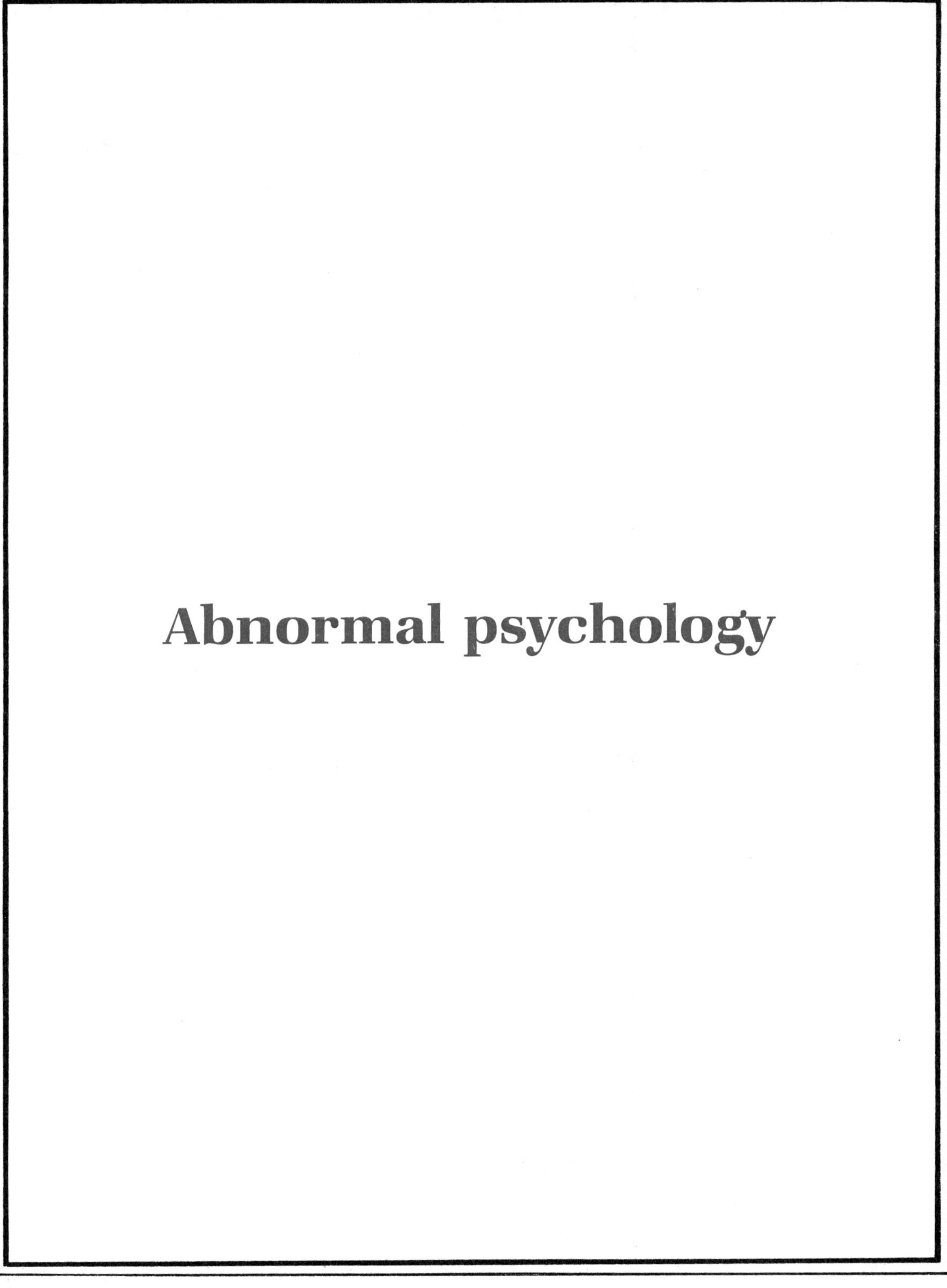

Abnormal psychology

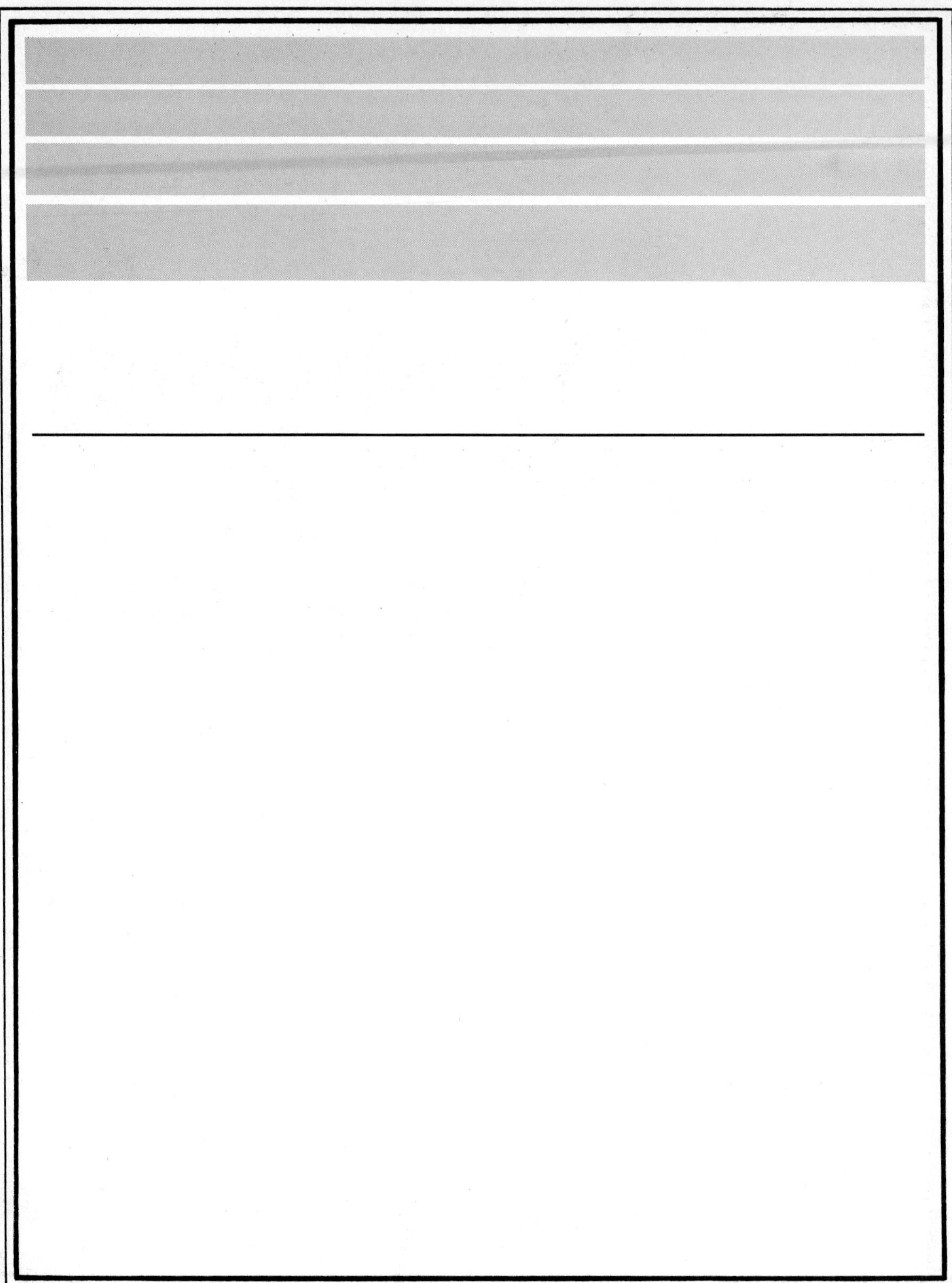

Abnormal Psychology

Joseph Mehr

Chief Psychologist
Elgin Mental Health Center

Elmhurst College

Holt, Rinehart and Winston

NEW YORK CHICAGO SAN FRANCISCO PHILADELPHIA
MONTREAL TORONTO LONDON SYDNEY
TOKYO MEXICO CITY RIO DE JANEIRO MADRID

Publisher: John L. Michel
Acquisitions Editor: Marie A. Schappert
Developmental Editor: Susan H. Hajjar
Senior Project Manager: Arlene D. Katz
Production Manager: Annette Mayeski
Art Director: Bob Kopelman
Managing Editor: Jeanette Ninas Johnson
Text Design: William H. Gray
Cover Design: Jack G. Tauss Associates

Library of Congress Cataloging in Publication Data
Mehr, Joseph, 1941–
Abnormal psychology.
Bibliography: p. 535
Includes index.
1. Psychology, Pathological. I. Title. [DNLM:
1. Psychopathology. 2. Mental disorders. WM 100
M498a]
RC454.M36 1983 616.89 82-21252
ISBN 0-03-056631-2

Address correspondence to:

383 Madison Avenue
New York, N.Y. 10017

Printed in the United States of America
Published simultaneously in Canada

4 5 6 7 032 9 8 7 6 5 4 3 2

CBS COLLEGE PUBLISHING
Holt, Rinehart and Winston
The Dryden Press
Saunders College Publishing

ACKNOWLEDGMENTS

Chapter 1

page 16 Figure 1.3. From *Fundamental Statistics In Psychology and Education* by J. P. Guilford. Copyright © 1956 McGraw-Hill Book Company. Used with the permission of McGraw-Hill Book Company.

Chapter 2

page 35 Figure 2.2. From *Brain Control* by E. S. Valenstein. Copyright © 1973 John Wiley and Sons. Used with the permission of Elliot S. Valenstein and John Wiley and Sons, Inc.

(Continued on p. 570)

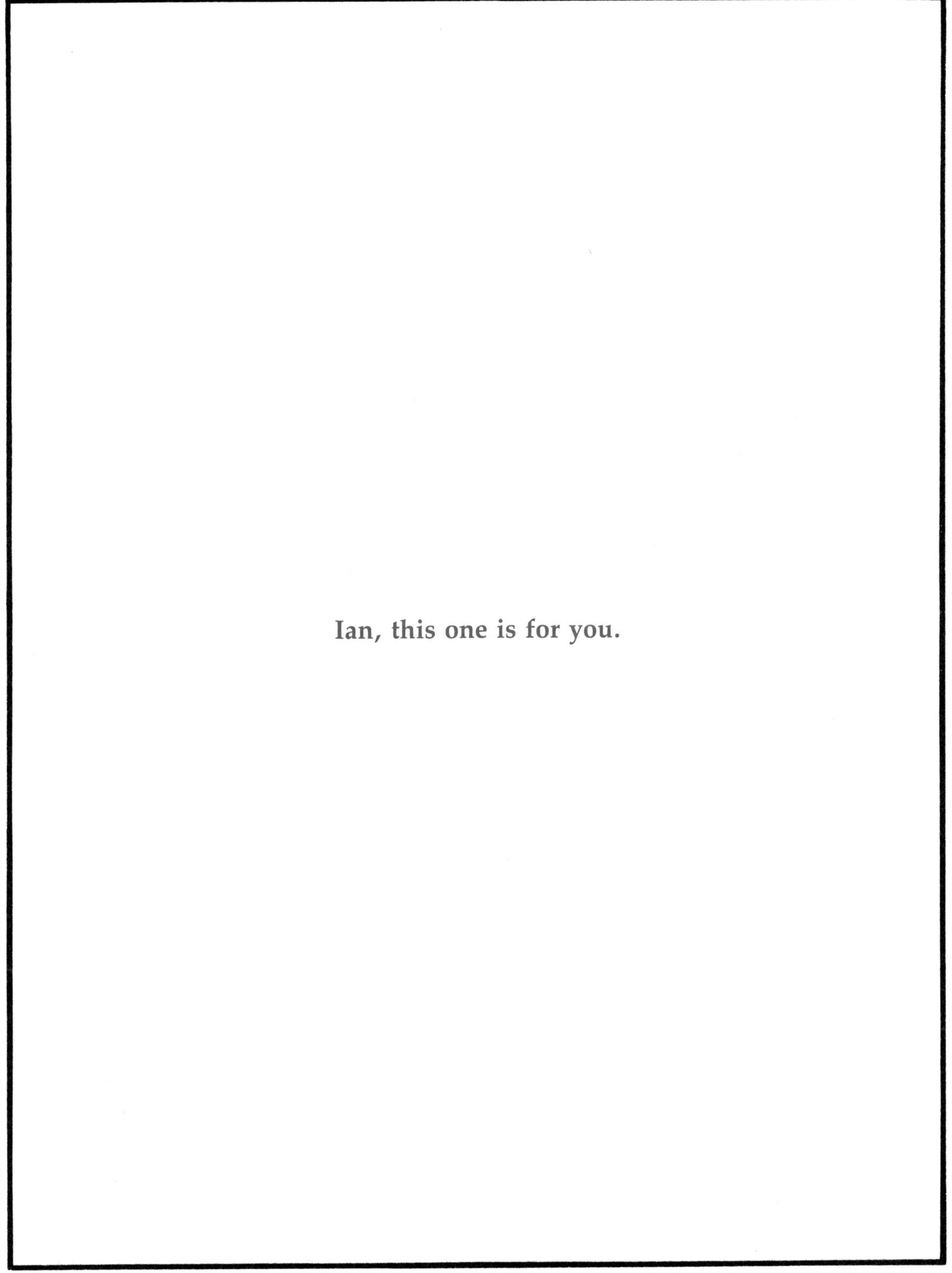

Ian, this one is for you.

Preface

Years of experience both as a classroom instructor and as a clinician in a mental health center have given me a rather useful double-vision. I've interacted with hundreds of troubled people, many of them caught up in the extremes of disordered behavior and personal crises; and I've also stood in front of hundreds of students who were struggling to memorize pages of data, symptoms, and theories about a subject called abnormal psychology.

This dual perspective has shown me that most texts on abnormal psychology fail to communicate to students that working with emotionally disturbed individuals can be a dramatically different experience from reading research studies or learning the theoretical orientations of practicing therapists. This "missing ingredient" in most texts is especially vital to those students who intend to work in clinical settings after school or even before they have completed their academic studies. It also shortchanges the nonmajor—for example, social work, criminal justice, and nursing or medical students—who may walk away from the course with a rather artificial and limited sense of the field.

Therefore when I began writing this text, my primary goal was to help students apply academic/theoretical concepts *accurately* to the real world. In line with this goal, I did not want to leave students wondering, after they read a chapter on a disorder, "What can you do for these problems?" For this reason, the text offers two-part coverage of treatment: each disorder chapter includes a full section on KEY TREATMENTS, graphically distinguished for easy reference. The reader may immediately learn the techniques and usefulness of specific treatment approaches for a given disorder *before* going on to the next chapter. The final part of the text provides a two-chapter evaluation of major treatment approaches and coverage of traditional and alternative systems. This organization also offers flexibility to instructors: they needn't wait until the end of the text to cover treatment and they have the option of dropping parts of the final two chapters if treatment issues are not important in their course.

The second goal in writing this text was to leave students knowing what they need to in the way of facts, and yet, puzzling about questions that even the experts cannot answer—now. I wanted to excite students about the possibilities for learning more about why people behave as they do. That, after all, is what education is about: learning to ask the important questions and then seeking the answers.

To achieve this second goal—which is, in effect, to make the text student-oriented—I've consciously built in a number of features that will prove helpful to instructors as well:

- a balanced presentation of the biological, psychodynamic, behavioral, humanistic, and sociocultural viewpoints in order to show how *various* forces interact to produce disorders and to avoid limiting instructors to a viewpoint they may disagree with
- coverage that is comprehensive and well-developed—that is, all major topics, research data, and current trends—without being encyclopedic
- a balance of phenomenological description, theory, research, and treatment in each chapter in order to give students a well-rounded understanding of the disorders
- consistent presentation of the basic distinctions, criteria, and terminology of DSM-III (*and* the problems associated with this system) so that students can learn the "language" currently used by the majority of clinicians in communicating and comparing information
- analysis of the limitations and implications of selected research in order to encourage critical thinking
- orderly presentation of topics, thorough explanation of terms and concepts, and careful and extensive use of examples so that even the most complex issues are accessible to students

FRAMEWORK

The text is organized so that it can easily be adapted to different course lengths and individual preference without a major change in the instructor's syllabus.

PART I sets the stage for studying disorders by exploring conceptions and definitions of abnormal behavior (including cultural relativism), major theoretical viewpoints which have influenced the diagnosis and treatment of abnormal behavior, and issues of classification and all major assessment techniques. Chapter 2 includes fictionalized vignettes to bring to life major historical conceptions of abnormal behavior.

PART II presents disorders traditionally associated with stress and anxiety, and covers the major theories and current research about the causes of these disorders. The chapter on Disorders of Psychophysiology requires no special background in physiology.

PART III deals with behaviors that are problems not only for the individual but which also can be of concern to society, including sexual deviations, substance abuse, and the antisocial personality. Chapter 11 includes up-to-date coverage of personality disorders (such as avoidant, borderline, narcissistic, and compulsive disorder) neglected in some other texts.

PART IV provides comprehensive coverage of the theory, research, and treatment of the schizophrenic disorders, including characteristic patterns of behavior, diagnosis, major types, genetic and biochemical theories, psychodynamic issues, and formulations using learning theory. Additionally, this part offers full chapter coverage of the paranoid disorders.

PART V explores the clinical features, theories, and treatment of the affective disorders and includes coverage of suicide and its prevention.

PART VI begins with disorders of childhood, follows with a full chapter on mental retardation (including issues related to adult retardation), and ends with a chapter on organic mental disorders that develop in adulthood.

PART VII concludes the text. The first chapter examines varieties of biological, intrapsychic, and behavioral (including cognitive) therapy approaches, reviews relevant research on their usefulness, and concludes with a section on the characteristics of effective therapists. The last chapter focuses on varieties of hospital treatment settings, legal issues related to those with disorders (including coverage of the insanity defense), alternatives to private practice and inpatient hospitalization, and problems associated with deinstitutionalization.

AIDS TO TEACHING AND LEARNING

I wanted to select pedagogical techniques and devices that would be useful and enhance the teaching/learning effectiveness of the text, rather than simply cluttering the text with distracting elements. Some of the following aids have proven useful in a variety of texts; others were derived from my own perception of student needs:

Part Openers These introductions provide students and instructors with an immediate overview of the chapters which follow and the rationale for grouping them.

Chapter Outlines Outlines of the major headings in the chapter give a sense of the scope of topics that the student will be expected to learn and provide a structure for reading and studying.

Case Studies Throughout the text, original and reprinted case studies provide a sense of variations within a given disorder and help to cultivate understanding and empathy for individuals manifesting disordered behavior.

Key Treatments These are distinct sections near the end of each disorder chapter that provide discussions of specific treatments immediately after coverage of clinical description, theories, and research about the disorder.

Chapter Summary All chapters include a numbered summary to reinforce learning of major themes, ideas, and concepts.

Key Terms Each chapter ends with a Key Term box to help familiarize students with new concepts and selected vocabulary items. Vocabulary terms are also *boldfaced* and defined within each chapter, as well as listed and defined in an end of text glossary.

Highlights Numbered boxed features, called Highlights, are judiciously used throughout the text. They provide background information, in-depth views, or interesting contemporary and historical issues related to the text proper.

Illustrations The text contains over 200 photos, figures, and tables intended to stimulate and facilitate learning. All figures and tables are cross-referenced in the text so that the student understands where and how they are relevant to what he or she is reading.

Glossary, Bibliography, and Name/Subject Indexes At end of text.

INSTRUCTOR'S MANUAL WITH TEST BANK

This text is complemented by a thorough, well-developed *Instructor's Manual with Test Bank* designed to help the instructor organize and effectively present the subject matter; to motivate students to learn and reflect upon information provided in the text; and to spark and enhance classroom discussion.

The *Instructor's Manual* consists of three parts: (1) Introductory materials; (2) a Chapter-by-Chapter review, including **Learning Objectives, Chapter Outline, Chapter Synopsis, Key Terms, Lecture Suggestions and Student Activities** (with references to research materials), **Recommended Additional Readings,** and an annotated list of **Audio-Visual Materials;** (3) 25–45 **Multiple Choice Questions** for each chapter with each question keyed to the appropriate page in the text.

A SPECIAL NOTE

Over twenty years ago, as a first year geology major (of all things!) I enrolled in a course in introductory psychology. I had almost no idea of what it was about other than the brief description given in the college catalogue. That course was taught by a brilliant, eccentric man whose lectures ranged from astronomy to music and from philosophy to death, sex, and taxes. His dramatic flair for teaching 300 students in an auditorium was awesome. Carl Smith, a Harvard graduate, acquaintance of B. F. Skinner, friend of Bertrand Russell, and graduate assistant to Henry Murray at the Harvard Psychological Clinic was instrumental in showing a naive midwestern adolescent that psychology was an incredibly fascinating and provocative subject. Carl made me ask questions and seek answers. A year later I had the good fortune to take several courses with Albert Hunsicker, a clinical psychologist par excellance. His acquaintance with the field, his insight, understanding, warmth, and brilliance impressed me as much as Carl Smith, though they were very different sorts of people.

Today, Hunsicker and Smith still serve as important models for my own career as a college instructor and a clinical psychologist. They instilled in me a fascination with the study of abnormal behavior. I hope this text serves that same end.

ACKNOWLEDGMENTS

A number of professional colleagues invested much time and hard work in assessing this text and contributing to its development at one or several points along the way. They offered guidance and valuable insights based on their experience as instructors as well as their in-depth understanding of the field. I wish it had been possible to implement all of their suggestions:

Harold Arkowitz, University of Arizona; Jeanne D. Brugger, Drexel University; Ronald G. Evans, Washburn University of Topeka; Robert W. Grossman, Kalamazoo College; Theodore Millon, University of Miami; Joseph J. Palladino, Indiana State University-Evansville; Barry D. Smith, University of Maryland. I owe a special note of thanks to William T. McReynolds, University of Tampa, for his sustained effort, from first through final drafts, in providing guidance not only about content but also about the quality of expression.

During the time it has taken to solidify my ideas into final form many other thanks have become due. I am grateful to the students who complained that the texts I was using were not interesting, since this led me to think about writing my own abnormal psychology text. I offer my thanks to Baxter Venable who actually started me writing the book and to Marie Schappert, Acquisitions Editor, who expertly guided the text to publication. Susan Hajjar, Developmental Editor, deserves more praise and appreciation than this brief space allows. Consistently encouraging as well as demanding, Susan brought a keen analytical ability to assessing the manuscript and the reviewer suggestions and an uncommon dedication and skill to teaching me how to express myself as clearly as I could. Arlene Katz, Senior Project Editor, skillfully maneuvered the text through the interminable final stage with its myriad production details and decisions. I must thank all the students in my classes who helped in many ways as I was writing the text. I am especially and deeply grateful to those who typed long hours for me: Imogene Diebert, a good friend who gave many hours of personal time in typing the early drafts; Nancy Harrison and Judy Lindquist who took over the pressured and tedious job of typing the final drafts. Finally, I cannot put into words the thanks I owe to my son Ian, who coped with my strange preoccupation with late hours, yellow writing pads, and 2½-hardness lead pencils.

Brief Contents

Contents

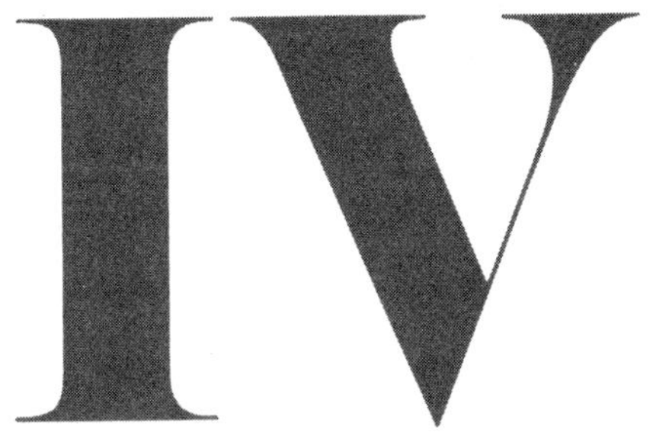

Schizophrenia and paranoid psychoses 285

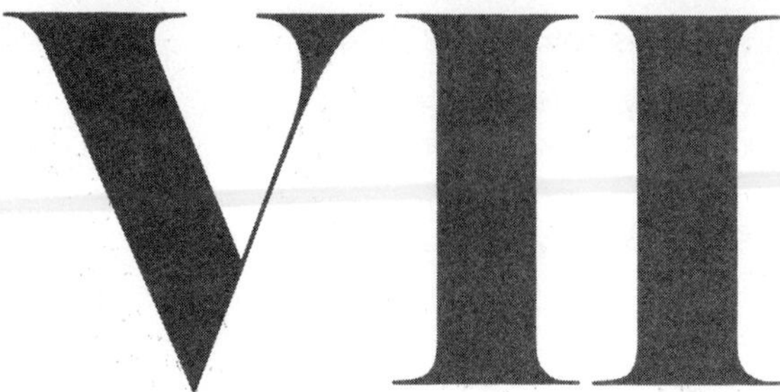

Therapy and treatment in the social context 465

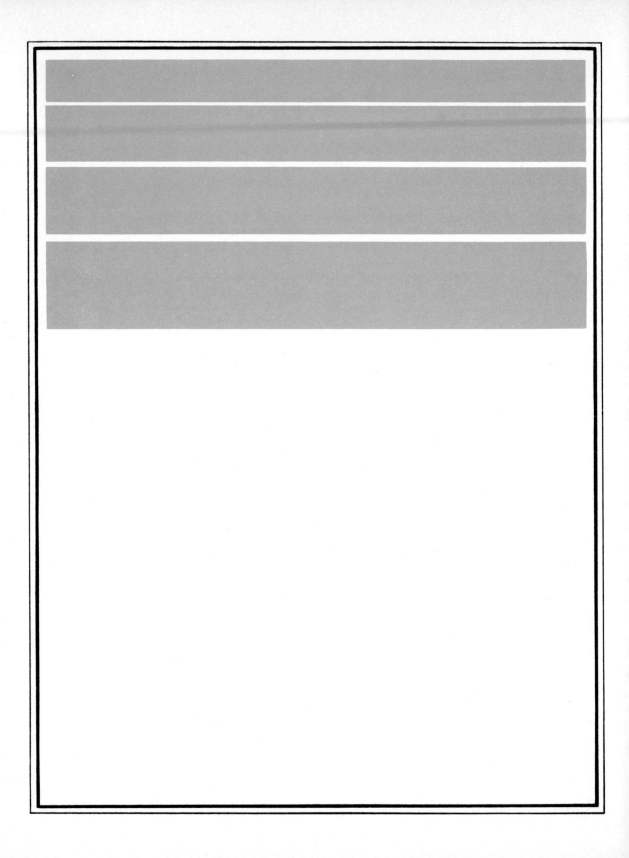

AN INTRODUCTION TO ABNORMAL BEHAVIOR

Abnormal psychology studies complex behaviors that have in some way become identified as abnormal. Part I introduces ideas and facts that will assist the reader to understand the complex behaviors covered in subsequent sections.

In Chapter 1, several ways of identifying behavior as abnormal are presented. Because various approaches to the identification of abnormal behavior exist, we may find disagreement about whether a specific behavior is abnormal. Chapter 1 also considers the extent to which abnormal behavior is a problem for our society, and ends with a presentation of formal procedures for studying behavior.

The field of study called abnormal psychology has not developed in a vacuum; there is a long tradition of concern about problem behavior. Chapter 2 examines the perspectives about abnormal behavior which have been held throughout history, and stresses three particularly important contemporary perspectives: the views that behavior is due to 1. inner psychological functioning, 2. learning, or 3. physiological factors. Chapter 2 emphasizes that views about the cause of abnormal behavior are influenced by the prevailing attitudes and beliefs held by a culture at a particular time.

In Chapter 3, modern perspectives about the development of behavior are presented in detail. These perspectives include Freud's psychoanalytic perspective, humanistic psychology, the learned behavior perspective, the physiological perspective, and the sociocultural perspective. Each of these perspectives has contributed to the understanding of abnormal behavior. In later chapters on specific abnormal behaviors, the contributions of these viewpoints will be presented.

The assessment and classification of abnormal behavior is an important activity in abnormal psychology. In Chapter 4, the purposes and techniques of assessment are presented. In addition, the benefits and problems in classifying abnormal behavior are considered, and a major current classification system called DSM-III is described. This classification system will often be used to organize the presentation of information about various behaviors in this text.

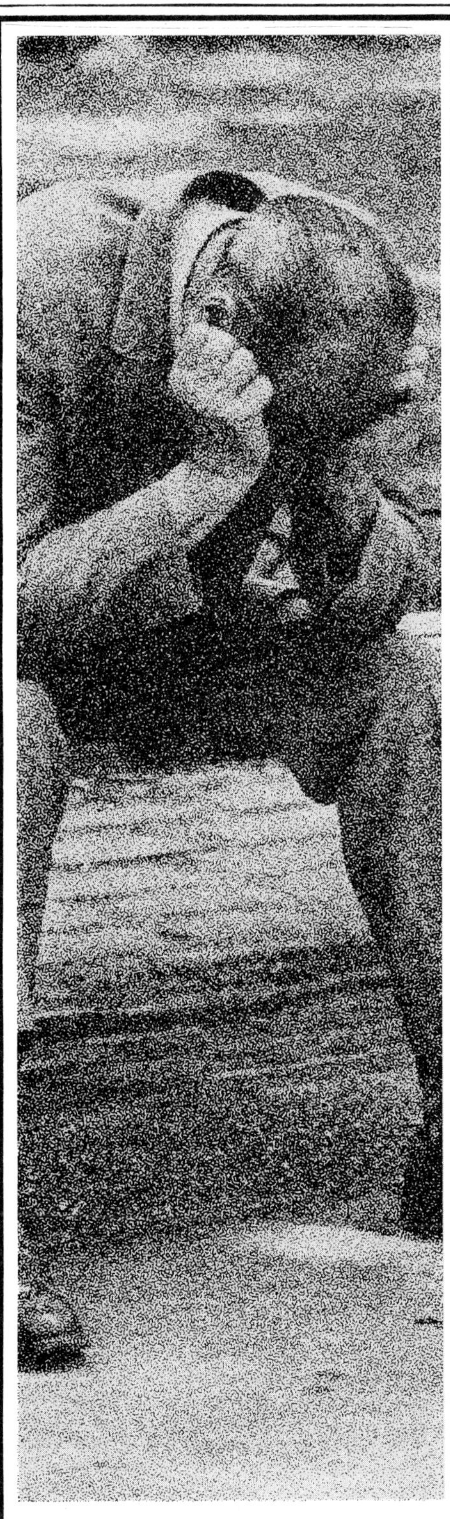

An overview of abnormal behavior

- Factors influencing the definition of abnormal behavior
- Abnormal people or abnormal behaviors?
- How big is the problem?
- The scientific study of abnormal behavior
- Orientation of the text
- Organization of the text
- Summary
- Key terms

When people behave as we expect them to, we rarely question the reasons behind their actions. But when others' behaviors seem unusual, surprising, or unpredictable, we begin to wonder, Why? Which of the following individuals behave in a way that leads you to question the reasons for their behavior:

1. An elderly widow stops attending a community socialization program after becoming unusually quiet and withdrawn for a few weeks. Upon visiting her boardinghouse, a social worker finds her to be fearful and hostile, shouting, swearing, and holding conversations with the television.
2. Soon after her husband abandons her, Mrs. H. stops eating and neglects her personal appearance. She becomes depressed, agitated, and cries almost constantly. Her landlord sees her aimlessly wandering the streets, shouting her husband's name. Wearing dirty, ragged clothing, she is hysterical and alternately rude or polite. Mrs. H. tells the landlord that if she cannot find her husband, "evil men will rape me."
3. Nine-year-old Billy panics at the idea of going to school. His father brings him to school, but he won't enter the building. Billy becomes nauseated, sobs, trembles, and feels like he cannot breathe. Unable to explain the sudden development of this fear to his distraught parents, Billy subsequently misses two months of classes and may be left back unless he begins attending school.
4. A middle-aged woman living alone barricades her hotel room, floods the floor with water, starts fires in wastebaskets, tears up money, and throws it out the window. After being evicted, she camps in the hotel lobby until ejected by the police. She hears "voices" telling her to do "bad" things; she says people are "out to get me" and that they follow her everywhere.
5. Mr. R. is young, single, and employed as an advertising copy editor. Others perceive him as happy and outgoing, but he feels shy and uncomfortable around others. He has a hard time asking women for dates and envies those who have the "gift of gab." He sees himself as passive and ineffectual, and wishes he could be different.
6. Mrs. M. is a 32-year-old mother of two young boys. She has a good marriage and lives comfortably from a material standpoint. However, she is unhappy and dissatisfied, feels that "something" is missing in her life. She no longer feels "close" to her husband. Lately, she alternates between daydreaming about having a career and feeling depressed.
7. Mr. K., 47 years old, has "retired" from a metropolitan fire department, in part because of his inability to remain sober for an extended time. Since his retirement, he has been unsuccessfully hospitalized in alcoholism treatment programs 21 times. He has frequently been arrested on misdemeanor charges. Friends and family expect him to end up on "Skid Row." He denies he has a drinking problem.

Some of the behaviors illustrated in these short cases may seem incomprehensible and unreasonable, and you might agree that "something must be wrong." Other behaviors are less dramatic, but still puzzling. Would you identify each of these individuals as **abnormal?** Do you think they identify themselves as abnormal? We could probably obtain a high level of agreement about the abnormality of some of these behaviors. Most people would probably agree that Mrs. H. (No. 2) engaged in abnormal behavior after her husband's desertion, although *she* might disagree. Less agreement is likely when people such as depressed Mrs. M. (No. 6) or shy young Mr. R. (No. 5) are considered. Their behaviors are less extreme and more familiar to us, but they did consider themselves to be abnormal (in the broadest sense) when they decided to seek help in changing their behaviors. Terms such as **emotional disorder** or emotional upset are often applied to these less extreme behaviors.

The field of **abnormal psychology** is concerned with a wide range of behaviors like those illustrated above. Professionals in this field try to find out why disturbed or disturbing behavior occurs; they also attempt to determine what can be done to prevent or alter such behavior. We care about abnormal behavior because of: 1. the internal misery it can bring to those who express it, 2. the problems of those who must have contact with it, and 3. the things we can learn about the study of human behavior in general.

In the search for answers to the questions of cause, prevention, and treatment, the student of abnormal psychology will encounter a broad range of behaviors—some very unusual, others quite familiar—because abnormality can be defined in a number of ways.

FACTORS INFLUENCING THE DEFINITION OF ABNORMAL BEHAVIOR

The typical person's identification of what is and what is not abnormal varies considerably upon his or her viewpoint. For example, some individuals might consider promiscuous sexual behavior abnormal because they think it is due to an extreme need for affection which cannot be satisfied by moderate sexual activity. An individual of deep religious faith might consider the behavior to be sinful, a sign of moral weakness, rather than as due to emotional disturbance. Others might consider the behavior to be quite normal because they believe that "sex is healthy, and our society is more tolerant of it now." To some extent, disagreement also exists among scientists and practitioners who study and work with **behavior disorders** (see Highlight 1.1). Mental health professionals also are influenced by their personal values. However, professionals' education and training emphasize some factors over others in the identification of behavior as abnormal. Among the factors that various experts see as important are: 1. a person's degree of subjective discomfort, 2. comparisons of the person's behavior to some ideal standard, 3. the statistical frequency of a behavior, and 4. the cultural context in which the behavior occurs.

Subjective Discomfort

Many people define or identify themselves as "abnormal" because of a subjective sense of personal discomfort. Feeling that one should be happier, less depressed, less anxious, or more independent can cause subjective distress. The subjective distress may become great enough to result in a self-perception of being abnormal or "different" from other people. This self-perception may motivate some persons to seek help from a mental health profes-

HIGHLIGHT 1.1
PROFESSIONALS WHO WORK WITH ABNORMAL BEHAVIOR

Most individuals recognize that abnormal behaviors can have multiple causes, so that those who seek treatment may benefit greatly from the training and expertise of professionals trained in differing fields. The major professionals one might encounter in clinical settings include the following:

1. *Psychiatrist.* Psychiatrists are physicians, with an M.D. degree from a medical school. Following four years of medical school, the individual obtains three and sometimes four more years of training in a psychiatric hospital or other mental health facility. The training consists of study and practice in diagnosis, psychotherapy, and use of medical techniques such as drug therapy in the treatment of abnormal behaviors. Since psychiatrists are physicians, they can prescribe medication.
2. *Clinical Psychologist.* This individual has a Ph.D. from a university. The doctoral training includes work in personality, diagnostic assessment, psychotherapy, and may also include courses in neuropsychology, **psychopathology,** behavior modification, physiology, and so on. The Ph.D. degree is awarded upon successful completion of course work, practicum experience, and a doctoral dissertation, which is an original research study. Thus, the clinical psychologist receives training not only in diagnosis and therapeutic techniques but also in the means necessary to conduct and evaluate research in areas relevant to the study of the causes, treatment, and prevention of abnormal behavior. The clinical psychologist spends at least one year in an internship, usually at a psychiatric hospital or other mental health setting such as a community mental health center.
3. *Psychiatric Social Worker.* The social worker may have a bachelor's, master's, or in some cases a doctoral degree. Most social workers employed as psychiatric social workers have a M.S.W. (master's in social work) degree.
4. *Psychoanalyst.* A psychoanalyst receives intensive training (including his or her own personal analysis) in the theoretical and therapeutic application of psychoanalysis. While most psychoanalysts have M.D. or Ph.D. degrees, neither is absolutely necessary. Sigmund Freud was quite explicit in stating that one need not be medically trained in order to be a psychoanalyst.

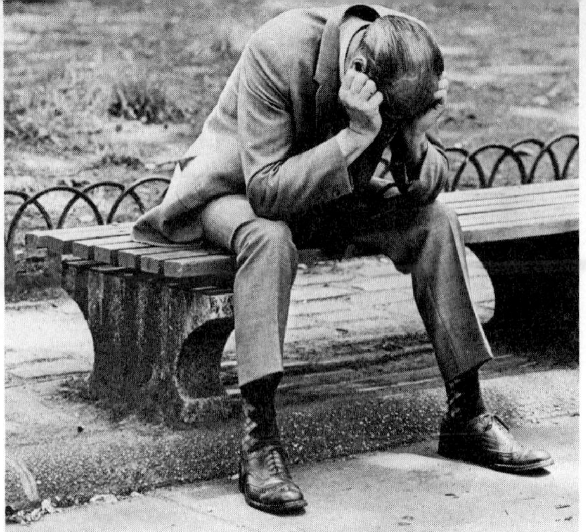

At times subjective discomfort may be shown in overt behavior.

sional, who may or may not confirm their self-perception.

Identifying oneself as abnormal (or upset) involves personal value judgments. That one's feelings, thoughts, or behaviors are "just not right." In the examples that opened this chapter, Mr. R., the shy young man, and Mrs. M., the depressed young mother, seem most representative of the subjective discomfort criteria for abnormality. In more extreme examples, the subjective discomfort may be visible to others. For example, a person's subjective depression may become apparent to others when the depressed person has difficulty concentrating at work, frequent crying episodes, or loss of appetite over a long period. As Mr. K.'s drinking illustrates, some people behave in ways that disturb others more than themselves. The criterion of subjective discomfort does not fit them. Some patients hospitalized in psychiatric institutions report no feelings of subjective discomfort, yet elements of their behavior were sufficiently **maladaptive** and disturbing to others to lead to the patients' institutionalization.

Comparison to an Ideal State

Some behavior may be identified as abnormal because it falls short of some ideal or optimal level of functioning. People commonly believe that the achievement of happiness is such an ideal state, but most experts see optimal functioning as more complex than reaching a goal like happiness. The specific definitions of an ideal state vary with the theoretical framework from which the expert views human behavior. However, these theorists share the view that if people have sufficient growth opportunities, an optimal level of functioning is within the potential of all human beings. By defining the attributes of optimum health or psychological functioning, these experts imply that falling short of these goals constitutes a serious problem. Marie Jahoda (1959) a social psychologist has summarized the major common elements in the definitions of optimal functioning proposed by a number of theorists (e.g., Allport, 1961; Maslow & Mittleman, 1951; C. R. Rogers, 1961; Shoben, 1957). The common elements include the following:

1. Attitudes towards the self. Most definitions of optimal functioning suggest that a person's self-concept should be accurate, and that people should be accepting of their view of themselves.
2. Growth, development, and self-actualization. Optimal functioning includes an ability to grow and to develop and to be invested in living and the future, rather than remaining static or living in the past.
3. Autonomy. The individual should be self-reliant and able to decide what best meets his or her own needs, rather than rely too heavily on the opinions of others.
4. Integration. A person should have a well-balanced personality and a sense of meaning in life. The person should not overemphasize some needs (e.g., power or security) over other needs (e.g., love and play).
5. Perception of reality. One must be free of distortions of reality, and be able to perceive one's real needs.
6. Environmental mastery. The person should have the ability to love, should be adequate in work and play, adequate in human relationships, and should be effective in problem solving.

The use of optimal functioning or an ideal state as a criterion against which to measure behavior has been criticized for several reasons. For example, when the definition of normality is based on what a person "should" be, value judgments become important factors (Horton, 1971). Who is to be the judge of what a person "should" be? In addition, many definitions of ideal functioning use modifying terms such as "adequate," "excessive," and "realistic." Such terms are open to interpretation, so that the definition's meaning will vary greatly from one user to another. How secure must one feel to have "adequate" feelings of security?

Definitions of an ideal level of functioning are often based on conceptions of personality which are neither well tested nor supported. In many cases, those who devise the criteria have not been interested in the experimental verification of their ideas. Rather, they are often interested in providing viewpoints different from prevailing notions of personality functioning.

In reading the list of common elements in definitions of optimal function, you may have developed a nagging doubt about how many people could meet these criteria. Indeed, one major criticism of these definitions as yardsticks of human behavior is that most people may never reach an idealized level of functioning (see Korchin, 1976). If most of us will never reach the idealized level of functioning, then it follows from this ideal viewpoint that a very large majority of us are, in fact, abnormal! An approach that would label so many of us abnormal because we do not reach an ideal level of behavior creates obvious problems for those who wish to use the approach.

The Statistical Approach

The underlying premise of the statistical approach is that the intensity, frequency, or type of behaviors or characteristics which are seen in most of the human population are **normal** (average), while behaviors or characteristics which occur in the minority are abnormal. From this perspective, abnormal behaviors differ from normal ones quantitatively, not qualitatively. For example, anger is normal until it becomes intense enough to be counterproductive. Anxiety is normal until it becomes intense enough to interfere with functioning. The converse also seems true. Low intensity of emotions can cause difficulties, too. If students experience no pretest anxiety, they are unlikely to study; and if individuals almost never become angry, they will probably be taken advantage of. It is not unusual to be sad or depressed occasionally, but if a person is depressed often or constantly, this is likely to be considered abnormal either by the person or by others. An individual who occasionally gets intoxicated is not particularly unusual; if he or she becomes inebriated several times each week, the label of abnormal could be applied.

The application of statistical definitions of abnormality involves the measurement of many behaviors in large groups of people. The results are then used to determine the distribution of the measurements. One common finding is that the measurements are distributed on a bell-shaped, or **normal probability curve.** For example, measurements of intelligence are distributed in the population in this fashion. Figure 1.1 represents the normal distribution of IQ (Intelligence Quotient) scores. Based on this distribution of scores, "normal" can be defined

Figure 1.1. A normal distribution, or bell-shaped curve.
This normal probability curve illustrates a statistical definition of normal (average) and abnormal intelligence. A Wechsler IQ of 70 is the cut-off point separating mental retardation from normal intelligence.

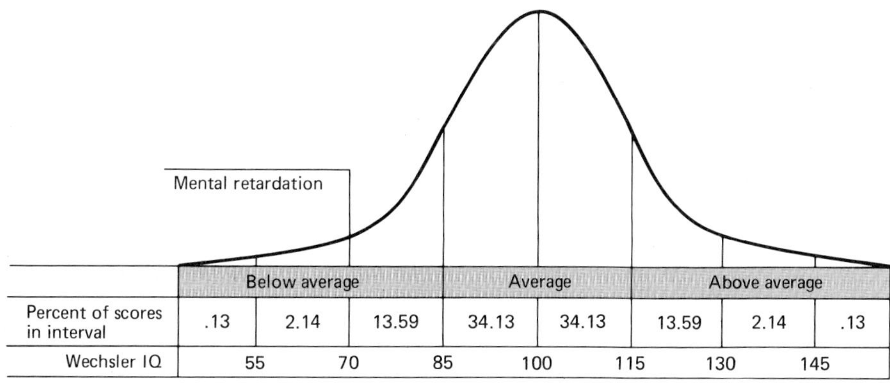

as an IQ of approximately 85–115, and abnormality can be defined as scores at the extremes of the curve: mental retardation as below 70, and the very superior as above 130. In this example, "abnormal intelligence" occurs at both extremes of the distribution and is present in almost 5 percent of the population.

If the thought of defining a desirable characteristic such as superior IQ as abnormal seems odd, you have identified one of the difficulties of the statistical approach. It does not provide a basis for differentiating between positive and negative behavior. Obviously, there is more to defining behaviors as abnormal than intensity or frequency. Some frequent behaviors are considered "abnormal" because of our social values, moral codes, and the behaviors' undesirable effects on those who display them. Furthermore, while many abnormal behaviors are infrequent, some infrequent behaviors are seen as highly positive aspects of humanity. In addition to high intelligence, other examples of infrequent but desirable characteristics include emotional warmth, self-sacrifice, and self-understanding.

The statistical approach also requires a judgment of which aspects of human behavior are "significant," and therefore subject to measurement, and a judgment of whether the behavior should be frequent or infrequent. In addition, in order to utilize this approach, we must be able to measure significant physical, psychological, behavioral, and social characteristics with a reasonable degree of accuracy. For the most part, particularly in the area of internal psychological processes, this is a very difficult task. However, presuming that the ability to measure these characteristics is sufficient (as in measuring intelligence), cut-off points which separate the range of normal functioning from abnormal functioning are then set (see Figure 1.1). The cut-off point which has been established to separate mental retardation from normal intelligence is an IQ of 70. Is an IQ of 65 really that different from an IQ of 75? Someone has set an artificial level above (or below) which the behavior receives a different label. Depending upon where the points are placed, individuals may be viewed differently (and treated differently), even though there may be little functional difference between them. The cut-off point for **mental retardation,** for example, could just as easily have been set at 55 as 70 (see Figure 1.1). We should remember no sharp clear-cut dividing lines exist between normal and abnormal behavior. The lines that do exist have been put there by someone.

Cultural Context

Some observers view the degree of abnormality or normality of behavior as dependent upon the types of behavior which are accepted or even promoted by the particular culture or society in which the individual lives. From this viewpoint of **cultural relativism,** abnormality depends on cultural context. Abnormality is culturally relative. Consider the following examples:

1. A girl is sitting in front of her home cutting intricate patterns into her flesh with a knife and rubbing mud and ashes into the open bleeding wounds.
2. A man convulses, falls to the ground, babbles in an incomprehensible language, and sees what he calls "demons" (which no one else can see) hovering over a bystander. He then engages in an argument with the demons and drives them away.
3. A man inserts thin rigid pieces of wire (almost four inches long) completely up the opening of his penis because God has told him that this act will give him strength.

Are any of these people manifesting abnormal behavior? When the cultural context of these individuals is considered, only the man in the third example is. In the first example, the girl is a member of the Korongo tribe of Africa, where scars are used to enhance beauty. In the second example, the man is a member of a fundamentalist Christian sect in the United States which values "visitations" of the Holy Spirit manifested in visions and "speaking in tongues." The man in the third example, however, is engaging in a behavior that violates the standards of his friends, relatives, and the community at large.

Our culture or society provides the fabric in which we live. When individuals gather in groups, certain patterns of conduct develop and become the standard for acceptable behavior within the group. These preferred patterns of behavior are called **norms.** When the patterns of conduct are made explicit, they are often formalized as rules or laws (Tapp & Levine, 1977). Other patterns of behavior are not formally prohibited, but are not considered appropriate. Scheff (1966) has described these behaviors as violating subtle or inexplicit rules. For example, no explicit rule or law prohibits one from inserting a wire up one's penis (in fact, some sanctioned medical procedures are roughly similar). However, this behavior appears to violate the rules of normative behavior in our culture.

From the cultural relativist's perspective, normality is behavior that is congruent with society's expectations or norms. Abnormality (or deviance) is behavior that varies sufficiently from the norms of the group so that, if known, it becomes a basis for negative sanctions (Wood, 1974). The sanctions may be formal such as legal action, or informal such as rejection by others. Since individuals belong to many different groups, a person may violate the norms of a larger group such as "society" (and be considered a deviant in that context) by adhering to the norms of a subcultural group. For example, most authorities agree that many criminals value law-breaking activities, and devalue "straight," or law-abiding, behavior. Within the criminal subculture, crime is normative, accepted, and promoted by one's peers.

Behaviors which are accepted in one culture may be considered abnormal if a person does them in a different cultural context. In the U.S., the cosmetic scarring on this Ugandan woman's body would be considered abnormal.

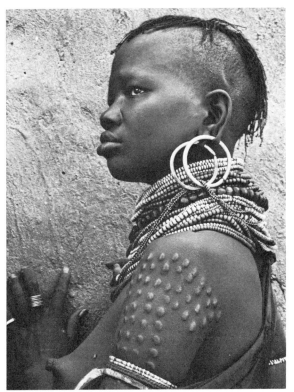

The view that behavior is normal or abnormal depending on its cultural context is supported by studies which have compared the norms of different cultural groups. Many studies have demonstrated that some behaviors considered abnormal or **deviant** in our culture are accepted and expected or required in other cultures. In addition, some of our normal behaviors are seen as abnormal by other cultures. Boas (1919) was the first to describe an example of such cultural reversal. Boas found that in order to gain prestige, tribal chiefs of the Canadian Northwest Coast Indians conducted a "potlatch" ceremony, in which they gave all their material possessions to their rivals. To these Indians, a typical United States citizen's interest in obtaining and possessing material goods would seem abnormal. Of course, in our culture, the behavior of these chiefs would be considered deviant.

Many other examples of cultural relativism exist. Benedict (1934a, 1934b) found that in the Zuni Indian culture, an individual with the initiative and drive common to our modern culture would be "branded as a witch and hung by his thumbs." Among some Plains Indians and Indians of the far Southwest, drug-induced hallucinatory states are common to religious experiences and accepted, valued, and sought, rather than treated as a sign of severe abnormality. In fact, members of these religious groups can legally possess and use chemical substances such as mescaline to induce such states. Recent studies support the idea that cultures differ in labeling behaviors as normal or abnormal. These studies (e.g., Kiev, 1969; Rubel, 1964; Yap, 1965) provide additional examples of cultural reversals.

A major problem in identifying behavior as normal or abnormal exclusively in terms of cultural context is that certain abnormal or deviant behaviors are found in virtually all cultures.

For example, no cultures (identified to date) are totally free of disorders such as anxiety or depression. While the incidence of these disorders varies from culture to culture, the presence of these disorders in all cultures suggests at least some behaviors we identify as abnormal are either partly "culture-free" or that all cultures view certain behaviors as unacceptable.

Cultural relativism also does not take into account the possibility that a whole society could be abnormal—a "sick society" (Naroll, 1969). A particular society's norms may be abnormal when viewed from a broader perspective. An example is the persecution and genocide of the Jews in Nazi Germany. In that setting, prejudiced behavior toward Jews was "normal," and those who did not participate in this behavior were labeled "deviant" or "abnormal." In Japan, suicide is viewed as an honorable course for defeated generals, captains of sinking ships, and officials who have betrayed the public trust. This custom is known as *hara-kiri.* During World War II, young Japanese aviators attempted to sink United States ships by crashing their planes onto the ships. Killing oneself in this fashion was viewed as a supreme sacrifice for the emperor. These *kamikaze* pilots were seen as engaging in an honorable task. While suicide is considered abnormal in most cultures, it is considered acceptable and even honorable under certain circumstances in Japan.

Which Definition Do We Use?

In our daily life, individuals are typically identified as abnormal through the application of a combination of the perspectives we have discussed, rather than a single one. When you label someone's behavior as "weird," "flaky," "hyper," "strung out," or **crazy,** or when you feel that something about your own behavior is not "right," these perspectives may come into play. Behaviors are labeled abnormal because: 1. the person exhibiting or experiencing the behavior feels it is a problem, 2. the individual fails to reach an optimal standard, 3. the behavior deviates from a statistical norm, or 4. the behavior violates cultural norms. Behavior that fits one or more of these criteria is troublesome either to the person with the behavior or to others, and thus may be called abnormal. This is the sense in which the term "abnormal" is applied to behavior in this text. While the strictest definition of abnormal means "away from the norm," some of the behaviors to be discussed occur with a high frequency. They are included because they lead to serious personal distress. Other behaviors are included because they are culturally or socially unacceptable, even though they do not cause the individual subjective distress.

ABNORMAL PEOPLE OR ABNORMAL BEHAVIORS?

The human behaviors that are called abnormal based on the criteria that have been formulated are usually perceived as negative. They cause the person or society a great deal of distress. In the following chapters, many case histories will be used to illustrate the painful consequences of disturbed behavior. Because of these consequences, it is customary to suggest or imply that such behaviors be changed, treated, or modified. In fact, most people with these disorders would rather behave differently, but some would not.

Human behavior is extremely complex, and there is much to learn about behaviors that are called abnormal. Consider the following three cases. Are these people abnormal? Do they need treatment? Would they be happier, more functional, and make greater contributions to society if their problem behaviors did not exist?

> An adolescent girl is placed in the custody of her grandmother. Her mother is separated from an alcoholic husband, who has since died. The girl is quite homely and rejected by her mother; at times the girl lies and steals. In her fantasies she lived as her father's housemistress, wishing she could take her mother's place. In spite of her father's alcoholism, the girl is very fond of him.
>
> The grandmother has not been able to manage her own children, and is determined to "do it right" with her granddaughter. She does not send the girl to elementary school, dresses her in strange clothing, and insists that the girl wear a back brace. The girl is not allowed to have playmates.
>
> In adulthood, the girl marries a lawyer who becomes extremely successful and prominent.

Their relationship is less than satisfactory from his perspective, and he later obtains a mistress. His mistress is his true love, but he does not obtain a divorce because he fears the effect it would have on his career. His wife adjusts to the situation, turning from the relationship to find satisfaction in other pursuits. Their marriage becomes a sham maintained primarily for social reasons.

A boy is developmentally slow, not speaking until age 4. He is a poor student, fails mathematics, has few friends, and seems to "live within himself." Teachers consider him a problem child. His father is ashamed of him because he lacks athletic ability.

The boy has many odd mannerisms. He makes up his own religion, and often sits chanting hymns to himself. His parents regard him as strange. When he is a senior in high school, a physician certifies that he has had a "nervous breakdown" so that he can leave school for six months.

As a young adult, this person works as a clerk for many years, living a very isolated life with few friends. He always seems preoccupied and distant, thinking about concepts that make very little sense to other people.

The son of socially prominent parents is overwhelmed by many extreme fears, yet he never discusses them with anyone. He is continually preoccupied with his physical and moral "weaknesses." He resolves to confront his fears through strength of will. To this end, he fights his fears by placing himself in situations where he must deal with them. Some of his attempts are bizarre. He fears rats, so he kills, skins, roasts, and eats one. He fears thunder and lightning, so during a violent summer storm, he ties himself into the upper branches of a tree to prove he can survive his fear. He combats fear after fear in this manner.

As an adult, he becomes a lawyer, a states' attorney, and an FBI agent. He gains prominence in his profession. He is admired for his straightforwardness, loyalty, and commitment to his country. He becomes an associate of high government officials, including the President of the United States, and seriously offers to assassinate several persons who he considers to be working against the interest of the country. He is convicted of criminal acts during the Watergate trials and spends more than four years in prison without squealing.

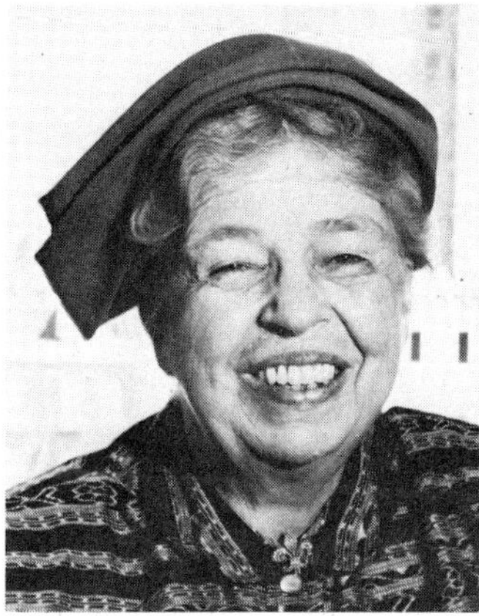
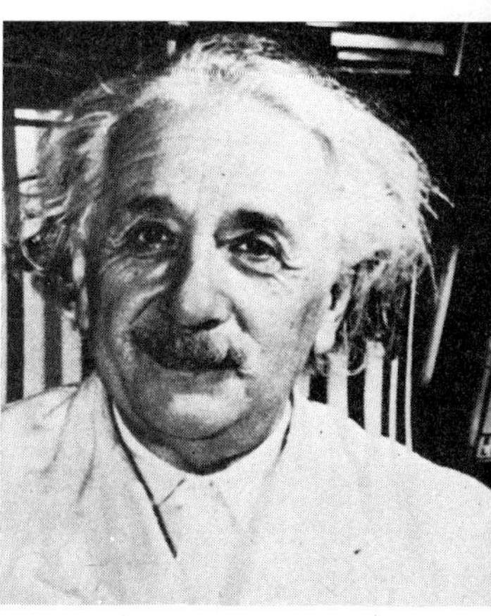

At times in their lives, Eleanor Roosevelt and Albert Einstein both behaved in ways which some clinicians would consider to be abnormal.

The first example is Eleanor Roosevelt, wife of President Franklin D. Roosevelt. She was a brilliant, tireless, empathetic crusader for the rights of others. The second example is Albert Einstein, the physicist who developed the theory of relativity, and who was regarded as a warm, friendly, but eccentric elder statesman of science. The third example is G. Gordon Liddy, a Watergate conspirator, admired by some as a man of conviction.

The behaviors exhibited by these three people would lead many mental health professionals and laypeople to label them as abnormal or disturbed. Yet in some ways, all have led extraordinarily productive lives. They illustrate the complexity of human behavior and the difficulty of finding simple conceptualizations in the field of abnormal psychology. Such examples emphasize that the presence of abnormal, disturbed, or troublesome behavior at some time in one's life does not necessarily imply that one cannot change or overcome the problem. When we think of people as abnormal, we have a tendency to see everything they do in a very negative light. Thinking of the behavior as abnormal helps us remember that no matter how disturbed the behavior, the person manifesting it is more like us than unlike us. The belief that people who manifest abnormal behavior are a minority very different from other persons is a common misconception. Some other typical misconceptions are presented in Highlight 1.2.

HIGHLIGHT 1.2
OUT OF FOCUS: TELEVISION'S MYTHS OF MENTAL ILLNESS

"I'd like to go on talking to you Flagg, but with your schizophrenia, I'd have to charge you double time." (Dr. Friedman, the psychiatrist on "M.A.S.H.")

A woman's corpse is found with an excessive amount of makeup, giving her face a mask-like appearance; it is the third such body found in three weeks. "Gentlemen we've got a psychopath loose on our island and I want him found," [declares Steve McGarrett of "Hawaii Five-O," who then seeks the assistance of a psychiatrist in apprehending the "psychopath."] The psychiatrist says, "He is young, probably a college drop-out from a broken home who, for some reason, harbors great hostility toward his mother, which he has never resolved. Perhaps she deserted him or his father when he was young. . . . Now, when he kills these women, he is really killing his mother. . . . He is probably impotent and drinks a good deal, mostly Bloody Marys. . . ."

The above examples both demonstrate the unique power of television to misinform the American public. Dr. Otto Wahl (1976), of George Mason University, has written about what he calls "TV myths about mental illness." Certainly, television's access to over 99 percent of the homes in the United States and the tremendous amount of time people spend in front of the television can affect their knowledge of **mental illness.** Too often the information conveyed is inaccurate.

Here are some of the myths which television seems to convey and even foster:

1. Psychiatric (and Psychological) Omnipotence. Psychiatrists who are consulted by television heroes for expert advice in tracking down criminals are always right on the mark. They seem able to deduce the perpetrator's age, motive, and innermost feelings from the barest shred of evidence. Does this happen in real life? Occasionally psychologists and psychiatrists are looked upon as people with "X-ray powers," powers to see others' deepest thoughts. This is simply not so. The belief in psychiatric omnipotence can cause two problems: People may not seek needed psychiatric assistance because they fear the discovery of their inner secrets; and this myth may lead some people to have totally unrealistic expectations about the curative powers of mental health professionals.
2. Schizophrenia is split personality. This myth is perhaps the single most common mental health misinformation held by the general population. The myth is fed continuously by television shows and the print media. Schizophrenia is *not* split personality. Split personality is actually a less serious disorder, and one that is quite rare. Schizophrenia is a psychotic disorder with symptoms such as delusions (fixed false beliefs), hallucinations (perceiving things that do not actually exist), and inappropriate affect. It is estimated that 1 percent of the population has been or will be schizophrenic. Schizophrenia is among the most common diagnoses of people admitted to psychiatric hospitals. This myth is so well entrenched in the minds of the public that even after taking several courses in which the myth is exploded, many students return to this mistaken belief.
3. The psychopathic killer. Many killers on television are labeled psychopathic, especially those who grossly distort reality. However, the true psychopath does not demonstrate the gross disturbance of thinking of the psychotic killer (who many television shows are probably actually trying to portray), nor does the psychopath have symptoms of anxiety. In fact, many psychopaths have an uncanny ability to make a good impression on others, have relatively good intelligence, and lack signs of nervousness. Unfortunately, the psychopath is also a thrill seeker who refuses to delay desired gratifications. This desire for immediate satisfaction, coupled with an inability to learn from past experience, seems responsible for the psychopath's behavior (which rarely includes premeditated, cold-blooded murder).
4. The mentally ill are dangerous. This myth is conveyed not only by television but also by print media. The thousands of mental patients who do not get into trouble with the law, do not harm others, and do not commit crimes are not news. The occasional mental patient who kills several people makes the front page of the newspapers and is the lead story on the TV news. Sometimes, the facts (carefully collected and analyzed) are no match for our preconceptions and misinterpretations. The data do not support the contention (Rabkin, 1979) that mental patients are seriously dangerous, yet the myth persists.

HOW BIG IS THE PROBLEM?

How common are abnormal behaviors? Scientists try to answer such questions by doing **epidemiological research** (the study of the incidence of disturbance or disease). If we use as the criterion for defining abnormal behavior a person's feeling of being "psychologically troubled" or an individual's identification by others as "disturbed" in thinking, feeling, or behaving, then the scope of abnormal behavior is quite large. In the well-regarded Mid-Manhattan Study, researchers studied a representative sample of residents of part of New York City. They found that 76–85 percent of the sample could be rated as having mild to incapacitating psychological symptoms of mental disturbance (Srole et al., 1962). A recent follow-up of the Mid-Manhattan Study investigated the presence of symptoms in the same subjects in 1974, 20 years after the initial study. The researchers found that 75 percent of the subjects continued to have mild to incapacitating symptoms of mental disturbances (Srole & Fischer, 1980). Subjects whose functioning was noticeably impaired, however, made up only about 12 percent of this group. In this study, Srole and Fischer were curious whether mental health was indeed poorer in the 1970s than in the 1950s, as some people have suggested. Srole and Fischer found no evidence that the general population's mental health had deteriorated, but there was also no evidence of improved mental health of the general populace over the 20-year period either. The numbers of people with mental disturbance in the general population had remained fairly stable.

Many estimates of the mental health needs of Americans have been made. For example, Regier, Goldberg, and Taube (1978) estimated that 15 percent (over 30 million) of Americans have emotional disorders with potentially serious consequences. This percentage was also used by the President's Commission on Mental Health (Mechanic, 1978) as an accurate estimate of the number of Americans in need of mental health services. The number of people with some type of abnormal behavior is quite large. When only four types of disorders are considered, the numbers give one pause for thought: schizophrenia, 2 million people; depression, 44 million people; alcohol and drug use, 20 million people; mental retardation, 6 million people.

THE SCIENTIFIC STUDY OF ABNORMAL BEHAVIOR

One reason that abnormal behavior is studied is because it affects so many of us. The cost in human suffering is immense, as are the economic costs. The direct and indirect costs of mental health care were estimated as close to 40 billion dollars in 1974 (Levine & Willver, 1976); Figure 1.2 provides a breakdown for that

Figure 1.2. The cost of mental illness—1974.

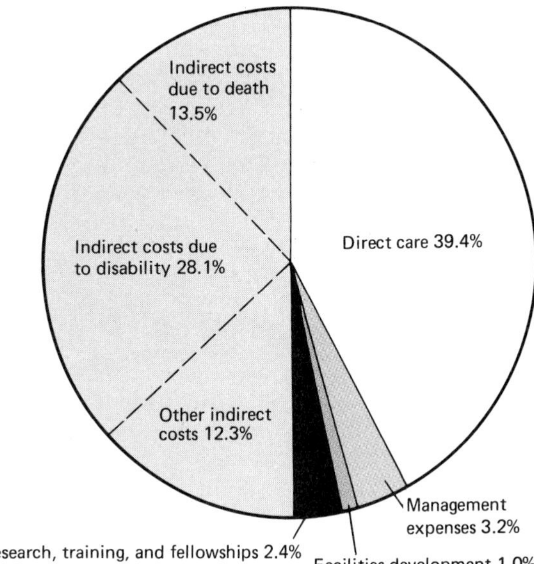

Total cost in (thousands)	$36,785,827
Direct care*	14,506,028
Research	607,003
Training and fellowships	284,842
Facilities development	385,230
Management expenses	1,167,298
Indirect costs	19,812,768
Due to death	4,942,320
Due to disability	10,345,951
Due to patient care activities	4,524,497

*Estimated at 17 billion for 1977

From: Statistical Note No. 125, Division of Biometry and Epidemiology, National Institute of Mental Health, Rockville, Md., 1977.

year. Beyond these issues, many of us find such behavior intrinsically interesting.

In Chapter 2, we will see that the search for answers to our questions about abnormal behavior has gone on throughout recorded history. Usually this search was characterized by subjectivity and was fraught with misconceptions. Today our approach to questions about abnormal behavior is characterized by a greater degree of objectivity and use of the tools of science.

The use of scientific tools permits us to be more confident that our facts and concepts are based as much as possible on the available evidence, rather than on preconceived notions. When the evidence must be interpreted, preconceptions may again influence our decisions and conclusions about abnormal behavior.

In the discussion of types of abnormal behavior in the remainder of the text, the data presented are based on a variety of investigative tools. These tools have different levels of credibility, or confidence. The more systematic our observations, the more confidence we can have in our results. The least systematic types of observations are casual and personal, the most systematic are controlled experiments. There are several levels in between.

The Case Study

Many clinicians use a **case study** approach. The psychologist or other mental health worker may use his or her experience with a series of people with similar behaviors as the data from which to generalize about such behaviors. This approach may provide rich descriptions of human functioning, and lead to broad theories of human behavior. A notable example is the work of the psychoanalyst Sigmund Freud.

Freud based his theories primarily on data he obtained from individuals he studied during therapy. He collected data from an individual, then considered the data's meaning in regard to the person's behavior. From his observations, he generated theories that he and others who followed him used to explain behaviors. Subsequent cases were analyzed in regard to the degree to which they supported or undermined the theoretical formulations. The case history method is best suited to the development of hypotheses about behavior, which can be later subjected to rigorous testing. Because of the lack of control over variables which may influence behavior, the case study approach cannot adequately demonstrate the soundness of a theory (see Highlight 1.3). The case study method is also limited, since the data used are often derived from clients' retrospective accounts (which may be unreliable) and the data's interpretation is subject to the clinician's preconceptions and subjectivity.

Correlational Research

A second widely used method to study abnormal behavior is correlational research, which attempts to determine if an association exists between two variables of interest. Suppose, for example, that several case studies of clients at a mental health center suggest that depression and loneliness are associated. We might wonder just how strong the association is.

To apply the correlational method, the researcher would select a sample of clients and administer tests designed to measure the variables of depression and loneliness. If 10 clients were selected and tested, the 10 pairs of scores (one score for depression and one score for loneliness for each subject) could be plotted on a scattergram, or **correlation chart** (see Figure 1.3). Figure 1.3 provides a visual illustration of some possible degrees of relationship between the two variables.

The researcher would then compute and report a descriptive statistic designed to indicate the degree of relationship. This descriptive statistic is known as a **correlation coefficient.** Correlation coefficients (labeled r) can have values from $+1.00$ to -1.00. The larger the value, the stronger the relationship. A correlation coefficient of zero indicates that the two variables are not related. The signs indicate the direction of the relationship. A plus sign in front of the correlation coefficient indicates a positive relationship: As scores on one variable increase in value, scores on the other variable also tend to increase in value. In Figure 1.3, the scattergram where $r = 1.00$ indicates that for each increase in level of loneliness, there is an equivalent increase in depression, a positive relationship. In the scattergram where $r = .76$, the relationship is not perfect but is still strong and in a positive direction. The scattergram where $r = .14$ illus-

HIGHLIGHT 1.3
LITTLE HANS: PROBLEMS IN THE USE OF CASE STUDIES

The problems inherent in the case study approach are illustrated in Freud's analysis of the case of Little Hans in the early 1900s, and the subsequent competing analysis generated by other theorists. Freud based his analysis on a great deal of written correspondence with Hans's father. At the age of 4 Hans developed a **phobia** (irrational fear) of horses. Through the use of case history materials provided by the father, Freud developed conclusions about why Hans's phobia had developed.

When Hans was about 3½ years old, his mother had caught him touching his penis. Around the turn of the century this behavior was very unacceptable, and Hans's mother threatened to have his penis "cut off" if he did it again. Later that summer, Hans behaved in such a way as to suggest to his father that Hans wanted to "seduce" his mother. After a bath, Hans had gleefully asked his mother to touch his penis because "it's great fun."

Freud viewed these accounts as data demonstrating that Hans was going through a stage of development when, Freud believed, children wish to sexually possess the parent of the opposite sex, and wish to see the parent of the same sex (in this case, the father) removed from the scene. During this period, Freud concluded, the child recognizes that the father will not tolerate such ideas, and sees the father as likely to cut off the penis which the child wishes the mother to touch and receive (remember what Hans's mother had said to him).

Freud speculated that Hans became anxious over his impulses because of this threat. Freud also concluded that rather than experience anxiety about these thoughts and feelings directly, Hans displaced the anxiety onto horses (the phobia), which symbolized his father. Horses are big, powerful, and their black muzzles and blinders could symbolize Hans's father's black mustache and glasses.

Hans's phobia first appeared while he was on a walk with his governess. A horse-drawn van had come thundering around a corner and overturned in front of them. Hans was very frightened and insisted on returning home to be held by his mother. After this event, he said he was afraid to go out of the house because a horse might hurt him or bite him. Hans's case provided the data from which Freud drew broad conclusions about the development of phobias. While analyzing later cases, Freud encountered data which he believed supported his earlier conclusions.

The problem with the case history approach is that the data are usually interpretable from a variety of perspectives. For example, the case of Little Hans has been interpreted by Wolpe and Rachman (1960) from an entirely different perspective. Using the data from Hans's case study, they suggest that Hans was a child who was easily stimulated emotionally. When the horse-drawn van thundered around the corner and overturned, they suggest that Hans became very frightened by the event, the noise, the confusion, the turmoil. Wolpe and Rachman propose that Hans was **conditioned** by this frightening event to react with a fear response to horses, since a large black horse was associated with this event. Only one experience was necessary for this conditioning, since Hans was intensely frightened by the event. The data generated by the case study of Little Hans support either view, and cannot be used to demonstrate that a theory is correct.

---

trates a positive but slight relationship. In the scattergram where $r = -.69$, the minus sign indicates a negative correlation coefficient, or reverse relationship: As scores on loneliness increase, scores on depression decrease.

Correlation coefficients do not necessarily demonstrate a causal relationship. In Figure 1.3, both depression and loneliness may be related to a third variable (e.g., level of stress or level of anxiety) which is the actual causal factor. However, a high correlation coefficient suggests the possibility of a causal relationship between measured variables.

Correlation research is considered more systematic than the case history approach, and this allows us to have more confidence in our results. Correlation research involves specification of variables, measurement, and a larger data base than the case history method.

Controlled Experimentation

The most powerful method available to researchers to establish cause-and-effect relationships is the *experimental method.* In this approach, the variables to be measured are specified with as much precision as possible,

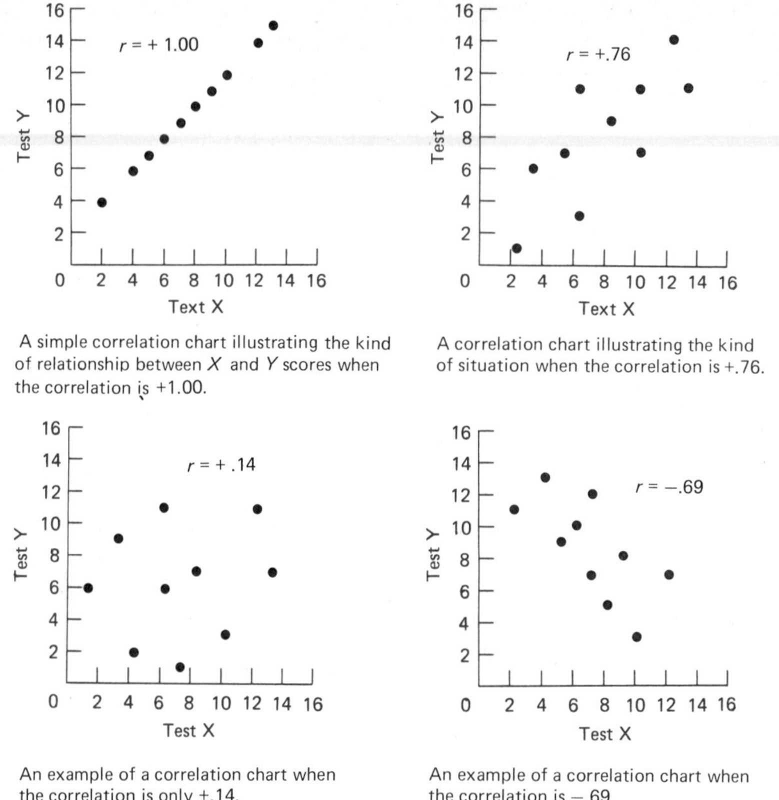

A simple correlation chart illustrating the kind of relationship between *X* and *Y* scores when the correlation is +1.00.

A correlation chart illustrating the kind of situation when the correlation is +.76.

An example of a correlation chart when the correlation is only +.14.

An example of a correlation chart when the correlation is −.69.

Figure 1.3. Hypothetical correlations between the variables of depression (test X) and loneliness (Test Y). From Guilford (1956, pp. 136–137).

and are measured as objectively as possible. Measuring instruments must be **reliable** (provide similar results at different times when used under the same circumstances) and **valid** (measure what they are supposed to measure).

Multiple Subject Experiments. In a typical example of the experimental method, subjects are chosen from a random sample (i.e., each member of the population has an equal chance of being picked for the experiment). For example, a researcher may be interested in determining if a new sleep-inducing drug will induce sleep in patients who report severe insomnia. Patients reporting severe insomnia would be the population of interest from which the researcher would randomly (by chance) select two groups: a **control group** and an **experimental group.** The process of randomization is designed to ensure that the two groups do not differ from one another at the start of the experiment. The experimenter then proceeds to provide the experimental group with the medication (this is called the treatment). The control group does not receive the treatment. Thus, any differences at the end of the experiment would be attributed to the drug, not to other factors. The "end" of the experiment comes when the researcher measures the **dependent variable.** In this case, the dependent variable may be the total time spent sleeping. Any difference in sleeping time between the two groups would thus be attributed to the treatment drug.

When selection of subjects cannot be random (as when comparing persons identified as abnormal to a group of persons who are normal), experimenters "match" the groups. First, the experimenter attempts to identify the variables that may affect the results, along with the variable to be studied. These additional variables (such as age, sex, social status) are then matched between groups. For example, each subject in the experimental group may be paired with a member of the control group whose age, sex, and social status are the same.

When the data from an experiment are obtained, they are subjected to a statistical analysis. Of major importance in such an analysis is the likelihood that the results could have been obtained by chance. In psychology, a *significant difference* is one which would have occurred by chance only 1 time in 20.

Single-Subject Experiments. A common type of study in abnormal psychology is the single-subject experiment, in which the experimental method is applied to the behavior of one individual. One such approach is called the ABAB, or **reversal design.** In this type of research, the behavior being studied is measured accurately for a time (condition A) and recorded. Then the treatment or experimental manipulation occurs during a time period (condition B) and the baseline behavior is again measured. During the second A condition, the treatment or experimental procedure is withheld or reversed, and the baseline behavior is again measured. Finally, the second B condition of treatment or experimental manipulation is again introduced (see Figure 1.4). If the behavior changes from the baseline (first A condition) measurement during the treatment or experimental period (first B condition); changes back during reversal (second A condition); and again changes in the second B condition in a direction similar to the first B condition, the evidence is strong that the treatment or experimental procedure produced the change.

Many different experimental approaches using single subjects and groups are used in research on abnormal behavior, and entire courses are devoted to these methods. Here, it is important to be aware that the experimental method requires that beliefs about human behavior be tested. This is done by formulating a **hypothesis,** a statement that if X happens, then Y will happen. An **independent variable** is then chosen (something related to X that we can change) and a dependent variable which

Figure 1.4. Single case ABAB design.
The effects of positive reinforcement of competing behaviors (standing still, sitting) on pacing in an adult male psychiatric patient are shown using an ABAB design.

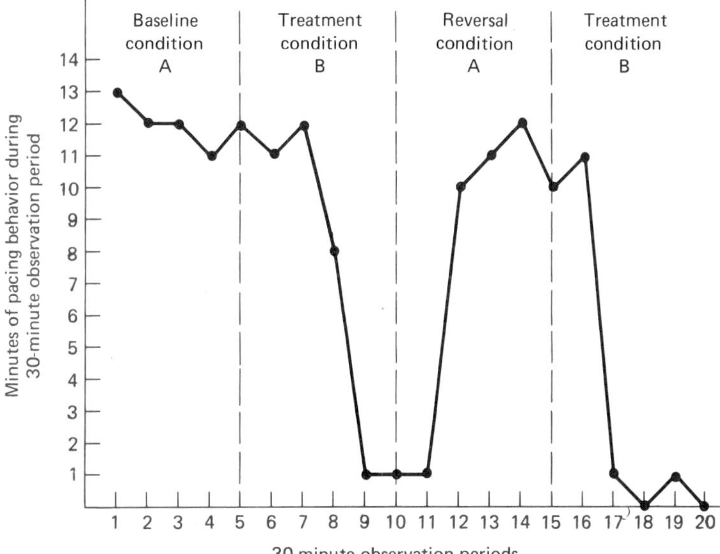

we can measure is identified (Y or something related to it). We then select an experimental group, for which we will change X, and a control group, in which we will not change X. We then measure Y in both groups. If Y changes in the experimental group after we have manipulated X, but does not change in the control group, we can attribute the change in Y to the manipulation of X (see Highlight 1.4).

When studies of abnormal behavior are organized along these lines, we tend to have much more confidence in the results. As research continues, the specificity of this approach allows other experimenters to repeat previous studies, providing either support or refutation of the earlier results. Such repetition gives us more confidence in previous researchers' conclusions or leads us to question the earlier data. The accumulation of knowledge about abnormal behavior sometimes involves great leaps of insight, but is more often characterized by a process of a few steps forward, one back, and then a few more forward.

While we can have a great deal of confidence in experimentally verified data, we need to remember that our data, no matter how good, are interpreted by human beings who bring preconceived notions and biases to the decision-making process. As we shall see in Chapter 2, on the history of perspectives on abnormal behavior, this problem has always been with us.

ORIENTATION OF THE TEXT

Like any other book, this text reflects the biases and perspectives of the author. Since I am a clinician, the text is very descriptive in terms of clinical data. It also covers a number of theoretical perspectives because, as a college instructor, I feel that students must be familiar with a variety of viewpoints about human behavior. As a clinician, I am concerned with helping others; thus, treatment is an important focus in many sections. Often some treatment systems are ineffective, or their efficiency is questionable, so a concern for the evaluation of treatment effectiveness is reflected in the writing.

As a clinician, I have contact with professionals from many disciplines who hold widely varying beliefs about the causes and treatments of abnormal behavior. This has made me acutely sensitive to the need for carefully collected data in regard to such behavior. For this reason, among others, I have tried to emphasize current research that bears significantly on the behaviors being discussed. In this text I have attempted to cover material which students will find interesting, which will answer some questions and raise others—material which will provide an understanding of the issues related to abnormal behavior, and provide the student with a basis for further study.

ORGANIZATION OF THE TEXT

This text is structured to assist your study of abnormal behavior. Part I consists of four chapters that will prepare you for the study of specific kinds of disordered behavior. Chapter 1 considers issues in the identification of abnormal behavior, and touches upon the scientific approach to its study. It is followed by chapters on the history of abnormal behavior, current theoretical models of behavior, and the issues of classification and assessment.

Part II begins the discussion of specific types of disordered behavior. It focuses on disorders which are primarily reactions to stress and anxiety. These chapters cover psychological reactions to severe environmental stress; psychophysiological disorders such as ulcers, asthma, and headaches; anxiety disorders; and somatoform and dissociative disorders such as multiple personalities. In all the disorder chapters, the text covers the characteristics of the disorders, considers causal factors, and examines key treatments. Treatment is considered from two perspectives. In each disorder chapter, key treatments for types of disorders are identified and discussed. However, in the final section of the book (Part VII), various treatment approaches are focused on, and the relative effectiveness of different approaches are examined.

Part III covers problems which are of social concern—sexual inadequacy and sexual "deviance," drug or substance abuse, and the personality disorders (enduring maladaptive personality traits). These disorders share a common feature. They consist of behaviors which are often not of great concern to the in-

HIGHLIGHT 1.4
TESTING A HYPOTHESIS

1. Formulate hypothesis. Medication A will increase time spent sleeping by insomniacs (if X, then Y).
2. Independent variable. Administration of medication A to insomniacs (X is presence or absence of medication).
3. Dependent variable. Amount of time spent sleeping (Y is the measurement of sleep time).
4. Compare results: The difference between A_1 minus B_1 is compared with the difference between A_2 minus B_2.

	Pretest[1]	*Independent Variable*	*Posttest*[1]
Experimental group	A_1	Treatment X applied	A_2
Control group	B_1	No treatment	B_2

[1]Y is measured at both pretest and posttest.

dividual who manifests them (except for sexual inadequacy), but society has identified them as special problems.

In Part IV, we cover the major psychotic behaviors of schizophrenia and the paranoid disorders. There are two chapters on schizophrenia. One covers the characteristics of schizophrenic behavior, and the other covers theories and research on causes and treatment. The chapter on paranoid disorders covers behaviors which are so severe they involve a loss of contact with reality and unjustified suspiciousness of others.

Part V is devoted to the affective disorders of depression and mania. The characteristics of these disorders are considered in one chapter. A second chapter deals with their theory, research, and treatment.

Part VI covers disorders of childhood and organic brain syndrome. The first chapter in this part considers typical disorders of childhood and also includes the very disabling childhood psychoses. It is followed by a chapter on mental retardation, which begins in childhood but is a lifelong disorder. The last chapter of this section covers organic disorders which first begin in adulthood and which have serious psychological and behavioral manifestations.

The last section of the text, Part VII, is concerned with society's formal responses to abnormal behavior. These chapters present what is happening in treatments in the United States today. The effectiveness of the most commonly used approaches and their rationale are covered extensively. The treatments offered in modern private mental hospitals, in public mental hospitals, and in the community are also covered. Rather than discuss the ideal situation, Part VII focuses on what can actually be done in these settings. The delivery of treatment services often falls short of our expectations. This is due to the limited resources available, and the constraints of many pressing ethical and legal issues that currently impact on the treatment and management of abnormal behavior.

Summary

1. Many kinds of behavior are identified as abnormal. Some of these behaviors are dramatic in their degree of disturbance. Others are obvious only to the person who has the problem.

2. Abnormal behavior is studied for at least three reasons: 1. the internal misery it can bring to those who express it, 2. the problems it presents to those who must have contact with it, and 3. what it can teach us about human behavior in general.

3. The definition of abnormal behavior is not clear-cut. Behaviors which one person might identify as abnormal may be seen as normal by another. Four criteria for defining abnormality have been identified: 1. subjective discomfort, 2. comparison with an ideal standard, 3. use of statistical methods, and 4. evaluation of the behavior in a cultural context. Most professionals make their decisions about the degree of abnormality of behavior using a combination of these criteria.

4. The view that people are abnormal tends to bias others' evaluation of all their behaviors. A more appropriate viewpoint is that specific behaviors are troublesome, not the individual's whole personality.

5. Although specific abnormal behaviors or disorders may have a low incidence, the total of all individuals who are psychologically troubled is quite large: At least 30 million Americans have been estimated to have serious behavioral problems.

6. The tools of science permit us to be more confident that our facts and concepts about abnormal behavior are based on actual evidence, rather than on preconceptions and biases.

7. The evidence derived from the scientific method varies in degree of credibility, depending on how systematic the approach is. The case study method can provide rich data for the development of hypotheses about behavior. Correlational research indicates the degree of association of variables, but cannot prove a causal relationship. Controlled experimentation with multiple or individual subjects is the most systematic type of data collection, and can provide information about causality.

8. Although the scientific method provides information that can be viewed with confidence, it is interpreted by people who have their own preconceived views about human behavior.

KEY TERMS

Abnormal. In its original usage, the term "abnormal" means simply "not normal" or "away from the norm." A more recent and commonly accepted definition is "maladaptive behavior detrimental to the individual and/or group." This recent definition adds the concept of a negative quality (i.e., the behavior is "detrimental"). In its original sense, "abnormal" can apply to positive behaviors such as high intelligence.

Behavior disorder. A relatively neutral term that indicates a problem in behavior. It does not imply any reason for the problem.

Crazy. A term used colloquially to describe extremely disturbed or strange behavior.

Deviant. Generally accepted as meaning "differing from accepted standards (norms)." It is synonymous with the original usage of "abnormal," and does not necessarily imply a negative quality in the behavior; for example, an individual who is brilliant is deviant in a positive direction.

Emotional disorder. A term used to label behavior that is due to disturbed emotions. It usually implies a less disturbed level of behavior than the term "mental illness."

Maladaptive. Indicates that a behavior is not adaptive. When exhibited, the behavior prevents the individual from adapting to the requirements of society in a manner that allows reasonable self-expression.

Mental illness. Although also used broadly to label disturbed behavior, this term implies that the person is suffering from a sickness, and has no more responsibility for the behavior than a patient has for the symptoms of cancer.

Psychopathology. The anatomic or functional manifestation of a disease of the mind. The term implies that such behaviors are a function of an illness.

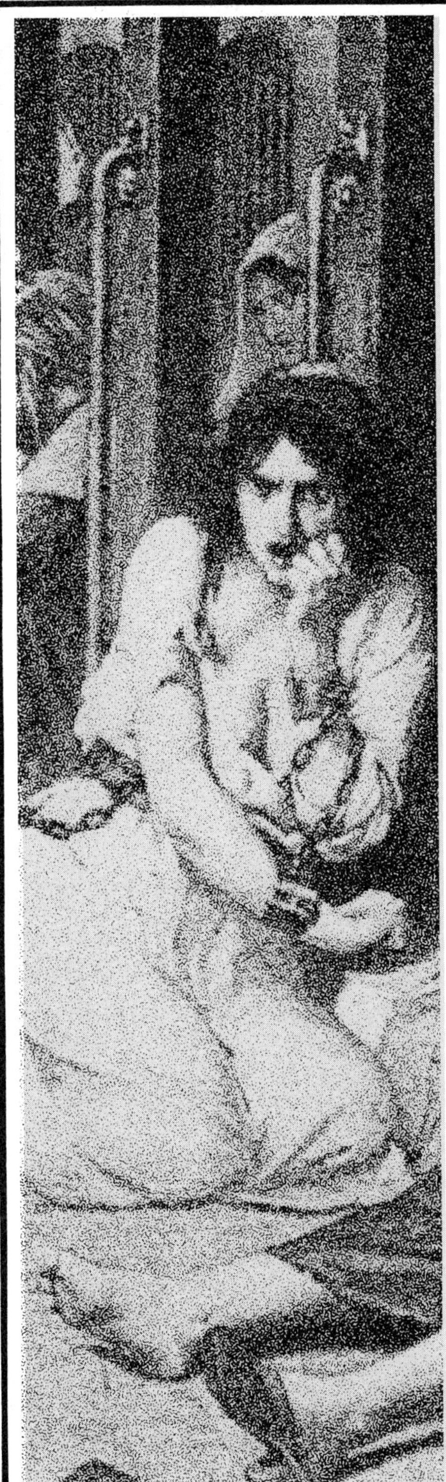

2

Historical perspectives on abnormal behavior

- Preliterate conceptions: spiritualistic possession
- The early Greeks: an organic viewpoint
- The Dark Ages: medieval demonology
- Witch hunts and abnormal behavior
- The rise and fall of humanitarian reasoning
- The recent past
- The organic approach
- The intrapsychic approaches and a major alternative
- The behavioral/learning theory approach
- Lessons for the present
- Summary
- Key terms

Abnormal behavior is not unique to modern times. It seems to have been of concern to societies even prior to recorded history. As historical conceptions of abnormal behaviors are examined, one conclusion becomes quite clear: The conceptions of abnormal behavior common during any historical period are more a function of the prevailing **Zeitgeist** ("spirit of the times") than of any set of carefully collected and demonstrated observations.

As we journey through history in this chapter, we will identify differing conceptions of abnormal behavior. Some eras of Western civilization had relatively consistent conceptions of why humans behave as they do. Although most of the conceptions identified were not "scientific" in the sense of being based on the scientific method (described in Chapter 1) or on concrete systematic data collection, they provided a framework for humans to perceive and to respond to their world.

The prescientific views of human behavior consisted primarily of untestable assumptions, which people believed simply had to be true. The belief in these assumptions was so strong that they were seen as simple truths. To question them was often to court disaster. Since these truths could not be questioned, they could not be tested and thus could not be disproved.

We will examine the prevailing conceptions of many different historical periods. During any period, many different assumptions may be held, and eras do overlap. For the purpose of clarity, eras will be treated as distinct, but we should remember that historical periods are not as neatly bounded by dates as many history texts would suggest. Figure 2.1 illustrates the conceptions of abnormal behavior discussed in this chapter, and the periods during which they were important. From today's perspective, many of these historical conceptions are clearly erroneous. They may seem absurd, humorous, wrong, perhaps even evil. What is important is that these conceptions of abnormal behavior had significant influences on what was done, by whom, and to whom. People of good intentions believed that they had the right answers about abnormal behavior.

Figure 2.1. Schematic Representation of viewpoints about abnormal behavior important throughout history

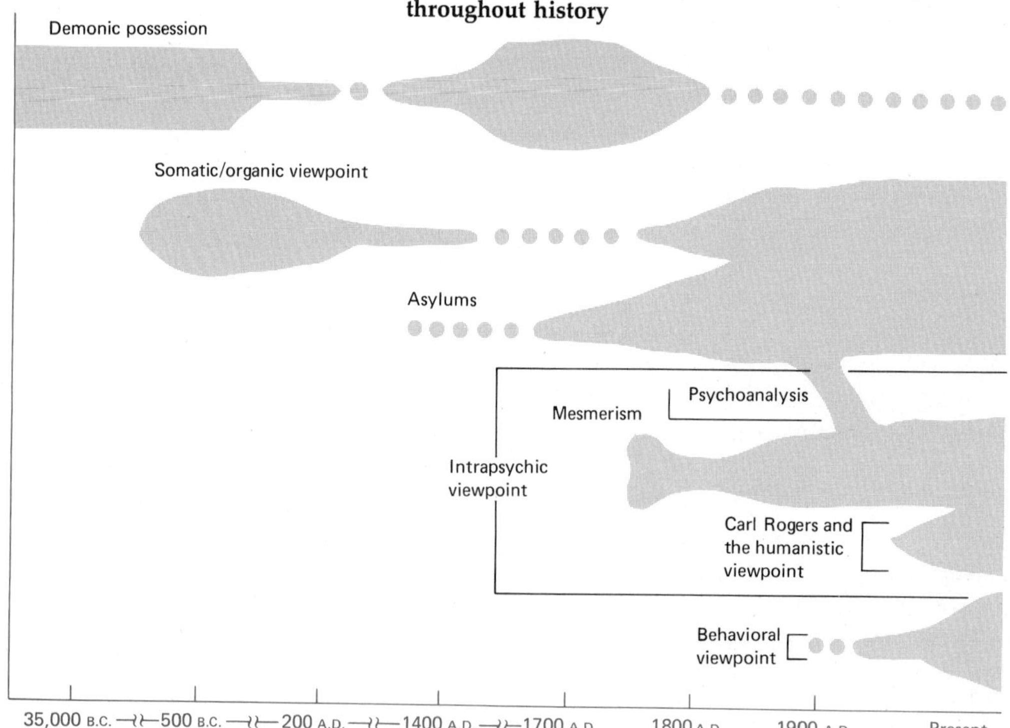

The student of abnormal behavior must consider a sobering question: Will the views about abnormal behavior taught today be valid when viewed from the perspectives of those who follow us?

PRELITERATE CONCEPTIONS: SPIRITUALISTIC POSSESSION

As he lay in the tall grass, Umtalla could smell the bison a short distance away. His tribesmen were near, but Umtalla would scatter the herd before they could stop him. His 19 seasons on the hunt made him rebel against what he was about to do, but the commanding voice of the bison spirit gave him no choice. He had many times told his brothers that the bison spirit had ordered him to keep them from slaying and eating the bison meat. But they scorned his warnings. Now it was too late. Umtalla would do as the bison spirit ordered. Tomorrow, he knew, his brothers would find him, hold him down, and with the sacred spear point they would release the bison spirit from his head: Then Umtalla would be free. But now thinking was hard, the bison spirit voice was loud! The herd must be scattered, now! Now!

How would the fictional Umtalla's tribe make sense of his behavior 35,000 years ago? Studies of anthropological evidence and cross-cultural studies of today's primitive societies suggest that tribal members would view Umtalla as being possessed by a spirit. Early societies probably tried to explain many unusual and even everyday occurrences, such as the rising and setting of the sun, by attributing them to god-like beings.

The "gift of prophecy," visions (hallucinations), speaking in gibberish, or other strange behaviors violating a clan or tribe's norms were probably attributed to possession of the person by a spirit. When such behaviors benefited the group (e.g., if a prophetic vision led the clan to a good hunting ground) the person was likely to be cared for and perhaps elevated to the rank of a spiritual leader. However, when the behavior was like Umtalla's and was troublesome to the group, more drastic remedies were probably tried.

Human remains have provided evidence that a procedure known as **trephining** was used in early societies to deal with disturbed people. In this procedure, a hole was chipped in the person's skull using a sharpened rock (in Umtalla's case, a sacred spear point). This procedure was apparently intended to release an evil spirit from the person's head, so that the subject would return to normal behavior. Many people who were trephined died from the massive injury. However, some lived for a number of years afterwards, as indicated by the bone growth found around the openings in some trephined skulls. If the procedure failed to modify behavior, the person was probably expelled from the tribe to live a solitary existence or perhaps was executed.

Possession by spirits as an explanation of disturbed behavior has a long history. Trephined remains have been found for periods that cover thousands of years. Even early literate societies such as the Babylonians, Egyptians, Hebrews, and Persians focused on spiritualistic explanations of abnormal behavior. For example, the Babylonians believed that the demon Idta caused emotional disorders. The Old Testament of the Bible says, "The Lord will smite thee with madness." A biblical passage which describes Saul's death implies that he suffered a depression caused by an evil spirit sent by the Lord. While depressed, Saul begged his servant to kill him. After the servant refused, Saul committed suicide.

THE EARLY GREEKS: AN ORGANIC VIEWPOINT

The trickle of blood from Damian's arm gently slowed. He rested quietly now. His flushed cheeks had become pale. To the eyes of the experienced physician this was a sure sign that the mania which had troubled Damian was over, at least for the time being. Before the bleeding, Damian had been so agitated that his friend Aretamus had feared for his very life.

"Will he recover?" asked Aretamus. The physician paused, thought for a moment before answering. "Young man, your friend was much too sanguine. Yes, he'll recover now that I've bled him. As long as his humors stay in balance, he should be well. If again they become disturbed, bring him to me immediately. Watch for the pinkish flush in his cheeks. That will be the danger signal."

If the Greek physician who treated Damian had lived about 400 years before Christ, he might have learned his profession from Hippocrates, a physician who challenged the belief in **demonic possession.** Hippocrates proposed that abnormal behavior was due to physical causes. He believed that intellectual activity was centered in the brain, not the heart (as others had proposed); and that disordered behavior was due to a physical disturbance of the brain, not to possession by a spirit. Hippocrates is credited as being one of the first to emphasize the *systematic* observation of the behavior or symptoms of the patient. As a result of his systematic observations, he was able to classify abnormal behavior into three major categories: mania (excitement), phrenitis (disorder of thinking), and melancholia (depression).

Hippocrates also believed that behavior was related to four **humors** (substances) in the body—blood, phlegm, yellow bile, and black bile. According to Hippocrates, behavioral traits (and subsequent abnormal behavior) depended on the dominance of the various humors or their combinations. If one had too much blood (sanguine, like Damian in the example), one would be giddy or feverish; too much blood and bile would result in excitation, while black bile would cause depression. In retrospect we know that this theory of abnormal behavior was wrong. However, the spirit of the times was such that systematic observation was widely embraced as a way of studying people's behavior.

Hippocrates' powers of observation were remarkable. They allowed him to identify a constellation of behaviors which are still occasionally seen. Until very recently these behaviors were called **hysteria,** the name given by Hippocrates. Hysteria was diagnosed in women and consisted of the appearance of symptoms such as paralysis, sensory deficits including blindness or deafness, and other physical symptoms with no *apparent* organic pathology.

Hippocrates' theory of the cause of hysteria was as incorrect as his ideas about the action of humors, but his emphasis on organic causes is important. According to Hippocrates, hysteria occurred because a women's uterus, or womb, needed to be filled by a pregnancy. If not pregnant, the uterus would wander about the body and finally become lodged in the part of the body in which the hysterical symptoms later appeared. The presence of the uterus was believed to cut off the flow of humors, resulting in the affliction.

The organic viewpoint promoted by Hippocrates was a convincing alternative to demonic possession. The Greek and Roman physicians who came after him accepted his view that disturbed behavior was due to physical disorders. Although beliefs in demonic possession continued to be common in the general population, treatment of abnormal behavior was based primarily on the physicians' organic views. Sanitoriums were established which focused on creating a humane, pleasant environment with music, good food, rest, massage, and other enjoyable activities. Some Roman physicians prescribed relaxation for disorders such as headaches, in many ways foreshadowing today's interest in relaxation approaches for similar disorders. However, less benign techniques such as bleeding, physical force, isolation, and purging were also used to treat disorders.

Why are the views of someone who has been dead for over 2000 years important today? Hippocrates' views represent the beginning of a conception of abnormal behavior that is very important today—the view that abnormal behavior is due to organic causes. Although its influence has waxed and waned over the 24 centuries since Hippocrates' day, this viewpoint has always influenced the thinking of some people (see Figure 2.1). Two thousand years later, Hippocrates' tradition of systematic observation and his emphasis on organic causes of behavior have again become a major viewpoint. But for centuries, his approach was eclipsed by a return to a belief in demonic possession.

THE DARK AGES: MEDIEVAL DEMONOLOGY

Father Ignatius had little taste for his supper of bread and cheese. He could not get the image of maid Beatrice out of his mind. Writhing and twisting on her pallet, she had shouted obscenities at him the whole time he had prayed for the Lord to cast the devil out of her

> soul. Oh, it was almost sinful that her parents had waited so long before calling him in. Much time had been wasted while the physic [physician] tried his bleeding, his potions. Did not the fools know that they had given the demon more time to gain hold? Now his rite of exorcism seemed to be fruitless as well! Father Ignatius shivered in the evening coolness. What else? What else could be done to fight the evil one's demons?

The early organic viewpoint of Greek and Roman physicians could not withstand a changing social scene. The fabric of Roman culture tore under the onslaught of wars with barbarian hordes from the north. Into this cultural vacuum came the Catholic Church. The development of Christianity was the most outstanding feature of the 1200 years after the fall of Rome in the fifth century A.D. In this early period, Christianity was extremely dogmatic and fundamentalist. The faithful were convinced that theirs was the one true route to salvation, and that rigid adherence to church teachings was necessary. Only a literal interpretation of the Bible was accepted, and the Bible was clear in its belief in demonic possession. The church was assailed by many forces: invasions by the "barbarians," the emergence of nationalistic states, socioeconomic changes including the invention of the printing press, and bubonic plague epidemics. Many felt that the destruction of civilization was near, and there was a strong conviction that the devil was the cause of much of this social upheaval (Cohn, 1970).

Involuntary Demonic Possession

By the eighth and ninth centuries, the clergy and populace had overwhelmingly returned to a belief that the devil could possess a person's soul. Once one was possessed, the individual's behavior, emotion, and thinking could be controlled by the devil or demons. However, possession by a demon was believed to be involuntary, against the subject's will. In an unguarded moment, the devil could enter someone and take over the soul. Some twentieth-century mannerisms can be traced back to this belief. For example, when we yawn in public, we cover our mouth. The custom arose to prevent entry by the devil; today it is a gesture of politeness. When someone sneezes, we say "Gesundheit" or "God bless you" as a polite convention. In the Dark Ages, these words were said quite seriously: "God, bless this soul which the devil may try to enter in this moment of weakness."

Once possessed, even involuntarily, the individual would engage in behavior in the service of Satan. The prevailing response to such abnormal behavior was **exorcism.** When possession was considered to be involuntary, exorcism was relatively benign, like that practiced by Father Ignatius in the example. Exorcism consisted of a series of prayers which called upon God to cast out the demons from the subject's soul.

While demonological possession grew as a conceptualization of abnormal behavior, the Greek tradition of natural causes continued to have a slight influence through the Middle Ages. In the thirteenth century, physicians were given the prestige of being called "doctor," a title implying that they were university educated. However, behavior disorders and physical illnesses were still treated with a great deal of superstition. During the early Middle Ages, a typical physician would prescribe herbs to treat physical problems, and other substances to fight witchcraft. For example, the type of seed called libcorn was supposed to cure spells cast by a witch (Zilboorge, 1941). Belief in demonic possession never completely eclipsed the ideas about natural causes for abnormal behavior (Neugebauer, 1979). However, in following centuries, the benign types of exorcism common in the early Middle Ages gave way to harsher attempts to cast out the devil as people encountered what appeared to be an increase in demonic possession.

Mass Madness

The thirteenth century was a time when mass madness seemed to sweep Europe. Whole towns would experience **tarantism,** or **St. Vitus's Dance.** These terms refer to a group disorder in which large numbers of people enter a disorganized state. They dance, jump, rave, and engage in other bizarre behaviors. The disorder swept from town to town, and at times thousands of people may have been affected. This strange phenomenon may have been due to people's feeling that they were losing control over their own survival. The period was a time of great stress. The countryside was being decimated by war, famine, and the deadly bubonic plague (Black Death). Faced with a poor chance of survival, people may have abandoned themselves to their impulses. However, the prevailing belief was that people were abandoning themselves to the devil!

WITCH HUNTS AND ABNORMAL BEHAVIOR

We bring the following charges against this woman, known to all as Mad Mary: The accused is known by her behavior to consort with the Prince of Darkness. She speaks in gibberish at times, and wanders the paths and lanes of the village at the witching hour. One villager has seen her speak to invisible demons. We have tried to drive her off with little success. Threats of stoning draw only her infernal screeching cackle. Most telling of all, since she has appeared in our village, three cows have gone dry, and one babe has been stillborn! This could be naught else but the work of Satan!

By the fifteenth century, the most powerful class of people (the clergy) were extremely concerned over the crumbling social order, the increases in mass madness, and an increase in questioning of the laws of the church. In 1484 Pope Innocent VIII decreed that witches exist and that they present a clear danger to the faithful; these witches and warlocks (male witches) were subverting the true faith and making people behave bizarrely. To disagree with this belief was heresy, and heretics were put to death. The decree emphasized the notion of voluntary, rather than involuntary, possession by demons. One could willingly give one's soul to the devil for power, wealth, or other favors.

The Witch Hunters

Encouraged by the Pope, the monks Johann Sprenger and Heinrich Kraemer wrote the *Malleus Maleficarum* (or *Hammer of Witches*) in 1486. The *Malleus* went through 30 editions in 200 years and became the ultimate authority on witchcraft, identifying witches, extracting confessions, and disposing of those found guilty. Catholicism and the new Protestant religions embraced the concept of witchcraft; and for over 300 years, witch trials and executions were common in Europe and the New World.

Those accused of witchcraft were often tortured until they confessed or died. Those who confessed and repented were strangled to death and then burned at the stake. Those who would not confess or repent, and who survived the tortures, were usually found guilty and burned alive.

Many of those accused of witchcraft had engaged in strange or deviant behavior. The accused were often women who did not conform to social expectations, or behaved bizarrely. Joan of Arc, for example, led men into battle for her king, and was inspired by visions that others could not see before she was burned as a witch. Some authorities such as Thomas Szasz (1970) suggest that witch burning was the main approach to dealing with deviance during this period.

Witchery or Illness?

During the 1500s, the nun Teresa of Avila, attempted to defend some nuns of her order who had been accused of witchcraft. She claimed that they were not possessed by the devil, but were behaving "as if sick." Her defense of her sister nuns was successful. Teresa seems to have meant her comments as a metaphor. However, in later years, the notion of abnormal behavior as a sickness was taken literally.

Teresa of Avila's defense of her nuns as sick, rather than possessed, may have met with acceptance because of a change in the spirit of the times. People were again adopting a view that at least some abnormal behavior was due to natural causes, not to demonic possession or witchcraft (Neugebauer, 1979). In 1563, for example, the physician Johann Weyer proclaimed that many of those burned at the stake were not possessed, but "deluded." In 1584, the Englishman Reginald Scot denied the existence of demons and other evil spirits; he asserted that those who behave abnormally are "but diseased wretches suffering from melancholy [depression] and their words, action, reasoning and gestures show that sickness has affected

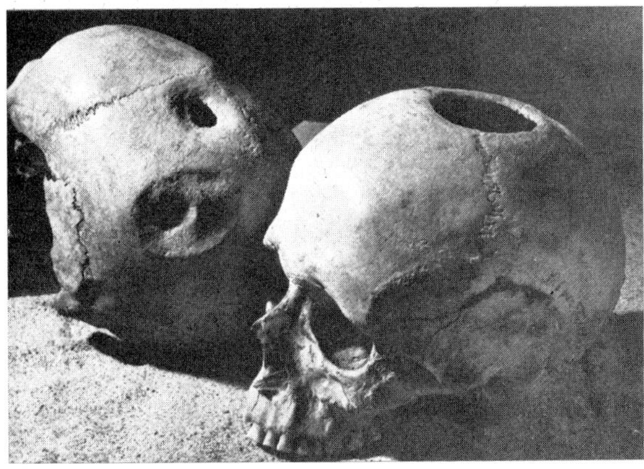

The holes in these skulls appear to have been made by trephining. Anthropologists speculate that the procedure was intended to release evil spirits from the victim's head. **(top)**

Hippocrates was a noted Greek physician. Today he is honored by being called the "Father of Medicine." **(bottom)**

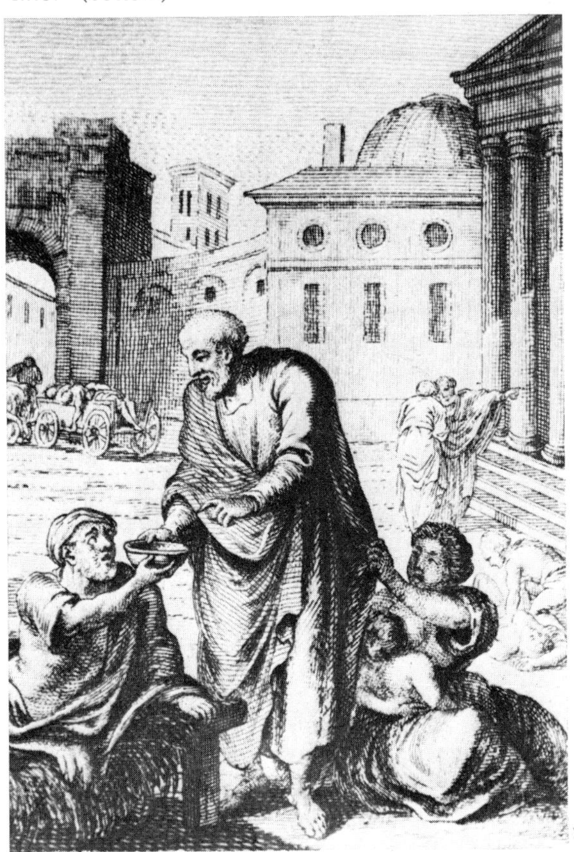

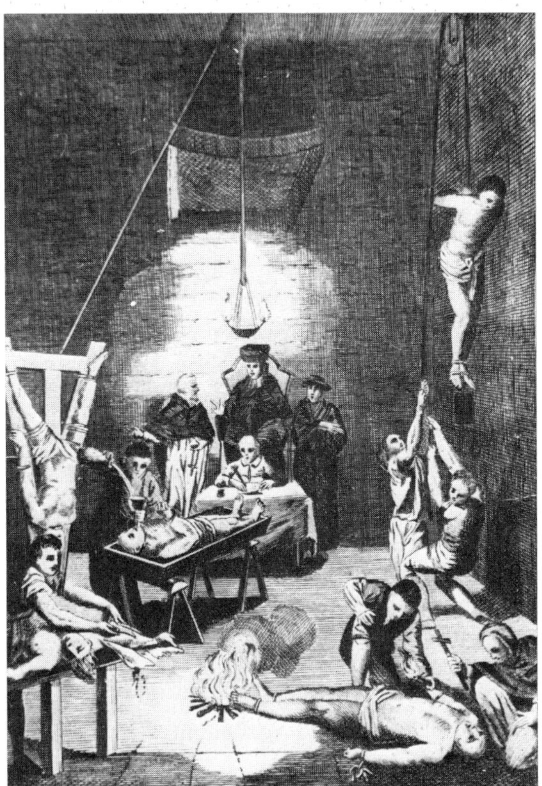

Who was most disturbed: the torturers or those tortured? The print above shows the various forms of torture used by members of the Inquisition. Below this is an engraving that illustrates a witch-burning.

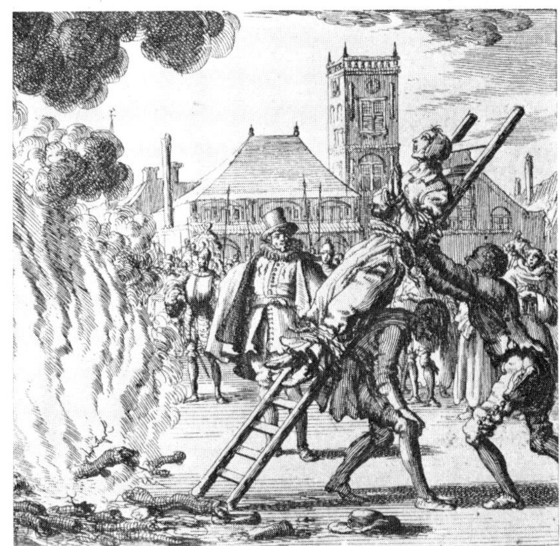

HIGHLIGHT 2.1
DEMONIC POSSESSION: STILL A VIEWPOINT IN THE 1980s?

Do some people still believe that disturbed behavior is due to demonic possession? Apparently, some do. Schendel and Kourany (1980) have reported five cases in which this belief was present. For example, they report the case of a 7-year-old boy who had been troublesome because of fighting, poor peer relations, and aggressiveness toward his mother:

> The parents divorced when he was less than a year old. The mother remarried and was having multiple marital and psychiatric problems. She reported that the patient's behavioral problems had become so bad that she tried "everything" to correct him but to no avail. Among those unsuccessful attempts she listed spanking, arguing, and punishing. . . . About 1 month prior to [the child's] admission [to a psychiatric hospital] she was told, and quickly believed, by her fellow Church of God members, that "demons have taken possession" of the boy and that they needed to be driven out. A church service was organized and the members of the congregation all prayed together and "drove the demons out of him." The boy was reported to have been "flung across the room by some force" when this happened. This "force" left a "mark" on his face. The boy mentioned that he "was glad that the demons were gone" and "saw angels after they left. . . ." (p. 120)

their brains and impaired their powers of judgement." The rationalism in these views was not readily accepted by the general population. For Weyer and Scot it was a personally dangerous stance to take. However, rationalism gradually grew stronger and led to a return to reason.

By the 1600s, witch hunting was beginning to decline. In Poland in 1793, the last officially sanctioned witch burning in Europe is reported to have occurred. But the model is not dead (see Highlight 2.1). Witch trials still occur in some less developed Christian countries (Baroja, 1964); and belief in demonic possession still influences some people's ideas about human behavior (Fields, 1976; Leon, 1975; Schendel & Kourany, 1980). Even in so-called modern countries, films such as *The Exorcist* seem to stir primitive fears in many of us.

THE RISE AND FALL OF HUMANITARIAN REASONING

During the 1600s, the scientific method began to emerge. This was the time of Galileo and Newton. The physician Thomas Sydenham unknowingly replicated Hippocrates' observations long lost in antiquity, and accurately described the clinical features of hysteria. By the 1700s, progress in the sciences and medicine was remarkable. Many theories were still incorrect, but the scientific spirit was growing. The three basic trends in the 1700s were rationalism, observation through experimentation, and classification. For example, in 1771 William Cullen used the term **neurosis** to describe behavioral disorders not accompanied by physical pathology, and described in detail what we now call an "anxiety attack." In Italy, Morgagni completed 800 autopsies on people who had manifested abnormal behavior, in an attempt to find brain pathology related to various categories of disorder.

Asylums: Segregation of the Mentally Ill

Though major advances were being made in all the sciences, no effective treatments for abnormal behavior existed. Severe mental disturbance was viewed as incurable, and the disorders were allowed to run their "natural" course. **Asylums** were opened as places where severely disturbed individuals could be kept while the disorder progressed. The notion of a place of asylum can be traced to the community of Gheel, Belgium, where as early as the twelfth century, townspeople took the behaviorally disturbed and mentally retarded into their homes. The practice continues in Gheel today, and the townspeople still provide housing, work, and care for disturbed individuals.

Asylum was also provided in special institutions, which later evolved into mental hospitals. As early as 1326, a *dollhaus* (madhouse) was opened in Germany. In 1403, the hospice at St. Mary of Bethlehem, London, had six men deprived of reason among its nine inmates. This hospice's name was shortened to "Bed'lam" in the speech of the general populace during the sixteenth century, and came to mean riotous activity. The first mental hospital in the New World opened in San Hipolito, Mexico, in 1565. Where asylums did not exist, disturbed individuals were often expelled from communities and consigned to a wandering life of rejection and poverty.

In the North American Colonies, the Pennsylvania Hospital, around 1756, provided a few cells for the mentally disturbed; and in 1773, the first Colonial hospital devoted to the mentally disordered opened in Williamsburg, Virginia. By the late 1700s most asylums, especially those in existence for some time, had few positive approaches to offer (Alexander & Selesnick, 1966). Selesnick (1968) presents the following description of asylums:

> Their cruel segregation and restraint was described by Johann Christian Reil (1759–1813), one of the most advanced psychiatrists of his era: "We incarcerate these miserable creatures as if they were criminals in abandoned jails, near to the lairs of owls in barren canyons beyond the city gates, or in damp dungeons of prisons, where never a pitying look of a humanitarian penetrates; and we let them, in chains, rot in their own excrement. Their fetters have eaten off the flesh of their bones, and their emaciated pale faces look expectantly toward the graves which will end their misery and cover up our shamefulness." Excited patients were locked naked into narrow closets and fed through holes from copperware attached to chains. Beatings were common and defended by shallow rationalizations. Strait jackets and chains attached to walls or beds were used to restrain patients, since the theory was that the more painful the restraint, the better the results, particularly with obstinate psychotics. The attendants were mostly sadistic individuals of low intelligence who could not find any other employment. "The roar of excited patients and the rattle of chains is heard day and night," says Reil, "and takes away from the newcomers the little sanity left to them." (p. 155)

Humanitarian Reform

The view that abnormal behavior is a function of disease, and a concern about the deplorable conditions in asylums, led to physicians being placed in charge of some of these institutions at the end of the eighteenth century. In 1787 Vincenzo Chiarugi became the first physician to head an Italian asylum (Kroll, 1973). Chiarugi contended that the insane should be treated with respect and understanding, an idea rarely held outside Gheel, Belgium. In the same spirit a few years later, the French physician Philippe Pinel became involved in improving conditions in several asylums in Paris. Zilboorge (1941) has quoted contemporary descriptions about what transpired when Pinel went to Bicetre, the asylum for men.

> A man, of athletic build, had been locked up in the Bicetre for ten years as a result of some accidents resulting from drinking. He was a soldier of the French Guard; dismissed from his regiment, he had been arrested in a brawl during which he had insisted on passing for a general. "Give me your hand," said Pinel to him, "you are a reasonable man, and if you behave well I shall take you in my employment." The man, whose name was Chevigne, at once became calm and docile.

The conditions in the Bicetre and the asylum for women at Salpetriere were grim. At Salpetriere, women were chained, poorly fed, and abused by their keepers. A famous painting depicts Pinel supervising the removal of chains from the female inmates.

While Pinel has received the lion's share of credit for these humanitarian reforms (he is called the "father of modern psychiatry"), more recent evidence (D. B. Weiner, 1979) indicates that he was following in the footsteps of the layperson Jean-Baptiste Pussin. Pussin, a former patient at the Hospice de Bicetre, found employment there and rose to the position of superintendent in 1784. By 1790, he was recognized for his humane treatment of the patients. In 1793 Pinel became physician at Bicetre and was introduced to Pussin's humanitarian leadership. When transferred to Salpetriere, Pinel continued Pussin's innovative approach and has been immortalized for his efforts. Later, Jean-Baptiste Pussin transferred to Salpetriere, where he and Pinel collaborated.

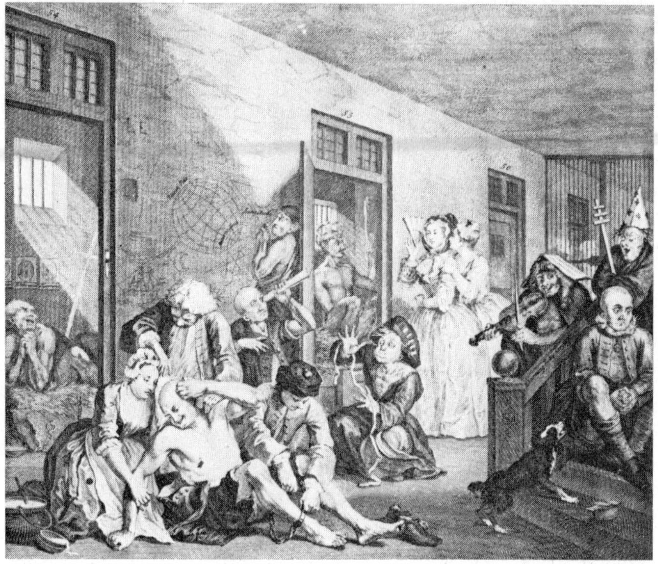

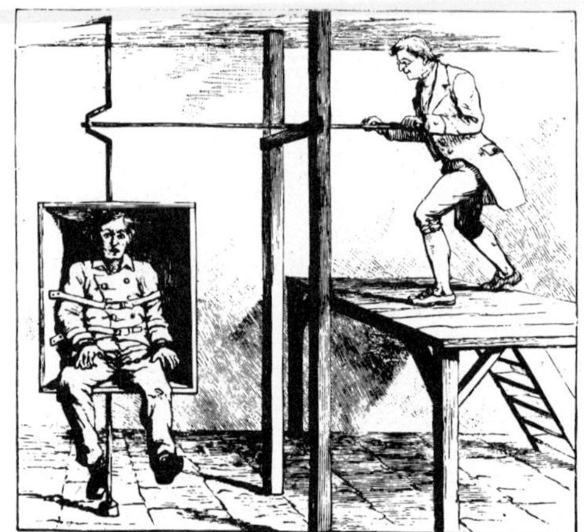

William Hogarth's "The Madhouse" depicts St. Mary's of Bethlehem ("Bed'lam"), after it was converted totally to an institution for the disturbed in 1547. **(top left)**

A device ("the rotator") whose purpose was to spin the person into unconsciousness. **(top right)**

Fleury's painting depicts Phillippe Pinel directing the removal of the chains and shackles from the female inmates at Salpetriere in Paris around 1796. **(bottom left)**

Rush's "tranquilizing" chair. **(bottom right)**

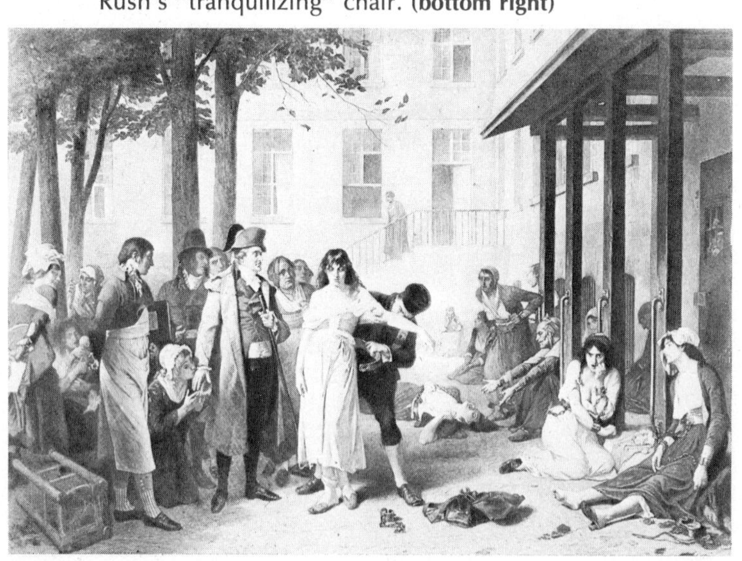

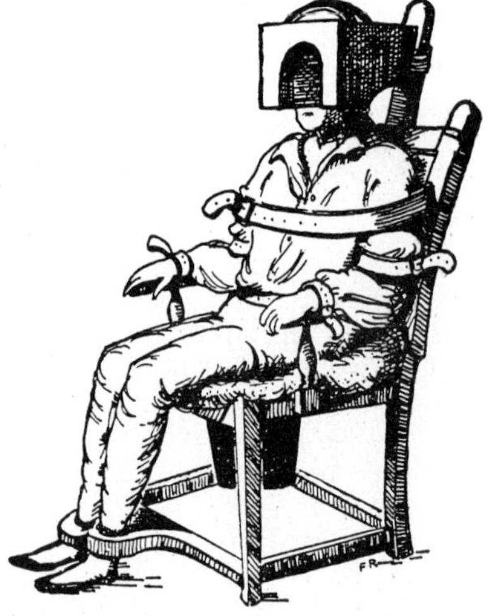

Though usually uncredited, Pussin was a critical influence on Pinel's thoughts and actions for many years.

Their innovations were not without criticism. Many thought that the inmates would run wild, killing, raping, and stealing. The French Revolutionary Committee thought Pinel was mad. In spite of critics, the notion that the mentally disturbed should be treated relatively humanely became much more common.

While Pinel cast off the chains in France, the Quaker William Tuke did the same in England; and in the newly formed United States, Benjamin Rush, a physician and signer of the Declaration of Independence, did likewise. Though more humane than their predecessors, both Pinel and Rush advocated the use of "terror" as a therapeutic tool. Rush used a rotator (a device to spin inmates until senseless) and invented a tranquilizing chair for agitated patients. In addition, he suggested the use of the straitjacket, deprivation of food, immersion in cold water, blood letting, solitary confinement, and prolonged darkness. In spite of these treatments, Rush has been called the "father of American psychiatry" because he improved the conditions in asylums, and was important in defining abnormal behavior as a medical problem. At this time physicians became a dominant force in conceptualizing and treating abnormal behavior.

Masturbatory Insanity: A Failure in Reasoning

"But Doctor, he was a good boy. He'd never do . . . that . . . to himself," Mrs. Edwards declared.

"My dear Mrs. Edwards, I assure you that he must have, and in fact is *still* doing it." To emphasize his point, Doctor Dorfman tapped his pipe upon the ashtray. "Your son has all the signs of masturbatory insanity. I'm afraid you must resign yourself to that fact. We shall do the best we can to keep him from harming himself any further, but we cannot watch him every moment. Unless we can keep your son from masturbating and spending his vital fluid, the prognosis will not be good."

The 1700s were probably an exciting and a frustrating time for people who held the view that abnormal behavior was a result of organic causes. This viewpoint was gaining increasing acceptance, and physicians were becoming more and more influential in dealing with abnormal behavior, as is illustrated by their gaining control over many asylums. Yet there was little that its proponents could do directly as a result of the organic viewpoint. After all, even laypeople such as Jean-Baptiste Pussin and William Tuke could institute humanitarian reforms. Proponents of the organic viewpoint were searching for a directly related theory and treatment approach. In 1758 they found it.

Tissot, a prominent European physician, proposed that loss of seminal fluid during masturbation resulted in a host of disorders, including criminality and insanity. He had observed (incorrectly) that many behaviorally disordered people masturbated with great frequency. He had also noted that the mentally disturbed behaved in much the same manner as some elderly people. That is, disturbed persons had memory problems, heard voices that were not really there, had poor judgment, and behaved in socially unacceptable ways. Tissot and others concluded that a "life force" must be used up too soon if one masturbates or engages in "too much" intercourse, and this lack of the life force would result in insanity. The treatment was obvious: "Excessive" sexual activity must be stopped. Benjamin Rush's tranquilizing chair was a favored form of restraint for those with masturbatory insanity (Gilman, 1982). Other, more severe treatments were surgical: severance of the dorsal nerve of the penis, or removal of the clitoris. The theory of masturbatory insanity was embraced by many people, including Benjamin Rush. From Rush's publication of *Medical Inquiries upon Diseases of the Mind* in 1812, through the early 1900s, few authorities disputed that habitual masturbation resulted in at least one type of insanity, and probably more.

This view's acceptance by psychiatrists (then known as "alienists") may have been related to their desire to be able to treat. At last they had found something they could deal with: masturbation. A patient who could be kept from masturbating would be "cured"; and if children could be prevented from beginning the habit, this type of insanity could be wiped out! The belief in the theory lasted into the early years of the twentieth century. Even today the beliefs survive in the street myths taught to many children and adolescents regarding what many people euphemistically call "playing with yourself."

From today's perspectives, this view of masturbation and its effects on behavior is clearly absurd, and illustrates a failure in the reasoning of people with good intentions. However, the acceptance of this theory and its associated treatment techniques illustrates the growing dominance of an organic approach to abnormal behavior.

The Decline of the Asylum

In the early nineteenth century, while the theory of masturbatory insanity gained broadened acceptance, the reforms initiated by Pussin, Pinel, Tuke, and Rush peaked in an approach called **moral treatment.** The more coercive treatments suggested by Pinel and Rush lost favor, and humanitarian aspects held sway. The asylums seem to have become *real* asylums—relatively pleasant places where disturbed people could seek relief. The physical settings were comfortable, staff were firm but pleasant, and an atmosphere of trust and acceptance was common (Repp, 1977). Asylums were small, usually having less than 200 residents, and discharge rates were reportedly high.

But most disturbed people were not admitted to such facilities, partly because of simple logistics (there were not enough facilities) and partly because of superintendents' reluctance to admit the poor. Mentally disturbed poor persons were kept in jails or poorhouses or were given to "keepers," who were paid a small sum for their maintenance. In either case, these poor souls were often beaten, starved; and in the winter, they often froze. Their living conditions were deplorable.

In the early 1840s the schoolteacher Dorothea Dix learned of these abuses while volunteering at the East Cambridge, Massachusetts, jail. Shocked at the conditions of the mentally disturbed in jails and aware of the humane treatment in asylums, she set out on a crusade for better conditions for all disturbed persons. Her attempts at reform struck a responsive chord with both the population and the government. During 40 years of active crusading, she was directly responsible for the creation of 30 new hospitals by state governments. She also led the reorganization of mental health care in Scotland, and initiated the opening of several hospitals in Europe. These were truly remarkable achievements.

For economic reasons, the new hospitals had large bed capacities when opened, and they grew larger as more and more poor were admitted. Sheer size would have caused a decrease in the effectiveness of moral treatment, but the problem was complicated by a lack of funds. These "paupers' palaces" (as they became known) evolved into custodial warehouses for the chronically disturbed.

The lack of active treatment in these facilities was apparently of secondary importance to Dix. Her primary interest was the physical well-being of the residents—clothing, warmth, and food. She was so dedicated to her cause that in 1854 she obtained passage of a bill through the United States Congress to have 12 million acres of public land set aside for the support of the "indigent insane" (Dain, 1964). The bill was subsequently vetoed by President Franklin Pierce. Her conception of disturbed individuals as helpless incurables whose physical needs should be provided above all else had run out of momentum.

THE RECENT PAST

Quest. Gentlemen, I have called you together because there seems to be some disagreement about the proper course of treatment for Mr. Johnson. At least we agree on his primary problems—hallucinations and social withdrawal. Dr. Smith, as a psychiatrist, what would you say?

Smith. Dr. Quest, it is quite obvious that Mr. Johnson is suffering from schizophrenia. The only possible course of treatment is electroconvulsive therapy to rapidly readjust the biochemicals in his brain. Anything less would be ineffective.

Brown. Excuse me, Dr. Smith. I'm Dr. Brown, a psychoanalyst. I find I must disagree with your assessment of the situation! Dr. Quest, while Dr. Smith's approach may work, we must keep in mind that psychoanalytic theory can explain the effects of shock therapy. The patient improves temporarily because his unconscious need to be punished has been satisfied. Lasting symptom reduction can only be obtained if Mr. Johnson enters long-term psychoanalysis to uncover and resolve his childhood fixations.

Jones. Doctors, please, why must we make these complex inferences about Mr. Johnson's biochemistry and unconscious processes? It's quite obvious that Mr. Johnson is engaging in behaviors which, though unusual, were learned because they were reinforced. Dr. Quest, based on my training as a behaviorally-oriented psychologist, I would suggest that the simplest and most effective approach would be to stop reinforcing these behaviors and to positively reinforce behaviors that are more socially acceptable.

Quest. Well, doctors, I'm not sure where to go from here. Each of you can present a convincing case for your viewpoint. However, these views are so divergent that I'm not sure how to integrate them. Perhaps the three of you can iron out some of these differences in the future, perhaps not. I *am* sure that we will meet again.

The fictional doctors Smith, Brown, and Jones represent three divergent views of human behavior which have become important since the 1800s. One is the focus on organic bases for abnormal behavior. The second is the viewpoint that abnormal behavior is due to psychological factors. It is sometimes referred to as the **intrapsychic** approach because it focuses on the working of the mind. Dr. Brown represents the intrapsychic approach called **psychoanalysis.** The early roots of the third viewpoint, the behavioral/learning perspective, can also be traced back to the 1800s. Each of these major conceptions of human behavior is based to some degree on a scientific approach to the study of disturbed functioning formulated in the 1800s. These approaches' early proponents advocated the systematic study and observation of human behavior. In the remainder of this chapter, each of these major conceptions of abnormal behavior will be traced from the turn of the century to current times.

THE ORGANIC APPROACH

Emil Kraepelin: Identifying Mental Illness

The view that disordered behavior was due to organic causes was vigorously promoted by an influential German physician named Emil Kraepelin. In the prevailing scientific spirit of the times, Kraepelin emphasized the classification of abnormal behaviors into discrete disorders. Each of these disorders according to Kraepelin had a distinct set of associated symptoms, and each disorder had a differing course and outcome. He identified two major syndromes (sets of symptoms), which he called manic-depressive psychosis and dementia praecox. Manic-depressive psychosis was believed by Kraepelin to be due to a problem of body metabolism, which led to alternating mood swings. Dementia praecox (what we now call schizophrenia) consisted of cognitive deterioration, delusions, and hallucinations and was thought to be due to a chemical imbalance that might be a result of heredity. Kraepelin was a respected scientist, and his advocacy of the position that behavior disorders were caused by physical problems of heredity and metabolism was of major importance in contributing to the emphasis on the organic approach to human problems.

Specific Treatment for a Specific Disorder

As Kraepelin was promoting the view that all abnormal behavior was a function of some as yet unproven physical disorder, research was being completed which gave some support to this notion. **General paresis,** a serious mental disorder, had been identified, and the symptoms were very accurately described in 1825 by the French physician A. J. Bayle. In 1879 Richard von Krafft-Ebing demonstrated that a significant relationship existed between **syphilis** and general paresis. During the following decade, an accurate test for the presence of syphilis in the blood was developed; and in 1913, the researchers Noguchi and Moore conclusively demonstrated by postmortem examination that the brains of those with general paresis had been invaded by the syphilitic organism.

The importance of such a discovery cannot be overestimated. At last, proof existed that at least one form of abnormal behavior was definitely the result of an organic problem. This discovery was a tremendous stimulus for major efforts to find organic causal factors for other behavior disorders. It provided empirical support for an organic viewpoint, and led to a massive search for medical treatments for a broad variety of abnormal behavior.

It was not long before a physical treatment for general paresis was found. In 1917 in Vienna, Julius Wagner-Jauregg found that fever had beneficial effects on people with paresis. Soon he was purposely infecting patients with malaria to obtain high fevers. These fevers did not cure the disease, but they did kill the syphilitic organism and prevent further deterioration. The **fever treatments** quickly became common. Through gross generalization, the attitude developed that if fever treatments worked with general paresis, then they were also worthwhile for other disorders. The enthusiasm for the approach, and the desire to be able to treat seemed to overwhelm the critical thinking of the experts. Wagner-Jauregg was honored with the Nobel Prize in 1927 for his discovery.

The Rush for the Cure

The success of the fever treatments with general paresis stimulated a massive interest in finding successful treatments for other disorders. For example, Manfred Sakel, a physician in Berlin had begun administering high dosages of insulin to excited psychotic patients in the belief that this would quiet them. Following insulin-induced coma, patients appeared to improve. This treatment, called **insulin shock,** became relatively common in spite of a vague rationale, inherent dangers, and expense. The technique required at least a 30–50-hour coma, highly skilled continuous nursing care, and included the potential hazards of irreversible coma, circulatory and respiratory collapse, and spontaneous "flashback" comas. About the same time, in 1933, Laszlo von Meduna, a Hungarian physician introduced **metrazol shock therapy.** After reading of studies that schizophrenia and epilepsy rarely occurred in the same person (the reports were in error), Meduna became convinced that the two disorders were incompatible. He concluded that a convulsive seizure would "cancel" schizophrenia in patients, and reported good results.

Sharing von Meduna's belief regarding schizophrenia and convulsive disorders, Ugo Cerletti and Lucio Bini administered the first **electroshock treatment** to a schizophrenic patient in Rome, Italy, in 1938. Cerletti conceived the idea of using electrical current on humans after learning that local slaughter houses stupefied agitated pigs by shocking them before putting them to death (Szasz, 1971). Bini, in fact, used experiments on pigs to determine nonfatal dosages of electricity for humans. The treatment consists of applying current to the temples of the patient, inducing a coma and convulsion. Common side effects of electroshock therapy, or **electroconvulsive therapy** (ECT) included fractures (resulting from the severe nature of the convulsion induced by the shock therapy) and memory loss. By 1941, the use of muscle-relaxant drugs was instituted to prevent fractures and ECT became an exceedingly common treatment. Its use declined somewhat after the mid-1950s, but it is still employed (Fink, 1979).

In the mid-1930s, an additional form of **somatic** (physical) treatment was introduced by the Portuguese physician Egas Moniz. Moniz introduced a surgical procedure known as a **lobotomy** (see Figure 2.2). He believed that "morbid ideas" stimulate and restimulate the neurons (nerve cells) in a cycle, and he felt that if he could interrupt this cycle, the unhealthy thoughts would stop. Moniz was aware that when certain brain fibers were severed in monkeys, they became docile; and he began to experiment with this procedure on humans. He performed the first frontal lobotomy on a psychiatric patient in 1935.

Because of its drastic nature, this type of brain surgery was originally advocated only as a "last resort." However, it soon became a common treatment, even in cases that one would have difficulty defining as last-resort types (Breggin, 1973). From 1935 to 1950, at least 40,000 known lobotomies were performed in the United States. The side effects included a loss of creativity and intellectual ability, the development of childlike behavior, loss of social sensitivity, and often a loss of bowel and bladder control. By the 1950s, such controversy

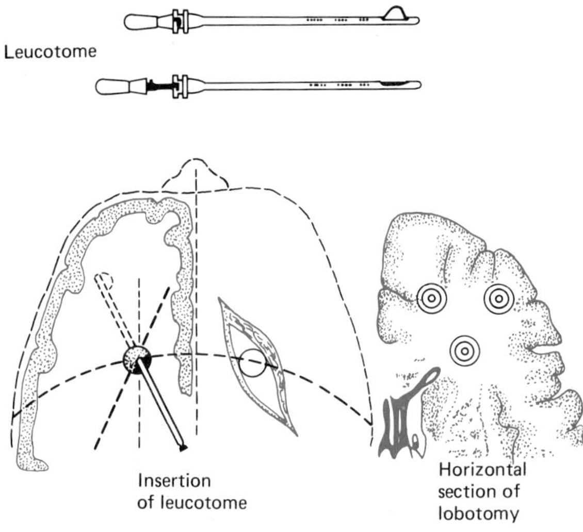

Figure 2.2.
Early lobotomies destroyed large amounts of brain tissue. In the "core" lobotomy procedure of Egas Moniz and Almeida Lima, the leucotome was inserted at different angles through a burr hole in the skull. When the leucotome was believed to be in place, the cutting wire was extruded and the instrument rotated. Three "cores" of destroyed nerve fibers in the frontal lobe resulted from the procedure.

From Valenstein (1973, p. 278).

had been generated by the procedure that the operations decreased tremendously.

Through the early 1950s, the search for an organic cause and cure preoccupied most researchers. Behavior changes which followed the use of the somatic therapies seemed to "prove" that disordered behavior was due to organic causes. Otherwise, why would the therapies help? It seemed obvious to organically oriented researchers that treatment must be affecting some unknown biochemical or neural fault. They just had not found out exactly what the organic cause was. A significant attitude that grew out of this approach was the belief that little could be done short of somatic therapies; yet increasing evidence showed that the somatic approaches were not as effective as had been hoped. There was a growing belief that the mentally disturbed should be kept locked away until the organic cause was found. It seemed futile to waste scarce resources on the mentally ill until an effective treatment could be found. Under these circumstances, conditions in institutions deteriorated.

In 1952, a major event occurred which contributed significantly to a decrease in hospital populations over the next quarter-century, and an increase in quality of care: The major tranquilizing drugs were discovered (National Institute of Mental Health, 1975). Even during early Greek civilization, substances (most notably opium) were known to have tranquilizing qualities. In the 1870s, chloral hydrate and the bromides were used to quiet psychotic patients. In fact, by 1928, one out of every five prescriptions was for bromide. Most tranquilizing drugs, however, also clouded one's consciousness or had other serious side effects. In 1952, the French psychiatrist Jean Delay and his co-worker Pierre Deniker reported on a drug that tranquilized **psychotic** patients (people not in contact with reality) with few apparent side effects: chlorpromazine. Within a short time, other tranquilizers and mood elevators were discovered; and by the late 1950s, most psychiatric patients were receiving one or more of the drugs on a regular basis. The chemical control of behavior exerted by these drugs allowed many patients to be discharged; and public hospital populations declined to approximately 200,000 by the late 1970s. While the drugs did not provide the hoped-for cure, continued use often helped to maintain discharged patients in the community.

The often dramatic effects of the **psychotropic** drugs on behavior gave added weight to the organic view of mental disorder. Since the development of the medications, the search for organic causes continues to be a major avenue of investigation. Researchers are exploring genetics, biochemistry, and neurophysiology in a continuing attempt to determine if organic disturbances are the primary factors in abnormal behavior. Is abnormal behavior actually a symptom of physical illness? Some organic theorists think so. Adherents of the two other major viewpoints disagree (see Highlight 2.2).

THE INTRAPSYCHIC APPROACHES AND A MAJOR ALTERNATIVE

Intrapsychic approaches view the inner psychological dynamics of the disturbed person as the most important factor in behavior. This

HIGHLIGHT 2.2
THE CLASH BETWEEN PSYCHOLOGY AND THE MEDICAL/DISEASE MODEL

During the recent past, the study of abnormal behavior has been fragmented by a clash between the three major viewpoints about abnormal behavior. Behaviorists, and psychologists who take an intrapsychic view are on one side. On the other are those who believe that mental disorder is due to organic causes. During the past decade, this has been decreasing as an issue, since we are becoming more and more aware that behavior is a function of an interaction of biological, psychological, and social variables.

But even today dogmatists from differing viewpoints have difficulty communicating and accepting each other's data. Psychologists are frustrated by the position of some organically oriented theorists (and vice versa). The organic viewpoint, or **medical disease model,** has special significance in the history of approaches to abnormal behavior.

The Medical/Disease Model

Begelman (1971) notes that there are, in fact, many medical models with different assumptions about disease etiology, symptomatology, and treatment. The narrowest of these models is usually discussed and criticized. This definition of abnormal behavior makes the following assumptions:

1. Abnormal behavior has an etiology consisting of an underlying physical condition such as tissue damage to the brain, malfunction of the neural processes, or other physiological disturbances of body tissues such as the endocrine system.
2. Abnormal behavior is a symptom of an underlying disease, and modification of symptoms is only a temporary measure: the *core disease* must be treated or the symptoms will return.
3. Diagnosis depends on accurate observation of symptoms, and accurate observations of the symptoms will ultimately lead to identification of the physical disorder.
4. Treatment of abnormal behavior involves treatment of a disease or illness. This root cause must be eradicated if the abnormal behavior (illness) is to be cured. Treatments should affect the underlying disease—change the biochemistry, remove the toxins.
5. Abnormal behavior is a physical illness that should be dealt with by medically trained personnel, using approaches which are the province of medical staff.

Conceptions of abnormal behavior such as the psychoanalytic view of Sigmund Freud, though not oriented around physical disorders, have many similarities to this model. Freud used the concepts of psychological disease and underlying cause with much the same effect in conceptualizing human behavior. He did, however, suggest that knowledge of medicine was not important for a therapist.

Criticisms of the Medical/Disease Model

Critics of the narrow medical model suggest the following:

1. The model tends to be dogmatic, and does not use our knowledge of interpersonal and social causes of behavior. Its assumptions about causes of human behavior are too limited, so that it does not adequately account for complex abnormal behavior for which no organic etiology can be found.
2. Helplessness in the subject is implied. One must wait to be treated, rather than *working* toward more appropriate behavior. Responsibility is taken away from the subject.
3. Available treatment strategies are limited. If this model is the focus of treatment, many effective techniques will not be used, since they were developed through the use of other models.

When rigidly defined, the medical/disease model can be set up and knocked down at will. However, some professionals still operate with this perspective. The criticisms of its conceptual narrowness apply to other models that operate within a limited framework. Dogmatism is certainly not limited to adherents of the medical/disease model.

viewpoint is often traced back to a flamboyant figure in the 1700s who held an unusual organic viewpoint about abnormal behavior and physical illness. Franz Anton Mesmer is an important figure in this approach not so much because of what he believed, but because of what he was able to do.

Mesmer: Organic Rationale, Psychological Effect

In 1778, the year that Phillippe Pinel came to Paris, Franz Anton Mesmer, an Austrian physician, also arrived there. While practicing medicine, Mesmer had concluded that illness was due to an absence of "magnetic fluid" in the patient. Mesmer thought this magnetic fluid was similar to the force of gravity, and believed that he must have more of this magnetic fluid than others, since he could "cure" his patients by stroking them and (he thought) passing some of his fluid to them. He called this ability **animal magnetism.**

Invited to come to Paris by King Louis XVI, Mesmer set up a practice and quickly became the darling of French high society. Mesmer opened a salon for the treatment of the sick, with astonishing success. He placed a *baquet* (trough) filled with magnets, mirrors and with projecting metal rods in his salon. The lighting was subdued, soft music played in the background, and the walls were covered with velvet draperies. The clients would be brought in, arranged around the trough, and would grasp the rods. After a wait of several minutes to build the tension, Mesmer would sweep into the room. He presented an imposing figure—tall, handsome, dressed in a lilac cloak and waving a yellow wand. Approaching the baquet, he would touch and stroke one client after another, until a "crisis" occurred. The crisis was manifested in the client by "involuntary" laughing, crying, convulsive contortions, or unconsciousness. After the treatment, the clients would feel relieved. Mesmer's success led to great notoriety, and he became the subject of much controversy.

Mesmer's approach was rejected by most of the medical community; and in 1784, the Academie des Sciences appointed Benjamin Franklin, the chemist Lavoisier, and others to a committee to investigate mesmerism. This committee concluded that mesmerism "does not exist and therefore cannot be useful, that the violent effects seen in public treatments result . . . from the imagination which is set into action . . . which . . . is the only thing which impressed us." Mesmer was labeled a charlatan, and the powerful effects of his treatment were dismissed. Not until 100 years later would Mesmer's technique be understood. Mesmer's animal magnetism was similar to a phenomenon called hypnotism in the 1800s.

In the late 1800s, several neurologists in France began to use hypnotism to study the disorder of hysteria. They found that many of the symptoms of hysteria would disappear in subjects under hypnosis. In addition, they noted that such hysterical symptoms as paralysis, deafness, and lack of physical sensitivity could be produced in "normal" subjects when they were hypnotized. While these French

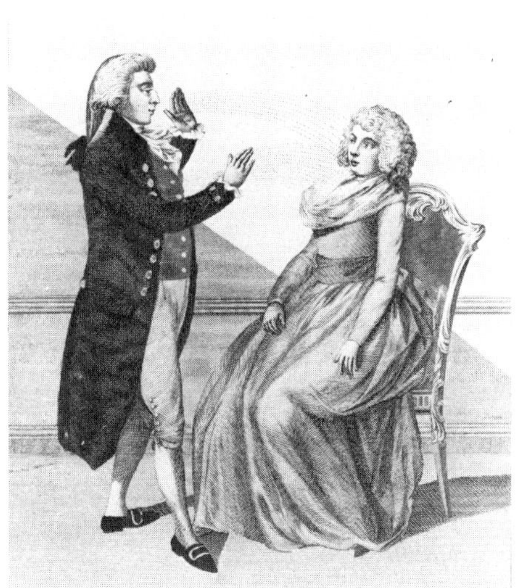

The late 18th century engraving by Dodd illustrates an "Animal Magnetizer" (Mesmerist) putting a patient into a "crisis." **(bottom left)**

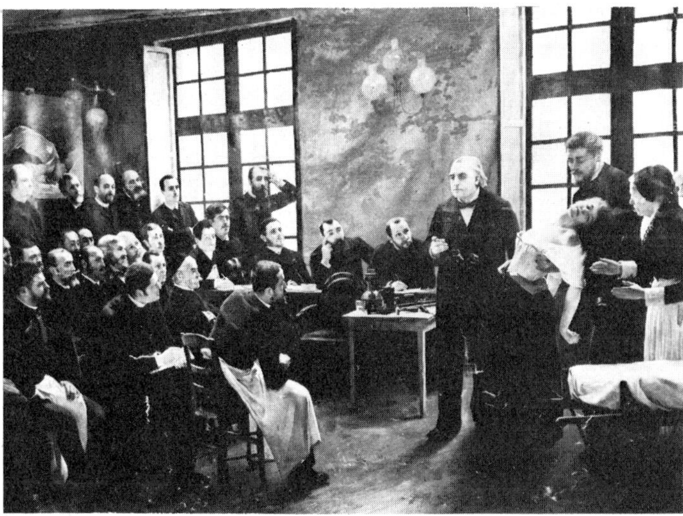

Charcot, a French neurologist demonstrates a hysterical disorder during a seminar in the late 1800s.

neurologists disagreed about the cause of hysteria, they had all observed the same phenomenon. It was becoming clear that not all disturbed human behavior could be related to organic causes.

Psychoanalysis

At this time, a young Viennese neurologist, Sigmund Freud, became interested in the study and treatment of hysteria. He eventually entered private practice with Joseph Breuer, an older friend and physician who utilized the hypnotic method. Breuer found that if hypnotized patients were encouraged to talk openly and emotionally about their problems, they felt relieved when awakened. The technique was called the **cathartic method,** and it led to the formulation of the concept of "unconscious processes." Freud later found that hypnosis was not necessary to the success of the catharsis. A random, free, unrestrained monologue by the patient had the same effect. Freud called this technique **free association,** and his method of analyzing and interpreting what the patient said was called "psychoanalysis."

With the publication in 1900 of his early work *The Interpretation of Dreams,* Freud (1938) began a career of developing and refining a revolutionary view of human maladaptation. He proposed that: 1. humans operate out of basic psychological instincts, 2. much abnormal behavior is an expression of repressed or unconscious sexual drives, and 3. behavior and personality traits are determined by the manner in which fixed stages of psychosexual development are resolved during childhood. These complicated concepts will be examined in more detail in later chapters.

Despite initial rejection because of Victorian attitudes toward the sexual emphasis of his ideas, Freud's theories gained wide acceptance. In 1909 he was invited to lecture at Clark University in the United States, and soon his theories began to be considered seriously by many important figures. By the 1920s and 1930s, Freud's ideas had become so well established that other fields were using his concepts as an integral part of their thinking. The anthropologist Margaret Mead, for example, began an ongoing attempt to integrate Freudian concepts into studies of primitive cultures.

Freud was unquestionably one of the great geniuses of our time; he made major contributions to our understanding of human behavior, society, and culture until his death in 1939. His theories are broadly accepted and serve as a cornerstone for many approaches to problems of human adaptation. His basic theories have been modified by others who followed him, but the field of psychoanalysis remains in touch with its origins. Today thousands of professionals in the fields of corrections, early education, mental health, public welfare, and the other problem areas have a psychoanalytic orientation. By the 1960s, psychoanalytic theory had become a dominant conception of human behavior, reflected in the popular media of newspapers, weekly magazines, radio, television, and movies.

Freud's ideas stimulated many other creative thinkers to develop intrapsychic viewpoints about abnormal behavior. By 1911, Alfred Adler, a student of Freud's, had split from the traditional psychoanalytic view. Adler felt that emphasis should be placed on studying the whole person, rather than isolated behaviors. In 1913, Carl Jung, also an early disciple of Freud, split from the strict Freudian approach because he disagreed with Freud's view that the sexual instinct was the primary motivator of behavior. However, Adler and Jung remained in the psychoanalytic tradition. A really significant alternative to Freud's concepts did not appear until the 1940s.

The Humanistic Viewpoint: A Phenomenological Approach

In 1942, an alternative viewpoint that became a significant competitor to psychoanalytic theory and treatment appeared with the publication of Carl Rogers's *Counseling and Psychotherapy.* With a background in theology, education, and clinical psychology, Rogers reacted negatively to the Freudian view of humanity as a base animal in need of socialization of instincts, and the subsequent authoritarian approach to treatment. Instead, Rogers saw humans as basically striving for good, and felt that each person had the potential for growth and development of a mature self. In essence, Rogers felt that abnormal behavior was an exaggeration of normal behavior, caused by a lack of congruence be-

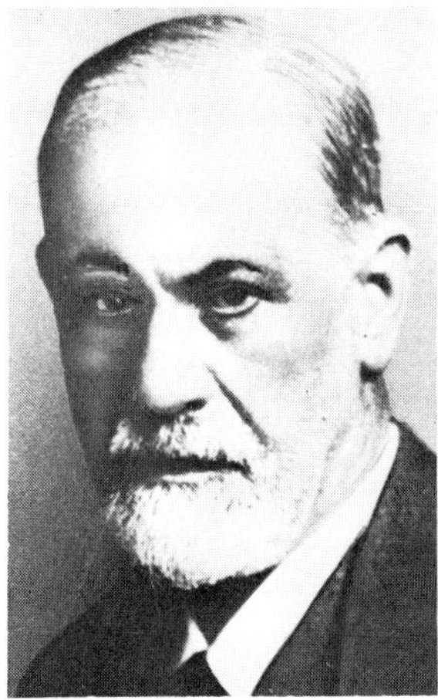
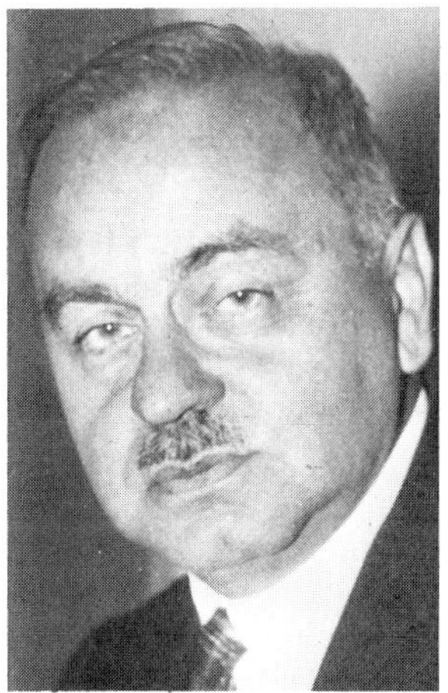
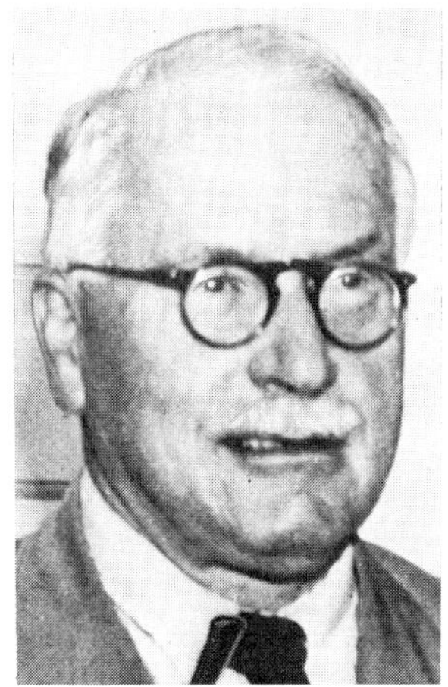
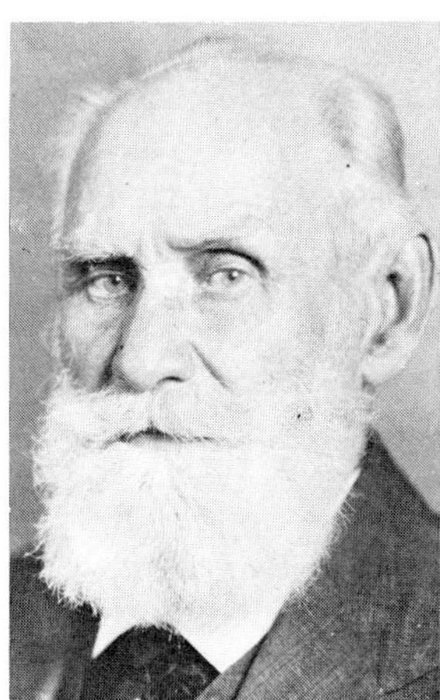

Sigmund Freud, (**top left**) the founder of the psychoanalysis, helped to revolutionize the way behavior is perceived. Carl Jung (**middle right**) and Alfred Adler (**middle left**) were early followers of Sigmund Freud. They both later developed their own divergent viewpoints about human behavior. Ivan Pavlov. (**top right**)

tween one's self-concept and experience. For Rogers, the therapist's purpose was to provide the setting in which clients could comfortably examine their problems in order to change their perceptions about their world and their place in it.

Rogers did not develop his approach in a vacuum. In the 1930s and 1940s, some of Rogers's contemporaries were developing theories and conceptualizations which were similarly oriented, and we can presume that some cross-fertilization of ideas occurred between them. Gordon Allport developed a **humanistic psychology.** It was called humanistic psychology because it has a heavy emphasis on personality as a unified, constantly changing and evolving entity, with the self-percept as an important aspect in motivation. This focus on conscious motivation was cemented in an early meeting with Freud, when Allport felt that Freud misinterpreted Allport's own motivation. Ryckman (1978) reports this event, which illustrates the conflict between different models of human behavior.

> When Allport arrived, Freud ushered him into his famous inner office and sat staring at him expectantly. Not expecting the silence and not knowing what to say, Allport thought fast and told him of an episode on a streetcar on his way to the office. He reported that he had seen a four-year-old boy who displayed a conspicuous dirt phobia. The boy kept saying to his mother, "I don't want to sit there . . . don't let that dirty man sit beside me," (Allport, 1968, p. 383). Since the mother was so clean and dominant looking, Allport assumed Freud would quickly see the point of the story . . . namely, that the boy's abhorrence of dirt was a result of his mother's obsession with cleanliness. Instead, when he had finished the story, Freud hesitated and said kindly, "And was that little boy you?" (Allport, 1968, p. 383). Allport, flabbergasted, realized that Freud was accustomed to thinking in terms of neurotic defenses, so that Allport's manifest motivation had completely escaped him. Allport reports that the experience taught him that depth psychology often plunged too deeply into the psyche and that psychologists might understand people better if they paid more attention to their manifest, conscious motives before probing into their unconscious natures. (p. 130)

Since the 1940s there has been a tremendous expansion in psychological conceptions of normal and abnormal behavior; however, the psychoanalytic and humanistic views remain among the most common. The popularity of these approaches may have much to do with people's conviction that we are more than a collection of molecules, and that our behavior is more than a series of biochemical reactions.

THE BEHAVIORAL/LEARNING THEORY APPROACH

A third view of abnormal behavior that has appeared primarily since the turn of the century is based on **learning theory.** This general approach has been subsumed under a variety of titles: behaviorism, behavior modification, behavioral theory, behavioral therapy. This viewpoint has been a distinct alternative to the Freudian, humanistic, and other intrapsychic views of human behavior. The common assumptions of the behavioral theories are that: 1. abnormal or disturbed behavior is learned, like any other behavior; 2. the principles of learning can be specified; and 3. one does not have to resort to elaborate mental constructs such as unconscious mental processes to explain behavior. The beginning of this approach can be traced back to the Russian physiologist Sechenov, who claimed in the mid-1800s that psychic activity depends entirely on external stimuli.

Conditioned Learning

Ivan Pavlov, another Russian physiologist, was aware of Sechenov's views, and by the turn of the twentieth century had accidentally discovered **classical conditioning.** Pavlov found that if he sounded a bell simultaneously with the delivery of a specified amount of powdered meat on a dog's tongue, and repeated the process at intervals, soon the sound of the bell alone, with no powdered meat, would produce a flow of saliva. The dog had been conditioned to respond to a new stimulus.

In the United States, the pioneer behaviorist John B. Watson originated a similar conceptual approach apparently unaware of Pavlov's work. Watson's view was that disturbed behavior is learned through association, or **conditioning.** In order to demonstrate this view, Watson (J. B. Watson & Rayner, 1920) completed the following classic experiment:

> John Watson's lecture and movies reported his observations and experiments at Johns Hopkins University and set forth his proposition that there were three basic emotions present at birth—fear, rage, and love—that were called out by specific but limited stimuli. More elaborate emotional responses were learned by association, or conditioning. To demonstrate his thesis, Watson chose 11 month old Albert (according to Watson, "a child with a stolid and phlegmatic disposition") as the subject of his conditioning experiment. As is well known, a loud sound, which called out the fear response, was coupled with Albert's positive response of reaching interestedly for a white rat of which he showed no fear.
>
> After several associations of the startling sound with the presentation of the rat, Albert not only withdrew in fright from the rat but the negative reaction to the rat eventually persisted without reinforcement of the loud sound. As far as we know, this was the first laboratory attempt to condition an emotion in a

Table 2.1
Historical highlights and their relationship to abnormal psychology

Highlight	*Relationship*
Trephining	First known attempts to change behavior of persons who had difficulty staying in the mainstream of their culture.
Hippocrates	First movement away from spiritualistic explanation of human behavior.
Dark Ages	Return to religious explanation for human behavior. Development of exorcistic treatment.
Age of Reason	Beginning of major medical model explanations of human behavior.
Humanitarian reform	Pinel and Tuke emphasize that humans should be treated as sick, not bad. Dorothea Dix crusades on behalf of the "insane," the poor, and criminals.
Recent history: fragmenting human behavior	Development of three schools of thought—the organic, the intrapsychic, and the behavioral—which use distinctly different models to attempt to explain and change human behavior.

> child. Transference had also occurred to a white rabbit, to other furry objects, and even to a Santa Claus mask with a white fuzzy beard! (M. C. Jones, 1974, p. 581)

This study had a major impact on psychology in the United States. It appeared to demonstrate that an emotional disorder (in this case, a phobia, or irrational fear) could be learned. It suggested that complex subjective concepts such as unconscious processes or drives towards self-growth were not necessary in order to explain behavior. Unfortunately, Watson's original study of Little Albert has been consistently misquoted in later texts, both through omissions and additions of "fact." While not minimizing Watson's study and its impact on the field of psychology, B. Harris (1979) has categorized the study as an "original myth." Harris believes that this study has been far more influential than its data warrant. The study is most important because it stimulated an emphasis on observable behavior and a rejection by some experts of unmeasurable internal events.

Instrumental and Operant Learning

After the identification of classical conditioning, a second type of learning was formulated: **instrumental learning.** A contemporary of Watson, Edward L. Thorndike studied the consequence of behavior. He formulated the **law of effect,** which states that behaviors followed by positive consequences are likely to be learned, and those followed by negative consequences are less likely to be learned. The term "instrumental learning" refers to the concept that the presence of the behavior is instrumental in whether or not it is learned. B. F. Skinner (1953) has followed the early work of Thorndike and applied the principles of instrumental learning to many types of human behavior. Skinner is a major proponent of **operant learning,** which asserts that psychologists must focus on observable behavior, rather than on mediating mental states.

Cognitive Learning

A third major behavioral approach does not reject the study of mediating mental states. In fact, the cognitive approach and **social learning theory** are quite interested in these mediating events. Albert Bandura (1969) studied the concept of modeling—how people learn by watching and imitating others. Other theorists have focused on internal factors such as beliefs and drives to explain human behavior. A "mediating" event such as a thought (cognition) may be activated by a stimulus, and then may initiate the behavior. The same stimulus may result in different behaviors, depending on the intervening internal events. **Cognitive theory** has become a popular approach for conceptualizing abnormal behavior. Treatment strategies for a variety of disorders (most notably depression) have been devised using this model (Huesmann, 1978).

The behavioral models have been cited by the National Institute of Mental Health (1975) as being one of the two major developments in the field during the past 25 years. The other is the utilization of the major tranquilizers. Both have become common in public institutions and private practice since the early 1960s.

Behavior therapy in its simplest form applies learning theory to the problem of changing behavior. The basic concept is that most behavior, adaptive or abnormal, is learned because it is reinforced. In order to reduce abnormal behavior, adaptive behavior is reinforced and maladaptive behavior is either not reinforced or is aversively reinforced. In this viewpoint behavior is focused on, not psychological dynamics or physiology.

LESSONS FOR THE PRESENT

In our historical odyssey, we have seen again and again how people's preconceptions about disturbed functioning affect their interpretation of the data available to them. The spirit of the times influences people's assumptions, and people's assumptions influence the spirit of the times in a mutually reinforcing process—broken on occasion by major social change.

Viewpoints about human behavior influence us in a variety of ways. They provide a broad perspective to assess which data about abnormal behavior are relevant and which are not. Viewpoints allow us to narrow our focus to issues that seem important. Unfortunately, our assumptions may lead us to ignore important data. Viewpoints also provide a framework for interpretation of data. Again, our preconceptions may lead us to an incorrect interpretation. It is difficult to accept data that refute our deeply held beliefs and assumptions; and once educated and trained in a particular model of psychopathology, we may have difficulty in breaking free and seeing behavior from a competing perspective.

Chapter 3 will present the current viewpoints about abnormal behavior in greater detail. As you read Chapter 3, remember what has happened throughout history (see Table 2.1). Culture and society interlock with past events to have a profound effect on what we believe is true. Are our "facts" today truer than those of yesterday? Perhaps some are, perhaps others are not. Involved as we are in the matrix of cultural, social, and political "reality," the truth is difficult to judge. History has taught us that our concepts about abnormal behavior have a powerful impact on our ability to be objective. History has also taught us to maintain a mild skepticism, to question, to demand proof. In the remainder of this text, we will explore current "truths" and the data that support or contradict them. Many of these "truths" will have historical staying power; others will not. The study of abnormal behavior remains a changing field.

Summary

1. The conceptions of abnormal behavior common during any historical period were more a function of the prevailing *Zeitgeist* ("spirit of the times") than of a set of carefully collected and demonstrated observations. People's assumptions were often so strong that people believed they were incontrovertible truths.

2. The earliest view of abnormal behavior involved a belief that spirits could take possession of people and control their behavior. Social responses to abnormal behavior were oriented to ridding people of the possessing spirit or demon.

3. The enlightenment of early Greek civilization allowed the acceptance of Hippocrates' somatic or organic view of abnormal behavior, which was important until the return of spiritualism. However, the repressive, disorganized social environment of medieval times and the fundamentalism of early Christianity contributed to a return to beliefs in demonic possession.

4. One response to disturbed behavior toward the end of the medieval era was witch hunting. Until some courageous individuals challenged this viewpoint, many disturbed individuals were executed because they engaged in socially unacceptable behavior.

5. The decline of a belief in witchcraft occurred concurrently with a new humanism in dealing with abnormal behavior. Asylums were opened, and the view that disturbed people were sick, rather than possessed, became more common. However, conditions in most asylums were poor.

6. The organic viewpoint of abnormal behavior as an illness was associated with the reform movements of Pussin, Pinel, Rush, and Tuke, which emphasized improving conditions in the asylums. If people were sick, they should be treated with care and concern, not punishment.

7. An emphasis on rationality in the 1800s did not always have positive outcomes. One failure in reasoning led to the belief that insanity was due to excessive sexual activity, particularly masturbation.

8. Moral treatment was the culmination of humanitarian rationalism. Treating disturbed individuals with dignity and acceptance was a praiseworthy approach. However, the expansion of asylums in order to serve the poor, which was advocated by Dorothea Dix, had an unexpected result: a decrease in the ability to provide moral treatment because of lack of resources.

9. The scientific spirit of the latter half of the 1800s and this century has led to the development of three major conceptions of abnormal behavior: 1. organic, 2. intrapsychic, and 3. behavioral/learning viewpoints.

10. Emil Kraepelin's identification of specific syndromes and the discovery of the organic cause of general paresis were two significant factors in the development of the modern organic (medical) viewpoint. In the 1900s several organic therapies were developed to treat disturbed behavior. Many were discarded as new information about abnormal behavior was generated.

11. Sigmund Freud developed the first major psychological alternative to the organic conception of abnormal behavior. Freud's emphasis on instincts and unconscious processes was rejected by Carl Rogers, an important figure in humanistic psychology.

12. The view that abnormal behavior is learned has gained prominence in the twentieth century. Various theorists have emphasized different types of learning. John Watson focused on conditioned learning, B. F. Skinner identified the reinforcement of behavior as most significant, and Albert Bandura emphasized modeling, imitation, and cognitive events.

13. The dominant viewpoints about abnormal behavior, and people's assumptions, have significant influences on which data are considered important and on how data are interpreted. To break free of conceptual biases and see behavior from a new perspective are difficult tasks. Through history, this has been a problem for people who wish to understand why people behave in particular ways. This problem haunts anyone who tries to make sense of abnormal behavior.

KEY TERMS

Asylum. A place of refuge and protection.

Cognitive. Pertaining to cognitions or mental activity.

Demonic possession. The taking over of a person's soul by the devil or a demon who can then control the person's behavior.

Exorcism. A religious rite intended to cast out the devil or demon from a person's soul.

Moral treatment. A treatment approach which emphasizes treating disturbed individuals with dignity and concern.

Psychotropic. Having an affinity for or effect on the mind.

Somatic. Referring to the soma, or body.

Syphilis. A veneral disease in which a parasitic organism enters the body and consumes body tissue.

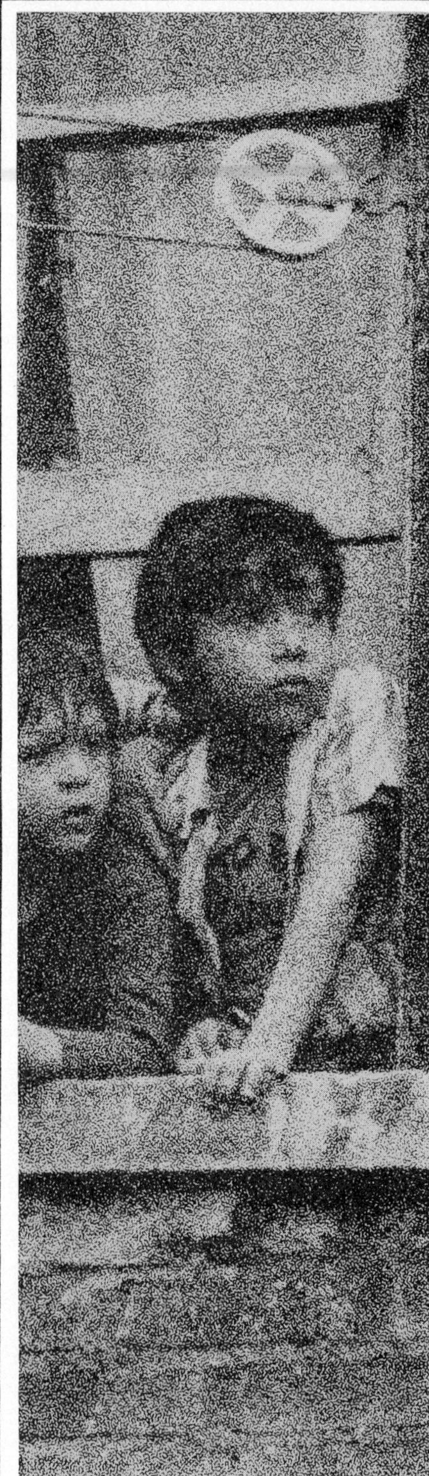

3

The etiology of behavior: current perspectives

- The psychoanalytic perspective
- The humanistic perspective
- The behavioral perspective
- The physiological perspective
- The sociocultural perspective
- A multifactorial viewpoint
- Summary
- Key terms

The history of abnormal behavior demonstrates that throughout the ages people have tried to make sense out of why people behave as they do. In order to make sense out of behavior, people make observations and try to organize them into a coherent whole. In the field of abnormal psychology the systematic process of formulating the apparent relationships or underlying principles of the observed phenomena of behavior is called theory building. When some verification of the relationships or principles exists, the formulation is called a **theory.**

In this chapter, theories about the cause (etiology) of abnormal behavior are presented in some detail. In later chapters on specific disorders, research that provides some verification of the theories is presented. One interesting aspect of theories of abnormal behaviors is their influence on the people who hold them. A theory about abnormal behavior tends to influence the way people interpret their perceptions, and organize their observations. The acceptance of a theory often results in the development of perspectives or viewpoints which influence how people interpret the general human condition. In this chapter, then, the major current perspectives about the etiology or development of human behavior are presented.

Five major perspectives about abnormal behavior seem particularly important today. Two emphasize the workings of the mind as the most important factor in behavior: the psychoanalytic theories, first developed by Sigmund Freud, and humanistic psychology. The third perspective emphasizes physiological factors in abnormal behavior. The fourth perspective focuses on ways in which abnormal behavior may be learned. These four perspectives were introduced in Chapter 2. The fifth perspective focuses on the impact of sociocultural factors on the etiology of abnormal behavior. The development of specific theories about how social factors can lead to abnormal behavior is a recent phenomenon, one not directly addressed in Chapter 2. However, social factors are indirectly important in Chapter 2 because of the significance of the spirit of the times on behavior in general.

As far as possible, each of the five perspectives will be presented in a similar format. The underlying concepts and principles regarding the development of behavior in general will be presented first. They will be followed by a consideration of the perspective's formulations of why some people manifest abnormal behavior. Each presentation then closes with an evaluation of the contributions and criticisms of the concepts and theories that make up the perspective.

THE PSYCHOANALYTIC PERSPECTIVE

> I had a dream last night. . . . I was in a long corridor, walking towards the end of it. I felt very small and weak. The walls looked soft, sort of mushy, and the floor was like . . . well, soft. I was going towards the end, and I didn't want to leave. Finally I went through the opening, and there was a beautiful naked woman with a great body. I wanted her and she wanted me. But as I moved towards her, everything changed. . . . I was just about to touch her and this huge man started yelling at me. It was crazy . . . he looked just like my principal . . . my grade school principal of all people . . . then I turned back and the woman was gone . . . but I heard her voice saying "turn back," so I did and the guy wasn't as big any more.

In the late 1800s and early 1900s, Sigmund Freud had startling insights about human behavior. He used these insights to develop a comprehensive theory of psychopathology and personality development. Freud had encouraged a number of his patients to talk about their problems. As his patients engaged in an unrestrained monologue, which Freud called free association, and related their dreams to him, Freud noted that they frequently brought up incidents that had apparently occurred long ago, in childhood. The free associations of his patients convinced Freud that childhood sexual impulses were at the root of the patients' problems. These unacceptable sexual impulses, Freud believed, were **unconscious,** not in the direct awareness of the patients. However, the unconscious impulses seemed to continue to influence the patients' behavior. Although Freud later modified many of his early beliefs, the notions of **unconscious processes, psychic determinism,** and childhood sexuality remained important (Freud, 1938).

Unconscious Processes, Psychic Determinism, and Childhood Sexuality

Freud was not the first to propose the concept of unconscious processes. However, he used the concept as a major facet of his theory. In Freud's view, unconscious mental processes were of fundamental importance in human behavior. Conscious awareness of one's true motivation was, from Freud's perspective, the exception rather than the rule. He saw most behavior as due to the action of mental processes that the person is not aware of. Further, Freud maintained a hypothesis of psychic determinism, which stated that all behavior is determined by past events. The concepts of unconscious processes and psychic determinism led to Freud's view that every behavior, thought, or emotion (including "accidental" slips of the tongue) had a cause that was not available to the person's conscious awareness. Thus, a person might believe and report disliking an employer because the employer has unrealistic expectations. Upon analysis, Freud might find that the person's difficulty with the supervisor was motivated by unconscious feelings about authority related to childhood relationships with a father. This example illustrates a third important facet of Freud's view; the importance of childhood experiences, especially those with instinctual sexual motivations.

As Freud tried to make sense of human behavior, he concluded that people are motivated by basic biological instincts. The **life instincts** (or "Eros") are the instincts for self-preservation and sexual drive. The instincts, especially the sexual ones, provide the energy for **libido,** or life force, which drives the person to search for gratification or pleasure. Freud called this drive for immediate gratification of instincts the **pleasure principle.** "Pleasure" is, in fact, what Freud meant by sexual gratification in children. The sexuality of infants, from this perspective, does not refer to an adult genital sexuality, but to physical pleasure. The pleasure principle is balanced by destructive instincts (Freud's followers later called them **"Thanatos"** or death instincts) that drive the individual toward the ultimate goal of life: death. These two opposing instinctual forces provide psychic energy to the organism; they are the propelling forces of behavior to which all action can be traced.

Structure and Function of the Personality

Freud conceptualized the personality as consisting of three major ongoing processes or systems, **id, ego,** and **superego** (see Figure 3.1). Though often spoken of as "parts" of the personality—as if they were actual places in the mind—these terms were Freud's labels for the types of functions involved in the personality.

The Id. The newborn infant operates primarily through id processes that function to satisfy instinctual impulses. The infant's behavior is a result of undifferentiated psychic energy and thus is amoral and selfish—a "seething cauldron" of primitive urges. An infant acts primarily on the pleasure principle. That is, it

Figure 3.1. Structure of the Personality and Level of Conscious Awareness.

Unconscious material in the id, ego, and superego influences peoples behavior without their awareness. Material in the preconscious has been forgotten, but can be recalled if enough effort is made. Aspects of ourselves which are available to our direct knowledge constitute material in the conscious level.

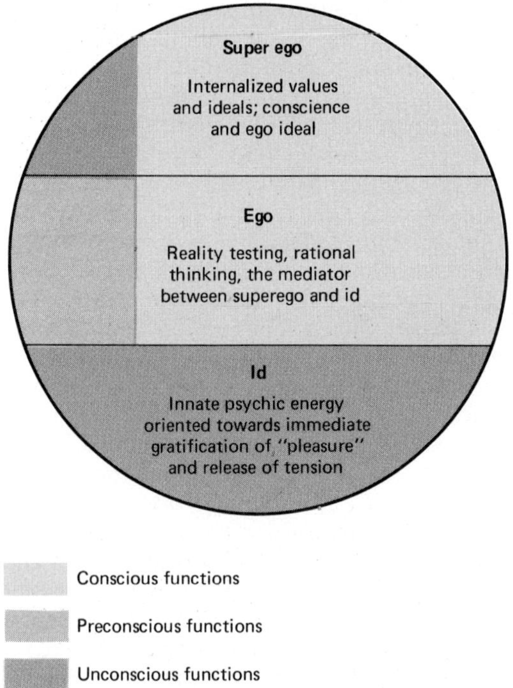

seeks immediate gratification, and tension levels increase dramatically if the child's instinctual need is not satisfied. At first, tension discharge is accomplished by reflex action and **primary process thinking.** Reflex actions such as sneezing and the startle reflex are obvious tension dischargers. Primary process thinking is more complex, and consists of the creation of a mental image of the need-satisfying event or object. In effect, this thinking is a wish-fulfilling hallucination. The hungry infant has a mental image of mother's breast which is momentarily satisfying. However, a mental image cannot satisfy as well as the real thing. When the wish-fulfilling mental image does not satisfy, the id provides energy for the functioning of the other two systems of personality, which begin to develop as the infant interacts with the outside world. This interaction must occur, since primary process thinking reduces tension only temporarily. An image of food does not satisfy as well as real food, so the tension will again increase until satisfied by the real event of eating.

The Ego. The ego processes develop during the interaction between the infant and the external environment. The developing infant is not allowed to satisfy its amoral impulses because it lives in a social matrix. Parents require the infant to obtain gratification through acceptable interaction with the real world. The ego processes that develop through this interaction function on the reality principle. The ego is characterized by **secondary process thinking** and **reality testing.** Secondary process thinking involves delay of immediate gratification until the setting is appropriate for the expression of the impulse. In reality testing, the individual devises a plan of action and tests it to see if it obtains the needed gratification. This ultimate gratification allows the seething id to be superceded by the ego functions. However, ego is in the service of id, since the ego's ultimate goal is satisfaction of the instinctual needs, albeit in socially acceptable ways. If the ego processes are inadequate in mediating between id process and environment, the id functions become or remain the main system for tension reduction: The individual is impulsive, self-centered, and unable to postpone gratification.

The Superego. The superego processes develop as a result of the rewards and punishments administered by parents to the developing child. These functions represent the internalized values and ideals of the parents and, to the extent that the parents share them, the values and ideals of society. These values and ideals are taken in by the child through identification with the parents. Two aspects of the superego functions have been identified: **conscience** and **ego ideal.** Thoughts, feelings, and behaviors which have been punished are internalized as conscience (e.g., "It's wrong to steal."). Thoughts, feelings, and behaviors which have been rewarded and approved by parental authority figures become incorporated as the ego ideal. When successful incorporation of these values occurs, the individual can substitute self-control for external control. The superego functions have three goals: 1. to inhibit id impulses when their expressions are condemned by society; 2. to substitute moralistic goals for the ego's realistic goals; and 3. to strive for perfection. The superego processes are in this regard no more rational than the id processes.

The processes of id, ego, and superego operate as a dynamic system. Id processes provide a reservoir of psychic energy and represent instinctual strivings; the superego processes provide strong control; and the ego functions mediate between the instinctual id and the repressive control of the superego. The ego functions are related to the real world. As an example, consider the sexual impulse. Operating on the pleasure principle, id processes seek immediate gratification of sexual urges. An individual with no superego or ego functions would satisfy the sexual urge immediately, with anyone or anything which happens to be present, with no concern for the setting. With no ego function, but with id impulses and a strong superego, individuals would be immobilized by a war within themselves in which the id would fight for expression, and the superego would demand suppression of the id impulses. According to Freud, if all three forces are in balance, the individual can experience the sexual impulse, recognize it, and through the ego express it in a socially acceptable way through marriage or another form of heterosexual consensual relationship. According to Freud, normality (which he called an "ideal fiction"), consists of balanced conflict between the id, ego, and superego. When these conflicting functions are not in balance, disturbed behavior occurs.

Psychosexual Stages of Development

In addition to creating models of the structure and function of personality, Freud proposed that personality development evolves through fixed **psychosexual stages.** In each stage, the expression of libido, or psychic energy, is localized in a specific area of the body through which the id impulses, or instincts, are gratified and socialized. Freud's studies of human behavior led him to propose five stages of development which follow each other in an invariant sequence, but are separated by vague dividing lines. These are called the **oral stage, anal stage, phallic stage, latency,** and **genital stage.**

The Oral Stage. From birth to approximately 1 or 1½ years of life, the mouth is the infant's principal source of gratification and interaction with the environment. Libido, or psychic energy, is focused in the oral zone, since this is the area in which the id impulses can be satisfied. Hunger raises tension levels, feeding reduces the tension of hunger. Even other infant discomforts such as coldness, wetness, and restlessness can be temporarily reduced by feeding. The infant, totally dependent upon a mother figure, is cradled, touched, and fed, and its dependency needs are met. As teeth sprout, oral aggressiveness in biting and chewing becomes erogenized (invested with libido). Sucking does the same for oral incorporation. Oral incorporativeness and oral aggression may become the basis for later personality traits, depending upon whether sufficient gratification was obtained and whether the infant was overindulged.

The Anal Stage. In Freud's lifetime and in ours, toilet training is an important milestone in children's lives. The expulsion of feces reduces tension in the lower bowel, and Freud viewed this as instinctual gratification. Toilet training during the second year of life was seen by Freud as the child's first decisive encounter with the regulation of an instinctual impulse. Handled properly, the child learns to postpone gratification until a more appropriate time and place. The socialization of these and other impulses become an important goal of the developing ego. When toilet training is not done well, the child may discover that holding back feces controls the parent or that inappropriate expulsion vents rage at the controls. These traits may continue symbolically in later life. The individual may be obstinate and stingy (holding back) or have an explosive temper. The critical aspect of the anal stage is impulse control.

The Phallic Stage. Around the age of 3, the penis and clitoris become the focus of libidinal energy. Freudian notions about the phallic stage of development remain controversial today, especially Freud's concepts of psychosexual development in females. During the phallic stage, the **Oedipal conflict** develops and must be resolved. At this point, the child develops a natural sexual attraction for the parent of the opposite sex and views the parent of the same sex as a competitor. The child has some awareness that incest is unacceptable, and the male child fears the father will harm him, and develops **castration anxiety.** The fear is specifically of castration, since the child's offending behavior was sexual. Castration anxiety results in the boy's repression of the sexual impulses toward mother and in identification with father as a protective measure. The child takes the position that "if I can't beat him, I'll join him." The repression of the Oedipus conflict is the final step in the development of the superego. The child internalizes the values and ideals of the parent (in this case, the father).

Freud saw a somewhat different process occurring in girls, which he attributed to **penis envy.** The girl discovers that the boy has a penis, but she does not, and holds her mother responsible for this "loss." In the daughter's primitive view, the mother must have removed the penis as punishment for the child's sexual feelings toward the father. As a result, the female child gives up some of her identification with the mother, represses her sexual feelings toward her father, but transfers her childish love to her father because he has the organ she wishes to have. Her feelings for men are mixed, a combination of love and envy. For women, the Oedipal conflict (also, in women, called the **Electra conflict**) results in a reduced identification with the mother as a love object, and a turning toward the father. The **incest taboo,** however, prevents the female child from actualizing the impulses toward the father, and they are later displaced onto other men, resulting (according to Freud) in a more appropriate heterosexual adjustment. This process is considered to be *normal* development in traditional psychoanalytic theory.

Latency. After the turmoil of the phallic stage and its Oedipal conflict, the child enters a stage of psychosexual quiet, at about the age of 7. Freud proposed that this was a period of plateau, lasting until puberty around the age of 12.

The Genital Stage. The increased activity of the sexual hormones at the onset of puberty ends the latency period. The heightened libido of adolescence reactivates Oedipal feelings, but if this conflict was successfully resolved during the phallic stage, the individual's sexual interests are transferred to members of the opposite sex outside the family unit. The reorienting of sexual interest leads to mature love, rather than selfish love. The self-centered (narcissistic) impulses of the oral, anal, and phallic stages fuse with mature genital impulses; thus, the individual becomes a socialized, reality-oriented adult with a relatively unique personality in which id, ego, and superego functions work in reasonable harmony. However, even in these conditions of reasonable harmony, the individual has to deal with anxiety.

Anxiety

Anxiety was a major phenomenon that Freud observed in the interplay between id, ego, and superego. Freud distinguished three types of anxiety: **reality anxiety, moral anxiety,** and **neurotic anxiety.** When ego functions are flooded with environmental stimulation that cannot be brought under control (i.e., real dangers), a person experiences objective, or reality anxiety. When one thinks or does something which violates a superego value or ideal (e.g., thinks of killing someone, or lies, or steals) moral anxiety is experienced as guilt. However, when the ego functions cannot cope with excessive stimulation from id impulses, the person feels neurotic anxiety because of the potential punishment for the expression of these socially unacceptable behaviors.

Freud considered the trauma of birth to be the prototype of anxiety. The newborn infant is flooded with stimulation that it cannot cope with, since it has just come from the sheltered existence of the uterus and amniotic fluid, in which all its needs were met. The newborn enters an immediate state of overexcitation. In later theorizing, Freud came to consider anxiety as a signal of impending overstimulation, a signal of a danger that would overwhelm ego functions. This anxiety functions as a drive, since the person seeks to decrease unpleasant tension. If and when the ego processes' more rational attempts to deal with the anxiety fail, less rational ego functions, which Freud called defense mechanisms, are brought into play to defend the self against the painful tension being experienced.

Defense Mechanisms

Freud placed the defense mechanisms on a continuum from more to less rational. The defense mechanisms of **identification, displacement,** and **sublimation** were seen by Freud as being relatively rational. Since Freud viewed most human behavior as irrational, he emphasized the importance of the less rational defense mechanisms, such as repression, in understanding human behavior. Before we cover repression and other irrational defenses, a description of the supposedly more rational defenses will show that they may also result in irrational behavior.

Successful use of the "rational" processes of identification, displacement, and sublimation allow the individual to resolve anxiety, conflict, and frustration. Freud considered these three processes to be the most healthy of the defense mechanisms. In identification, individuals take features of others' personalities into their own. In effect, people take in as part of themselves the anxiety-reducing behavior of others, usually people who have great significance, such as parents. This process is not in the individual's conscious awareness. A person's final personality is an accumulation of many identifications made during the life span, but most importantly during early childhood.

Like identification, displacement also normally functions to reduce tension or anxiety. When the target of an instinctual impulse is blocked by external barriers or internal barriers (what Freud called anticathexis), the impulse is displaced to another target (object). A common example is an aggressive impulse toward one's boss which cannot be expressed because of fear of retribution. The fear of retribution may be a result of an external threat (barrier) such as the danger of being fired; or the fear may be due to internal threats such as a childhood fear of father, which is activated by authority figures such as a boss. Because the aggressive impulse cannot be directly expressed, it is displaced to a more acceptable (less anxiety-provoking) target: One yells at the kids. However, Freud proposed that action toward the substituted target is not as satisfying as toward the original, and residual anxiety may build over time: One kicks the cat, also! Even then the action is probably not satisfying, and a more-or-less permanent motivating pool of aggressive impulse remains to influence the individual's behavior.

A third defense mechanism, sublimation is considered to be fairly healthy because of its supposed contributions to society. In this process, unacceptable impulses are transformed into socially acceptable behaviors such as artistic creativity. Freud, for example, studied the life of the Renaissance artist and creative genius Leonardo da Vinci and deduced that da Vinci was so productive because he was sublimating unacceptable homosexual impulses. (Freud's sweeping conclusion about da Vinci have been criticized by others.)

When identification, displacement, and sublimation are ineffective in reducing anxiety, and the anxiety grows to excessive proportions, the ego may utilize the less rational defense mechanisms. Freud identified several defense mechanisms with two characteristics in common: 1. they distort reality, and 2. they operate unconsciously, out of the person's awareness. The most common of these mechanisms are repression, regression, reaction formation, projection, and rationalization.

Repression. Freud saw **repression** as the most basic and important ego defense mechanism. An undesirable impulse, threatened by punishment, is kept from entering consciousness by being repressed into the unconscious, out of the individual's awareness. Repression is ineffective, however. The id impulses are strong and threaten to break through into behavior either directly or symbolically. Once unpleasant, threatening, or repulsive experiences have been repressed, they cannot be brought back into conscious awareness in their original form. If they do come back, they are changed or disguised to protect the person from recognizing them. For this reason, Freud was very interested in the symbolic meaning of behavior and dreams.

Regression. In normal development, the individual must successfully pass through a series of developmental stages. On this journey, the individual may not completely resolve certain developmental tasks at a particular stage, leaving residual problems. At a later age, overwhelming anxiety may be "handled" by returning to behaviors more characteristic of an earlier developmental stage (i.e., the person "regresses"). Common examples of **regression** to the oral stage, for example, include cigarette smoking, eating, and alcohol ingestion—all of which can reduce anxiety. Regression is usually not total, and not all of the individual's behavior is characteristic of the earlier stage of development.

Reaction Formation. Freud has pointed out that ambivalence (having two conflicting feelings, thoughts, or impulses toward the same object) is quite common. In **reaction formation** such conflict is handled by repressing the more unacceptable impulse and overemphasizing the acceptable one. For example, an individual threatened by the breakthrough of dangerous sexual impulses may repress sexual feelings and guard against them by becoming overly moralistic. Thus, a Freudian would see prudishness as an attempt to avoid the anxiety caused by the fear of punishment for one's sexuality.

Projection. In **projection,** the anxiety over an unacceptable id impulse is avoided by externalizing the impulse onto another person. For example, a person with id impulses of rage may project them onto another person or group of persons, and perceive these others as threatening and dangerous.

Rationalization. Individuals who rationalize misperceive their own motive. They give "good" reasons for their behavior, rather than the real reasons. When the id impulse breaks through into behavior, the ego disguises the content of the thought and turns it into a more acceptable notion. An example might be the parent who physically punishes a child and then says, "I did it for your own good." There is usually an element of truth in the **rationalization** which makes it sound plausible.

These defense mechanisms are operative in both normal and abnormal behavior. Freud would say that they are neither positive nor negative, but may be simply more or less effective.

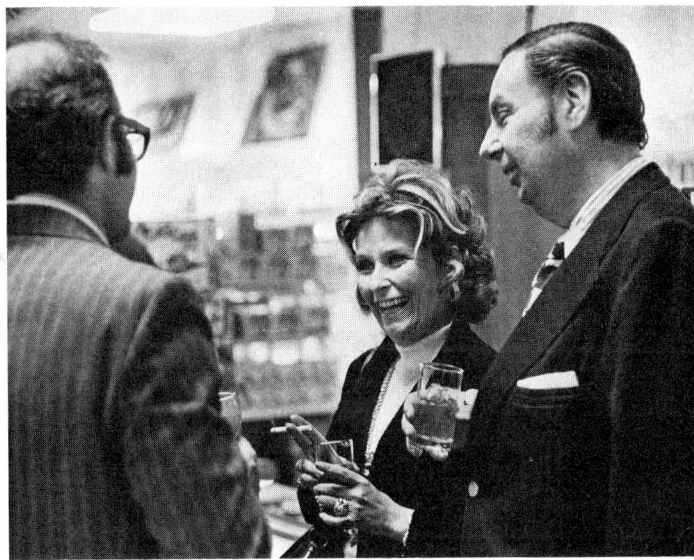

Freud proposed that under conditions of anxiety, some adults regress to behaviors which were satisfying at earlier stages of development. For example, Freudians would regard drinking and smoking as regressions to the oral stage.

Later Psychoanalytic Theorists: The Neo-Freudians

Freud was a seminal thinker and creative theorist. His concepts were so startling for the time that many rejected them and were outraged at his boldness. However, others were drawn to him and became his students, beginning a line of "theoretical descendants" which continues to exist. Most of Freud's first students rivaled him in their ability to develop theories of human behavior. As they reached disagreement with him, they often "left the fold" to develop their own major conceptual frameworks. These theorists are known as **neo-Freudians.**

Carl Jung. Carl Jung was among the first to break away from Freud. Their parting was unpleasant, since Freud strongly opposed Jung's decreased emphasis on the importance of childhood sexuality. Jung emphasized the person's future goals and desires. Jung also proposed the concept of a **collective unconscious,** a storehouse of racial memories which he believed to be transmitted genetically. Jung's focus on these memories led to an interest in the symbolism of dream content as a way of interpreting the impact of the collective unconscious on people's current behaviors. Jung's concepts are even less amenable to rigorous definition than Freud's, and almost no research has been done on Jung's ideas.

Alfred Adler. Alfred Adler, another student of Freud's, also deviated from the master. Adler believed that Freud's emphasis on internal dynamics was too limited. Unlike Freud, he took the position that social interaction was a critical factor in human development, and that a striving for superiority is a primary motivation. Adler felt that this "will to power" was a reaction to the inferiority that the child develops out of a recognition of its relative weakness vis-à-vis the parents. A common example of this process is that of President Theodore Roosevelt, who was a sickly child who overcame his weakness through great effort. He "overcompensated" and became a cowboy, soldier, hunter, and famous politician. Adler's view of humans was quite positive in terms of his belief that they could overcome great odds. He emphasized social engineering in his "individual psychology" and remains a popular theorist among educators of children.

Karen Horney. From the vantage point of the 1980s, Freud's ideas about the psychology of women may seem chauvinistic. Karen Horney was a neo-Freudian who rejected Freud's views about women long before the women's rights movement was fashionable. She denied that female personality development had anything to do with penis envy. Instead, Horney proposed that the primary issue for *both* men and women is the development of a sense of security. If the child's sense of security is upset by parental overprotection or rejection, the child will develop "basic anxiety." In order to deal with this basic anxiety, the person develops needs which lead to problem behaviors. Karen Horney placed these problematic needs in three general categories: the need to move against people (e.g., aggression), the need to move away from people (e.g., withdrawal or social isolation) and the need to move toward people (e.g., overdependence on others).

Erik Erikson. Erik Erikson is a very popular neo-Freudian. His theories reflect an increasing emphasis on environment as a factor in personality development. Erikson is an "ego psychologist." In other words, his emphasis in personality development is on the mediating functions of the ego as they deal with the problem of need satisfaction in a complex social environment. Erikson is perhaps best known for his reconception of developmental stages. In contrast to Freud, who believed that personality development was essentially complete by the end of childhood, Erikson proposed that personality development is a lifelong process (Erikson, 1964). His concept of developmental stages focuses on life tasks that must be resolved, rather than on psychosexual development as do Freud's. Erikson's view of life as a series of developmental hurdles, with solutions that determine later personality, are representative of an important conceptualization in the psychology of personality development.

When Things Go Wrong: Psychoanalytic Views

According to traditional psychoanalytic theory, when the superego, ego, and id are well developed as a function of appropriate resolution of the psychosexual stages of development, the individual has a well-functioning personality. However, ineffective resolution of the developmental stages leads to problems in later life. If the child is either overindulged or suffers excessive frustration, the ego may not develop enough to effectively mediate between the unconscious id impulses and external reality. When extreme frustration is present, the id impulses are rarely satisfied, and are left at a high drive level. Energy must then be expended in the defense mechanisms to keep the impulses repressed. The ego is then depleted and is less effective in dealing with external reality. However, the defense mechanisms are relatively ineffective, and the residual impulses continue to threaten to break through. The person then experiences the danger signal of neurotic anxiety. When the developmental stages are characterized by overindulgence, the id impulses are expressed and easily satisfied, and the ego functions do not develop sufficient strength. In effect, the functions are not tested through experience, and cannot develop appropriate reality-testing skills. Either overindulgence or excessive frustration results in fixation at the developmental stage at which it occurs. Later, the adult ego is weak, and anxiety may be resolved by regression to the behavior that reduced anxiety at the earlier stage. The anxious person who is fixated at the oral stage, for example, may reduce anxiety by smoking, drinking, or eating—adult behaviors that symbolically represent the anxiety-reducing oral behaviors in infancy.

The superego processes may also lead to problem behaviors if the Oedipal conflict is not resolved. The unresolved sexual impulses toward the opposite-sex parent, and the aggressive impulses toward the same-sex parent may lead to feelings of inferiority and guilt because of violation of superego values and ideals (see Figure 3.2). On the other hand, when the societal values, ideals, and prohibitions have not been introjected (taken in by the child) during the developmental stages (possibly because the parents' values were too lenient), the superego development is not sufficient and the individual has a "weak conscience" and no moral self-control. Such individuals feel no remorse, guilt, or anxiety when they break rules or hurt others.

According to psychoanalytic theory, the more severe forms of disorders (psychoses) are

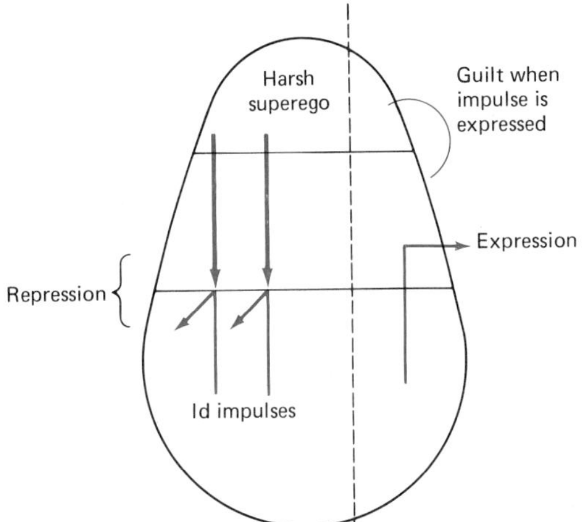

Figure 3.2. Conflict between the superego and id. The harsh superego forces id impulses to be repressed. If these impulses are expressed, a harsh superego punishes the ego, creating guilt.

a function of childhood experiences in the first few years of life, when trust and survival are paramount issues. The individual who is delusional and hallucinates has an extremely weakened ego, which cannot prevent unconscious material from breaking through into consciousness. The irrationality of psychotic thinking and behavior is representative of the primary process thinking that characterizes the unconscious mind.

Comments on the Psychoanalytic Perspective

A significant problem of the psychoanalytic approaches is that their concepts are extremely inferential. The theorists have observed behavior and inferred underlying constructs (e.g., like the unconscious) and processes which are extraordinarily difficult to measure, if they can be measured at all. In addition, these grand and elaborate theories are based on a case history method of investigation. The population sample studied is extremely small. For example, while Freud was an astute observer of human behavior both in and out of his consulting room, it is doubtful that he actually treated more than a few dozen people in his lifetime. This estimate is based on the fact that psychoanalysis of one individual takes many years (perhaps 10–15), and an analyst usually has only 8–10 patients at any one time. From the very limited data base of his own dreams and the treatment of a small number of middle- and upper-class citizens of Vienna in the early 1900s, Freud generalized his theories to a world of billions of people in many diverse cultures.

The concepts of the psychoanalytic framework are extremely metaphorical. They are difficult to specify objectively, and formulation of a researchable hypothesis is difficult. Thus, little corroborating research data exist to support the existence of many of Freud's concepts. Researchers keep trying. Lloyd Silverman (1976), for example, reported on the results of 10 years of laboratory studies on an important psychoanalytic concept: the activation of psychopathology by unconscious libidinal and aggressive wishes. He reports that these studies support the conclusion that unconscious libidinal and aggressive wishes affect the manifestation of abnormal behavior both in regard to type of pathology and degree.

Heilbrun (1980) attempted to replicate Silverman's results using a slightly modified design (which favored positive results), but was unable to demonstrate similar results and conclusions. The negative results of Heilbrun's experiment throw doubt on Silverman's conclusions.

The conflicting findings of these two research reports illustrate the problems in the experimental validation of psychoanalytic theory: for every piece of supporting research, one can find an equally well-designed study that refutes the first study's conclusions. At this point, psychoanalytic concepts still appear unverifiable through the experimental method. They remain concepts that are primarily supported because they make sense to their advocates, and seem helpful to some people in conceptualizing human behavior. Perhaps in the near future, some researcher will find a way to test these concepts and resolve the issue.

Even without a great deal of empirical proof, psychoanalytic theory has contributed a great deal to our thinking on personality development. Concepts such as the unconscious processes, psychosexual stages of development, infantile sexuality, id, ego, superego, and the defense mechanisms are widely adopted. In spite of being based on a small population studied through the case study approach, and in spite of its speculative nature, psychoanalytic theory has been a major stimulus for empirical research into human behavior—either attempts to prove the concepts right or wrong, or to demonstrate more functional systems can explain abnormal behavior.

THE HUMANISTIC PERSPECTIVE

> I'm 43 years old, I've got a wife and three kids, and we get along fine. My law practice is booming, I play golf with my dad, love my mother and I've got two cars and a boat. I've achieved everything I really ever wanted. . . . So tell me—why am I bored? Why am I having an affair with a 20-year-old kid who couldn't add 2 and 2? And why do I feel so damn guilty about it? Damn it! Why don't I like myself?

Chapter 2 noted that in the 1940s, a view of behavior arose which rejected the pessimistic determinism of Freudian psychoanalysis. This alternative perspective on human behavior has become known as **humanistic psychology.** Since then, humanistic psychology has also been seen as an alternative to what some consider the mechanistic determinism of learning theory conceptions of behavior. Thus, the humanistic perspective has been called a "third force" in psychology.

The proponents of the humanistic approaches emphasize the subjective nature of human existence. Carl Rogers, a spokesman for this perspective, has said, "Man lives essentially in his own personal and subjective world, and even his most objective functioning . . . is the result of subjective purpose and subjective choice" (C. R. Rogers, 1959). In order to fully understand a person's behavior, one must understand the person's subjective world. Like psychoanalytic theory, humanistic approaches focus on the inner person. However, they do not emphasize instincts, unconscious processes, and psychic determinism.

Humanistic psychologists believe that behavior is predominantly organized around the positive motive of self-fulfillment; the need to develop one's potentiality to the fullest. More than many others, humanistic psychologists have explored the concepts of optimal levels of personality functioning (presented in Chapter 1). Humanistic psychology is a major conceptual model in the field of psychotherapy, and many psychologists operate from this framework. Two psychologists considered primary theorists in this approach are Abraham Maslow and Carl Rogers.

Maslow's Concept of a Hierarchy of Needs

Maslow (1970) recognized that a variety of needs motivate and direct human behavior, and suggested that these needs are ordered in a hierarchy from basic needs to those which are manifestations of the highest human potential. Maslow's hierarchy has become widely accepted as a model of this concept. He suggested that two types of needs motivate us: deficiency needs and growth needs. Deficiency needs, from the most to least powerful, include physiological drives, safety, belongingness, love needs, and esteem needs. Growth needs include the **self-actualization motive** and cognitive understanding. Self-actualization is the attainment of one's full intellectual, emotional, and behaviorial potential. In Maslow's context, cognitive understanding means to understand people in a nonjudgmental way, with a recognition of the demands of reality.

Maslow uses the term "deficiency needs" to identify needs that have priority only when they are not satisfied. That is, if a person's safety needs are not met, the person will focus on satisfying these needs to the exclusion of others higher in the hierarchy. Stranded in a car in the midst of a winter blizzard, a person will be motivated to find shelter. The need to be loved will be a secondary concern. If safety needs are satisfied, but the need for love is not, the person will strive to find satisfaction of love before satisfying the need for self-esteem. In order to achieve love, the person may engage in behavior that reduces self-esteem (e.g., begging for someone's love). Each level of need must be satisfied before the next can take precedence. Only when all the deficiency needs are satisfied are we motivated to move toward self-actualization and cognitive understanding, the growth needs (see Figure 3.3).

The needs of self-actualization and cognitive understanding are difficult to satisfy, and most individuals do not reach these goals. People may not achieve these levels of function because they live in an environment that continually frustrates the deficiency needs, thus, the person never reaches a point where the growth needs can take priority. Obviously, a minimal level of physical security must be present if adequate personality development is to occur. Existence in rat-infested urban slums, drug-ridden neighborhoods, or a ramshackle Appalachian cabin will have adverse effects on satisfaction of the basic needs; and the higher needs will not assume priority. Such environments have an effect on intellectual levels in some children (Benda et al., 1963; Heber, 1970). Deprivation of security needs may result in an adult who appears to be overwhelmingly concerned with material gain, rather than maximization of the self-concept.

Even in environments at least as moderately need-fulfilling as those of the middle-class United States, self-actualization is often delayed or prevented by subtle environmental effects. Discrimination against women, for example, is often identified as a factor that prevents them from achieving their full potential. In our modern society, it seems difficult to satisfy the needs of belonging, love, and self-esteem, which must be satisfied before self-actualization can occur. This is why humanistic psychotherapists often focus on the issues of belonging, love, and the self-concept in psychotherapy. The concept of "self" is the focus of the other major humanist, Carl Rogers.

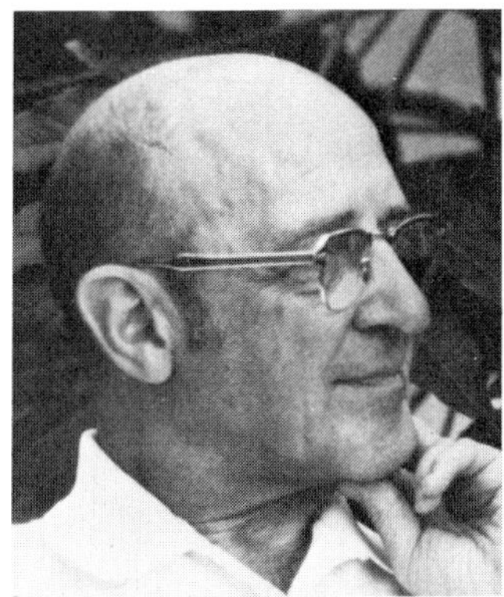

Carl Rogers, born 1902, American psychologist and humanist.

Carl Rogers's: Humanistic Self-Concept Theories

Carl Roger's view of personality functioning has three conceptual ingredients: 1. the **organism,** 2. the **phenomenal field,** and 3. the self. By organism, Rogers means the total individual, including thoughts, feelings, perceptions of the external world, and sensory or visceral experiences not clearly available to the person's awareness. The phenomenal field includes experiences and perceptions that the person is focusing on at any given moment. Some of these perceptions and experiences become defined by the person as stable attributes of the self and come to constitute the **self-concept.**

Figure 3.3. Maslow's hierarchy of needs

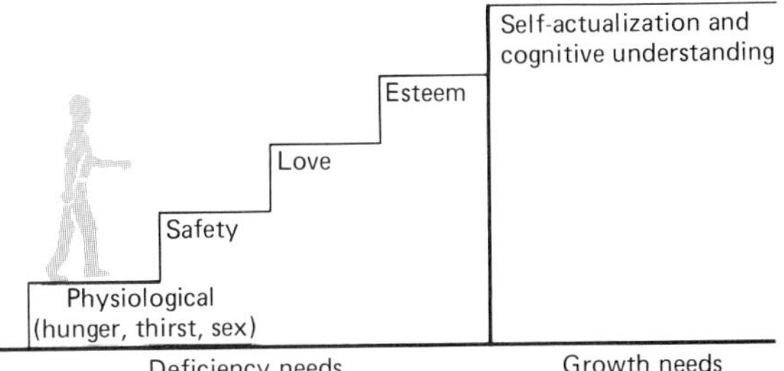

In Carl Rogers's view (as in Maslow's), human behavior has one basic motive: to actualize, enhance, and maintain the organism. This motive acts as a drive toward development, autonomy, and maturation, and is present in all organic life, though in humans it may be hidden by many layers of psychological defenses (C. R. Rogers, 1951, 1961). The individual personality is unique; although one may share broad aspects of existence with others, each person has his or her own phenomenal field and self-concept.

Humanistic psychologists see the self-concept as the integrating core of personality, around which our experiences are organized and interpreted (May, 1973; C. R. Rogers, 1961). Most people think about this "self" when they speak of "personality." The "I" includes how we see ourselves, how others see us, and how we would like to be seen by ourselves and by others. Through experience, people come to see themselves in a particular way; each person develops unique attitudes, beliefs, and feelings about him- or herself, about others, and about the world and his or her place in it. People make assumptions about how things are, how they can be, and how they should be. People's concepts of self, the world, and their place in it are seen by humanistic psychologists as important factors in personality development, since these concepts appear to influence how people perceive experiences and how they behave.

Personality Development

According to Carl Rogers, at birth the infant has **organic wisdom,** the ability to value its experiences as good or not good, depending on the degree to which they meet the basic actualizing, growth motive. As the tendency toward growth and actualization is expressed, the infant begins to differentiate the "I" or "me" as a distinct part of its experience. Some aspects of the developing concept of self may be perceived sharply (consciously) or cloudily (even unconsciously, below conscious awareness). These perceptions are given positive or negative values. These values may be experienced directly by the organism or introjected (taken in) from others such as parents, teachers, sibs, and friends. However, values introjected from others tend to distort the self-concept, since they often require the individual to ignore inner feelings. For example, the child who learns that anger is not valued, may sometimes experience events that lead to angry feelings. When such discrepancies exist between genuine values (angry feelings) and introjected values (anger is bad), conflict ensues and the individual feels tense, uncomfortable, and dissatisfied.

As experiences occur, the organism may either: 1. perceive, symbolize, and organize them into the self-structure; 2. ignore them because they are not perceived as having a relationship to the self; or 3. deny the symbolization because the experience is *inconsistent* with the self-percept. Denial often occurs through distorted perception. For example, if one's self-concept values success, then poor performance on a test may be inaccurately perceived as a function of poor testing conditions rather than as caused by one's own lack of understanding of the material being tested. In some cases, behavior may be brought about by experiences and needs which are totally denied symbolization: They are not "owned" by the self. In instances when self-consistency is violated, the individual usually disowns the behavior by conceptualizing it as "not like me" or as being "carried away." These descriptions of perceptual distortion and disowning of behavior may sound familiar to you. They are Rogers's way of thinking about some of the behaviors that Freud called defense mechanisms.

As the awareness of self emerges, emotion facilitates goal-directed behavior. Emotion is always positive from Rogers's perspective. It causes difficulty only when the self-concept is distorted. When the person is effectively in touch with the actualization motive and the self is not distorted, the emotions and self-concept both are consistent or "congruent." The person can engage in optimal self-actualization. However, if the self-concept is distorted, then actualization of distorted aspects of the self-concept may lead to problem behavior.

Rogers suggests that as the self-concept forms, people develop both a "need for positive regard" (which may be either innate or learned—Rogers was not sure) and "a need for self-regard." The need for positive regard may become strong enough to take precedence over one's own values if the self-concept has been based on others' values. When this occurs, the person acquires a **condition of worth,** a sense that the regard of others and one's own regard for self depend primarily on the approval of other people. However, if a person has experienced "unconditional positive regard" (i.e., positive regard independent of any conditions), the needs for positive regard and self-regard would be satisfied. This ideal condition rarely exists; it is a state, Rogers believes, which must be worked toward at all times.

The Rogerian conception of personality development is essentially an optimistic one. The basic motive is actualization of the total organism and growth; and the personality, though generally consistent, can change as the self-concept perceives a changing environment. However, distortions of the self-concept or incongruence can lead to tension, anxiety, denial, and other extremely maladaptive behaviors.

When Things Go Wrong: The Humanistic Perspective

Carl Rogers has said, "Psychological maladjustment exists when the organism [person] denies to awareness significant sensory and visceral experiences which consequently are not symbolized and organized into the gestalt [pattern] of the self-structure. When this situation exists, there is basic or potential psychological tension" (C. R. Rogers, 1951). When one's behavior and experiences do not mesh with the way one sees oneself, there is a lack of "congruence" which must be dealt with somehow. Often, the process of dealing with inconsistency involves further distortion or denial, and subsequently even more behavior that does not fit the individual's perception of self and the way others see her or him. For example, children who fail at a task may experience their parents as having rejected them for their failure. They may then come to see themselves as people who are not able to succeed. When faced with future tasks, they may give up or avoid the tasks completely because they know that they "can't do that." This reinforces their growing view of themselves as "failures" or "helpless" or "inadequate." Their self-concept may in later years promote helpless behavior. Then, when placed in a situation where they *have* to cope or where others' expectations are very high, they may experience a great deal of anxiety over the lack of fit between how they see themselves (as helpless) and the expectation (to be able to cope). The sense of anxiety or tension may lead them to experience the lack of fit between self-concept and experience as a threat to the consistency of the self-concept. To deal with the threat, the self-structure becomes even more rigidly invested in maintaining the self-image and, therefore, becomes more incongruent and more maladjusted.

From the perspective of humanistic theory, self-concepts tend to filter perceptions so that they confirm the person's view of the self. An individual who has a self-concept that centers on helplessness or inability to cope will deny or distort the perception of his or her own independent or coping behavior. The individual will perceive these behaviors in a way that supports the self-concept of helplessness. Perceptions become symbolized in a manner that supports the original self-concept of helplessness when, in fact, the person (and each of us) is at times helpless, and at other times independent and self-reliant.

Humanistic psychologists believe that positive self-concepts can develop through counseling. The humanistic psychologist who treats disturbed individuals attempts to provide a setting of unconditional positive regard, understanding, and an absence of conditions of worth. In this setting, the "helpless" adult, through positive experience, can begin to modify critical aspects of the self-concept so that she or he can begin to experience the self as competent, not helpless (Depue & Monroe, 1978).

Comments on the Humanistic Perspective

The humanistic perspective, represented by Maslow's and Rogers's views, has attained broad popularity among both the general public and psychologists. However, Rogers and Maslow have little to say about how specific behaviors are learned, and they do not consider the question of developmental sequences in growth and maturation. The humanistic perspectives (especially Rogers's) have stimulated a great deal of research on personality, personality change, and psychotherapy (Ryckman, 1978). Much of this research has attempted to identify the characteristics of an effective therapeutic relationship, and will be discussed in Chapter 20.

The most significant criticism of the humanistic theories is that they are extremely subjective and inferential. They lack precision. Just as in the psychoanalytic model, concepts tend to be broad, ill defined, and metaphorical. Concepts such as self-actualization, cognitive understanding, organic wisdom, and congruence are no more concrete or objective than unconscious processes, ego, or repression.

Humanistic psychologists' theories may also be criticized in terms of narrow scope. Although humanistic psychological concepts seem to "fit" mildly disturbed individuals, the concepts inadequately describe and explain more severe forms of disorders. The perspective appears most appropriate when applied to problems of mild dissatisfaction, anxiety, and unhappiness rather than to extremely troublesome behaviors. The fact that humanistic psychology's concepts make sense when applied to problems of personal dissatisfaction may explain its popularity with the moderately well-to-do individual who wants to raise his "consciousness" or "do her own thing." Perhaps humanistic psychology's major contribution is its emphasis that people are not static, but are in a continual process of growth and change. Its focus on the self-concept is also important, in that the conscious self is seen as a major determinant of behavior, an issue generally neglected by psychoanalytically oriented theorists and by many behaviorists. The humanistic approach remains a major force in psychology today.

THE BEHAVIORAL PERSPECTIVE

> You know, I could always handle my booze. I remember when I was little, my dad would give me a sip of beer now and then. . . . I guess I just had good training! Hell, drinking's part of growing up. Nothing like a few sips of suds to liven up a party. Everyone I know drinks, except some real creepy types; they're no fun.

Just as many variations of psychoanalytic theories and many variations of humanistic theories exist, several theories of human behavior are based on the concept of learning. The term "learning theory" is usually applied to approaches which have their roots in the experimental laboratory tradition of psychology, and which tend to focus more on observable behavior than intrapsychic events. An overview of the historical developments of these viewpoints has been presented in Chapter 2. Now the views on personality development and behavior of four viewpoints will be examined in greater detail: classical conditioning, the operant approach, the social learning approach, and cognitive behaviorism.

Classical Conditioning

A major concept of learning theory is that behavior can be "conditioned." This concept can perhaps best be illustrated by expanding upon the description of Ivan Pavlov's classic **conditioning** experiment, which was mentioned in Chapter 2. Pavlov placed a dog in an elaborate apparatus in order to study its digestive processes. During the course of the studies, the dog was given meat powder to induce salivation. After a number of trials Pavlov discovered that the dog began to salivate *prior* to the presentation of the powder. Salivation in the absence of meat powder occurred in conjunction with a variety of events: when the dog saw its feeder enter the room, when it heard the technician's footsteps, or even when it was placed in the harness at the beginning of later trials.

Pavlov began then to systematically study this phenomenon. Using the harness and a device to measure salivation, he presented meat powder to a series of dogs, and demonstrated that they salivated automatically when the powder was placed in their mouths. Later, a tone was sounded behind the animals, and the meat powder was placed in their mouths. Again salivation occurred automatically. The tone was paired with meat powder in this manner in a series of presentations. Finally, the tone was sounded alone and salivation occurred even when the meat powder was not presented.

In this model of learning, the meat powder which automatically induces salivation is called the **unconditioned stimulus** (UCS), and the response of salivation is the **unconditioned response** (UCR) (see Table 3.1).

The tone, when it begins to elicit the salivation response becomes the **conditioned stimulus** (CS). At this point, we can call the salivation, when elicited by the tone, **conditioned response** (CR). Pavlov went on to discover the process of **extinction.** If the tone continued to

Table 3.1
The classical conditioning model of Pavlov[1]

Situation	*Stimulus*		*Response*
Original Situation	S_1 (Food)	⟶	R_1 (Salivation)
Paired Stimulus Situation	$S_1 + S_2$ (Food) (Bell)	⟶	R_1 (Salivation)
Postconditioning Situation	S_2 (Bell)	⟶	R_2 (Salivation)

[1]Key: S_1 = unconditioned stimulus (UCS), S_2 = conditioned stimulus (CS), R_1 = unconditioned response (UCR), R_2 = conditioned response (CR).

be sounded repeatedly over a long period of time, the conditioned response would diminish. Finally, the tone could be sounded and no salivation would occur. The behavior had been "extinguished."

Pavlov's discovery was an important precursor to the development of more complicated concepts related to the acquisition of behavior. However, some theorists have applied his concepts directly to the understanding of behavior, especially to behaviors such as anger, fear, and anxiety, which we call emotions. We will return to this issue when we discuss the relationship of learning theory to abnormal behavior.

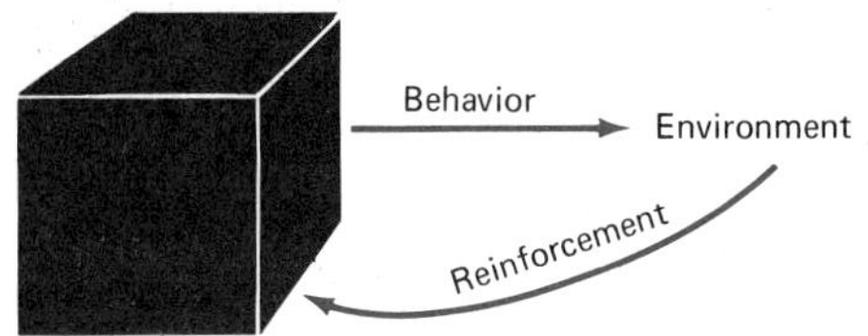

Figure 3.4. The mind as a black box. The radical behaviorist says that since we cannot objectively *measure* what goes on in people's minds, the mind is like a black box whose contents cannot be determined. Thus, we should base our views of behavior on what we can measure with some accuracy: behavior and environment.

Operant Learning

B. F. Skinner (1938) has what some have called a "radical behaviorist" approach to human behavior. His position is that we can study only what is observable, (i.e., behavior). The mental states that others have identified as leading to behavior cannot be seen, touched, or smelled and therefore cannot be measured or objectively studied (see Figure 3.4). Skinner, however, is not as radical as some believe. Though he does not accept the concept of a personality or a self that guides and directs behavior, he does not deny that mental events exist, nor that the person has many innate characteristics, which are not learned, such as temperament (B. F. Skinner, 1953, 1974). However, Skinner asserts that these mentalistic events and internal characteristics are simply beyond our capability for objective assessment. From the operant behaviorist's perspective, personality is the unique set (repertoire) of behaviors learned by an individual who has a unique genetic endowment and unique environmental conditions.

Skinner's predecessors studied how behavior becomes more probable, depending upon its effects on the environment. If the consequences are negative, the behavior is less likely to occur. From Skinner's perspective, behavior "operates" on the environment. Its manifestation is "instrumental" in whether the organism will have the opportunity for positive or negative reinforcement.

It is important to examine the term **reinforcement.** We often think of reinforcement as being synonymous with reward, in the sense of a pleasant consequence. Common positive reinforcers which seem pleasant include money, tasty food, and the approval of other people. In **operant learning,** however, a "positive" reinforcer is not necessarily pleasant. Positive reinforcement is defined simply as an event that increases the probability of the occurrence of a behavior.

Some positive reinforcers may seem unpleasant. A child, for example, may have a temper tantrum, and the consequence may be that the parent spanks the child. If we were measuring the frequency of temper tantrums, we might then discover that their frequency decreases. The spanking appears to have been a punishment and probably was experienced as unpleasant by the child. What if the tantrums increased after spanking? The increase in frequency would tell the operant behaviorist that the spanking was a positive reinforcer. How could this be? Each blow is painful, and the child still cries! We must assume that the spanking has some positively reinforcing consequence. The behaviorist may find that during a temper tantrum the child receives a great deal of attention from the parent; but when the child behaves, the parent is inattentive. We might conclude that the painful, negative consequence of spanking is less important to the child than the presence of attention from the parent. This attention is the positive reinforcer. This example illustrates not only the definition of positive reinforcement but also several other characteristics of the operant approach: 1. a reliance on objective data (frequency counts in this case), 2. a focus on behavior rather than subjective states (such as pain), and 3. a rela-

Table 3.2
Examples of operant consequences

Situation	*Sequence*		*Consequence*
Positive Reinforcement	Operant behavior →	Reinforcement →	Probability of behavior increases
	Temper tantrum →	Parental attention →	More tantrums
Negative Reinforcement	Operant behavior →	Negative reinforcement (termination of aversive stimulus) →	Probability of behavior increases
	Picking up clothing →	Roommate stops nagging →	Picking up clothing occurs more frequently
Withdrawal of Positive Reinforcement	Operant behavior →	Withdrawal of reinforcement →	Probability of behavior decreases
	Child swears at parent →	Parent takes toys away →	Swearing decreases
Punishment	Operant behavior →	Punishment →	Probability of behavior decreases
	Child swears →	Parent slaps →	Swearing decreases
Extinction	Operant behavior →	Extinction →	Probability of behavior decreases
	Temper tantrum →	Parent ignores tantrum →	Tantrums decrease

tive avoidance of subjective judgments about internal states.

Other consequences of behavior which have been studied by operant behaviorists (see Table 3.2) include the following:

1. Negative Reinforcement. The probability of a behavior's recurrence is increased by terminating an aversive stimulus. For example, suppose that your roommate nags you for leaving clothes on the floor, and you finally pick up the clothes (behavior). Your roommate stops complaining (termination of an aversive stimulus, or negative reinforcement). It becomes more likely that you will pick up your clothes if they are on the floor in the future.
2. Withdrawal of a Positive Reinforcer. A behavior occurs (a child swears at a parent) and a reinforcer is withdrawn (child's toys are taken away).
3. Punishment. The consequence of a behavior is an aversive stimulus. A child swears at a parent, the parent slaps him. Punishment is a common negative, unpleasant, or aversive consequence in our society. Unfortunately, when it is withdrawn, the punished behavior is likely to reappear (B. F. Skinner, 1938, 1953). In addition, punishment may result in emotional responses that are incompatible with appropriate behavior. In this example, the slap may lead to fear and avoidance of conversation with the parent—results not intended.
4. Extinction. A more effective consequence in the long term which will reduce the probability of behavior is extinction, or the absence of reinforcement. However, if a behavior is not reinforced for a number of occurrences, then is accidentally reinforced, then is extinguished again, then is reinforced, and so on, an **intermittent schedule of reinforcement** results, and the behavior becomes extremely resistant to extinction.

Skinner has identified various reinforcement schedules: continuous (reinforcement after each response) and such intermittent schedules as fixed ratio (reinforcement after a fixed number of responses), fixed interval (reinforcement after elapsed time such as 10 seconds, 60 minutes, 2 weeks), and variable ratio (reinforcement following different numbers of responses, i.e., after 5, 3, 10, 6 responses). Real life examples of intermittent schedules are piecework pay (fixed ratio), hourly pay (fixed interval), and slot machine payoffs (variable ratio). As noted in the description of extinction, an intermittent schedule of reinforcement is extremely resistant to extinction.

Another important concept in operant learning is the **discriminative stimulus.** When reinforcement occurs, some stimuli present become associated with the reinforcing event. These discriminative stimuli act as cues. For example, when a person walks into a dining room and sees the table set for a meal, the presence of the place settings acts as a cue that dinner is about to be served. On the other hand, if the table is not set and no food odors are present, these stimuli may be cues to ask if dinner is to be eaten in a restaurant. Some simple discriminative cues in everyday life include alarm clocks, stop signs, smiles, and frowns. Each of these cues is associated with behaviors that may or may not be reinforced.

The development of complex behaviors involves a process of **shaping,** also known as "successive approximation" or "chaining." All behaviors are composed of a series of pieces of behaviors. When we are learning to act in a particular way, we rarely learn in one attempt. We learn small bits which are reinforced and then chained together by reinforcing larger and larger groupings of these bits of behaviors. When we make errors, they are not reinforced, and correct responses are. Over time the complex behavior is "shaped" by the reinforcement of successively closer approximations of the desired end result.

For an operant behaviorist such as Skinner, personality is the sum total of observable behavior developed according to the learning principles outlined above. In addition, the individual learns to become an active manipulator of the environment to gain positive reinforcement and remove aversive stimuli. People even learn to manipulate themselves to obtain control of the environment. For example, they may learn to induce emotional changes such as "psyching themselves up." Skinner does not see humans as totally passive machines responding automatically to environmental stimuli, even though he does argue that all behavior is determined, not autonomous. Behavior, Skinner says, is not a function of "free will." Operant behaviorists do not utilize the concepts of drive, need, belief, attitude, instinct, and other "mentalisms" so prevalent in other theories, since they feel these concepts are not required to explain and predict behavior.

Social Learning and Cognitive Learning

The social learning approach to personality development takes a less radical stand than operant behaviorists on the issue of mental activity. Theorists such as Albert Bandura (1971, 1977) have investigated the effects of both environmental reinforcers and internal processes. Internal processes are covert, but are viewed as measurable and subject to manipulation. They can, for example, be measured by clients' self-reports or by using various psychological tests. Social learning theorists would grant that this type of measurement is less objective than is desirable, but it can be done. Social learning theorists view internal mediating events as primarily learned, and do not consider concepts such as innate needs and drives of great importance.

Since humans are the most cognitive of organisms, imaginal representations and symbols can be used to direct behavior. Although reinforcement of behavior by external events is important for learning (just as in the operant tradition), behavior is regulated to a significant degree by "anticipated outcomes." In effect, people are able to imagine or symbolize the future, and direct their behavior to enhance reinforcement or avoid painful consequences.

Observational Learning. Social learning theorists depart from the operant approach in proposing that through modeling, or **observational learning,** people can also learn without external reinforcement. Bandura (1977) suggests that observational learning can occur because people make a mental or cognitive image of behavior which can later be copied in physical behavior. In this process, trial and error play a negligible role, although reinforced practice refines the behavioral skills. Learning behaviors through modeling or imitation is extremely important in human development. Social learning theorists believe that the complexity of human behavior precludes the shaping of each single response through differential reinforcement. Some other learning process such as modeling *must* be operative, from their perspective.

Effective modeling depends on many factors. Among those which have been demonstrated are sex of the model and observer (the learner)

(Bandura, Ross, & Ross, 1963). Other things being equal, boys learn more effectively from males, and girls from females. The model's level of nurturance (or caring) and the model's power over the modeler are also important (Grusec & Mischel, 1966). A parent is a more powerful and (probably) a more nurturing model than a neighbor, so a child is more likely to model the parent's behavior. The model's similarity to the observer in terms of social characteristics also appears important (Rosenkrans, 1967). A psychologist is more likely to model the work behavior of other psychologists than the behavior of a long-haul trucker.

Modeling becomes even more complex a process when one realizes that more than one model may be observed, and modeled behaviors may conflict. The greater the consistency between models, the more likely the behavior will be consistently modeled. Behaviors are modeled (learned) when they are observed to gain reinforcement for others (vicarious reinforcement), and when they gain reinforcement for the observer who manifests them.

Little concern has been expressed by social learning theorists toward unlearned aspects of personality development, although they have acknowledged that such factors affect personality. Biological, genetic, and somatic aspects of the individual are not seen as unimportant, but the focus remains on learned behavior.

From a social learning perspective, personality develops from birth, when the infant learns new behaviors through direct reinforcement; but the infant quickly begins to imitate or model the behavior of parents. For example, even very young children will imitate parents' facial expressions (such as smiling), and parents give a great deal of social reinforcement to their infant when it smiles back. Inaccurate imitations may be shaped by parents (or other significant persons) through small steps to increase the accuracy, and some imitations may be punished ("Do as I say, not as I do") or simply not reinforced, and may drop out of the behavior repertoire. As the cognitive process develops, anticipated outcomes (called "expectations" by Julian Rotter; Rotter & Hochreich, 1975) begin to regulate behavior and internal control begins to develop.

Since many disturbed behaviors seem to involve a "lack of control," social learning theorists consider the learning of internal control important. From their perspective, self-control is learned and is primarily cognitive. Individuals learn to consider the consequences of their

Stereotypic sex roles may be modeled very early. Little girls are likely to model femininity; little boys are likely to model stereotypic male behavior.

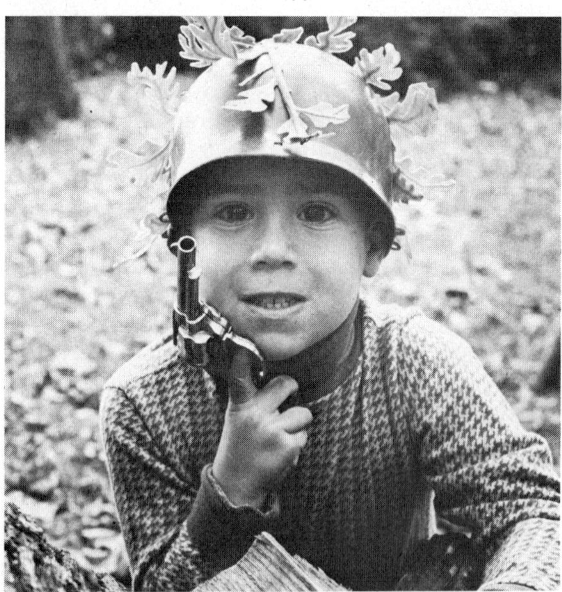

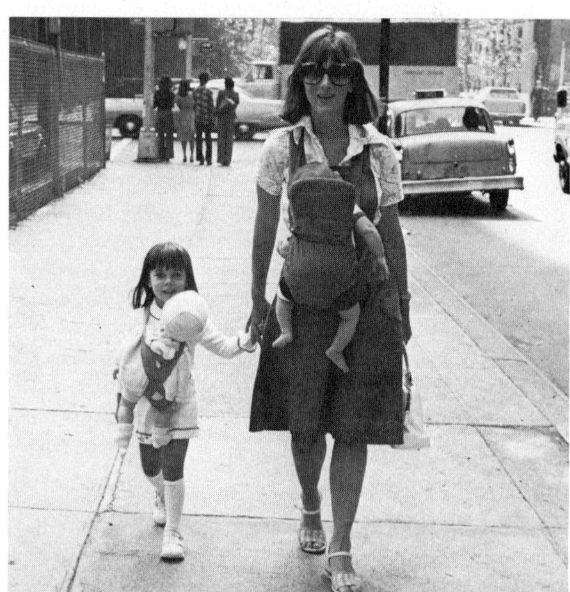

behavior and may inhibit their response (resist temptation) if they anticipate negative outcomes (Bandura, 1978). This anticipation of consequence is dependent on the observation of models throughout one's lifetime. Impulsiveness (nondelay of reinforcement) or lack of control is a function of modeling similar behaviors in parents and peers, not of id impulses breaking through—as the psychoanalysts would conceptualize it.

Self-reinforcement also seems to be learned through modeling and has an important impact on behavior. If one's models self-reinforce with "things" (treats) or self-approval only after reaching high levels of achievement, the observer tends to do the same. If the standards of achievement are too high, the infrequency of reinforcement may adversely affect the cognitive mediating process (the individual may learn that "I'm no good" or "I can't do it"). Individuals have different personalities because of the unique learning experiences, unique models, and unique environments they have experienced and the unique internal cognitive processes they have developed.

Cognitive Learning. The increasing emphasis on the importance of such cognitive factors as thoughts, talking to oneself, mental images, self-evaluation, feelings, memories, and beliefs is a relatively new development in learning theorists' views about human behavior. The learning that these factors mediate is called **cognitive learning.** People who *focus* on the importance of these factors in the learning of behavior are often called cognitive learning theorists. However, the dividing line between social learning theory and cognitive learning theory is not clear-cut. Albert Bandura, for example, is important in both perspectives.

Cognitive learning theorists believe that classical conditioning, operant conditioning, and observational learning are important in the development of behavior; but for a full understanding of why people behave as they do, one must also take into account the person's inner experiences, or **cognitions** (Mischel, 1973, 1976). Among the variables seen as important are: 1. encoding—how people selectively attend to specific aspects of their environment; 2. expectancies—what outcomes people expect,

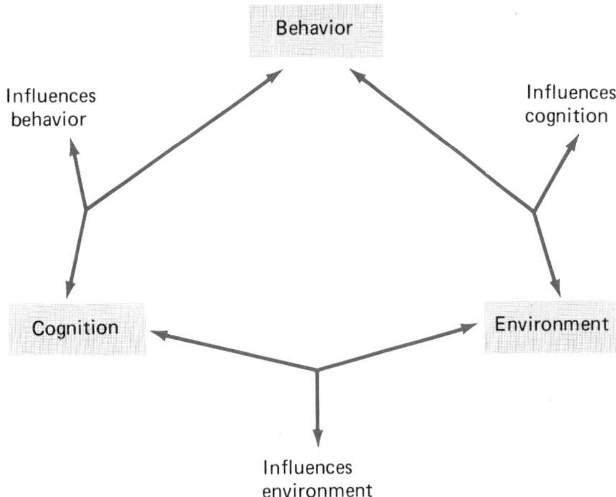

Figure 3.5. Reciprocal determinism.

both in terms of what their behavior can achieve and what they expect to be the results of events in their environment; 3. the values that people attach to outcomes, or the "subjective stimulus values" in Mischel's terms; and 4. the goals and standards which people set for themselves.

The increasing emphasis on the cognitive factors in learned behavior has resulted in a more comprehensive view of behavior on the part of many learning theorists. Bandura (1978), for example, sees behavior as due to a process of reciprocal determinism. Specific acts or ways of behaving that have been learned through reinforcement are influenced *by* the environment and cognitions; behaviors act *on* the environment and also influence cognition; and cognitions affect how people perceive the environment and how they behave (see Figure 3.5). Under certain circumstances, one factor may clearly dominate the others, but usually cognitions, strengths of learned behaviors, and environment are all factors that must be considered if one is to understand why people behave in particular ways.

When Things Go Wrong: The Behavioral Perspective

Learning theorists suggest that abnormal behaviors are learned exactly as we learn normal behaviors. Abnormality may consist of behavioral deficits (i.e., behaviors we should have learned but did not) or excesses (behaviors we should not have learned, but did). A behavioral deficit, for example, would be a lack of social skills, which results in social withdrawal and isolation. A behavioral excess would be a strong fear response to relatively neutral stimuli such as spiders (usually called a phobia).

In the most basic conceptualization, "abnormal" behavior (or simply "behavior") is elicited by a stimulus, spontaneously emitted, or modeled. It is then reinforced by its instrumental effects or through self-reinforcement. The behavior is then more likely to occur in the future. Behavioral deficits occur when the behaviors manifested are not reinforced, or when the behaviors have never been manifested. This conceptualization appears deceptively simple, even when the factors of varying reinforcement schedules, stimulus-and-response generalization, discrimination, shaping, response hierarchies, punishment, and cognitive mediation are considered in detail, as they were in relation to normal personality development.

Some behaviorists include additional variables. B. A. Maher (1966) suggests that a simple learned behavioral model must be tempered by consideration of three aspects: 1. past learning in similar circumstances, 2. current motivational states and their attendant effects on sensitivity to environmental stimuli, and 3. individual biological differences which may be either genetic or due to physiological disorders. Furthermore, an emphasis on the introspective approach in behaviorism is gaining momentum, and the simple stimulus-response-reinforcement concepts of the strict behaviorists are being broadened by many researchers (Bandura, 1982); (Lieberman, 1979). Leonard Krasner (1978) has suggested that behavioral principles will at some point be integrated (as Maher suggests) with many concepts of the other approaches into a broad-based science of human behavior. Others (Wolpe, 1978) are less sanguine about the benefits of returning to what B. F. Skinner called mentalistic concepts, and remains committed to an approach that deals primarily with observable behavior.

Comments on the Behavioral Perspective

There is little doubt that classical conditioning occurs in humans. This is particularly important in the association of the psychophysiological reactions of anxiety to various stimuli. The classical conditioning model would be extremely limited in scope, though, if used in isolation from other behavioral models. Operant behaviorism adds another dimension to the conceptualization of human behavior. Its focus on observable behaviors, accurate measurement, and prediction of behavior has been and is a significant counterpoint to the subjective and inferential theories of psychoanalysis and humanistic psychology. The operant behaviorists have been extremely concerned with the use of the scientific method, and have focused on eminently testable concepts. This is a point strongly in operant behaviorism's favor.

From a negative perspective, operant behaviorism is much too reductionistic in the sense that all behavior is reduced to simple stimulus-response connections involving observable behavior. This view does not deal with internal events, which each of us knows occur. While this position is understandable from the perspective of accurate science, it falls short when we try to explain the broad range of human behavior.

Though not as precise as operant behaviorism, social learning theory is much more comprehensive, and it is more precise than psychoanalysis and humanistic theories. Impressive research supports its formulations (e.g., Bandura, 1977, 1982). However, internal cognitive mediators cannot yet be measured with the precision that most overt behaviors can. Its broadness tends to make social learning theory more liable to the problems of subjectivity, overgeneralization, and a lower ability to accurately predict behavior.

In general, learning theories of personality development can be described as well founded empirically. Their concepts tend to be more related to observable behavior, and therefore more measurable. Their major drawback may be their lack of comprehensiveness and their narrowness of focus. The response to this criticism is that further research may broaden the theories' applicability. A major criticism often expressed is that the learning theories have too little to say about issues such as innate aspects of the individual. It seems unreasonable to presume that the infant is strictly a blank slate upon which only the environment will write. We must join with Mischel (1976) in emphasizing that an interactional model must be applied to the study of human behavior before behavior can be well understood.

THE PHYSIOLOGICAL PERSPECTIVE

> A 52-year-old housewife was admitted with a history of recurrent episodes of depression of sufficient severity to require hospitalization. The original onset was characterized by a period of several weeks of severe frontal headache, for which no cause could be found and which disappeared with the onset of the first depressive episode. The depressive episodes varied in length from a few weeks to two months. With the fourth episode in five years, the patient began to demonstrate evidence of increased intracranial pressure [increased pressure in the skull]. A neurological examination suggested the presence of [a tumor in the front of the brain on the right side]. After removal of the [tumor], the mental symptoms disappeared and did not recur. Thus, the mental symptoms appear to have been definitely correlated with the presence of [a] cerebral [tumor]. (Waggoner, 1967)

The historical material in Chapter 2 has revealed the long tradition of searching for physiological correlates of human behavior. At one extreme, advocates propose that virtually all abnormal behavior can be reduced to malfunctions of the physiology of the body (Abood, 1959); an example is the so-called medical/disease model, reviewed in Chapter 2.

A less extreme physiological viewpoint suggests that disturbed behavior is partly a result of a disturbance in one or more physiological processes. There is, in fact, ample evidence that many behavior disorders are partly due to physiological issues. Yet for many other disorders, there is little evidence of specific physiological factors. In a broad sense, all human behavior is influenced by physiology, since behavior takes place within a physiological organism. Subsequent chapters on specific abnormal behaviors will show that physiological factors contribute to the development of many behavioral disorders.

Heredity

Few behavior disorders are directly inherited, although many authorities consider genetic influences quite significant in human functioning (e.g., see D. Freedman, 1979). With the exception of identical twins, every person has a unique genetic makeup, which is inherited from one's biological parents (see Figure 3.6). The **genes** (biochemical messengers) are contained in **chromosomes** (parts of the cell body), and are made up of molecules of **DNA** (deoxyribonucleic acid), which carry the genetic code and pass it on to every cell of the body.

The 23 chromosomes a person receives from each parent pair up in the union of the father's sperm cell and the mother's egg cell. The subsequent 23 *pairs* of chromosomes and the genes they carry comprise the **genotype** of the individual. Some characteristics such as eye color are almost totally determined by the coding of the genes. However, most characteristics are the result of a combination of genetic code and the impact of environment and comprise the

Figure 3.6. Genetic transmission by dominant and recessive genes.

Inheritance of dominant genes: If one parent shows the trait, an average of one in two children will show the trait. If both parents show the trait, all children will show the trait. Inheritance of recessive genes: For the trait to appear, both parents must carry a recessive gene. An average of one in four children will inherit a recessive gene from each parent and manifest the trait; two in four will inherit one recessive gene and will *carry* but not manifest the trait; and one in four will not inherit the gene.

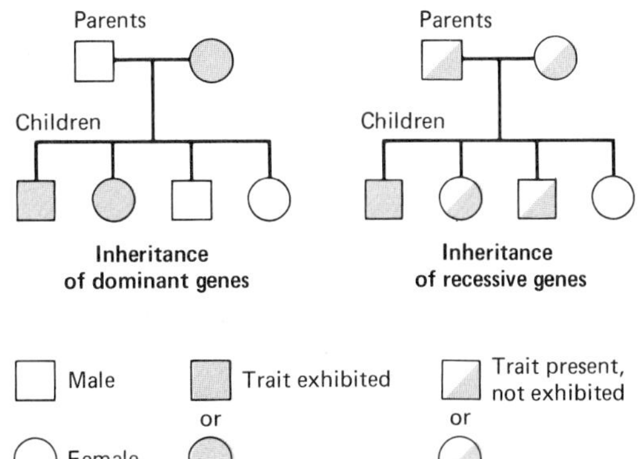

phenotype. For example, height is partly determined by the genetic code. However, someone extremely ill nourished as a growing child may end up shorter than if the nourishment had been adequate. At the other extreme, no matter *how good* one's nourishment, one will reach a genetically programmed height limit and grow no farther. For example, a malnourished child's genotype may predispose the child to average height. However, the child's phenotype (actual behavioral-physical characteristics) is a result of environmental influences, and is one of short stature.

The characteristic of height can also be used to demonstrate how genetic endowment can affect human behavior in a broader sense. If a male's genetic endowment results in an adult height of five feet, six inches, he is extremely unlikely to make a profession of basketball, even though he may play the game very well. If the same male's adult height were seven feet, two inches, however, and he had developed a high level of proficiency at the game, his occupational choice might include that profession. The genes would not have *made* him choose basketball, but they would have provided the correct makeup to allow the choice to be possible.

In subsequent chapters on specific behavioral disorders, hereditary influences on the development of abnormality will be examined. The available evidence suggests that many disorders have a genetic component (Fieve, Rosenthal, & Brill, 1975). We shall find that heredity is an important issue in the study of such disorders as schizophrenia, depression, anxiety, and mental retardation. Two evidence-gathering procedures commonly used to study the degree of genetic influence on disordered behavior are twin studies and adoption studies.

Twin Studies. Two types of twins have been used for genetic research, identical (or monozygotic) and fraternal (or dizygotic) twins. Identical twins result from the splitting of one fertilized egg and have exactly the same genetic makeup. Fraternal twins result from the fertilization of two eggs by two different sperm cells at the same time. Thus, fraternal twins are no more alike genetically than nontwin siblings.

Since twins are usually raised together, it seems logical to assume that they experience the same environment. Thus, if there is greater behavioral similarity between identical twins than there is between fraternal twins, the greater similarity should be due to the impact of the former's identical genes. This degree of similarity is called "concordance." For example, if we find high concordance for schizophrenia between identical twins, and low concordance for schizophrenia between fraternal twins, we would conclude that a genetic factor is operating in schizophrenia. This finding in studies of schizophrenia is, in fact, common. However, the conclusion about genetic influence in such studies are compromised because the twins have been raised together. Even though the twins share the same family, their environments may *still* be different. For example, the parents may treat one twin differently than the other. In an attempt to control for environmental factors even more systematically, some researchers have studied adopted children.

Adoption Research. In adoption research, people who have been separated from their biological parents shortly after birth and raised by foster parents are studied. To study schizophrenia, for example, these studies examine the behavior of adopted children whose biological parents did not show any evidence of schizophrenia, and children whose biological parents (one or both) did show evidence of the disorder. If heredity is important in the development of schizophrenia, we would expect the children in the latter group, rather than the former, to show a higher incidence of schizophrenia as adults. A presumption is made, of course, that the environments of the two groups of subjects in the foster home settings are not significantly different.

When Things Go Wrong

Physiological Dysfunction. A problem in the genetic code may lead to a physiological dysfunction which results in abnormal behavior. However, physiological dysfunction may also result from other factors. A great deal of research has examined other factors in addition to heredity. Simply to determine that a disorder is genetically influenced is certainly not enough, since this leaves few options to eliminate the problem other than selective breeding—a "solution" with many ethical and moral problems. Instead, many researchers have focused on determining what the physiological problem may be, and on trying to develop procedures to rectify the dysfunction.

As we shall see in subsequent chapters, some theorists and researchers have focused on the study of the biochemistry of the human organisms in the hope of determining what physiological faults might exist which lead to abnormal behavior (Kety, 1975). Three bodily systems that have received particular attention are the endocrine system, the autonomic nervous system, and the central nervous system.

The Endocrine System. The endocrine system consists of several glands that secrete **hormones.** Hormones are complex chemical messengers which influence a variety of physiological processes. For example, hormones are extremely important in how our bodies respond to stress. Some disorders of behavior are directly attributable to a malfunction of this system. An oversecretion of the hormone thyroxin, for example, results in an increase in body metabolism, leading to irritability, jitteriness, and a sense of apprehension.

The Autonomic Nervous System. Like the endocrine system, the autonomic nervous system is important in the body's response to stress. The autonomic nervous system functions will be examined in detail in Part II (Chapters 5–8).

The Central Nervous System. The biochemistry of the central nervous system has received a great deal of study. Much of the information on the biochemical aspects of behavior has evolved out of studies on the effects of drugs on humans and animals. As specific disorders are discussed in later chapters, these areas of investigation will be examined more fully. The biochemistry of the central nervous system appears to be a particularly important factor in disorders that involve extreme distortions of perception and emotion. In recent years, research on the biochemistry of brain function has made tremendous advances (see Highlight 3.1).

HIGHLIGHT 3.1
NEW TECHNOLOGY FOR STUDYING THE CENTRAL NERVOUS SYSTEM

How does one study the ongoing biochemical processes of the human brain? Most approaches are extremely indirect, such as the measurement of chemicals in the blood which are the end product of brain metabolism, or studies of the effects of the administration of various drugs. An exciting new technique called the PETT scan may provide much more direct information than has previously been available.

The PETT (for positron emission trans-axial tomography) scan is a color or black-and-white reconstruction of x-ray pictures which show different patterns of glucose utilization —an index of brain activity—in different parts of the brain, depending on the subject's mental state and behavior. It enables scientists to follow moment-to-moment biochemical changes in the brain that could never be charted before. The widely used CAT (computerized axial tomography) scan only shows the brain's anatomy. The PETT scan records the fate of a radioactively tagged substance that has been injected in the subject's blood and has entered his brain; it thus reveals the varying strength of biochemical processes that occur in different areas of the brain.

When a monkey raises its left hand, for instance, its brain activity can be traced, with a PETT scan, through different areas of the monkey's right hemisphere, cerebellum, and spinal cord. A rat having its whiskers stroked will produce different brain patterns according to which of five separate whiskers is actually touched. Last summer [1980], researchers at the National Institute of Mental Health saw the auditory cortex of a schizophrenic patient light up on the screen in what may have been "the first physiological evidence of voices [auditory hallucinations] in a schizophrenic," according to Monte Buchsbaum, chief of NIMH's section on clinical psychophysiology.

Eventually, the scan may be used to observe what happens in the brain during such emotional moments as when a person breaks into tears. It may reveal what happens when a person's attention shifts. It may also offer clues to the deeper mysteries of how people learn and how they remember. (Pines, 1981, p. 6)

Brain Injury. Physical damage to the brain can have a variety of profound effects on human behavior, depending on the locale and extent of damage. Many of us have had experiences with people who have physical and behavioral problems after suffering a stroke (rupture of a blood vessel in the brain) or similar brain damage. A host of agents have been identified which can damage the brain, including poisons, high temperatures (from infections), tumors, and lack of oxygen. When the primary causal agent identified is one of these, the disordered behavior is usually called an organic mental disease.

Comments on the Physiological Perspective

As noted in the presentation of the medical/disease model in Chapter 2, a focus on abnormal behavior as a function of entirely physical causes is much too simplistic to do justice to the wide range of behaviors which are bothersome to individuals and society. At the same time, some behavioral disorders are primarily a function of physiological malfunctions. In other disorders, the cause is not so clear. Even where a clear physiological cause for disordered behavior is present, the characteristic manifestation of the behavior is often dependent upon psychological and social factors which impact upon the individual.

THE SOCIOCULTURAL PERSPECTIVE

Lawyer. How long have you been a gang member, Johnny?
John. Six years, ever since I was 14.
Lawyer. Well, you're not a juvenile anymore. It is going to go hard on you.
John. I can handle it. Avengers can handle any shit the joint [prison] puts out.
Lawyer. You sound tough, but not remorseful. What about the shopkeeper you snuffed?
John. Tough! That old jerk had it coming. He been bleedin us for years! Let him rot in his grave!

To what extent does one's society or culture affect the development of behavior we consider abnormal? We have already seen in Chapter 1 that society or culture influences which behaviors are defined as abnormal. In addition, society or culture also determines which behaviors are available to be learned. Chapter 1 indicated that differences between cultures have led to the concept of "cultural relativism." Abnormality is relative to the norms of the culture in which the behavior is exhibited.

The existence of disorders unique to specific cultures suggests that cultural factors may be more important in the development of some behaviors than physiological factors, intrapsychic dynamics, or simple reinforcement. However, while some disorders are culture bound, most appear to be cross-cultural. For example, the primary symptoms of schizophrenia are relatively stable across most cultures. Even in extremely primitive rural areas, psychotic behavior usually stands out. Could some theories about the impact of society on behavior account for the psychopathologies seen in virtually all cultures? Some theorists have proposed that at least some severely abnormal behavior can be explained on the basis of sociocultural factors without the need to consider other causes.

When Things Go Wrong: Sociocultural Perspectives

Abnormal Behavior as Role Enactment. Sarbin (1969) views most abnormal behaviors as a function of social **role enactment.** Behavior is due to the individual's enactment of roles which are expected by others in complementary relationships. Individuals behave "abnormally" because they are expected to do so. For example, the loss of social skills often seen in severely disturbed persons may occur, not because of some intrinsic disorder, but because a "mental patient" or "crazy person" is not expected to maintain social skills. Gruenberg (1967) has also suggested that "chronic" mental patients, to a large extent, behave as they do because mental health professionals and community members expect such individuals to be dependent and apathetic, lacking in motivation, careless of self-care skills, generally annoying, and sometimes dangerous. Thus, **role expectations** contribute to problem behaviors.

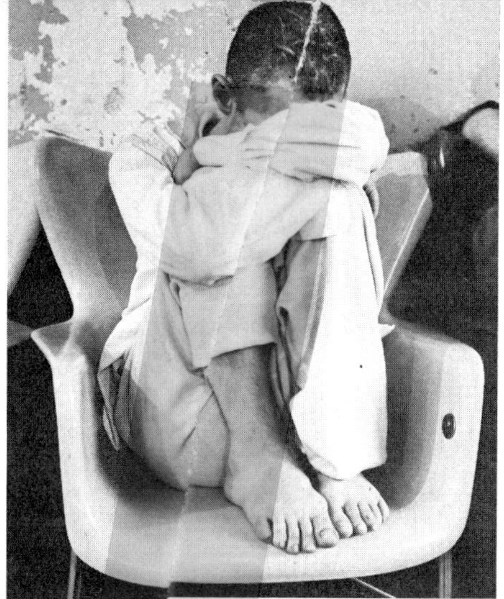

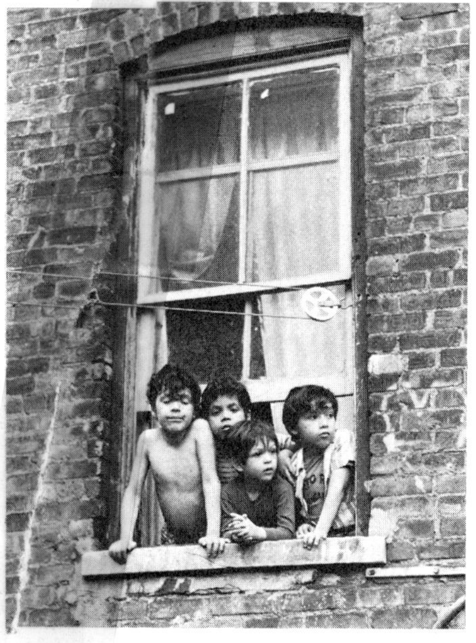

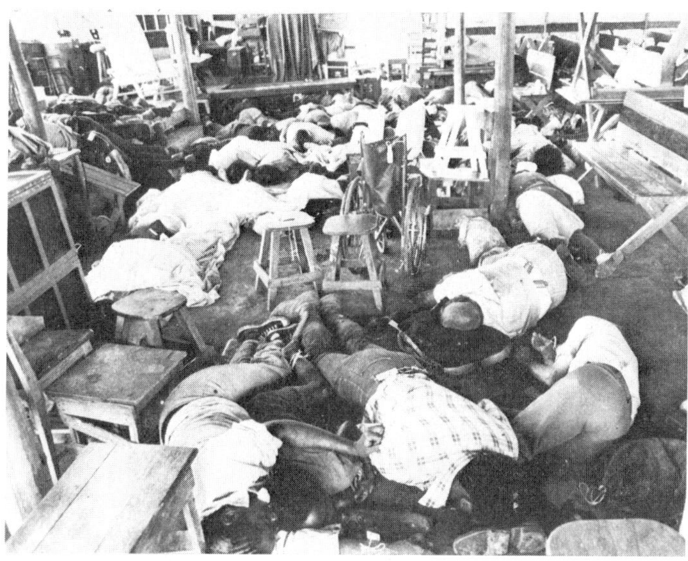

Some authorities have suggested that many of the behaviors characteristic of chronic schizophrenia may be due to the impact of others expecting that the behavior will be present, rather than due to the presence of "mental illness" caused by physiological or psychodynamic factors. Is this man shoeless because he is mentally disturbed, because no one expects him to wear shoes, or because he has no shoes? **(top left)**

Living in a poverty-stricken environment can have profound effects on human behavior. **(bottom left)**

Jim Jones was the leader of a religious group who led his followers to a "new life" in the country of Guyana. His power over the members of his group was so great that in 1978 he was able to convince hundreds of them to commit suicide and to persuade his close "disciples" to murder hundreds of others. Reverend Jones also took his own life during the mass suicide. **(top)**

Scheff (1966, 1975) holds a similar view in what he calls **societal-reaction theory.** He suggests that there are two kinds of deviance: primary and secondary. When individuals first violate a societal rule or custom by behaving oddly, this is primary deviance. However, if such individuals are then labeled "ill" or abnormal, and learn to label themselves this way, subsequent abnormal behavior occurs because the individuals behave "as if sick." They behave this way because of their own and others' expectations of how persons carrying such labels should behave. The behavior is secondary to society's expectations, and is secondary deviance.

Social Class and Discrimination. An additional sociocultural factor that appears significant is the stress of "fringe life" (i.e., membership in a social, economic, racial, political, religious, or other group that experiences difficult acceptance, perhaps even persecution, by the cultural majority). Many studies have indicated that rates of abnormal behavior are higher in groups living in changing deteriorated neighborhoods in urban areas (e.g., L. Levy & Rowitz, 1974). However, some researchers have suggested that this result is due to the drifting of disturbed persons into lower socioeconomic classes, since they cannot support themselves (Dunham, 1965; Levy &

Rowitz, 1973). The black psychiatrists Greer and Cobbs (1968) have proposed that black males must maintain an unusual level of suspiciousness of others (mild paranoia) to survive in a predominately white society filled with both subtle and blatant discriminatory attitudes. Research has consistently found that membership in the lower socioeconomic class is associated with a high incidence of poor physical health, material deprivation, familial disintegration, and other stressful living conditions (Srole et al., 1978).

A complicating factor is that within a larger society, such as the United States, subcultures may sanction or promote behaviors that the majority of the population perceives as disturbed. Not many years ago, for example, the minister Jim Jones convinced about 900 of his followers to move with him to a South American country and set up a religious enclave. This subculture ended in mass suicides and possible homicides of hundreds of men, women, and children. The subcultural expectations must have been very intense to result in so many people's acceptance of death. Less dramatically, the antisocial behavior of juvenile gang members appears to be at least partly due to the individual's acceptance of the gang's subcultural expectations. These expectations may well be a response to factors involved with membership in a social class or group which experiences significant rejection by the majority.

Comments on the Sociocultural Perspective

Obviously, sociocultural factors influence the absence or presence of disturbed behavior. In the case of severely persecutory situations, these factors might be considered causal, at least in the sense that the disturbed behavior would not have occurred in the absence of persecution. The prime example of such persecution and its effects is probably seen in the aftereffects of imprisonment in World War II Nazi concentration camps on those who survived. (The effect of this experience is examined in Chapter 5.) More generally, sociocultural factors' most significant effect may be on such manifestations of disordered behavior as the content of delusions or false beliefs, content of hallucinations, precipitants of anxiety, and types of social norm–violating behavior. The impact of sociocultural factors on psychopathology is quite certain. However, as J. S. Strauss (1979) has pointed out, a concrete conceptual structure for organizing and integrating data on how social and cultural factors affect disturbed behavior is still needed. An exclusive reliance on a sociocultural (or other) model to explain disordered behavior is not possible.

A MULTIFACTORIAL VIEWPOINT

In this chapter, five ways of conceptualizing the etiology of normal and abnormal behavior have been presented. A question that cannot be answered is, Which is the best one? Instead, we should ask, What can we learn about human behavior from the application of each of these approaches?

In reviewing possible factors that influence the development of normal and abnormal behavior, we have seen that competing notions exist, and each viewpoint has supportive research with varying levels of methodological soundness. Each approach has a few dogmatists who believe they have *the* answer, rather than part of the answer. If we ask, "What causes abnormal behavior?" the answer may too often be only one of the following: "biochemical disturbance," "unresolved Oedipal conflict," "distorted self-concept," "learned behavior," or "social role functioning." Inherent in this polemical approach are the dangers of a lack of breadth in the conceptualization of human behavior, and a likelihood that one may ignore important factors that impact on the development of abnormality. These risks do not mean that specific theory building, the formulation of specific predictions based on theories, and experimental testing of the predictions should not occur. At this stage of development of a science of human behavior, such activities are critical.

While specific theories are important, the broadest understanding of abnormal behavior comes from an integration of many theories, and from the subsequent research that the theories have generated. Enough is known to emphasize that human behavior is a function of an interaction of many factors, including, but not limited to, what we bring with us into the world in terms of our heredity, what we learn, our physiological makeup, our personality, and certainly our sociocultural environment.

A concept important in this regard is diathesis-stress interaction. A **diathesis** is defined broadly as a predisposition to respond in a particular way. From the diathesis-stress approach, we can view the development of abnormal behavior as a function of a diathesis, or set of predisposing factors, activated under conditions of stress. If the diathesis is slight, extremely high levels of stress must exist before the abnormal behavior occurs. If the diathesis is strong, low stress may result in the abnormality. If the diathesis is absent, the abnormality will never occur (see Figure 3.7). As an example, consider the development of schizophrenic behavior. If an inherited physiological predisposition must exist in people who develop schizophrenia (as much of the research indicates), then people who have this diathesis are more likely to develop schizophrenic behavior than people who do not have the diathesis. The former will be more vulnerable to the disorder than the latter. In the chapters on specific disorders, behavior will be examined from a variety of perspectives such as the relevant personality factors, physiological predispositions, learning, and sociocultural issues, since any human behavior may be a function of many factors.

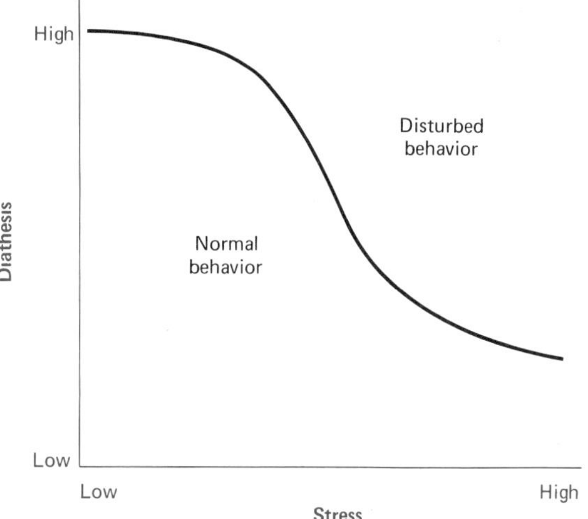

Figure 3.7. The hypothetical relationship between degree of diathesis and degree of stress. Diathesis may be biological, psychological, learned, or sociocultural.

Summary

1. Five perspectives on the etiology of behavior are of major importance today: the psychoanalytic perspective, the humanistic perspective, the behavioral/learning perspective, the physiological perspective, and the sociocultural perspective.

2. The psychoanalytic perspective proposes that behavior is determined primarily by unconscious processes that aim to satisfy instincts.

3. The instincts become socialized as the child moves through fixed psychosexual stages of development: the oral stage, the anal stage, the phallic stage, latency, and the genital stage. These stages of development are named after the areas of functioning which are important for gratification in the various phases of childhood.

4. Freud distinguished three structures of personality which have different and sometimes competing functions: the id, which represents instinctual, unconscious strivings; the superego, which consists of internalized values, goals, and prohibitions; and the ego, which mediates between the competing functions of id and superego and the demands of reality.

5. According to Freud, neurotic anxiety is a sign of the impending breakthrough of unacceptable instinctual impulses, and leads to the use of more or less effective defense mechanisms intended to protect the individual from the danger of socially unacceptable behavior, thoughts, and feelings.

6. A third force in psychology, humanistic psychology, is an alternative to the determinism of both the psychoanalytic and behaviorist views. Abraham Maslow identified a hierarchy of needs which are split into deficiency needs and growth needs. The deficiency needs (which include safety, love, and esteem) must be satisfied in addition to physiological needs before the person can satisfy the needs of self-actualization and cognitive understanding. Carl Rogers, like Maslow, sees people as motivated by positive strivings toward actualization.

7. According to Rogers, each individual has a unique "phenomenal field": a perception of the world as the individual experiences it, and of his or her own place in it. The self-concept, or way people experience themselves, is the most important factor in determining how people behave. When the self-concept is distorted by imposed "conditions of worth" the person may behave in ways that lead to anxiety or other interpersonal difficulties.

8. A major perspective of human behavior is that all behavior, both normal and abnormal, is learned. This perspective encompasses a range of views. Some theorists focus on conditioning as an important factor in the development of behaviors and emotions. Operant behaviorists avoid "mentalistic" concepts, and emphasize behavior and its effects on the environment. Changes in environment subsequent to behavior may reinforce the behavior. Reinforcement may be positive, increasing the probability of the behavior. It may be negative, increasing the probability of the behavior because an aversive stimulus is terminated. If reinforcement does not occur, the behavior is extinguished and no longer occurs. The occurrence of an aversive stimulus is called punishment, and usually decreases the probability of the behavior.

9. The learning perspective also includes social learning theory, which emphasizes that behavior can be learned through observation of others. In observational learning, direct environmental reinforcement of the individual's behavior is not essential. The reinforcement may be cognitive. However, conditioning and operant reinforcement are still important to the social learning theorist. The emphasis on internal mediators by social learning theorists has led to a greater emphasis on cognitive learning by some theorists. The integration of cognitive variables, behavior, and environment has been described as "reciprocal determinism," in which each factor interacts with the other to produce complex behavior.

10. The physiological perspective on the etiology of abnormal behavior has a long historical tradition. Extremists in this perspective view all abnormal behavior as a result primarily of disruption of physiological functioning. A less extreme view suggests that behavior is at least partly influenced by physiological factors. The physiological perspective emphasizes that behavior is a function of a physiological organism. People's genetic makeup (genotype) interacts with environmental factors to produce specific behavioral or physical characteristics (phenotype). The influence of heredity on physical and behavioral characteristics has been typically studied in twin and adoption research. Physiological dysfunctions that affect behavior may occur in the endocrine system, the central or the autonomic nervous system, or may be due to brain injury.

11. A fifth perspective on the etiology of abnormal behavior focuses on the effects of sociocultural acceptance of deviant behavior and social expectations. From this perspective, abnormal behavior may occur as an enactment of an expected social role such as "being mentally ill" or "being schizophrenic." Thus, abnormal behavior may be due to societal reactions to unusual behavior. The sociocultural perspective also emphasizes that some abnormal behavior may be a reaction to membership in persecuted minorities, or to specific values of subcultural groups.

12. Each of the five perspectives influences the thinking of large numbers of researchers and clinicians in the field of abnormal psychology, and each perspective has been criticized by adherents of the other perspectives. The psychoanalytic perspective offers broad conceptualizations of human behavior, but its underlying principles are hard to prove or disprove because they are difficult to measure. Humanistic psychology offers a positive view of the intrinsic motivation of humans, and emphasizes the importance of conscious aspects of personality. However, this perspective is also inferential and subjective. The perspective that human behavior is primarily learned places more emphasis on objective definition and testing of principles, but tends to be limited in scope. The physiological perspective neglects psychological variables, but demonstrates that physiological factors can have an important impact on behavior. The sociocultural perspective neglects psychological and biological differences between individuals, but demonstrates that behavior is influenced by sociocultural factors.

13. At this point, the question of which perspective is the better one cannot be answered. Instead, the student of abnormal psychology must ask what can be learned about human behavior from an application of each of these approaches. The broadest understanding of abnormal behavior comes from an integration of these perspectives. Human behavior is a function of an interaction of many factors. People have diatheses, or predispositions to respond in particular ways, which can be activated under certain conditions. The predispositions may be biological, psychological, learned, or sociocultural. In subsequent chapters, the importance of the varying perspectives on the etiology of specific disorder will be presented and evaluated.

KEY TERMS

Cognitive learning. Learning mediated by psychological events.
Collective unconscious. Carl Jung's term for racial memories of which people are not consciously aware.
Conditioning. A process in which a stimulus is paired with a response and, after several trials, the stimulus can evoke the response.
Conditions of worth. Conditions that significant people such as parents place on the behavior of others, and which become important in determining a sense of self-worth.
Diathesis. A predisposition to behave in a particular way under certain conditions.
Discriminative stimulus. A stimulus that acts as a cue to a behavior (an operant).
Genotype. The genetic makeup that the individual inherits from his or her biological parents.
Neurotic anxiety. Anxiety which is a signal of the impending overstimulation of id impulses.
Observational learning. A form of learning in which one person imitates the behavior of another; also called "modeling."
Operant learning. A form of learning in which a response is followed by reinforcement; also called "operant" or "instrumental conditioning."
Organic wisdom. A term of Carl Rogers which indicates a basic awareness of the organism (person) of what is good for it. This awareness is below the level of consciousness.
Phenomenal field. The subjective experience of the environment and the person's relationship to it.
Pleasure principle. Freudian principle that the id acts to immediately gratify instinctual impulses with no regard for reality.
Primary process thinking. Primitive thinking that is not based on the rules of logic; characteristic of the id.
Psychic determinism. The view that all behavior is ultimately determined by unconscious processes.
Phenotype. The individual's physical or behavioral characteristics which are the result of an interaction of heredity and environment.
Reinforcement. Any event which increases the probability of a response.
Role enactment. The enacting of a social role such as the role of spouse, doctor, child, criminal, or "crazy person."
Role expectation. The overt and covert expectations which people hold about the enactment of social roles; for example, the expectations about the type of behaviors that constitute "being a good mother."
Secondary process thinking. Logical thinking which is characteristic of the ego or conscious personality.
Self-actualization motive. The need to achieve one's full potential.
Shaping. A process of operant conditioning which involves reinforcing successively closer approximations of a desired behavior.
Unconscious process. Any mental process that is not available to the person's conscious awareness.

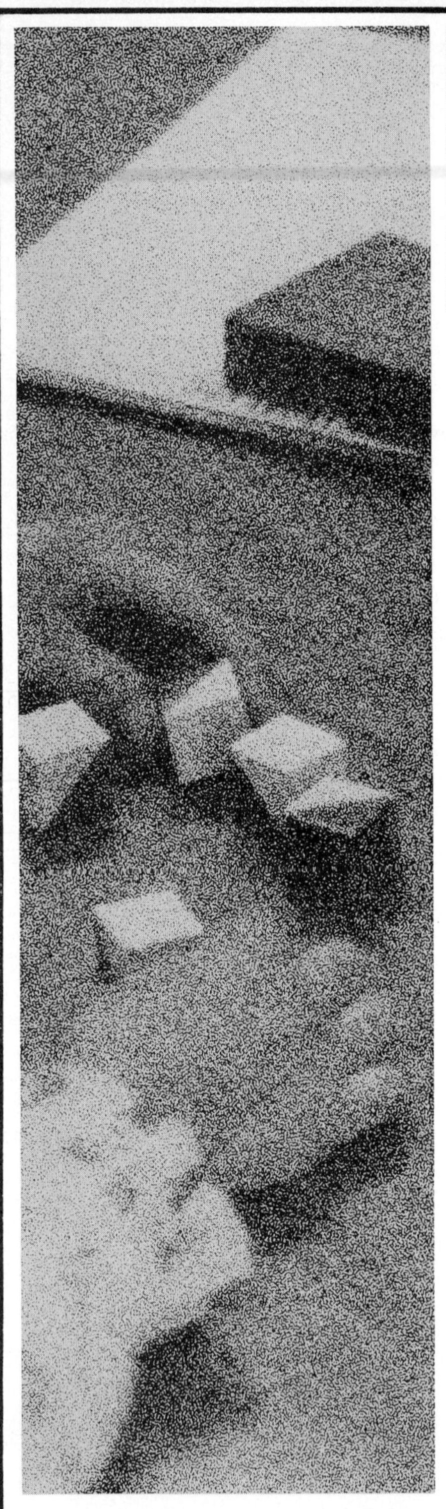

4

The assessment and classification of behavior

- Assessing human behavior
- Classification of human behavior
- A common classification system: DSM-III
- Summary
- Key terms

Darryl had been admitted to the hospital the evening before, and was now being interviewed by a clinical psychologist, Dr. Lawson. Dr. Lawson had already talked to Darryl's wife and parents, and obtained as much information about Darryl's behavior as he could. He had asked Darryl's relatives about Darryl's childhood adjustment, educational, marital, and work history, and behavior during the past few years.

Dr. Lawson was now asking Darryl many of the same questions, and was paying special attention to the way Darryl responded: how rapidly or slowly Darryl talked, whether he fidgeted or stared into space, and whether he looked sad or angry. Dr. Lawson also was interested in whether Darryl was aware of where he was and whether he could think clearly and speak logically. As the interview progressed, it became obvious that Darryl was very depressed. However, other bits and pieces of information led Dr. Lawson to think that Darryl's problem was more than just depression.

As the interview drew to a close, Dr. Lawson decided that he wanted to know more about Darryl. He decided on the following day to spend several hours observing Darryl's behavior in the environment of the ward. Later that afternoon he would schedule Darryl for a series of psychological tests. Once Dr. Lawson had all the information he felt was necessary, he would complete several tasks. First, he would use the results of his assessment of Darryl to formulate a *diagnosis,* a statement of the type of disorder that Darryl has. Second, Dr. Lawson would formulate a treatment plan for Darryl based on a broad understanding of what led to Darryl's behavior, information about current events in Darryl's life, and on Dr. Lawson's training and experience with other people who had problems like Darryl's. Within a few days Dr. Lawson would complete an intensive assessment and classification of Darryl's problems.

Dr. Lawson is following in the footsteps of many before him. As in most endeavors involving enormously complex data, those who have studied disturbed functioning have tried to group sets of behaviors according to common characteristics to simplify their task of study and understanding. The process of classification is not unique to the study of abnormal behavior. Physicists classify substances according to atomic weight, chemists classify according to whether a substance is an acid or a base, and biologists classify according to whether a living organism is plant or animal, mammal or nonmammal.

The attempt to develop a classification system for abnormal behaviors has a long history. Chapter 2 showed that Hippocrates' personality types were an early effort in this direction, and Emil Kraepelin's identification of specific disorders in the late 1800s formed the basis for modern classification systems. In the past few decades, investigators concerned with abnormal behavior have developed classification systems of quite complex natures. For most students of abnormal behavior, classification of the immense range of abnormal behavior promises to simplify their task of understanding its causes, character, and treatment.

The specific procedure, focus, and goal of classification, however, have been the subjects of intense criticism. Some critics question whether we should attempt to classify at all. Others think that classification can be useful, but the current approach to the classification of abnormal behavior is so flawed that it hinders, rather than helps, our attempt to understand and deal with disturbed functioning.

When a classification system is developed and used, its utility is partly dependent upon the collection of information. This process of information collection, or *assessment,* provides the information needed in order to classify disorders into their appropriate categories. Assessment, however, does not have to be used only to classify. It may be used to gain greater understanding of an individual's assets, deficits, and potentials, without assigning a label to the person. This chapter examines the procedures currently used to obtain the information used to classify disorders into various categories, or to obtain a greater understanding of an individual's functioning. The current major classification system also will be presented, and the benefits and problems of classification will be covered.

ASSESSING HUMAN BEHAVIOR

The study of human behavior has a long tradition of measurement and assessment. Whether one intends to classify behavior or individuals into differential categories, or whether one's aim is an in-depth understanding of a single unique individual, assessment provides the information necessary to achieve the goal. Some psychologists, primarily those with a humanistic psychology framework, have little interest in the formal assessment and classification of human behavior. However, most psychologists (like Dr. Lawson) believe that classification or diagnosis (the formulation of the problem) and treatment planning are enhanced by the availability of specific information about the subject's behavior. Clinicians need to know as much as possible about a client in order to adequately clarify the issues likely to be raised during treatment.

Information is obtained by a variety of assessment approaches, including interviews, psychological testing, interviews of friends and relatives, and direct observation of behavior. These assessment approaches range from informal, unstructured conversational interviews to very formal, structured tests. The information gathered often depends on the theoretical assumptions of the assessor. For example, a psychoanalytic psychologist might be interested in assessing dream content as a representation of unconscious symbolization, while an operant behavioral clinician would be more interested in assessing environmental reinforcement contingencies.

When clinicians make assessments, they usually attend to an extremely broad range of behaviors. At times, the client's problem behavior is so well defined that the assessment can be quite limited. However, when a major disorder is suspected (as in Darryl's case), and the clinician must produce a comprehensive assessment and description of the individual's functioning, a combination of assessment techniques is likely to be used.

Assessments of psychological and behavioral functioning are usually completed by one or more mental health professionals: psychologists, social workers, psychiatric nurses, or psychiatrists. Techniques used by these professionals vary, but include interviewing, data gathering from friends and relatives, behavioral assessments, and psychological tests.

The Clinical Interview

An interview is a more or less structured conversation with a particular goal. In the **clinical interview,** the goal is usually to identify the problems that the client is experiencing, to determine which factors have led to the development of the problems, the severity of the problems, and to provide data that can be used to formulate approaches for dealing with the problems. Often, the clinical interview is the only assessment approach used.

The style of the interviewer and the content of an interview may vary according to the interviewer's theoretical background. Psychodynamically oriented interviewers are likely to focus on past life experiences, while behaviorists are more likely to focus on current life circumstances. Most clinicians, regardless of theoretical background, will try to obtain as much information as possible.

Areas explored in a clinical interview usually include the individual's current life setting, specific problem behaviors; a chronology of problem development; description of past and present treatment; and an assessment of the individual's physical characteristics, emotional state, self-description, and intellectual functioning. The interviewer wants to find out as much as possible about social factors such as group memberships, family structure and relationships, education, type of work, and community involvement. In addition, the clinician is interested in possible precipitating factors such as the individual's perception of levels of stress, and any recent life changes such as losses, physical illness, and marriage.

In other words, in the clinical interview, one wants to find as much information as possible about the individual which is relevant to the problem behavior. In practice, interviewers often depart from such a format as the need arises. In the following excerpt, a very disturbed man has difficulty entering into a relationship with the interviewer. At first the patient's anger is quite obvious, and the interviewer (I) realizes that a highly structured approach will do more harm than good. He focuses on keeping the patient (P) involved and succeeds in getting him to open up slightly. In response to a question, the interviewer reassures him that he is on the patient's side. Finally, the patient is ready to reveal more information about himself:

I. Mr. Jones, would you sit down?
P. No.
I. Ah, it would make this more comfortable. . . .
P. Forget it!!
I. The staff asked me to talk to you about . . .
P. Screw you and the staff! (Pacing back and forth)
I. We need to know a little more . . .
P. Well, you can forget it. I said "forget it," buster!
I. You're pretty angry about some . . .
P. You damn right . . . they're all lying about me, saying bad things (stops, stares out window), bastards. . . .
I. Who?
P. Don't know . . . (cocks head, still staring out window).
I. You don't know?
P. Yuh . . . (whispers) radio.
I. What about the radio?
P. Japs made a special one. . . . It's really strong.
I. How strong?
P. It gets people to do things (shares this with interviewer in a conspiratorial tone).
I. How?
P. Radio waves . . . make you do what you don't want to.
I. They do it to you?
P. Uh . . . (nods "yes" and sits down).
I. Like what?
P. (Long pause.)
I. What do they make you do?
P. Are you an American?
I. I'm on your side . . . What do they make you do?
P. Aw . . . it's not good. I don't want to talk about it (looks very downcast).
I. It bothers you?
P. Ah . . . crap!
I. Why don't you tell me about it?

Many factors can influence the clinical interview process. An interviewer must be sensitive to the emotional factors in the interview setting. In the example above, the patient was very angry at the beginning; and until this anger abated, he was not able to volunteer much information. If other people had been present, the patient may have been less able to open up to the interviewer. Such situational factors may be extremely important to the success of the interview process. The interviewer's characteristics are also important. Suppose that the examiner had been of Japanese descent in our example? Would this have helped or hindered the patient's ability to relate to him?

In addition to information gathered from the client, third-party information may also be gathered in an interview format. Relatives, such as parents, siblings, or spouses, are most likely to be interviewed, although friends, employers, or police sometimes also have relevant information. Third-party information can provide more understanding of the reliability of the subject's responses in the clinical interview process. In Dr. Lawson's interview with Darryl, (at the beginning of the chapter) much of the information given by Darryl was later confirmed by Darryl's wife and parents.

The accuracy of the clinical interview can be affected by many factors. Some important factors include the environment in which an interview is conducted, the skill of the interviewer, the cooperativeness of the subject, the subject's perceptions of the interviewer, and the structure of the interview. Several studies have demonstrated that structured, standardized interviews are much more reliable than unstructured interviews (Matarazzo, 1978; Weitzel et al. 1973).

Behavioral Assessment

The clinical interview is a structured situation in which behavior is observed. Other types of **behavioral assessment** may also be used, ranging from informal observations in the natural setting to highly structured task situations in which formal ratings are made on specified behaviors. In the case of Darryl, Dr. Lawson observed Darryl's behavior on the hospital ward for several hours. Dr. Lawson could have used one of many scales which have been published and used extensively in behavioral assessment. The use of such a scale would have helped make Dr. Lawson's observation more objective and standardized.

Behavioral Interviewing. Assessments of specific behaviors often occur in a **behavioral interview.** In this procedure, the interview focuses on specific problem behaviors and their frequency (such as anxiety attacks). Like a typical clinical interview, a behavioral interview attempts to clarify the development of the disorder, but the focus is on behavior and the learning process which led to it. Thus, the behavioral interview centers on the environment in which the behavior occurred, the reinforcers in the environment, the persons who might be involved in reinforcement, and possible modifications of the environment which can be made to change the reinforcement contingencies (Hersen & Bellack, 1976).

Rating Scales. An example of a **rating scale** is MACC-II, (Motility, Affect, Cooperation, and Communication-II) which assesses mood, cooperation, communication, and social contact (Ellsworth, 1971). The scale has 16 items which are rated from 1 to 5 after direct contact with or observation of the patient. The following sample item from MACC-II measures social contact.

Is he well informed about others with whom he comes in contact?

1. Shows no evidence of knowing any of the persons around him.
2. Sometimes knows to whom you are referring when you use a person's name.
3. Usually knows to whom you are referring when you use another person's name.
4. Knows and usually calls by name most of the persons around him.
5. Knows and usually calls by name almost all of the persons he comes in contact with.

An advantage of scales such as the MACC-II is that their structure adds to their level of **reliability.** For example, trained raters can reach high levels of agreement when repeated ratings are compared using the MACC-II.

Baseline Observations. Behavioral assessment may be much more structured and objective

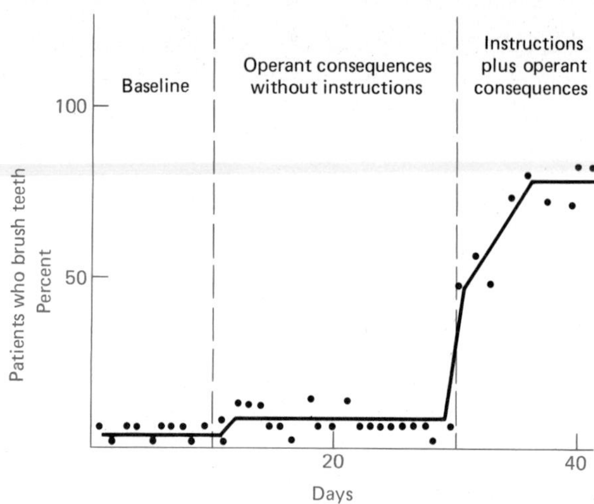

Figure 4.1 Behavioral Observation. Behavior observations are often plotted on a graph as in the example above. This graph charts the percent of patients in a group who manifest a baseline behavior, the increase in percentage of those who display the behavior when positively reinforced without instructions, and the change in frequency when verbal instructions were combined with the reinforcement.

than a rating scale such as the MACC-II. One type of very structured objective assessment is **baseline observation.** In this procedure, a specific behavior is identified for measurement. In Figure 4.1, the behavior measured consists of tooth brushing. In this example, the behavior is assessed for a group of patients. The frequency is counted, and the percentage of patients manifesting the behavior is recorded for each morning. The environment is then manipulated: The patients are positively reinforced for the behavior, but are not given any instructions. For 20 days, the percentage of patients manifesting the behavior is recorded. Finally the third condition is measured: Reinforcement is combined with instructions to the patients for 10 days and the frequency of the behavior is counted and the percentages recorded. Such behavioral assessments require exact definitions of the behavior to be assessed, and very consistent observations.

Physiological Measurement. An area of assessment that has recently gained prominence is psychophysiological functioning. Some psychologists now use equipment that measures the physiological events common in emotional reactions, such as change in breathing rate, heartbeat, blood pressure, and electrical conductivity of the skin. These measurements provide information on physiological activity and its relationship to subjective reports of emotional arousal. The assessment of physiological functioning has become particularly important for disorders that appear to be related to anxiety and stress.

Behavioral assessment approaches tend to be more reliable than more subjective clinical procedures. Still several variables affect the utility of the assessment procedures. The techniques vary in their objectiveness (Goldfried & Kent, 1972). The measurement of behavioral baselines (illustrated in Figure 4.1) is extremely objective, while MACC-II is much more judgmentally subjective. The simple presence of an observer, even in an objective technique such as baseline observation, may result in such a change of the behavior in the subject that an assessment of typical behavior is not possible (R. Rosenthal, 1967). People often behave differently when aware that they are being monitored and when aware of the expectations of the observer. In spite of these problems, the reliability of structured behavioral assessment is impressive, and the contributions of this approach are becoming increasingly recognized as its techniques attain wider usage.

Psychological Testing

During the afternoon following Darryl's interview, he was scheduled to meet Dr. Lawson for a psychological testing session. The session took slightly over three hours, and Dr. Lawson administered three psychological tests to Darryl. The tests Dr. Lawson selected were a test of intellectual functioning, a personality test, and a test sensitive to organic brain dysfunction.

As in other assessment approaches, the primary purpose of using psychological tests is to obtain information that will aid the clinician and the client. Tests are often used in conjunction with the clinical interview, because of the belief that the tests will provide a more detailed assessment of the client's assets, deficits, and potentials. In contrast to most interviews, tests are more structured and quantifiable. In addition, tests are efficient and can provide a great deal of information with less expenditure of

The clinical interview is among the most common of assessment approaches used in obtaining information on which to base a diagnosis. **(bottom left)**

Behavioral assessment can involve the measurement of physiological variables, such as brain waves. Photo shows a electroencephalograph (EEG) machine, used to record brain wave patterns. **(bottom right)**

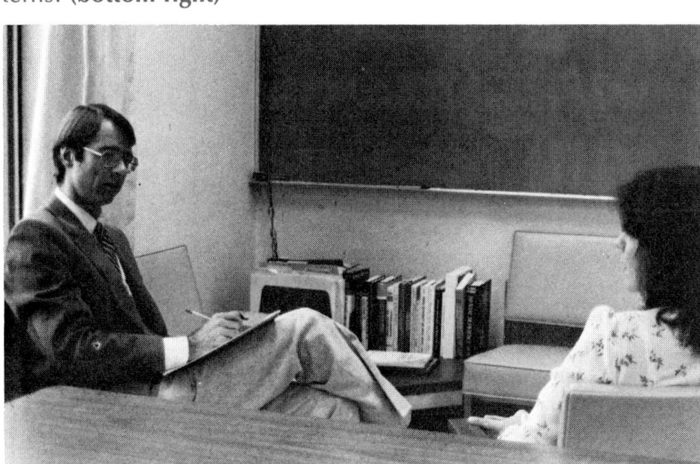

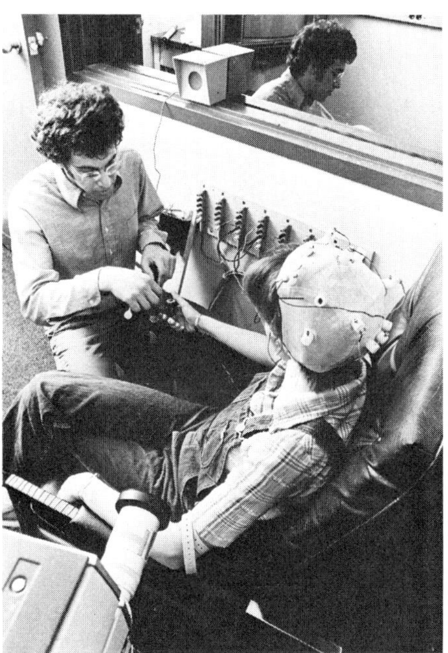

time and effort than many other assessment approaches (Maloney & Ward, 1976).

Intellectual Assessment. Around the turn of the twentieth century, interest in intellectual development led to a need for a procedure to measure this factor. In response to this need, the French physician and psychologist Alfred Binet developed an **intelligence test,** which was revised in 1916 to become the Stanford-Binet Intelligence Scale. The Stanford-Binet yields scores of "mental age" such as "6 years 6 months" which are converted to an IQ by the formula $IQ = \frac{MA}{CA} \times 100$. In this formula, the mental age (MA) is divided by the chronological age (CA) and multiplied by 100. For example, an MA of 6 years 6 months in a person with a chronological age of 5 years 6 months results in an IQ of 111. While the revised Stanford-Binet continues to be a frequently used measure of individual intellectual functioning, alternative intelligence tests have been developed. One commonly used alternative is the Wechsler Adult Intelligence Scale (WAIS), developed by David Wechsler, who was dissatisfied with the Stanford-Binet. Wechsler felt that the single global score provided by the Stanford-Binet was not sufficient. He believed that intelligence is composed of separate abilities which combine to form a global capacity to act purposefully, think rationally, and deal effectively with the environment (Wechsler, 1971). He developed the WAIS so that more data could be derived than a single global score. The WAIS has become extremely popular because of the additional information that it supplies, and was revised in 1981 (WAIS-R).

The Wechsler Adult Intelligence Scale—Revised (WAIS-R) consists of 11 subtests and is individually administered. Six subtests comprise the Verbal Scale, and five make up the performance scale. The test provides three major assessments: Verbal IQ, the Performance

Table 4.1
WAIS-R subtests, abilities measured, and items similar to those used

WAIS-R subtests	*Abilities measured*	*Items similar to those used*
Verbal subtests		
Information	General information on culture, contemporary affairs, science	Where does milk come from?
Comprehension	Ability to make practical judgment and to generalize	Why do we wash dishes?
Arithmetic	Ability to concentrate, memory, and problem solving	How much are 7 cents and 13 cents?
Similarities	Verbal comprehension, ability to make associations	How are a chicken and an eagle alike?
Digit span	Auditory perception, attention, and memory	After hearing a series of numbers, the subject repeats them from memory (3–7–1–6)
Vocabulary	General intelligence	What does summer mean?
Performance subtests		
Digit symbol	Visual acuity, speed, and motor coordination	Subject must substitute symbols for digits (paper-and-pencil test)
Picture completion	Attention to detail and concentration	Subject must look at line drawings and find the missing detail.
Block design	Nonverbal test of perception, concept formation, and visual-motor coordination	Using multicolored blocks, subject must reconstruct two-color designs from pictures.
Picture arrangement	Comprehension and social judgment	Subject assembles panels, (like in a cartoon series) in order, so that a story is told.
Object assembly	Problem solving, visual perception, sensorimotor feedback	A jigsaw puzzle of simple figures (for example, a human form, a horse, a house).

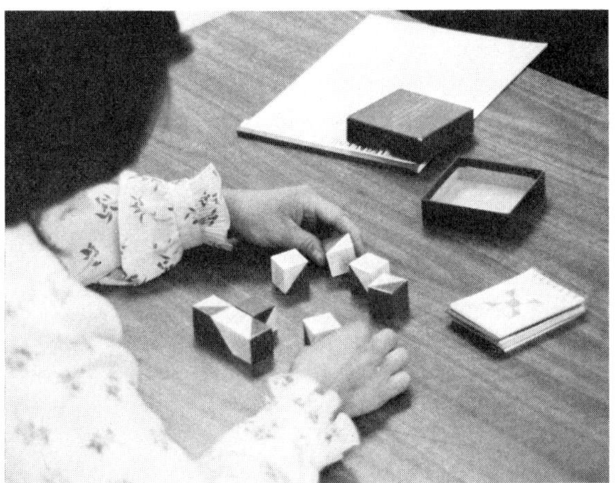

In the block design subtest of the WAIS-R, the subject must use multicolored blocks to copy a design from a picture.

IQ, and the Full Scale IQ. Many psychologists prefer the WAIS-R to other individually administered tests of intelligence, since the strengths and deficits on the subtests can be used in describing the functioning of the individual. The various subtests, the areas they measure, and test items similar to those used in the WAIS-R are given in Table 4.1. The WISC-R (Wechsler Intelligence Scale for Children—Revised) is a similar test, available for use with children. Table 4.1 shows that a broad variety of areas are assessed and assumed to reflect levels of intellectual ability and achievement.

An ongoing controversy is whether such tests accurately assess intelligence. Some aspects of these types of tests are actually achievement tests, which assess how well one has learned what is considered important in middle-class United States culture (Miele, 1979). As an example of the impact of possible cultural bias on the validity of such tests, consider the child raised in a ghetto environment where schools are poor and "book learning" is not valued. This individual might perform quite poorly on the WAIS-R and yet have high native intelligence (i.e., be "street smart"). David Wechsler (1971) points out that "the abilities called for to perform these tasks do not, per se, constitute intelligence or even represent the only way in which it may express itself." He notes, however, that intelligence tests are useful because they correlate with widely accepted criteria of intelligent behavior such as school performance. Yet these correlations are not as great as one might expect. The criticisms of intelligence testing are covered in more detail in Chapter 19, on mental retardation.

Psychologists use the data from intelligence tests for various purposes. For example, this information is critical in terms of differential classification of mental retardation. These tests may also give clues to the existence of organic brain damage, and may lead to further examination for the problem. Information about intellectual assets and deficits may also be important in treatment recommendations. The more complex verbal therapies seem to require a relatively adequate intellectual level for best results. A person with a high performance IQ but a low verbal IQ would probably not do well in such therapies; and a psychologist might make such a prediction for this individual, based on WAIS-R subtest scores. This was one reason why Dr. Lawson wanted to evaluate Darryl's intellectual functioning. Intelligence testing may be done for many other specific purposes, but the test is frequently administered with other assessments to provide as well-rounded an assessment as possible—also one of Dr. Lawson's goals. When a broad assessment is desired, the WAIS-R is often given in conjunction with tests of personality such as projective assessments.

Projective Personality Assessment. The assessment of personality through **projective tests** is based on the assumption that individuals reveal something about their inner person in their responses to unstructured tasks. When tasks are ambiguous, people's behavior or responses are presumably influenced primarily by what goes on inside them (personality variables) because little guiding information is available in the environment. The more unstructured the environmental stimuli, the more likely the individual will be to "project" personal factors into the response. In addition, when structure is vague, and there are no obviously "right" or "wrong" answers, it is thought that the subject has less chance to "fake" or to present a socially acceptable facade.

The childhood amusement of seeing "pictures in the clouds" is an example of the process of projection. The cloud may have no concretely defined shape, yet its ambiguous shape may be reminiscent of something to the onlooker. One child may "see" a threatening monster; another may "see" a flower. Projective theory suggests that the difference in the children's perceptions of the same stimuli is a function of differences in their personality variables.

Rorschach inkblots. In 1921, Herman Rorschach, a Swiss psychiatrist, published the Rorschach Psychodiagnostik Test. The Rorschach consists of 10 cards, or "plates." Each card contains an almost symmetrical printed inkblot (see Figure 4.2). Five of the blots are printed in shades of black and gray; 2 are mainly black, with splotches of red; and 3 consist of a variety of pastel colors. The subject is instructed to look at the blot and tell the examiner what it looks like or is reminiscent of. Cards are viewed one at a time, and the subject's responses are recorded verbatim by the examiner. After all 10 cards have been administered and the responses recorded, the examiner again presents each card during an inquiry phase. During this phase, the examiner reviews each response with the subject to determine the stimuli's location on the card, and to obtain data on what influenced the subject's response. Typically, subjects give a total of 25 to 30 responses, although fewer responses may be seen, as are totals of over 100 responses.

Figure 4.2.
The subject being given a Rorschach card tells the examiner what the inkblot appears to look like.

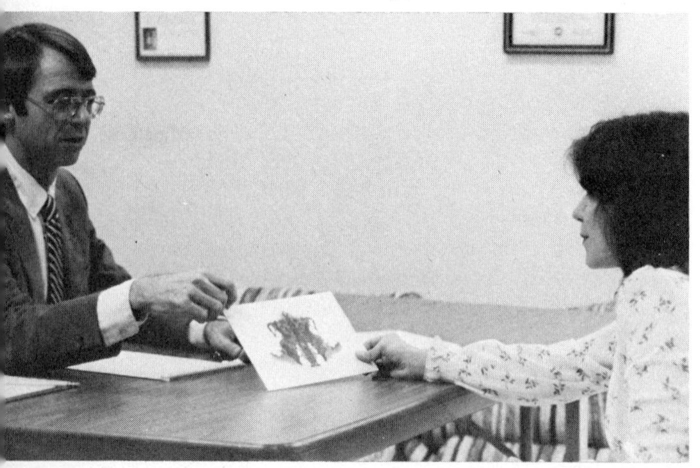

Different complex scoring systems have been developed for use with the Rorschach. The scoring of individual responses can be quite reliably done by different trained examiners. That is, two psychologists who have been trained in the same scoring procedure are very likely to score each response in the same way (Exner, 1974, 1978). Thus, we would expect that the overall personality assessments of psychologists using the Rorschach would be fairly reliable. This is often not the case.

In clinical practice, personality assessments based on the Rorschach tend to have low reliability. To a large extent, this is because many psychologists rely on a subjective, psychodynamically based content analysis of the Rorschach. Even when the psychologist has used a formal scoring system, a content analysis may increase the subjectivity of the final personality description. In content analysis, the content of a response is presumed to be symbolic of some aspect of the client's personality. For example, if a subject gives several responses that involve the content of eyes, this is presumed to be suggestive of paranoia. Anatomy responses (such as ribs, lungs, hearts) imply that the individual is overly concerned with physical health. Analyses of this type are so subjective that some critics have claimed that they have no empirical basis (L. J. Chapman & Chapman, 1969).

Despite the criticisms leveled at it, the Rorschach continues to be popular. Its use had declined, but the efforts of John Exner (1974, 1978) to increase its reliability and **validity** have made many psychologists feel that the Rorschach can be a valuable tool. A psychologist who is well trained in administration and competent in interpretation is able to provide a complex and detailed Rorschach assessment of personality that is impressive in breadth (e.g., see Piotrowski, 1982). Though the subjectivity of the Rorschach continues to be criticized, the detail, depth, and breadth of the results make large amounts of information available for the clinician's use in the processes of diagnosis, treatment planning, and understanding the personality functioning of the subject. Thus,

HIGHLIGHT 4.1
TAT CARD, SAMPLE STORY, AND CLINICAL INTERPRETATION

Subject's Story

Why . . . the young woman doesn't know what to do about the old crone. They've just had an argument. The old lady is feeling very smug and satisfied. She's got the younger one just where she wants her . . . in her control. The young woman is very angry; this always happens to her. People manipulate her . . . make her do things. She hates it. She's going to get rid of the old woman. I mean . . . get away from her. But it won't work. Someone else will come along to try to control her. She can't escape from it.

Interpretation

The subject (a 32-year-old woman) feels controlled by others, and resents their influence. She feels powerless and helpless in avoiding the control of others. She perceives others as purposely manipulating her and tries to deal with her anger by escape, but recognizes the futility of her attempts. Her sense of being controlled, the helplessness she experiences, and her anger are consistent with paranoid-like behavior and with the major themes in her other stories.

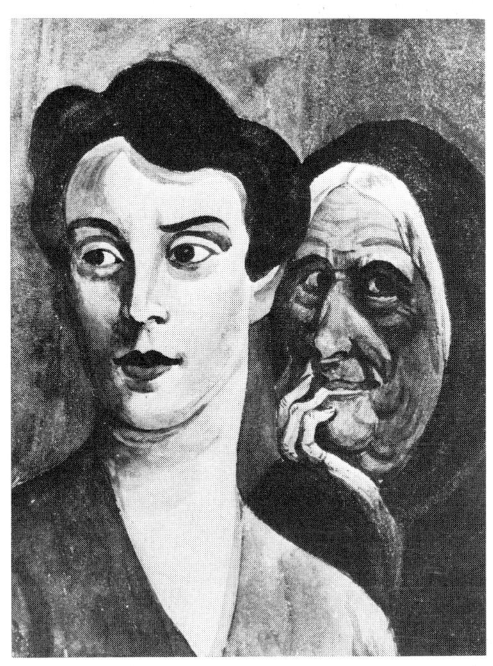

though criticisms of the subjectivity of the Rorschach are justifiable, it is still an important tool of many psychologists.

Thematic apperception test. The TAT (Thematic Apperception Test) consists of over two dozen pictures and one blank card. Most psychologists administer a subset of these cards to a subject. The selection depends upon the subject's age, sex, and other variables. Most pictures portray humans in interactive scenes of varying ambiguity. Subjects are instructed to tell a story about the scene, including what went on before, what is happening now, and what the outcome will be. The subject's narrative response is recorded verbatim by the examiner.

A commonly used standard scoring system for the TAT does not exist. Some psychologists evaluate the themes of the symbolic content. Others treat the stories as directly reflecting the subject's conflicts, motivations, and aspirations. Some do a formal analysis of the needs expressed in the story, such as the needs for achievement, dominance, aggression, or dependence. This latter approach is based on the concepts of Henry Murray (1938), the TAT's originator.

In responding to TAT cards, the subject creates a fantasy based on stimuli with which the experimenter is familiar, and has used before. The subject is assumed to identify with the figures in the pictures, seeing some as himself or herself, and others as important figures in his or her life. The subject's story reflects the projection of the subject's own personality variables, and the examiner has the task of interpreting the critical, often symbolic, projected communications. The psychologist's interpretations may be quite subjective, and their usefulness depends upon the experience of the examiner. In Highlight 4.1, a TAT card is shown, with a subject's story and a summarized interpretation of its meaning by a psychologist.

The lack of validity and reliability criticized in the Rorschach have also been applied to the TAT. However, the TAT has recently demonstrated possibly important clinical usefulness. An interesting example is provided in a study of the relationship of the need for power to the disorder of hypertension (high blood pressure). In a major study by D. C. McClelland (1975), examiners trained in a structured scoring technique achieved interrater reliabilities of .90 on the TAT. Even more remarkably, McClelland found that TAT scores at age 30 on the need for power could predict high or low blood pressure in men at age 51. Such studies provide evidence that with further refinement, projective tests such as TAT could become even more accurate and useful.

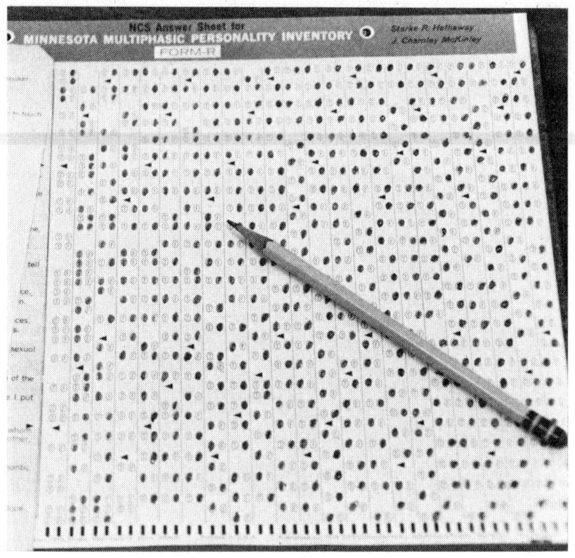

The MMPI is a personality inventory. Since it is a paper-pencil test, it can be given to single individuals or to groups.

Personality Inventories. Some clinicians use "objective" tests such as **personality inventories** to measure personality and clinical variables. These inventories usually have people respond to a series of written statements (such as "I like fast cars") by answering either "true," "false," or indicating that they are unsure. The tests are considered objective, partly because the statements are much less ambiguous than the stimuli in a projective test. In addition, the process through which the tests are developed is much less reliant upon the speculative theorizing and clinical inference which characterizes the early development of the projective technique.

Although many **objective personality tests** have been developed, the Minnesota Multiphasic Personality Inventory (MMPI) remains among the most popular in clinical and research settings (J. R. Graham, 1978). For example, Dahlstrom (1974) reports that at least 6000 studies using this instrument had been published by the mid 1970s.

Minnesota Multiphasic Personality Inventory. The 566-item MMPI was developed in 1943 (Hathaway & McKinley, 1943). The test constructors gathered many items that could be answered "true," "false," or "cannot say." These items were grouped into clinical scales, depending on how well responses to the items distinguished various groups of patients identified as belonging to a particular diagnostic category from patient groups and people who were not psychiatric patients. The items cover a wide range of areas including fears, social interests, sexual behavior, and physical health. Some sample items are the following: "I am likely not to speak to people until they speak to me," "I have very few fears compared to my friends," "Sexual things disgust me," "I loved my father." The result of this effort was the identification of nine clinical scales, each related to a different disorder.

Four additional scales were developed somewhat differently. The Lie Scale (L) contains 15 items which measure the subject's denial of common frailties: for example, one item is "I never tell a lie." A "true" response to this item raises suspicion about the openness of the subject's self-report. The Frequency Scale (F) contains items which, if endorsed, indicate that the subject was careless or confused about taking the test. The Correction Scale (K) measures defensiveness, and the Question Scale (?) measures evasiveness. The complete list of scales and the original interpretation of elevated scores appear in Table 4.2 (Gynther & Gynther, 1976).

Table 4.2
MMPI scales and original interpretations of elevated scores

Title	Abbreviation	Scale number	Interpretation
Lie	L	—	Denial of common frailties
Question	?	—	Evasiveness
Frequency	F	—	Invalidity of profile
Correction	K	—	Defensive, evasive
Hypochondriasis	Hs	1	Emphasis on physical complaints
Depression	D	2	Unhappy, depressed
Hysteria	Hy	3	Hysterical symptomatology
Psychopathic deviancy	Pd	4	Lack of social conformity; often in trouble with law
Masculinity-femininity	Mf	5	Effeminate (males); masculine orientation (females)
Paranoia	Pa	6	Suspicious
Psychasthenia	Pt	7	Worried, anxious
Schizophrenia	Sc	8	Withdrawn; bizarre thinking
Hypomania	Ma	9	Impulsive; expansive
Social introversion-extroversion	Si	0	Introverted, shy

Originally, a person was classified according to his or her highest scale elevation; however, it quickly became apparent that the relationship among scale scores was of great significance. Current interpretation primarily evaluates typical "profiles" (relative elevations of more than one scale) seen in various psychiatric or other reference populations. Recently, a number of computer programs for scoring and interpretation of the MMPI have become available. It is now possible to submit MMPI answer sheets to several centers around the country and, for a fee, receive a relatively complex report written by a computer. Figure 4.3 shows a MMPI scale score profile, from which a clinician would make a personality assessment.

The MMPI has several clinical uses. Like other psychological tests, it is used to identify the appropriate categorization of clients. It may also be used for treatment planning and the development of recommendations. In clinical research the MMPI is particularly useful because of its standardization, ease of administration, and reputation for reliability. The MMPI is highly efficient in terms of human labor and costs, particularly when the assessments are scored, interpreted, and typed by a computer.

The MMPI is not without problems. The sampling procedures used in its development have been sharply criticized. Norman (1972) has pointed out that the sample of patients and the nonpatient controls did not represent a broad cross-section of either group. In addition, the definition of the diagnostic categories used as reference groups were vague and may have contained subjects who were not representative of the specific disorders.

In spite of these criticisms, the MMPI remains one of the more reliable and useful personality tests. A recent study found considerable stability in MMPI profiles of individuals

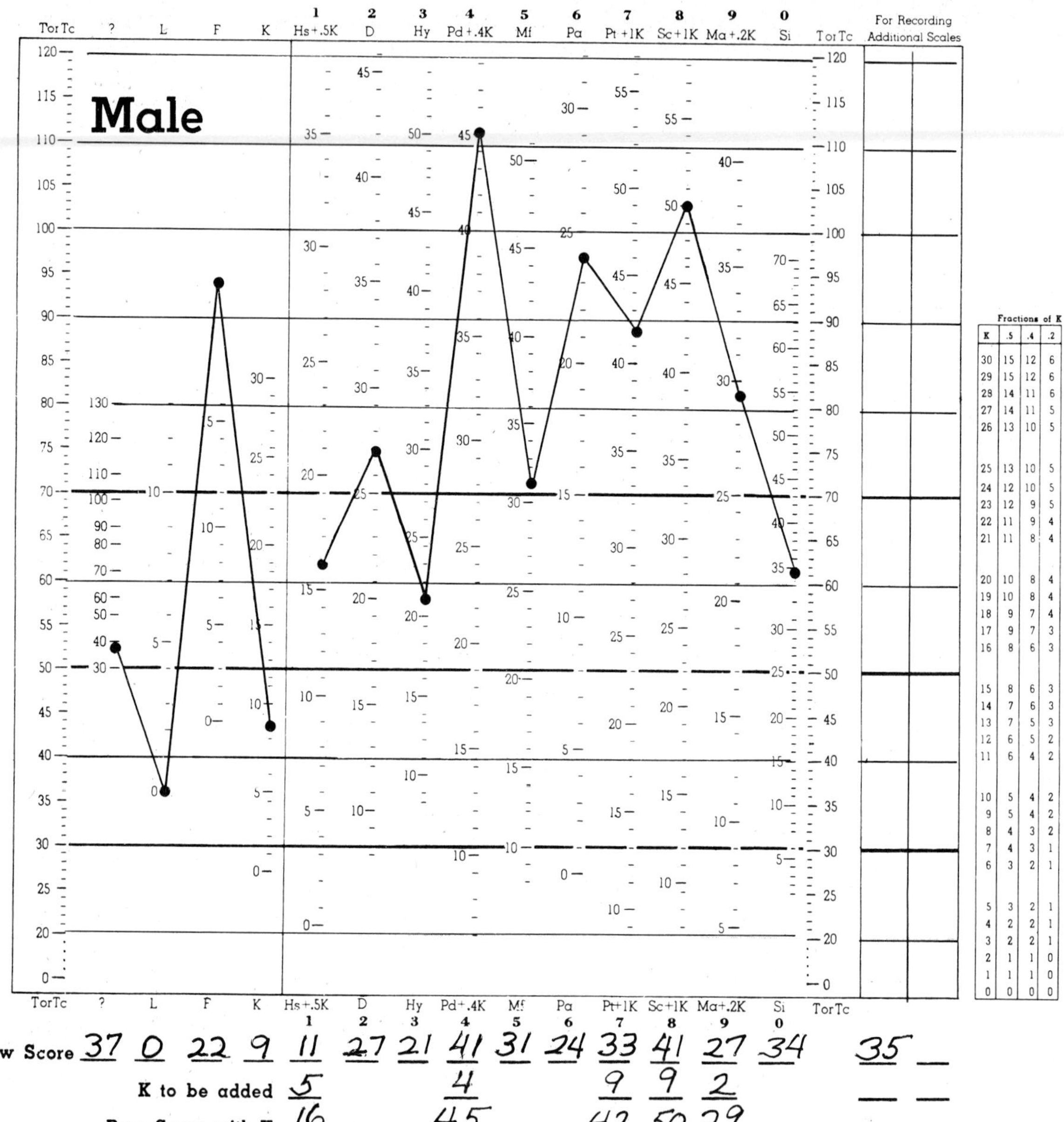

K	.5	.4	.2
30	15	12	6
29	15	12	6
28	14	11	6
27	14	11	5
26	13	10	5
25	13	10	5
24	12	10	5
23	12	9	5
22	11	9	4
21	11	8	4
20	10	8	4
19	10	8	4
18	9	7	4
17	9	7	3
16	8	6	3
15	8	6	3
14	7	6	3
13	7	5	3
12	6	5	2
11	6	4	2
10	5	4	2
9	5	4	2
8	4	3	2
7	4	3	1
6	3	2	1
5	3	2	1
4	2	2	1
3	2	2	1
2	1	1	0
1	1	1	0
0	0	0	0

Figure 4.3 MMPI profile and brief interpretation.
This 20-year-old white male, who was arrested on charges of rape and assault, shows the possibility of feigned illness with the intent to confuse the examiner. Nevertheless, from this profile configuration, it can also be safely assumed that the patient is going through a period of rebellion against authority and traditional values and mores. In addition, he can be described as unpredictable, adventurous, impulsive, nonconforming, and lacking affect in situations where emotional response is considered appropriate. He also is suffering from impaired social relations, emotional coldness, and indifference to praise or criticism (i.e., he is generally lacking in favorable psychological features).

tested repeatedly over a 30-year period while they aged from an average of 49 to 77 years (Leon et al., 1979). Changes in scores were consistent with changes that would be expected in people as they aged. The clinical validity of the MMPI has also been found to be high. For example, H. A. Skinner and Jackson (1978) have found that the MMPI was accurate 76 percent of the time in differentiating between severely and moderately disturbed clinical groups. Hathaway (1972), one of the test's originators, has pointed out that the MMPI's primary utility lies in obtaining a large amount of data with a minimal expenditure of energy.

Tests of Neurological Functioning. Neurological functions have demonstrable brain behavior relationships; these functions are disturbed when there is a brain dysfunction. In Chapter 19, on organic mental disorder (brain syndrome), we shall see that many of these functions can also be disturbed by psychological causes. In clinical practice, a question often asked is whether a particular behavior or set of behaviors is due to an identifiable organic brain dysfunction or to other factors. The answer to this question may have important consequences for the treatment of the patient. Even life-or-death consequences may be involved. For example, an individual may manifest disturbed behavior that appears psychological, but is the result of a brain tumor. If the patient is treated for a psychological problem, the tumor may not be discovered until it has become so advanced that medical treatment is not possible, and the patient is likely to die. If the correct diagnosis is made early enough, the tumor may be treatable, and the patient may recover.

Several procedures are available to assess such cases: X rays, electroencephalograms (EEGs), and other highly sophisticated medical procedures such as the positron emission (PETT) scan (discussed in Highlight 3.1). However, some brain anomalies are not detectable by these approaches. Brain anomalies that are detectable by these techniques, and some that are not, can often be detected using neuropsychological tests. Lezak (1976) has reviewed over 200 tests used for this purpose. One of the more promising **neuropsychological batteries** is the Halstead-Reitan.

The Halstead-Reitan Battery. Ralph Reitan (Reitan & Davison, 1974) has modified the work of the psychologist Ward Halstead and has developed a test series that appears quite valuable in neurological assessment. This extensive assessment procedure involves the administration of a number of different tests. The final result is an assessment of functioning on various perceptual, motor, and cognitive (thinking) tasks including concept formation, the sense of touch, auditory concentration, perception of verbal stimuli, physical motor speed, intelligence, and memory. The Halstead-Reitan Battery is composed of many tests primarily because accurate diagnosis of brain dysfunction involves the assessment of patterns of behavior on a variety of tasks. For example, an individual's difficulty in the visual recognition of familiar objects may suggest damage to a specific part of the visual cortex. Difficulty in speech, such as the inability to name objects, suggests damage to a part of the brain called Broca's area. An assessment of known brain-behavior relationships and the pattern of response to such tests allows many inferences to be made about the absence or presence of brain damage, the extent of damage, and the localization of damage.

The reported success of this battery has been impressive. Filskov and Goldstein (1974) have reported that the Halstead-Reitan has a higher accuracy rate for determining type and location of brain pathology than medical procedures, such as EEG's and X rays. The approach is extremely useful, particularly when used with other assessment techniques such as traditional neurological evaluations.

Effective use of the Halstead-Reitan Battery requires extensive training and experience and a great deal of specialized knowledge. Psychologists who specialize in the study of brain-behavior relationships are called **neuropsychologists.** Neuropsychology is not a specialty of the average clinical psychologist, and most clinicians have not been trained in the use of the Halstead-Reitan. In actual clinical practice, most psychologists use their general clinical knowledge and the WAIS-R as a rough screening device for organic brain disorder. If organic pathology is suspected, the time and expense of a referral to a specialist for further assessment with the Halstead-Reitan is justified.

The Psychological Battery and the Case Conference

In the preceding material each assessment instrument has been reviewed individually. However, in the case that opened this chapter, Dr. Lawson did not rely on a single assessment device. The patient, Darryl, was assessed with a variety of approaches determined by the type of information Dr. Lawson desired. Like most psychologists, Dr. Lawson used a clinical interview, an intelligence test, a test of personality (either projective or objective), and a screening test for organicity. If a specific diagnostic problem such as an organic one had been indicated, a more extensive test (e.g., the Halstead-Reitan) could have been administered.

The results from several assessment devices are usually integrated into a psychological report. Such a report usually presents identifying data, and states the referral problem and the tests used. The body of the report consists of a narrative section, which provides the testing results and interpretation, and ends with recommendations. In such a report, the clinician strives to present as comprehensive a picture of the subject as possible, including deficits and assets.

In Darryl's case, Dr. Lawson presented the results of the assessment at a case conference with other professionals who were involved with Darryl's assessment and treatment. In a case conference, there is a sharing of information and clinical opinion, which will influence the professionals' final recommendations for treatment of the client. In some settings, the client is invited to join in the discussions of the assessments and recommendations.

In most situations, the integrated case conference discussion results in the categorization of a client into a specific diagnostic category. Different clinicians will use this **diagnosis** to different degrees. Some will conceive of the diagnosis as a label that "pigeonholes" the person, something best avoided. Other clinicians will use the diagnosis as a vehicle of communication and as a way to organize their thinking about the client. These professionals may be more concerned about subsequent, more detailed analyses of specific behaviors and the procedures for treating these behaviors. Other clinicians will find that the formal diagnosis is critical in suggesting the initial treatments to be used. At the conference on Darryl, Dr. Lawson presented information which led to similar discussions in Darryl's case. The information and decision are summarized below:

> Dr. Lawson had found out a number of significant pieces of information about Darryl. He reported that intelligence testing revealed that Darryl had superior intelligence and good verbal skills. Personality testing indicated that Darryl was usually quiet and a loner. However, he was also introspective, concerned with his own motivations; and he wanted to know more about why he thought, felt, and behaved as he did. Dr. Lawson concluded from this and other information that Darryl had the potential to benefit from psychotherapy.
>
> Dr. Lawson's interview of Darryl and his relatives revealed that Darryl had had episodes of depression before, and he also had had periods of extreme elation and impulsive behavior. There was some indication that these alternating moods were precipitated by marital difficulties. The degree of these mood swings and evidence from the psychological tests indicated that Darryl was suffering from a major problem called bipolar affective disorder. Based on this diagnostic classification and other information, the treatment team decided that Darryl should be given medication to reduce his depression. They also suggested that as his depression lifted, Darryl should be given another medication called lithium, which is often effective in preventing or reducing the elation and impulsiveness that caused Darryl difficulty. These medications would be given, but Darryl would also be treated with psychotherapy to help him understand and deal with his marital problems.

In Darryl's case, the extensive evaluation conducted over a period of days led to an in-depth understanding of Darryl's functioning, a specific diagnosis, and treatment recommendations that promised a positive outcome. However, in many cases, the outcome is not clear-cut. Assessment techniques present problems in reliability and accuracy. Clinicians' inferences about the behaviors of people are sometimes subjective and influenced by the clinicians' personal biases.

The diagnosis given to Darryl, bipolar affective disorder, comes from a widely used classification system. In Darryl's case, the diagnosis led to treatment recommendations specific to this particular disorder. The end result of the assessment completed on Darryl had clinical utility, placing him in a specific diagnostic category. However, in the field of abnormal psychology, the classification of human behavior has positive and negative aspects.

CLASSIFICATION OF HUMAN BEHAVIOR

Potential Benefits

The use of a system for classifying abnormal behavior must be of some worth if time and energy are to be invested in it. Mental health professionals expect to gain positive benefits from effective assessment and classification, in spite of the inadequacies of the systems available.

Organization of Information. The use of a classification system allows information and data to be organized so that they are easier to understand. And classification is a necessary aspect of sound research: When one uses research methodology to study abnormal behavior, the behaviors must be clearly specified, since individuals and groups are contrasted on specific variables.

Darryl benefited from years of research that sought, with some accuracy, to classify individuals into relatively distinct groups. Some of this research, has revealed that people with the disorder that Darryl had can benefit more from antidepressant medication and lithium than from other types of medication. If a classification system had not differentiated bipolar affective disorder from other disorders, it would have been much more difficult to discover the differential effect of treatment on certain disorders.

Generalization. An effective classification system allows us to generalize. Suppose a grouping of behaviors are found to consistently appear together. For example, perhaps almost every individual encountered who is depressed also has difficulty sleeping, has a poor self-concept, and has few social contacts. As confidence is gained that this pattern of behaviors is usually seen in depressed individuals, conclusions can be generalized from the group studied to other people who are depressed. We may be able to generalize about the causes of depression, the best treatments, and the likely outcomes. Our ability to generalize from our limited sample may allow us to predict behavior. If an individual is depressed, has a poor self-concept, and few social contacts, we can predict that sleeping difficulty is also likely. However, generalization is a two-edged sword. If a classification system is inaccurate, the generalizations may be in error.

Shorthand Communication. If an individual can be identified as belonging to a specific category for which other professionals know the characteristics necessary for membership, then a great deal of information can be communicated in a few words. If a psychologist states that "John manifests paranoid behavior," something quite different is being communicated about John's behavior than if the psychologist had said "John is depressed." If there is consensus about the features of depression and paranoid behavior, it is not necessary to list and describe each and every behavior in order to communicate them to another person.

Potential Problems

Biases. Classification assists us in organizing our thinking. However, since classification systems are often based on specific models of behavior, the organization of the system may bias our thinking. For example, if our classification system assumes that disturbed behavior is a disease, we are not likely to look for alternative conceptualizations of abnormal behaviors. We may become locked into viewing problems as diseases, conceptualizing behaviors as symptoms, clustering symptoms into syndromes, searching for underlying causes, and applying a medical model of treatment.

Loss of Information. While classification assists the process of generalization, generalization may result in the loss of information. The uniqueness of the individual is lost, for example, when a diagnosis such as paranoid schizophrenia is made. Such a diagnosis tells much about some characteristics, but little about others. We would not know that the person is a loving parent, bright, a good golfer, a doctor, personable, or concerned for the welfare of a spouse—facts that may be relevant to an understanding of the problems the person is experiencing. Our process of shorthand communication may be short on some information!

In addition to these potentially negative consequences of classification, discrete categories may tend to obscure the range of human behavior. People are often seen as either belonging or not belonging to a specific category. One is either a schizophrenic or depressive, disturbed or normal. Most clinicians are well aware of the range of human behavior. However, once a clinician has placed a person into a specific category, the diagnostic label can result in undesirable secondary effects (see Highlights 4.2 and 4.3).

Requirements for an Ideal Classification System

The adequacy of a classification system depends on a number of factors: 1. there must be reasonable **homogeneity** within categories, and

HIGHLIGHT 4.2
THE NEGATIVE EFFECTS OF LABELING

When an individual is "labeled," or receives a classification or diagnosis, there may be effects that are not intended. For example, consider the label "schizophrenic." Each of us has many preconceptions about people who are so labeled. We might expect that such a person has bizarre behaviors, is unable to maintain a job or care for a family, is dangerous, and needs to be locked up for his or her "own good." In any individual case or in most cases, such expectations may not be valid; but they are likely to influence how we perceive and react to the individual. Our expectations may also influence the labeled person's behavior. If we expect individuals to be bizarre, and we respond according to our expectations, these persons are more likely to behave in a way that conforms to our expectations—they are more likely to be bizarre!

Thomas Szasz (1961, 1970), a psychiatrist, and Nicholas Kittrie (1971), a professor of law, have both criticized the diagnostic system because of its stigmatizing effects. Once labeled with a category of severe mental disturbance, people may have difficulty finding jobs and places to live; their civil rights may be violated in the name of treatment. This stigmatization because of a psychiatric label appears to be sometimes used purposely to destroy the credibility of political dissenters. In 1979, a Russian Army general was found mentally ill after he began to dissent with the political powers in the Soviet Union. The Russian psychiatrists who examined him found that he was suffering from "chronic paranoia"; three United States psychiatrists found him to be "perfectly sane." Psychiatrist Alan Stone, of Harvard, concluded that this case confirms that psychiatry (and by extension, psychology) is sometimes used as a tool of political repression (*Elgin Daily Courier-News,* 1979). We would like to believe that such events are rare in the United States, but Szasz (1970) has identified a few cases in our own country which may be somewhat similar. In 1964, for example, opponents of one presidential candidate diagnosed him as a "paranoid schizophrenic." The label did not do the candidate any good!

Labels may have more pervasive, less dramatic effects on clinicians' perceptions, which in the long run may be more significant. Langer and Abelson (1974) conducted a study that demonstrates how labels may affect clinicians' perceptions. They compared two groups of clinicians, one group trained in a psychodynamic perspective, and the other trained in a behavioral perspective. Each group was shown a videotape of an individual being interviewed. Half of each group was told the person was a job applicant; the other half was told the person was a "patient." At the end of the videotape, each clinician completed a questionnaire rating the interviewee. The results demonstrated that the behaviorists' ratings were very similar, whether they thought the man was a job applicant or a patient. In contrast, the psychodynamically oriented clinicians rated the subject as significantly more disturbed when he was labeled as a patient. Apparently, their perception of the person as a psychiatric patient added something negative to their assessment of the data. The concern over the negative effects of labeling is obviously justified. However, most clinicians feel that further refinement of classification systems may help to decrease at least some of these labeling effects.

HIGHLIGHT 4.3
PERSONAL IMPACTS OF LABELING

The personal impact of psychiatric labeling is demonstrated in the following excerpt from the article "First Person Account: After the Funny Farm," written by an anonymous mental health professional who was hospitalized for mental illness. In this excerpt, the author describes the subtle and not so subtle discrimination she encountered after discharge.

> Mental handicap creates new "stalls" for those traumatized by hospitalization for mental illness, just as it does for those who are crippled physically. . . .
>
> For me, the scene has been repeated in many different settings: a supervisor who viewed my work and abilities as outstanding and my rate of productivity as very high before my illness, but who recommended disability retirement when I was depressed and less productive; a university that graduated me with high honors, admitted me into its graduate program with outstanding recommendation, and then sent me a form letter in response to my request for readmission (following my illness) saying, "You do not meet our admission requirements"; and community mental health agencies that rejected my offers to be of assistance because I "scared" mental health professionals. (Anonymous, 1980, pp. 545–546)

heterogeneity between categories; 2. the system must yield reliable differentiations; 3. the categories should be relatively stable; and 4. the categories should have validity.

Homogeneity/Heterogeneity. Each diagnostic category should be composed of elements which do not appear in other categories: the category should have homogeneity. When elements appear in more than one class, there is heterogeneity. The elements should allow one to discriminate between categories. Most classification systems vary significantly from this ideal. Some studies have demonstrated a broad overlap of many characteristics among the categories of the *Diagnostic and Statistical Manual* of the American Psychiatric Association, the classification system used by many mental health professionals. Though this system has recently been revised, a study conducted prior to the revision illustrates the problem. In a study of 793 patients diagnosed as either manic-depressive, neurotic, schizophrenic, or as having a character disorder, Zigler and Phillips (1969), found that hallucinations were reported in 11 percent of manic-depressive patients, 4 percent of neurotic patients, 35 percent of schizophrenic patients, and 12 percent of patients with character disorders. The overlap of hallucinatory behavior in these categories indicates that the categories are not homogeneous. Ideally, we would not want such a situation to exist in a classification system. But overlap compromises the system without necessarily destroying the system's usefulness.

Psychologist Nancy Cantor and colleagues (1980) have suggested that diagnosis (or categorization) of abnormal behavior should be viewed as an approach in which "prototypes" are developed. From their perspective, an absolute lack of overlap among categories is not necessary. In **prototype classification,** a disorder such as depression is described by a cluster of behaviors (a prototype) which can be used to define the disorder, even though some of the behaviors may appear as part of another disorder (see Figure 4.4). Cantor et al. illustrate this concept with the following example: The features that make up the category of birds include "feathered," "winged," "flies," and "sings." Feathered and winged are necessary features (all birds are feathered and winged). But while most birds fly and sing, many do not. These features are only correlated with the category of birds. In DSM-III (1980), a common current classification system, the categories are similar to this prototype system of classification: Some features of a category are necessary, others are correlated, and the defining characteristics are clusters of behaviors.

Reliability. An adequate classification system must result in reliable categorization. A diagnostician should classify an individual in the

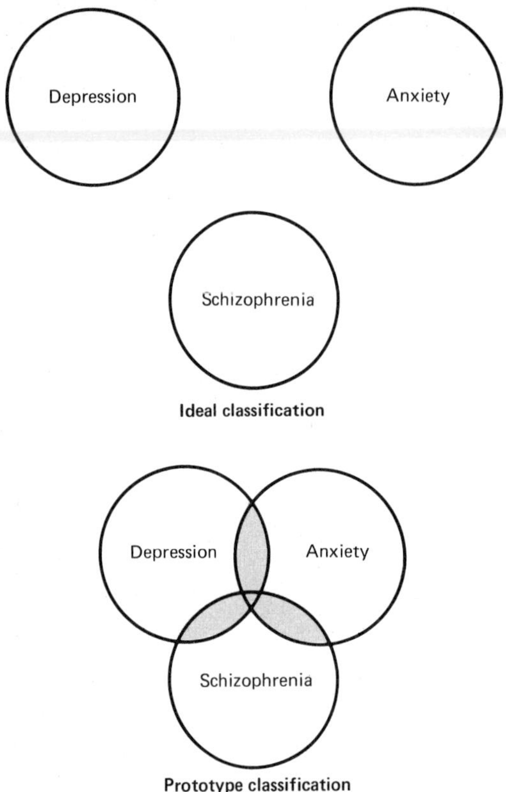

Figure 4.4. Ideal vs. Prototype Classification. Homogeneity within a class is required for an ideal classification. Heterogeneity within a class is acceptable for a prototype classification. There may be overlap among diagnostic groups in prototype classification; but if a significant proportion of symptoms do not overlap, diagnosis or classification can still be valid and reliable.

same category at different times (assuming that the subject's behaviors have not changed). In addition, different diagnosticians who have access to the same data should agree on the category in which a subject should be placed. Most studies have indicated that this level of agreement is relatively low when standard diagnostic categories are used (J. Greenberg, 1977). A study by A. T. Beck et al. (1962), for example, indicates that interdiagnostician agreement on diagnoses of patients varied from 63 percent on neurotic depression to 38 percent on specific personality trait disturbances. However, when the categories were more general and included only psychosis, neurosis, and character disorder, the agreement reached 70 percent.

Recent revisions of the diagnostic categories that Beck and colleagues studied promise to increase agreement levels by increasing the exactness of each category's criteria. The more inexact the criteria, the less likely two individuals are to agree whether a specific behavior meets the definition (Winoker, 1977). Other factors also influence the accuracy of diagnosis and interrater (between examiners) reliability. Subjects may give different data to different examiners, either on purpose, because of the setting, because they have changed, or because of differences in the examiners. Examiners may be trained differently, or may have different levels of competence. However, Kendall (1975) in reviewing studies of DSM-II (1968), a diagnostic classification system used until 1980, concluded that 60 percent of the disagreements between diagnosticians were due to the internal problems of the *classification* system, rather than to problems of the person making the diagnosis.

Stability. Categories must be stable over time. Of course, diagnoses of individuals may change over time with treatment or because of other factors. However, if diagnostic categories change in prevalence over historical periods, this may indicate that they reflect more about society's perception of behavior than about the disorder itself. In fact, to some extent, this seems to occur. J. D. Blum (1978), for example, found major changes in the diagnosed incidence of affective disorders (threefold increase), neurotic disorders (major decrease), and schizophrenia (significant increase) from 1954 to 1974. He discovered that changes in symptoms or behavior could not fully explain the differences, and concluded that interpretation of behavior was relative to the historical period. Such studies raise questions about the validity of diagnostic categories. If the disorder's behaviors or symptoms do not change significantly, but the diagnosis does, does the diagnostic category really exist outside of the perception of the diagnostician?

Validity. In the context of a classification or diagnostic system, we can view the issue of validity from two perspectives: Do the categories really exist? Are they useful? No one seriously rejects the notion that the behaviors that make up the symptoms of the various categories exist. However, some individuals feel that to call these behaviors "disorders," "illnesses," or "diseases," misrepresents reality. Thomas Szasz (1961, 1970), for example, says these behaviors are "problems in living" that do not fall into discrete categories. The more radical behaviorists take a similar view, arguing that each behavior has a unique learning history, so that traditional categorization can add little to our understanding. Most clinicians, however, would argue that clusters of behaviors exist, whether or not one calls them diseases.

Certainly, categories can be useful. In Darryl's case, Dr. Lawson and colleagues found that being able to diagnose Darryl's problem was a great help in planning treatment. The benefits of classification in organizing information, making generalizations, and facilitating communication have led most clinicians to accept the necessity of a classification system. At the same time, most clinicians are painfully aware of the shortcomings of current classification systems. Although the potential benefits of an accurate, valid classification system have not been fully achieved, it seems better to try to improve classification systems than to dispense with them.

A COMMON CLASSIFICATION SYSTEM: DSM-III

In 1952, the American Psychiatric Association formalized a **diagnostic nomenclature** (a system of classification of abnormal behavior) by the publication of the *Diagnostic and Statistical Manual of Mental Disorders* (DSM-I, 1952). This first edition was based on an assumption that abnormal behavior was a reaction to psychological, social, and biological factors. In its second edition (DSM-II, 1968), the classification system was changed to reflect the growing conviction of the psychiatric profession that disordered behavior was a disease rather than a reaction to psychological, social, and biological factors. (As noted, this is a conviction not shared by most psychologists.) This particular conception of disordered behavior (the medical/disease model) has been detailed in Chapters 2 and 3.

In the first two editions of the DSM classification system, the criteria for the diagnostic categories were vague and unclear (Winoker, 1977). However, they were quickly accepted by professionals from many disciplines as the diagnostic standard. DSM-I and DSM-II suffered from a lack of homogeneity within categories, low reliability, lack of stability, and lack of validity. However, these problems were outweighed by the need for a uniform system of classification, and DSM-I and DSM-II were available to fill the vacuum. No alternative systems that have been offered have found the broad acceptance of DSM systems promoted by the American Psychiatric Association.

The valid criticisms and dissatisfactions expressed about DSM-II led finally to a major revision of the system. In 1974, the American Psychiatric Association began development of the third edition, DSM-III. The task force and advisory committees which worked on the revision were large, totaling almost 200 members. Although these groups were composed mainly of psychiatrists, a significant number of representatives from psychology, social work, and the other mental health clinical and research fields were also involved. Many professional organizations acted as reviewers of prepublication drafts. From late 1977 to late 1979, a series of field trials used the new materials, and subsequent modifications were made. The final product was completed and published in 1980.

The *Diagnostic and Statistical Manual,* third edition (DSM-III, 1980), lists and describes over 200 specific diagnostic categories or disorders (see Highlight 4.4). Its descriptive approach does not assume that sharp boundaries must exist among diagnostic entities. The manual's designers assume that individuals identified as belonging in a particular category will manifest at least the defining criteria of the category. DSM-III is a prototype classification approach, similar to that described by Cantor and colleagues (1980). While there are many similarities in the categories of DSM-III and DSM-II, there also are some significant differences. Some disorders listed in DSM-II are no longer

HIGHLIGHT 4.4
SAMPLE DISORDERS LISTED IN DSM-III

The list of disorders in the *Diagnostic and Statistical Manual* has been expanded from approximately 150 in DSM-II (1968) to over 200 in DSM-III (1980). The major category headings in DSM-III and a few examples of disorders in each category are listed below:

1. Disorders Usually First Evident in Infancy, Childhood, or Adolescence.
   Separation Anxiety
   Stuttering
   Infantile Autism
2. Organic Mental Disorders
   Senile Dementia with Delirium
   Organic Personality Disorder
3. Substance Use Disorder
   Alcohol Abuse
   Cocaine Abuse
4. Schizophrenic Disorders
   Catatonic Type
   Paranoid Type
5. Paranoid Disorders
   Paranoid State
6. Psychotic Disorders not Elsewhere Classified
   Schizophreniform Disorder
7. Affective Disorders
   Bipolar Affective Disorder, Mixed
   Major Depression
8. Anxiety Disorders
   Phobic Disorder
   Anxiety State
9. Somatoform Disorders
   Conversion Disorder
   Hypochondriasis
10. Dissociative Disorders
    Psychogenic Amnesia
    Multiple Personality
11. Psychosexual Disorders
    Exhibitionism
    Inhibited Sexual Desire
12. Disorders of Impulse Control
    Kleptomania
    Isolated Explosive Disorder
13. Adjustment Disorder
    With Depressed Mood
    With Anxious Mood
14. Psychological Factors Affecting Physical Condition
15. Personality Disorders (Axis II)
    Antisocial
    Dependent

included; and some new categories have been added to DSM-III. These changes will be addressed in Chapters 5–19, which deal with specific abnormal behaviors.

One very important change in DSM-III is an increase in the specificity of criteria for each class of disorders. A second important change is the use of a **multiaxial diagnostic system.** The increase in specificity of defining criteria for a disorder (depression) is illustrated in Highlight 4.5. Notice also that the DSM-II diagnosis of depression includes the term **neurosis,** which originally implied an etiology, or causal process, specific to psychoanalytic theory. However, many people started to use the term simply for descriptive purposes, with no intention of implying a specific etiology. The inconsistency in usage of the term resulted in its being dropped from DSM-III. The symptom complexes usually associated with "neurosis" are included in other categories. Also note that the DSM-II definition of depression makes specific statements about causal connections (e.g., "due to an internal conflict . . . loss of a loved object or cherished possession"). The DSM-III description contains no such references. The designers of DSM-III have tried to avoid basing their system on any one theoretical perspective.

Multiaxial Diagnosis

DSM-III uses a multiaxial approach to diagnosis. Five different axes (dimensions) are assessed when making a diagnosis. The following list includes examples of how this system would be applied to Darryl's case by Dr. Lawson.

1. Axis I (The clinical syndrome): This is the major disorder that the individual is manifesting at the current time. For example, Darryl's case diag-

HIGHLIGHT 4.5
DIFFERENT DIAGNOSTIC CRITERIA IN DSM-II AND DSM-III

The following excerpts from DSM-II and DSM-III illustrate the increased specificity and concreteness of DSM-III.

DSM-II: Depressive Neurosis

This disorder is manifested by an excessive reaction of depression due to an internal conflict or to an identifiable event such as the loss of a love object or cherished possession. It is to be distinguished from Involutional melancholia and Manic-depressive illness. Reactive depressions or Depressive reactions are to be classified here. (DSM-II, 1968, p. 40)

DSM-III: Depressive Episode

A. Dysphoric mood or loss of interest or pleasure in all or almost all usual activities and pastimes. The dysphoric mood is characterized by symptoms such as the following: depressed, sad, blue, hopeless, low, down in the dumps, irritable. The mood disturbance must be prominent and relatively persistent, but not necessarily the most dominant symptom, and does not include momentary shifts from one dysphoric mood to another dysphoric mood, e.g., anxiety to depression to anger, such as are seen in states of acute psychotic turmoil. . . .

B. At least four of the following symptoms have each been present nearly every day for a period of at least two weeks. . . .

1) Poor appetite or significant weight loss or increased appetite or weight gain.
2) Insommia or hypersomnia [sleeping too much.].
3) Psychomotor agitation or retardation (but not mere subjective feelings of restlessness or being slowed down). . . .
4) Loss of interest or pleasure in usual activities, or decrease in sexual drive not limited to a period when delusional or hallucinating.
5) Loss of energy; fatigue.
6) Feelings of self-reproach or excessive or inappropriate guilt (either may be delusional).
7) Complaints or evidence of diminished ability to think or concentrate, such as slow thinking, or indecisiveness not associated with marked loosening of associations or incoherence.
8) Recurrent thoughts of death, suicidal ideation, wishes to be dead, or suicide attempt. (DSM-III, 1980, pp. 213–214)

nosis on this axis would be "bipolar disorder, depressed."

2. Axis II (Personality disorders or specific developmental disorders): This axis allows the diagnosis of a preexisting disorder which may have contributed to the development of the primary syndrome, or which may be of significance after resolution of the primary syndrome. Dr. Lawson found that before having major emotional problems, Darryl had had an "avoidant personality disorder."
3. Axis III (Any existing physical disorder): An example would be essential hypertension. Darryl had no diagnosis on this axis.
4. Axis IV (Rating of previous psychosocial stressors on a scale of 1-none to 7-catastrophic): Psychosocial stressors include events such as marital discord, unemployment, and natural disasters. For example, Darryl had experienced marital discord of moderate severity, which would be rated 4 on this axis.
5. Axis V (Rating of highest adaptive level during the past year): If superior, the rating is 1; if grossly impaired, the rating is 7. Dr. Lawson found that Darryl had a fair level of adaptation at some times during the past year, and gave Darryl a rating of 4.

The replacement of the classification system of DSM-II, in which only the information on Axis I would be listed, by DSM-III's multiaxial system will allow much more information to be routinely communicated.

General Criticisms of DSM-III

Although DSM-III has attempted to consider the concerns of critics (e.g., Feighner, 1979; M. A. Taylor & Heiser, 1971) who have argued for a descriptive, atheoretical approach to the classification of disturbed human functioning, many criticisms applicable to DSM-I and DSM-II still apply. For example, the fact that DSM-

III has redefined several disorders raises the question whether the categories describe stable entities. Gergen (1973) argues that classification should focus on the enduring phenomena such as behaviors, rather than on conceptual entities such as "diseases," which may be considered pathological only because of a prevailing cultural belief at a particular time. As a case in point, we can consider homosexuality. In early editions of DSM, published at a time when sexual attitudes were very constricted, homosexuality was considered a mental disorder. Today sexual attitudes are more liberal, and homosexuality is diagnosed in DSM-III as a mental disorder only if the homosexual persistently desires to be heterosexual.

McLemore and Benjamin (1979) have described the shortcomings of DSM-III as including a continued reliance on impressionistic clinical judgment, continued use of an implicit illness model, and what they consider to be almost total neglect of social-psychological variables and interpersonal behavior. They argue that abnormal behavior is primarily an issue of problematic interpersonal relationships, and classification ought to focus on problem interactions, rather than on the internal pathology of the individual. While DSM-III tries to include issues of psychosocial functioning and adaptation, it seems to ignore the fact that problems may occur in a relationship between two people, rather than be vested within an individual.

Impressionistic clinical judgment still remains a primary problem in the use of DSM-III. The types of ratings used on Axes IV and V are extremely global and sensitive to a great deal of subjective judgment. This subjectivity is likely to result in a lack of reliability. The DSM-III system still lacks a process for the rigorous and systematic description of social behavior that many feel is critical for the effective definition and treatment of disordered functioning.

The diagnostic reliability of DSM-III appears more adequate than that of previous editions. In early field trials (Spitzer & Forman, 1979; Spitzer, Forman, & Nee, 1979), 274 clinicians were paired and made diagnoses on a total of 281 patients. Most clinicians assessed 2 patients each. A prepublication draft of DSM-III was used as the standard for the evaluations. The results of these field trials have been described by the evaluators as encouraging (see Table 4.3). The authors concluded that the results were generally better than typically reported reliabilities for DSM-I and DSM-II. However, other studies have been less positive. Mezzich and Mezzich (1979) found a poor degree of agreement between clinicians using DSM-III criteria on diagnoses of childhood and adolescent behavior disorders. At best, only 4 out of 10 clinicians agreed on the diagnoses of childhood disorders using the DSM-III criteria. DSM-III has not totally solved the problem of the lack of reliability of diagnoses. However, studies conducted after DSM-III has been more widely used and clinicians have gained more experience, may indicate greater reliability (Scheftner, 1980).

Psychologists and DSM-III

DSM-I, DSM-II, and the current DSM-III have been criticized for their implicit (if not explicit) acceptance of the medical/disease model, to the exclusion of other theoretical frameworks. In spite of a relatively atheoretical approach in early versions, the framers of DSM-III were criticized for maintaining that abnormal behavior is an "illness" or "disease" in the individual, with primary internal causes of a physiological or psychological nature. While pointing out that many of the revisions in DSM-III are positive, Schacht and Nathan (1977) are concerned about these implicit disease assump-

Table 4.3
Sample levels of agreement of diagnosticians on diagnoses using DSM-III criteria

Disorder	*Level of agreement*[1]
Psychotic disorders	
Schizophrenia	.82
Major affective disorders	.70
Schizoaffective disorders	.56
Nonpsychotic disorders	
Adjustment disorders	.74
Anxiety disorders	.74
Personality disorders	.54

Based on Spitzer et al. (1979).

[1]Pairs of diagnosticians had equal access to all relevant data, but did not discuss the materials with each other prior to formulating the diagnosis. An agreement level of .70 or above indicates reasonably high agreement.

tions. Schacht and Nathan suggest that a major problem with the prepublication version of DSM-III was that it continued to define abnormal behavior as exclusively in the province of the medical profession, to the exclusion of psychology. Advocates of DSM-III have responded that the final, published version of DSM-III (1980) was revised to avoid this emphasis (Spitzer, Williams, & Skodol, 1980).

McReynolds (1980) has criticized the implicit assumptions of a disease model, and has expressed concern about the inclusion of many additional syndromes under the term "mental disorders." He expresses concern about some newly included "disorders" of childhood. For example, DSM-III (1980) lists a new disorder called "developmental arithmetic disorder." McReynolds thinks that little is gained from labeling a problem such as poor math ability a mental disorder. What will be the effect on children who are labeled as having a psychiatric disorder because they have difficulty reading, pronouncing words, or doing mathematics?

DSM-III and This Text

In Chapters 5–19, many types of disordered behavior will be discussed. In most instances, the descriptions of specific symptom clusters and the terms used to label abnormal behaviors will parallel DSM-III terminology. The few departures from DSM-III will be noted. The reason for using DSM-III criteria for disorders is simple: The vast majority of clinicians—regardless of their professional identity as psychologists, social workers, or psychiatrists—use DSM-III as their classification system. In order to communicate and compare information, the student of abnormal psychology must know DSM-III's "language."

Summary

1. In order to understand abnormal behavior, psychologists use a variety of procedures to assess people's functioning. These procedures include interviews, direct observation of behavior, and psychological tests.

2. The clinical interview is a more or less structured conversation in which a clinician attempts to find out relevant information about a client's history, current behavior, and emotional state. The accuracy of information gained in an interview depends on many situational and interpersonal factors.

3. Behavioral assessment is one of the most structured techniques for gaining information from a client. It may include an interview which focuses on specific problem behaviors, their frequency, and the reinforcement contingencies that maintain the behavior. Other behavioral assessment techniques include rating scales, baseline observations, and physiological measurements.

4. Psychological testing includes intellectual assessment, personality assessment and tests of neurological functioning. The Stanford-Binet intelligence test yields a global IQ. The Wechsler Adult Intelligence Scale, in contrast, allows the comparison of the individual's various scores on subscales, which measure a range of functions and abilities.

5. Projective personality tests consist of relatively ambiguous tasks which allow a person to project the inner self into the activity. The examiner uses these revealing responses to interpret the subject's behavior.

6. The Rorschach consists of 10 inkblots. The person describes what the inkblots remind him or her of. The Rorschach has been criticized as unreliable and its validity has been questioned, but many psychologists believe that the Rorschach is an accurate and comprehensive test of personality functioning.

7. The Thematic Apperception Test consists of pictures about which the client is to make up stories. The TAT has recently been demonstrated to have very good predictive ability for some types of behaviors.

8. The Minnesota Multiphasic Personality Inventory is one of the most widely used personality inventories. In the MMPI, people answer a series of questions about themselves, and their answers are compared to norms developed on known groups believed to be representative of particular types of personalities.

9. The Halstead-Reitan Battery is a series of tests designed to measure various brain-behavior relationships. It seems to be a highly effective procedure for assessing deficits caused by organic brain dysfunction.

10. Psychologists use psychological tests for several purposes. The information is used to enhance understanding of a client's personality functioning and to plan treatment strategies. In addition, the information derived from many types of assessment is used in conjunction with the results of psychological tests to derive a diagnosis or classify a person according to an established system.

11. Classification systems offer many benefits to those who wish to understand abnormal behavior. Classification 1. organizes information so that it makes sense, 2. allows us to generalize from limited data to larger groups of people, and 3. acts as a shorthand communication system.

12. Classification also has potential hazards. It may bias one's perceptions, and has a tendency to lose details of information.

13. The ideal classification system would have reliability, homogeneity within classes, and categories that are stable and valid. A prototype classification system does not fully meet the requirement of homogeneity within classes, but can be reliable, stable, and valid.

14. The most commonly used classification system for abnormal behavior was developed under the sponsorship of the American Psychiatric Association, but has been adopted by clinicians and researchers from many disciplines. Its latest revision (DSM-III, 1980) includes many newly described behaviors. DSM-III is a multiaxial system; individuals are classified on five axes.

15. DSM-III utilizes much more specific criteria in its descriptions of disorders than past editions (DSM-I and DSM-II). The increased specificity of the criteria should enhance this classification system's reliability, utility, and validity.

16. The DSM approach to classification has been heavily criticized as unreliable, and lacking in validity. In spite of the recent revisions of the system, some professionals (especially in psychology) still feel that the DSM-III approach has significant faults.

17. Although clinicians recognize that DSM-III is not perfect, it continues to be the most widely used classification system for abnormal behavior in the United States. This state of affairs is likely to continue until a significant alternative becomes available. Because of DSM-III's broad acceptance, its criteria and terminology are used in discussing most disorders in subsequent chapters.

KEY TERMS

Homogeneity. A characteristic of an ideal classification system. A single category should have homogeneity (its elements should not appear in other categories).

Heterogeneity. A characteristic of an ideal classification system. The group of categories should have heterogeneity (they should each be different from the others and not overlap).

Objective personality test. A test of personality which is constructed so that the task can be measured with relative objectivity and the results of the testing can be interpreted by comparing it to established norms derived from administration of the test to large samples of people.

Personality inventory. A relatively objective personality test which consists of a series of a standard questions that are usually answered, "true," "false," or "don't know."

Projective test. A personality test constructed so that the subject must respond to relatively unstructured, ambiguous stimuli. The subjects' responses are believed to be determined more by their inner personality dynamics than by the test stimuli, thus revealing important aspects of the person's inner life.

Prototype classification. A type of classification system in which some overlap between categories is expected. However, classification can still be accurate and reliable, since the classification is based on clusters of elements characteristic of only one category.

Psychological battery. A group of tests combined to yield information about a variety of aspects of the individual.

Reliability. The degree to which a test, measurement, or classification system yields the same information each time it is applied to the same data.

Validity. The extent to which a type of measurement measures what it is supposed to measure.

PSYCHOLOGICAL AND PHYSICAL REACTIONS TO STRESS AND ANXIETY

This section presents disorders traditionally associated with stress and anxiety. The feeling of being under pressure and the discomfort of anxiety are sensations that most of us have experienced to some degree in our lives. For some people, stress or anxiety is experienced so intensely or so chronically that it results in important problems in managing day-to-day behavior.

In Chapter 5, psychological and behavioral reactions to major stress are presented. Each of us can easily imagine that under some severe stress, we might "break down." For some of us, the level of stress might have to be very great. For others, the stressor might not appear to be very severe when observed objectively, yet the person's reaction indicates that the event was experienced as very stressful. Some people experience common events such as getting married, entering school, losing a job, or having a prolonged illness as particularly stressful and have great difficulty adjusting to them. Other events are extremely stressful for almost everyone. Few people are able to handle major stresses such as war and natural disasters with no aftereffects in their behavior.

Chapter 6 focuses on disorders believed to be related to physiological reactions to stress. In a stressful situation, we often feel fearful, anxious, or angry. Our body physiologically gears itself to "fight or flee." Major sudden stress can have very serious consequences on the physical well-being of an individual, but a more common situation is the experience of chronic low level stress, which may lead to physical ailments. In Chapter 6, the physiological processes involved in the fight-or-flee response are examined in detail, and their relationship to the development of physical illness is considered.

Chapter 7 considers psychological disorders that are characterized by the presence of disabling anxiety or that appear to function to avoid the experience of anxiety. As in the physiological disorders in Chapter 6, the fight-or-flee response seems to be an important aspect of the anxiety disorders. Individuals who have an anxiety disorder experience a disturbance in behavior in their day-to-day living at a level greater than would be expected of most people.

Chapter 8 is devoted to somatoform and dissociative disorders, which have traditionally been associated with the avoidance of anxiety-provoking experiences. The somatoform disorders mimic physical disorders, but do not involve underlying organic change or damage like the psychophysiological disorders. The individual behaves *as if* paralyzed, blind, deaf, and so on, but no physical damage can be found to account for the disability. The dissociative disorders interfere with the maintenance of conscious awareness of behavior. Individuals do not seem to be aware of what they are doing at the moment, or of what they have done at some past time.

In Part II, and in the following sections, many specific disorders will be described. The major theories about the etiologies of these disorders will be presented, with emphasis on the contributions of the psychoanalytic, biological, and learning theory approaches to these disorders. The contributions of current research on the disorders will be presented. The chapters will usually close with a special section on key therapies for the treatment of the chapter's disorders, so that this important topic will not be postponed. The last part of the text will provide a review of the major treatment approaches and an evaluation of the overall effectiveness of the therapies.

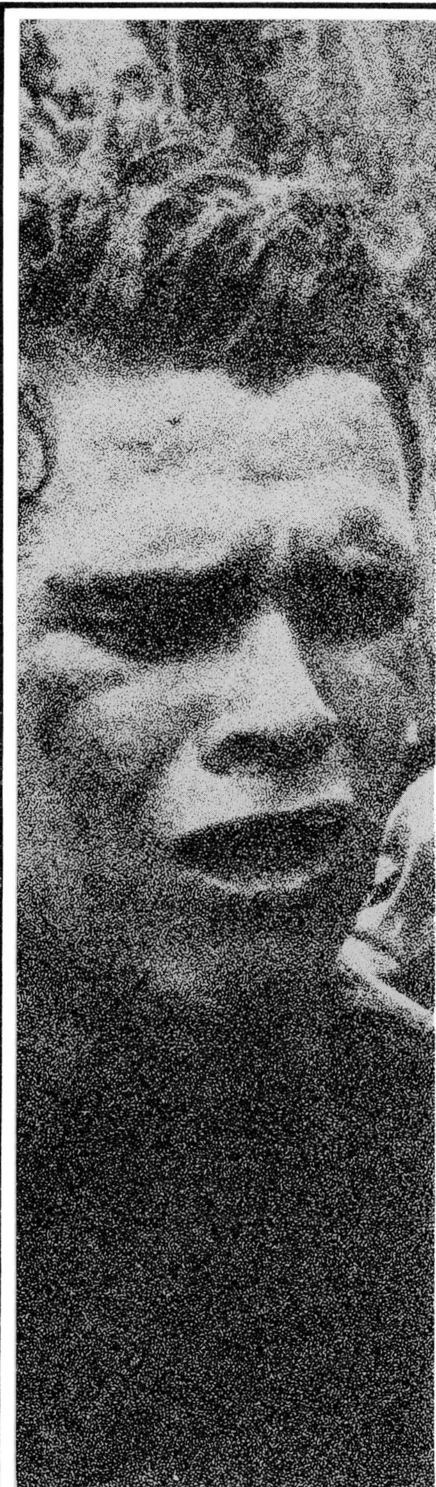

5

Psychological and behavioral problems in adjusting to major stress

- Coping with stress
- Characteristics of adjustment reactions and crisis states
- Typical crisis or stress situations
- Chronic intense stress
- Acute major disaster states
- Summing up
- Key treatments
- Summary
- Key terms

When an individual encounters a situation which places demands on physical or psychological functioning, it is called stress. What is a "normal" reaction to stress? We would not expect that most people could face any and every extreme stress calmly, adequately, and with no adverse effects. Still, we expect that most everyday, common stresses can be faced with little difficulty. When individuals manifest disturbed behavior while under stress, when they can't "cope," we consider a number of factors before deciding how serious their problem may be. Is the stress very mild, or is it extreme? Is the level of stress the most important factor in the disturbed behavior? Could a previous emotional disorder have led to the person's behavioral problems? If stress is mild, a previous emotional disorder is likely to be at the root of the problem. If the person seems to have been well adjusted and free of emotional problems, but has recently been in a stress situation, the behavioral disorder is likely to be due to the stress. That even the most adaptive and stable individual may "break down" under conditions of severe stress is widely accepted today.

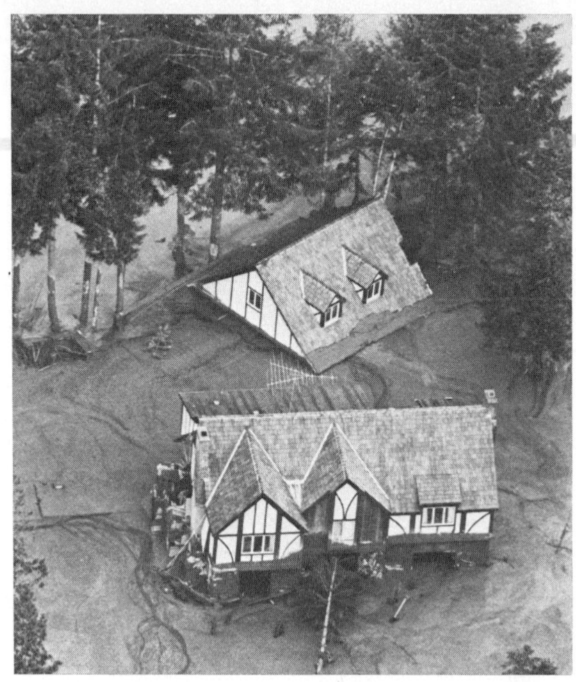

The eruption of the Mount St. Helens volcano in 1980 in the state of Washington resulted in damage to life and property that may require years of adjustment by the inhabitants of the area.

Imagine, for example, that on May 18, 1980, you were vacationing at a campsite on the slopes of Mt. St. Helens in the state of Washington. On that date, a volcanic eruption destroyed a large area of land and forest, killing 63 people and injuring others. Many of the dead have never been found. What would it have been like to be there and survive? Imagine yourself there. A deafening roar, the earth shaking, day turning into night from the falling ash, the air almost unbreathable from gases, extreme heat, roads blocked—helpless against the threat of injury or death, you think only of escape. Abandoning your camp, you try to walk out; your car will not run. In terror for your life, you and your companions start for safety, which you hope exists miles away through the wilderness. After marching continuously for 36 hours, you are finally found and rescued; but a vivid memory remains of your companions being swept away by a flood of mud as you all tried to cross a ravine, their screams echoing in your ears. You are certain that they are dead and their bodies maimed, but they are never found. Few of us would handle such an experience well; we would manifest disturbed behavior almost immediately, and perhaps for some time after. The disturbed behavior would be called a **posttraumatic stress disorder** because the stressor is outside the range of normal human experience.

The stress which leads to disordered behavior need not be so cataclysmic. Consider the individual who faces a series of stresses, each of which might be handled well alone but which together lead to a breakdown of one's ability to cope. Imagine that as a senior in college, your father dies suddenly. Preoccupied, your study habits slip and you receive the first "F" of your college career on a midterm exam, in a course you need in order to graduate. While you are depressed over your father's death and anxious about your grades, your lover tells you the relationship is over, that you will never see each other again except as acquaintances. Your former lover then begins to date your "best friend." On spring break, your car is stolen and wrecked, and you discover that you have no insurance. How would you react? Most of us would have a great deal of difficulty dealing with all these stresses at once, some of us might even have problems dealing with one of them. Behavioral disorder that occurs in this type of situation is called an **adjustment disorder,** since it prevents adequate adjustment to the life stresses.

In these two types of disorder the disturbed behavior results primarily from the individual's inability to cope with a stressful event. Once the stress is gone, the disturbed behavior often goes away. The functioning of individuals who have other disorders (such as longstanding depression) may also deteriorate under stress. We are more concerned here with the reaction of "normal" people to major stresses. That is, we are concerned with the reactions to stress of people who have no previous mental or emotional disorder. Adjustment disorder and post-traumatic stress disorder primarily represent disordered functioning in otherwise normal people.

The stresses with which we all must cope are numerous (e.g., Coelho & Adams, 1974). Some examples include marriage, illness, death of loved ones, school transitions, puberty, loss of parents during childhood, and retirement. You can probably think of many more. In addition there are the more catastrophic stresses of natural disasters such as floods, fires, tornadoes, hurricanes, and earthquakes. Some stresses are chronic such as imprisonment in penal institutions, concentration camps, prisoner-of-war camps, and the stresses of combat. Although catastrophic and chronic stress events are rare (though more frequent than we desire), they are significant sources of behavioral disturbance and provide us with opportunities for studying human reactions to major stress. Many of the findings from such studies are applicable to our everyday life.

What makes an event stressful? Bowers and Kelly (1979) cite four characteristics of stressful events often noted in the literature.

1. People feel a sense of a loss of control of the events in their lives. They feel helpless to change what is going on or to successfully intervene in the process.
2. There is an anticipation or occurrence of physical or psychological pain. For example, the individual fears being injured or killed (as in a disaster) or is threatened with a loss of self-esteem (as in a divorce).
3. There is a loss of social or emotional support. In a disaster, friends and relatives may be missing or killed. Less dramatic events such as divorce, job loss, or marriage may separate individuals from family members and old friends.
4. The event or some aspect of it is perceived as unpleasant or aversive, and the individual tries to actively avoid it.

Whether someone experiences an event as stressful depends both on the character of the event and the characteristics of the individual (Dohrenwend, 1973; May & Sprague, 1976). A vacation, a marriage, or the birth of a child may be desired, looked forward to, and yet may be stressful because of the adjustive demands that the person experiences. On a family "vacation," a wife and mother may have more work than at home. Marriage places new responsibilities and demands on both partners. A new infant requires many different adjustments in family relationships, and increases the responsibilities of the parents. Individuals who have good coping ability can experience such events with little perception of stress, or can feel stressed but handle the difficulties.

COPING WITH STRESS

If we were to study people who seem able to cope with potential stress events such as job loss, divorce, or going away to school, what would we expect to find? Individuals who have good coping skills are usually good problem solvers. They engage in task-oriented behaviors such as breaking the problem into its component parts, and solving a part at a time. They try to anticipate the outcome of their actions. New behaviors are rehearsed and practiced before being tried. **Adaptive behavior** involves the use of information. Good coping skills require accurate perceptions and active attempts to find new information. Problems must be kept in conscious awareness, not denied or avoided. Adequate copers manage their feelings about the stressful situation and reduce tensions by sharing feelings with people who are important to them. They seek out people who are supportive of the coping behavior and who are willing to help. Caring, supportive people who are important to the person who is struggling with a potential stress situation form a **psychosocial support system.**

Meichenbaum, Turk, and Burstein (1975) have emphasized cognitive factors in adjustment to stress. Effective worrying, for example, allows one to plan techniques to meet the stress. It seems to lower a person's sensitivity to the emotional reactions attendant upon the occurrence of the event. Fenz (1975) compared novice parachutists (on their first several jumps) with experienced parachutists. He found that novices tried unsuccessfully to defend against fear with denial, and perceptual distortion (i.e., not perceiving anxiety-provoking stimuli). They tended to worry about the injuries they *might* receive. Experienced parachutists focused on decreasing their physiological reactions to the jump experience (jitteriness, churning stomach, pounding heart) while remaining aware of the potential danger. Effective worrying allowed them to develop contingencies to prevent something from going wrong. For example, they packed their chutes with special care and reviewed emergency procedures. The novices engaged in **ruminative thinking** (worrying) about the negative aspects of the event, without effective thought about positive solutions; these behaviors increased fear and hindered effective coping. For example, the novices were likely to be preoccupied with the thought that the chute would not open. The experienced parachutists had learned how to cope with a stressful situation cognitively, behaviorally, and emotionally.

When Coping Breaks Down

One's adjustment to stressful experiences appears to depend upon several factors. When adjustment reactions occur, they seem to be related both to the individual's available coping resources and the level of stress encountered. The coping resources include physical condition (or predispositions), the presence or absence of other psychological disorders, learned coping skills, and the presence or absence of emotional support systems.

Some individuals respond to stress with greater **autonomic nervous system** reactivity (Lacey, 1967), which may interfere with coping ability even for relatively low levels of stress (this will be explored in the following chapters). Physical exhaustion or illness can be a cause (as well as a result) of a decrease in coping ability. The presence of other psychological disorders, such as a depression, may exaggerate a response to stress, magnify the perception of stress, or hinder the development of coping strategies (Merbaum & Hefez, 1976). Some learned behaviors may interfere with the development of adequate coping skills. For example, Seligman (1973) has identified the phenomenon of **learned helplessness.** Individuals may learn that they are helpless to control their own fate or to solve problems. This sense of helplessness pervades their behavior, so that in the face of stress they stop their problem-solving behaviors after only a few ineffective attempts.

The availability of psychosocial support systems has been considered important by many investigators. For example, James Pennebaker and Darren Newtson of the University of Virginia, in a study of the Mt. St. Helens eruption found different psychological reactions in persons living in various communities surrounding the volcano. The differences depended to some extent on the degree to which the communities organized a response to the disaster (Schaar, 1980). The more the townspeople drew together and organized to deal with the disaster, the better they were able to handle the stress. In towns with no organization for dealing with the volcanic aftermath, adjustment was more difficult. Stress seems easier to handle when we can face it with the psychological and social support of others.

Level of stress is an obvious factor in the failure of adjustment mechanisms. The perception of stress depends to some extent on personal variables. Some events may be so cataclysmic that all but the most unusual person react as if under overwhelming stress, for example, in a Vietnam firefight or internment in a concentration camp. Other events such as moving from one home to another appear to be relatively mild stressors. However, the individual's vulnerability may result in the event being experienced as a very stressful transitional state, and an adjustment disorder may develop.

CHARACTERISTICS OF ADJUSTMENT REACTIONS AND CRISIS STATES

When stress is overwhelming a number of behaviors may appear. Common behaviors include depressed mood, anxiety, disordered conduct such as vandalism or violence, work or academic inhibition, and withdrawal from contact with others. Under extreme stress, such grossly disturbed behavior as hallucinations and delusions (fixed false beliefs) may occur (Goldstein, 1976).

Studies of people responding to major stress or crisis have identified a commonly seen crisis pattern of behavior (see Figures 5.1). "Crisis" has been defined by Caplan (1964) as "a short period of psychological disequilibrium in a person who confronts a hazardous circumstance that for him constitutes an important problem which he can for the time being neither escape nor solve with his customary problem-solving resources."

Before a crisis occurs, most individuals maintain an adjustment level that varies only slightly over time. However, as a crisis impacts on the person, the person's usual coping mechanisms fail and behavior becomes relatively disorganized and ineffective in solving problems. This is known as **crisis decompensation.** Individuals who experience crisis decompensation as a result of stress eventually "bottom out," or reach a lowered level of functioning. However, crisis states seem to be self-limiting so that this period of decompensation is followed by a resolution phase. Following the resolution, the person once again enters a steady adjustment state, which has only slight variations in levels of effectiveness over time. Most significantly, the postcrisis adjustment level may be at a higher functioning level than the precrisis state, a lower level than the precrisis state, or at the same level as the precrisis state.

After the impact of the crisis, the period of decompensation may be characterized by the following behaviors:

1. The individual may be preoccupied.
2. Guilt may be experienced over one's inability to resolve the problem.
3. Hostility is often felt toward others or toward the "world" in general.
4. Physical distress may be experienced—nervousness, stomachaches, inability to sleep.
5. Established patterns of conduct may change, personal hygiene may slip, routines may be disrupted.
6. The person may become apathetic and not seem to care.
7. There may be aimless activity, which is not goal directed.
8. Relationships with others change; the individual may become more dependent or withdrawn.

Figure 5.1 Crisis phase sequence.
Adapted with permission of Robert J. Brady Co., Bowie, Md., 20715, from 1975 copyrighted work titled, "Emergency Psychiatric Care: Management of Mental Health Crisis."

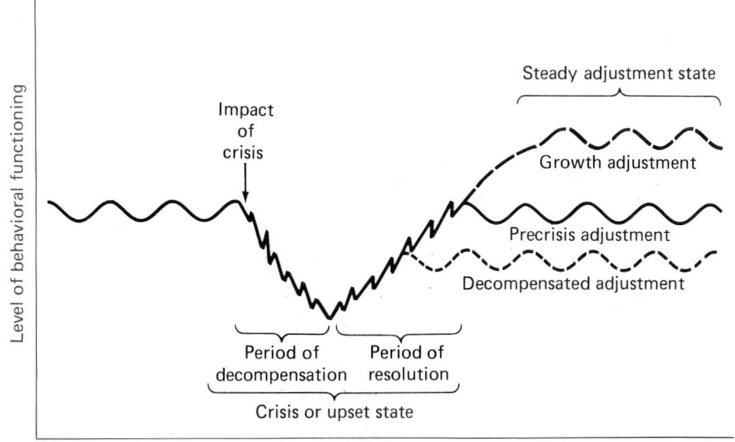

9. Behavior detrimental to the person's self-interest may appear.

Parad and Resnik (1975) have described decompensation in terms of the subjective feelings of individuals in crisis. They are bewildered about how they feel: "I never felt this way before." They feel in danger, "I feel so nervous and scared—something terrible is going to happen." They feel frustration, "I feel stuck—nothing I do seems to help." They are desperate, "I've got to do something," or apathetic, "What's the use—nothing can help me." They feel helpless, "I can't manage this myself," and have a sense of urgency, "I need help *now*." They feel discomfort, "I feel miserable, so restless and unsettled."

When a high level of stress is chronic, the actual decompensation may occur suddenly due to a precipitating event (like a divorce or a job loss). In situations of acute-onset stress, which later becomes chronic, such as internment in a prisoner-of-war or concentration camp or limb amputation, these symptoms of decompensation may become less obvious but remain severely incapacitating. The decompensation may be primarily manifested in behaviors such as withdrawal, apathy, or depression. The precise symptomatology of an adjustment reaction depends on both personal and situational variables, including the nature of the crisis or stress.

TYPICAL CRISIS OR STRESS SITUATIONS

Common Crises

It is relatively easy to appreciate how the severe stresses of a disaster may result in disturbed behavior. However, stresses and stress reactions occur on a continuum from severe to mild. Even everyday events may become crises. Many essentially normal people find it difficult to adjust to common crises, and exhibit varying levels of disturbed functioning. The level of stress which common events place on people varies.

Marital and Family Problems. The human relationships of marriage and family are often fraught with difficulty. Divorce, often the end result of such problems, is recognized as a stressful event. The dissolution or change in role relationships, new challenges, and the impact on self-esteem for one or both divorced spouses often lead to personal difficulty. In addition, children frequently develop maladaptive behaviors in response to the dissolution of their parents' marriage. This crisis is particularly common: The incidence of divorce from 1867 to 1970 increased more than tenfold. From 1970 to 1980, an estimated 10 million divorces occurred. Although some divorces may end a bad, even abusing relationship, most divorces have positive and negative results. For most people, divorce signifies failure in an extremely important relationship.

At the age of 32, John married Ann, a 29-year-old school teacher. The first year and a half of the marriage appeared to be relatively uneventful. By their second anniversary, things were no longer going well. Ann told John that she felt that the marriage was not working. She felt tied down by John's desire that she spend all her time with him. Ann begain going "out with the girls" several times a week. During the next year, Ann and John fought more and more often. As the problems escalated, they finally came to a mutual decision to divorce.

John felt bad about the upcoming divorce. During a separation while waiting for the divorce to become final, he was preoccupied by thoughts about how he had failed as a husband. All he seemed able to do was to think about Ann. As the filing of the final divorce papers came near, he became very depressed. He was unable to complete his work satisfactorily and dropped out of an evening graduate course that he had been taking. His unusual behavior alarmed his parents, who had never seen him become depressed over setbacks before. They encouraged him to enter counseling to "get his head straight." In counseling sessions, John finally expressed his anger at Ann for "dumping him" and his sense of helplessness about the situation: "Nothing I did, none of the changes I made, seemed to make any difference to her."

Over six months John's depression lifted, and he began to date again. He was no longer preoccupied with "what [he] did wrong" in his marriage to Ann. He was again able to work energetically and competently. Three years later John married again, and he has had a successful relationship with his second wife for the past seven years.

Some family-related behaviors may be both a source and result of stress. Harbin and Madden (1979) cite the case of a 17-year-old boy who would take decorative swords from the wall of his parents' home, destroy their furniture, and make threatening gestures when they tried to stop him. This behavior often occurred when he was stressed by factors outside the home, as when he had problems with his girlfriend. The parents were extremely stressed by his behavior and overwhelmed by their inability to deal with it. Another example of extreme family stress which often leads to an adjustment reaction is child or spouse abuse (Ackley, 1977; Flynn, 1977). These behaviors are far more common than many think (see Highlight 5.1). Gelles (1972), for example, found that spouse abuse occurred in over one-third of a randomly selected group of 40 families. In addition to the abuser and the abused person, other family members tend to have adjustment reactions to the stress of this situation.

School. The first day at school is often a stressful experience for many children, who may respond by withdrawal, anxiety, and resistance. The competitive school environment, with its threat of failure, also can have significant effects on the child (Morse, 1967). As many college students know, the freshman's experience of separation (and freedom) from home, parents, and old friends often leads to "homesickness" (withdrawal, sadness or depression, lack of motivation) and, less obviously, to behavior such as drug usage, drinking, and frantic social activity.

Death of a Loved One. We all face the prospect of the death of someone to whom we are emotionally tied, a "loved one." Even when one protests that a parent or sib is hated, the feelings are usually not clear-cut, and when death occurs, adjustment reactions are still possible. The usual loss reaction is called **uncomplicated bereavement** in DSM-III and includes normal sadness. In less normal reactions, depression and despair are frequent in the survivor, as are guilt or anger about things done or not done by the time of the death. The reaction may not occur immediately after the death, but rarely happens later than the first two or three months. Stoical acceptance, denial, or avoidance of feelings may lead to a prolonged reaction to the death. One possible reaction involves behaving as if the person were still alive, for example, maintaining a bedroom as a "shrine." Another possible reaction is depression, which if not worked through, may last for many months or years and finally require hospitalization (Becker, 1974; Kubler-Ross, 1969). Reactions of this severity are the exception, not the rule, when a loved one dies.

HIGHLIGHT 5.1
INTRAFAMILIAL VIOLENCE: ADJUSTMENT REACTION?

Family life is often beset by internal crises in the personal relationships and external ones, such as loss of economic resources. Evidence exists that aggressive behavior is partly a function of the frustration of behavior directed towards goals (Kutash, Schlesinger, & Associates, 1978). In recent years, violence within families has been found to be much more common than anyone suspected. Wolkenstein (1976) reports that reliable estimates place the incidence of unreported child abuse at 2.5 *million* cases per year! Flynn (1977) reports studies finding spouse abuse in 40 percent of randomly selected families, and in 16 percent of college students' families. Spouse abuse victims are usually wives, but cases of abused husbands are now more frequently being reported. Recently, focus has been placed on the physical abuse of parents by children (Harbin & Madden, 1979). An estimated 10 percent of all children between the ages of 3–18 have physically attacked their parents, and Steinmetz and Strauss (1974) have reported the abuse of elderly parents by their adult children. Does the apparently widespread incidence of intrafamilial violence suggest that it is a reaction to familial stress, a result of innate instincts toward human violence, or is due to psychopathology?

Criminal Victimization. Millions of crimes are committed every year, and many individuals are victims. The victims of muggings and beatings, the relatives of those murdered, and victims of rape commonly have significant adjustment reactions to the event. LeJeune and Alex (1973) found that mugging victims developed fears of being alone on the streets, had nightmares, and some male victims became sexually impotent. Burgess (1975) has identified adjustment reactions in families where a member had died by homicide. An acute grief reaction was combined with the long-term problem of dealing with the violent loss of a family member. Survivors' reactions were usually characterized by fear, anger, and nightmares. It has been commonly observed that many rape victims suffer serious psychological consequences from the attack (see Chapter 9).

The effects of criminal victimization are illustrated by the long-term effects of a well-known mass kidnapping (Terr, 1981). In July 1976, a school bus containing 26 children aged 5–14 and a bus driver was highjacked by three masked men. The children were driven around for 11 hours in darkened enclosed vans and then transferred to a truck trailer, which was buried underground. Sixteen hours later, two of the older children were able to dig an escape route. The kidnappers were never caught. Twenty-three of the 26 children were studied, and each of the 23 manifested disturbing behaviors in the year afterward. Twenty-one of the children developed unusual fears of mundane experience (e.g., anxiety attacks when riding in the family car). All the children feared another kidnapping attempt, and became extremely suspicious and frightened of any event that reminded them of the ordeal.

> Mandy, 7, twice screamed that her little brother had been kidnapped, when he was actually playing next door or trying on clothes in a store dressing room. Exactly 1 year after the kidnapping, Johnny, 11, refused to sleep in his bedroom for many nights because he believed the ceiling was collapsing.
>
> Sammy, 10, experienced two panicky episodes, according to his mother. "Before Christmas during vacation he was biking with a friend [in the] sandhills. A station wagon, two guys, and a dog were there. He abandoned his bike and ran home. He said he didn't want to be kidnapped again. He cried a lot. I advised him not to panic and run. . . . Just before the fair in May there were strangers on the road, and he gave up biking there and refused to go further." (Terr, 1981, pp. 18, 19)

The reactions of these children parallel the reactions of adults who have been criminally victimized in a stressful manner. Lifton and Olson (1976) have described the effects of sudden life-endangering stress as a "shattering of the illusion of invulnerability." The person suddenly comes to a realization that "it can happen to me."

Employment. While the stresses of employment may result in adjustment disorders, chronic unemployment is a more significant factor. The chronically unemployed tend to feel defeated. Constant rejection by employers often leads to a sense of apathy: Why bother? Many people find unemployment compensation or the receipt of welfare money very damaging to their self-concept. They often react with anger and rage at a system that allows this situation to exist. Many urban riots (Detroit, Watts, Miami) may have been a form of adjustment reaction to the stresses of poverty and to life outside the mainstream.

Retirement. The major transition from gainful employment to retirement, and the advance into late life involves many stresses. Though retirement means less job stress, retirees often feel useless, engage in boring makeshift activities, and encounter a loss of status and buying power. Tyhurst (1957) has found that most retirees have a honeymoon period, when they attempt to live out the retirement myth of happy leisure, but soon find their new "freedom" unsatisfying. They often become depressed and anxious. Dean Morse, an economist, and Susan Gray, a sociologist (Cory, 1980), have found in a study of 1000 retirees that over 40 percent returned to paid work because of dissatisfaction with retired life. The development of new meaningful activities can resolve this phase, but some retirees become chronically dissatisfied with their routine life and feel unable to do anything about it.

In addition to the loss of meaning that retirement has for some people, almost every older person must face other losses involved in aging: Physical abilities decline, friends die, children leave and are busy with their own lives. In our culture, the elderly are often seen as a burden and consigned to an isolated, lonely existence. Perhaps it is not surprising that depression is the most common reaction of the elderly to this situation (Vaillant, 1977).

Poor Health. Any major illness may lead to an adjustment reaction either in the ill or disabled person or in family members who must cope with the subsequent problems. To adjust to partial or total disability is very difficult. Adams and Lindemann (1974) point out that depression, anxiety, and extreme psychological defensiveness are often seen in disabled people. The sense of self as "permanently different" (e.g., paralyzed, disfigured, bedridden) is difficult to accept. The old basis for self-respect, self-confidence, and self-esteem has changed.

CHRONIC INTENSE STRESS

The recognition that situational stress can lead to significant behavioral and emotional disturbance is in large part due to studies of large groups of individuals who have experienced severe stresses. Two situations have received special attention: the chronic stress of armed combat and enemy capture and the imprisonment of civilians in concentration camps. Millions of people have had these experiences in this century.

Combat

Since World War I, when the term "shell shock" was used to describe severe reactions to

The stresses and dangers of combat environments affect civilians as well as soldiers. These men were taking news photos in El Salvador during the civil strife in 1980.

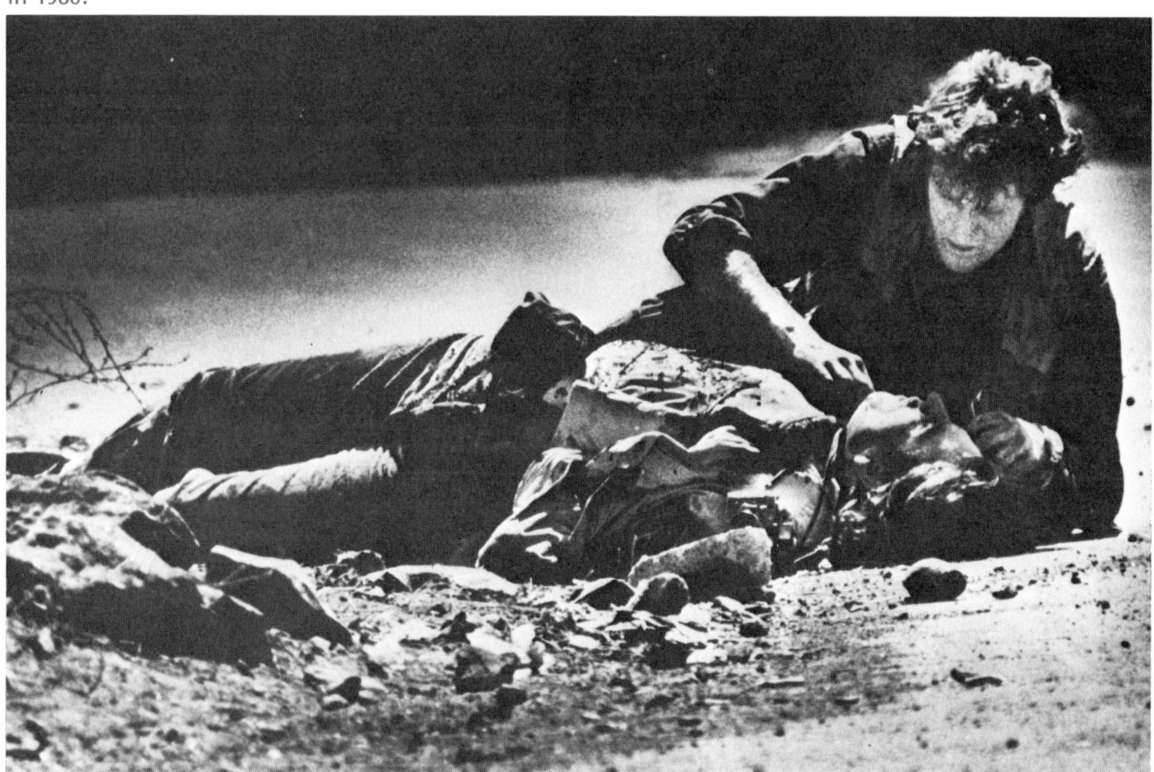

combat, war has provided a laboratory for the study of the effects of stress on human behavior. In World War II, "combat exhaustion" or "combat fatigue" (other terms for posttraumatic stress disorder) caused the greatest loss of manpower. In the Korean Conflict, the frequency of these disorders was less, but ranged from approximately 4 to 6 percent (Bell, 1958). In the Vietnam war, the incidence of acute stress reactions was 1.5 percent (Allerton, 1970; Block, 1969). The decline in percentage may represent improved or perhaps different conditions in the Vietnam war (Kormos, 1978), compared to World War II. A psychiatrist who served in Vietnam treating American troops reported that "It was good duty; we had fresh pineapple and milk every morning." Still, Wallen (1969) found that the psychological test results of many supposedly nonpsychiatric medical patients in the military who had become ill in Vietnam showed acute emotional turmoil, instability, and insecurity. The major impact of combat duty in Vietnam seems to have been delayed until the men were mustered out. Shatan (1973, 1978) reported that in 1972, of the 300,000 Vietnam veterans in New York City, 50,000 were unemployed, 5,000 were on welfare, and 30,000 were on drugs. Yager (1976) found that violence was a major problem for some postcombat Vietnam veterans who were considered maladjusted:

> Soldier A, who had no previous history of problems with either military or civilian authority, attacked his commanding officer, punched him several times, and heaved him over a desk following a series of escalating minor incidents in the unit. According to the soldier, the officer repeatedly misperceived events and had irrevocably characterized him as a troublemaker. Just prior to the attack the officer had berated and humiliated the soldier in front of the entire company, and was in the process of arranging for the soldier to be sent to the stockade. (p. 1334).

Anecdotal accounts must be viewed with caution, however. Borus (1974) has pointed out that many studies of Vietnam combat veterans focused on men already identified as maladjusted because of their war experience, or on combat veterans who had or developed significant antiwar attitudes. Most of these studies had no control groups. In his own studies he found no differences in level of maladjustment between Vietnam combat veterans and noncombat veterans who served at the same time. However, 23 percent of a group of 577 combat veterans and 172 noncombat veterans manifested maladjustment during an average five and one-half months in the United States prior to discharge. Borus has suggested that controlled long-range follow-up is needed to determine the actual extent of maladjustment that is due to Vietnam *combat* experience. More recent studies have indicated that many Vietnam veterans did not manifest combat-related stress reactions until many months (even up to a year) after their return to the United States (Williams, 1980); they had a delayed stress reaction (now called a delayed posttraumatic stress disorder). When the symptoms appear, their severity is related to the amount and intensity of combat the individual participated in (Figley, 1978). Currently, over 500,000 Vietnam veterans have serious behavioral problems related to their Vietnam experience. The seriousness of the problem is illustrated by the finding that more Vietnam combat veterans have died since the war by suicide than were killed in combat (Williams, 1979).

The symptoms of an adjustment reaction to combat stress are quite similar to the symptoms of crisis described earlier. The symptoms seem to develop sequentially from an initial irritability to hypersensitivity, jumpiness, and startle reactions. Sleeplessness then develops, followed by fatigue. This stage may last for long periods until some acutely stressful event precipitates the final adjustment reaction. Goodwin (1980) indicates that the following disturbances are commonly seen in Vietnam veterans with chronic stress reactions:

1. Depression. The veteran who experienced the death of a comrade is likely to develop depression. The depression is often associated with a feeling of helplessness over the futility of fighting a war that was not supported at home.
2. Isolation. Veterans often feel isolated from nonveteran peers, friends, and family. They feel that only another Vietnam veteran can understand what they have been through. The sometimes open hostility of civilians who opposed the war

is very unlike the reaction to veterans of previous wars, who are hailed as "heroes."

3. Rage. Many Vietnam veterans feel anger, even rage, at "the system" and the people who put them in an intolerable no-win situation. Most do not act out the rage, but are frightened that it will "break through" into their behavior.
4. Survival Guilt. Many veterans feel **survival guilt** because they survived, and friends or comrades died. They feel that if they had behaved differently, the others might have lived.
5. Anxiety. Many settings can evoke anxiety in these veterans: people walking behind them on the street, standing in an exposed place, a loud noise. Though these men know their anxiety is irrational, they respond to these stimuli as if they were still in combat.
6. Sleep Disturbances. The period before sleep is often filled with anxiety-provoking memories of Vietnam. During sleep, many have nightmares about combat experiences.
7. Intrusive Thoughts. Daytime events often trigger unpleasant thoughts (and associated emotions). A helicopter flying overhead, for example, may trigger **intrusive thoughts** or memories of a violent firefight, and feelings of panic or rage.
8. Avoidance of Feelings. Many veterans describe themselves as emotionally dead. They feel no love, no caring, no joy. They seem to have pushed away all feeling in order to avoid feeling pain.

A major difference between combat and other major stress situations is that in war a soldier is expected to kill the enemy. The necessity of this action, so contradictory to what most of us are taught all our lives, often leads to problematic reactions such as the general emotional "numbing" process which often occurs in warfare (Lifton, 1972). The enemy must be reduced to nonhumanity to reduce the soldier's guilt of killing. Later, the ex-soldier may have intense guilt feelings, anxiety, and depression when the defense of seeing others as nonhumans breaks down.

> Tom remembers: "I was a helicopter doorgunner. . . . All I want now is to forget the look on their faces as we shot them down . . . to forget what death spasms look like, to forget what it feels like when your hooch is blown apart. They may suffer the defeat, but I'll never forget my pleasure in killing my first 16-year-old 'Commie for Christ.' I carried out the orders. I carried the guns." . . . His nightmares were unaffected except by his own treatment: [In order to sleep well] every night, after work, he hurtled along the local freeways on his motorbike for hours; when he tumbled into bed, exhausted, he knew he would sleep without nightmares.
>
> Don sat mutely, eyes glazed, for six slow months. Even under his comrades' sympathetic prodding, he insisted he didn't want to tell "one more war story." When the others persisted, he finally poured out the story of his best friend's death in 'Nam. To console his friend's mother, he regularly reassured her that her son had died in his arms—instantly, painlessly. He had never revealed the truth, that after being mortally wounded his buddy had taken four wretched days to die. Until he unburdened himself of this cruel experience, Don said he felt as if that day's suffering had still not ended, as if his friend had taken an eternity to die. The shame of being alive when his comrade had died had frozen him into silence, and fixed his eyes forever on the past. (Shatan, 1973, p. 642)

Combat reactions lasting into civilian life are not unique to the Veitnam experience. Brill and Beebe (Brill, 1967) followed up discharged World War II soldiers who, while on active duty, had been hospitalized or lost duty-time

The stress of combat can cause an intense emotional reaction.

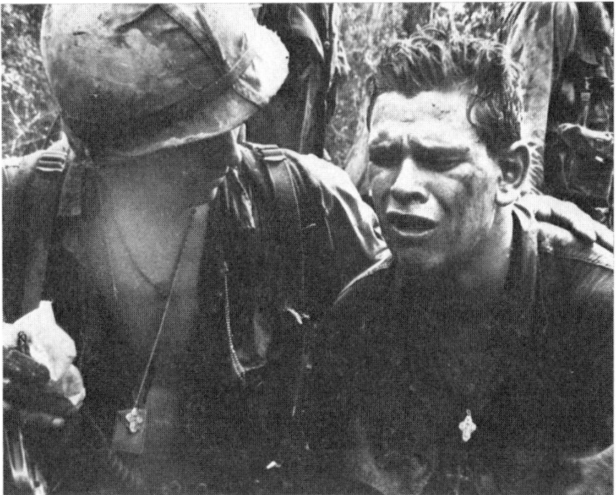

because of psychological reactions to combat stress. They found that five to six years later, 90 percent still had some symptoms of the reaction. The most common residual symptoms included irritability, anxiety, restlessness, headaches, and stomach disorder complaints. Employment was impossible for 14 percent because of residual symptoms. Twenty percent of the total were moderately disabled and 8 percent were severely disabled. If these percentages are generalizable to the 850,000 men from whom the small sample was drawn, the toll of combat stress in World War II was significant.

Prisoner-of-War and Concentration Camps

During most wars, some soldiers are captured and held prisoner in guarded camps, and civilians may be placed in work camps, internment camps, or even in death camps. Internment in such a situation results in extreme stress, and often in severe acute and chronic adjustment reactions. Physical hardship may be severe. In World War II 50 percent of United States soldiers in Japanese prisoner-of-war (POW) camps died before release. Farber, Harlow, and West (1956) describe the "DDD" syndrome (debility, dependency, dread) apparent in POWs in the Korean Conflict. It included debility due to semistarvation, fatigue, and disease; dependency on captors due to separation from comrades; and dread due to fear of death, pain from torture, and endless imprisonment. For many POWs, anxiety and depression were constant companions; others became emotionally isolated to avoid such feelings; and some simply gave up and died. Even in Vietcong POW camps, where Americans appeared to handle the stresses better because of modifications in their training, some captives retreated into death (Kushner, 1973).

Recent research (Hall & Malone, 1976; Hunter, 1978) indicates that most returned POWs have difficulties in mental functions including time distortions and confusion, depressive symptoms, fears and anxieties, nightmares, **flashbacks** (reexperiencing past perceptions and emotions), and mood swings. Marital adjustment problems were quite prevalent, with the divorce rate for POWs at 26.9 percent two years after their return. While many of these problems were slowly resolved over several years, some difficulties may be long lasting.

Some studies indicate that some POWs feel that they have changed for the better during the POW experience. Schein, Cooley, and Singer (1960) found that 21 percent of American POWs in the Korean Conflict felt they benefited from learning to deal with the experience. More recently, Sledge, Boydstein, and Rabe (1980) found that over 61 percent of a large sample of American POWs released from Vietcong camps felt in retrospect that they had grown from coping with such adversity. Sledge and his colleagues sent structured questionnaires to 251 ex-POWs who were still on active duty and to 415 non-POW controls who were matched on variables such as age, type of combat duty, and military rank during combat. Ninety percent of both groups completed and returned the questionnaire. Twice as many POWs as non-POWs felt that they had subjectively benefited from their wartime experience. The POWs felt that the harshness of their experience changed their personal values, so that they could communicate better with others, had greater self-understanding, and more patience with others.

The findings of this survey focused on ex-POWs subjective evaluations and did not compare these subjective reports with the incidence of stress disorders in the subjects. The subjects may have experienced stress-related reactions in spite of their subjective evaluations. Furthermore, only POWs on active duty were surveyed. POWs who were no longer on active duty may have had quite different subjective evaluations of whether they had benefited from their POW experience. Extreme stress may lead to adjustment reactions and a new perspective about oneself. People may feel that they have grown through adversity, but still have problems adjusting after the stress.

Few experiences are more chronically stressful than existence in a POW camp. However, the Nazi concentration camps of World War II seem to have been even more stressful than the

POW camps. Over 6 million people (mainly Jews) were systematically tortured and killed in these camps.

Within the camps, reactions of apathy, withdrawal, and emotional repression were common (Chodoff, 1970). Many inmates refused to believe that friends and relatives who suddenly disappeared had been gassed and cremated; they denied that the smoke they saw was from the cremations. Bruno Bettelheim (1943, 1960) has described many disturbed inmate behaviors such as extreme regression, stealing, hoarding, and identification with the aggressors. A few inmates became "capos" and worked for the Nazis to gain favored status (see Highlight 5.2). The hopelessness and helplessness of the situation appears to have led many to give up or, at the other extreme, to almost complete psychological denial (Dimsdale, 1974). There were few opportunities to engage in socially responsible and personally useful tasks, behaviors which Rachman (1978) has suggested help people to cope with continued threat.

Among survivors, long-term emotional disability is common. Hoppe (1971) found that of 190 survivors of camps and other types of Nazi persecution, 70 percent had a chronic depressive reaction, 23 percent showed combined depression and aggression, and 2 percent had developed a schizophrenic reaction during the persecution. Mattusek (1971) found that many survivors displayed chronic adjustment reactions long after release from the camps. His findings suggest that all survivors have these symptoms, even when they do not report them. Berger (1977) has found additional symptoms of chronic guilt and self-loathing, inability to cope with anger, chronic depression, impoverished relations with others, and continued apathy—all of which may appear years later. He calls this the **survivor syndrome.**

Some death camp survivors seem to have no obvious symptomatology. They seemed over

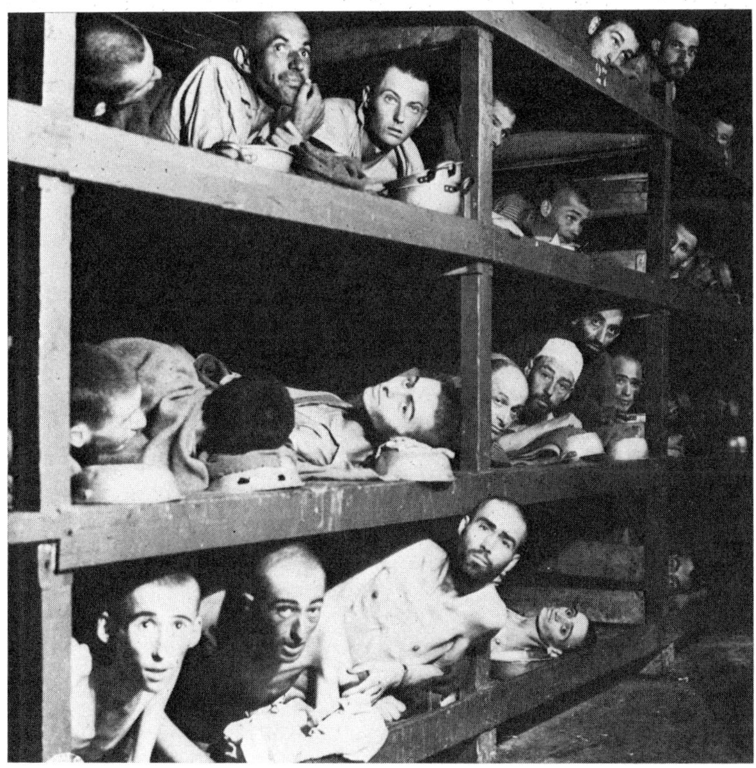

This photo shows prisoners of the Nazi concentration camp in Buchenwald, Germany, during World War II. Prisoners of such camps suffered extraordinary psychological and physical hardships. Many survivors have likely suffered chronic psychological reactions.

HIGHLIGHT 5.2
THE CONCENTRATION CAMP—WHAT WAS IT LIKE?

During 1938–1939, Bruno Bettelheim was held as a prisoner in both Dachau and Buchenwald, Nazi concentration camps. He was fortunate to obtain his release and escape to England. Three years later, he dealt with his feelings about his experience by writing an article for a professional journal about his observations as a psychiatrist/psychoanalyst while in the camp. Even at that point the article was as impersonal as possible, Bettelheim referring to himself in the third person as "he" rather than in the first person as "I," perhaps to continue to keep the horror at a distance.

After his arrest, he spent several days in prison, then was brought to camp. The following material has been adapted from his account, with the pronouns changed to the first person:

> I can vividly recall my extreme weariness resulting from a bayonet wound I received early in the course of transportation and from a heavy blow on the head. Both injuries led to the loss of a considerable amount of blood, and made me groggy. I wondered all the time that man can endure so much without committing suicide or going insane. . . . I have no doubt that I was able to endure the transportation, and all that followed [beatings, being stripped naked, laughed at, and ridiculed by guards], because right from the beginning I became convinced that these horrible and degrading experiences somehow did not happen to "me" as a subject but only to "me" as an object. . . . All the thoughts and emotions which I had during the transportation were extremely detached . . . with a conviction that "this cannot be true, such things just do not happen.". . .
>
> On a terribly cold winter night when a snowstorm was blowing, we were punished by being forced to stand at attention without overcoats—we never wore any—for hours. This after having worked for more than twelve hours in the open, and having received hardly any food. After more than 80 of us had died, and several hundred had their extremities so badly frozen that they had later to be amputated, we were permitted to return to the barracks. . . . The yearly mortality rate was close to 20 percent. [This was before the systematic killing of prisoners began!] This high death rate was mostly due to the large number of new prisoners [each year] who did not survive the first few weeks in the camp, either because they did not care to survive by means of adapting themselves to the life in camp or because they were unable to do so. . . . Old prisoners did not like to be reminded of their families and former friends. When they spoke about them, it was in a very detached way. . . . We were forced to soil ourselves. . . . In the camp, defecation . . . was strictly regulated. . . . It seemed to give pleasure to the guards to hold the power of granting or withholding the permission to visit the latrines. . . . We were forced to dig holes in the ground with our bare hands, even though tools were available. (Bettelheim, 1943).

Bettelheim goes on to describe many of the disturbed adjustments which prisoners made to the camp environment in order to survive. He was able to cope to some degree (although the setting had profound effects upon him) by focusing all his energy on remembering every detail, studying other prisoners, and planning how he would assess and describe the experience from a psychological perspective when released. In effect, he clung to his identity as a behavioral scientist creating a scientific task for himself, in order to retain as much of his identity and self-esteem as possible. These are activities which Rachman (1978) has identified as useful for dealing with such situations. Bettelheim's release preceded the ultimate horror of the Nazi extermination process, which they called the "Final Solution."

the years to have been able to recover from the stresses of the experience. For example, camp survivors who emigrated to Israel may have worked through many of their repressed feelings and experiences in the aggressive development of a new nation (Winick, 1968). More recent work suggests this is not so. Dor-Shav (1978) extensively studied 42 camp survivors and 20 controls in Israel. Using several psychological tests, she found that even the 42 survivors who had no obvious symptomatology 25 years after their internment still felt long-lasting effects. They were more limited in imagination, less creative, not open with others, aloof, had poorer emotional control, were more conservative, and took fewer risks than the matched controls. In addition, they were dependent on others for a sense of safety and security, but were less able to emotionally "connect" with others. Dor-Shav speculated that this detachment might be due to a fear of psychic hurt if the others disappeared from their life, a scenario very common in the death camps. The extreme threat and stress of life in the camps appears to have had universally negative lasting effects on all those who experienced it, no matter how good their coping ability before internment.

Less dramatically stressful imprisonment situations may have similar effects on human adjustment, which make the retrospective study and understanding of the concentration camps valuable. For example, Alexander Solzhenitsyn (1968) has described the fatalism and despair in Soviet labor camps for political prisoners. It remains to be seen what reactions develop in the 52 United States hostages held prisoner for 14 months from late 1979 to early 1981, first by Iranian militants and later by the new Iranian government. Preliminary accounts in the news media suggest that some hostages developed stress reactions in captivity, and some have had behavioral difficulties since their return to the United States.

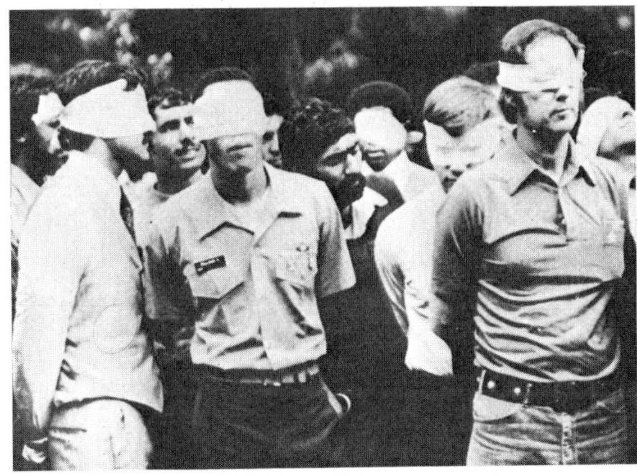

The Americans held hostage for 14 months in Iran were subject to both acute and chronic stress. It is likely that some will manifest stress reactions of lengthy duration.

ACUTE MAJOR DISASTER STATES

Short of war, perhaps the most objectively stressful experience may be that of a major natural disaster. Tornadoes, floods, earthquakes, hurricanes, and even volcanic eruptions are such threats. Additional disasters are related to human works: airplane crashes, train wrecks, explosions, fires, shipwrecks. Human disasters have been studied for quite some time. An early major study was conducted by Erich Lindemann (1944), who examined the surviving victims, and the relatives of the 492 dead, of the 1942 Cocoanut Grove night club fire in Boston. Half of the survivors required psychological treatment, and many family members had difficulty dealing with the sudden death of a loved one. Lindemann found, as have others, that some individuals *appear* to adjust remarkably well immediately after a major trauma, but manifestation of the adjustment reaction is only delayed:

> A girl of 17 lost both parents and her boy friend in the fire and was herself burned severely, with marked involvement of the lungs. Throughout her stay in the hospital her attitude was that of cheerful acceptance without any sign of . . . distress. When she was discharged at the end of three weeks she appeared cheerful, talked rapidly, with a considerable flow of ideas, seemed eager to return home and to assume the role of parent for her two younger siblings. Except for slight feelings of "lonesomeness," she complained of no distress.
>
> This period of griefless acceptance continued for the next two months, even when the household was dispersed and her younger siblings were placed in other homes. Not until the end of the tenth week did she begin to show a true state of grief with marked feelings of depression, intestinal emptiness, tightness in her throat, frequent crying, and vivid preoccupation with her deceased parents. (Lindemann, 1944, p. 144)

Unfortunately, there are no lack of disasters to study. Farberow (1977), for example, reviewed studies of 10 disasters occurring between 1971 and 1976. All these studies revealed that lasting adjustment problems related to the

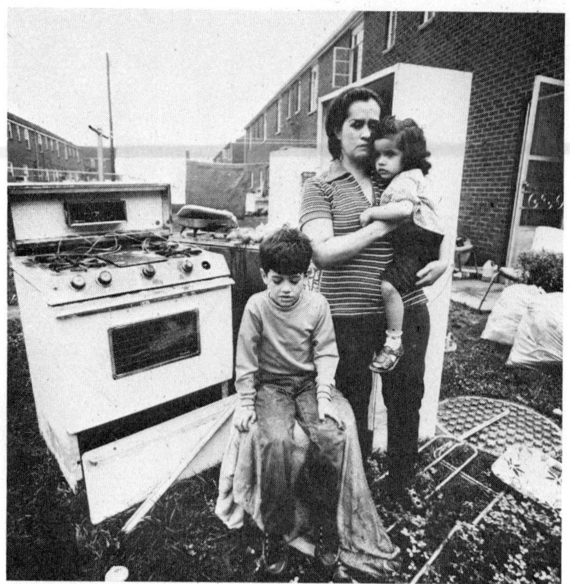

The mother and children in this photo were victims of a major flood. They appear depressed, withdrawn, and apathetic, all signs of crisis decompensation.

disaster experience were present in a large proportion of the people involved. Most research indicates that 45 to 55 percent of a group subjected to disaster stress will manifest symptoms of psychological or behavioral disturbance (Chamberlin, 1980). However, these percentages may be conservative. In a study of the aftermath of the Xenia, Ohio, tornado of April 3, 1974, Taylor (1976) found that only 9 percent of the survivors felt emotional distress immediately after the tornado. However, a large proportion of the victims developed problematic symptomatology at a later point (Figure 5.2). The 91 percent who felt no emotional distress immediately after the tornado may have, in fact, been emotionally "numb," a common reaction in disaster experiences.

Most disaster victims act neither heroically, nor do they panic. McDavid and Harari (1968) have pointed out that panic usually only occurs when: 1. a group is directly endangered; 2. escape is possible, but the escape route appears soon to be unavailable; 3. the group has no prearranged plan for dealing with the disaster. Friedman and Linn (1957), two psychiatrists present on a rescue ship immediately after the collision of two ocean liners (the *Andrea Doria* and the *Stockholm*) were able to observe the reactions of the survivors (52 were killed, 1600 rescued). They noted that there was little panic, but most survivors experienced temporary **emotional numbness.** As this numbness wore off, they became suggestible, passive, and their emotional range was constricted. Later, the survivors seemed to need to tell the story of their experience over and over, apparently to resolve the feelings they had repressed (see Highlight 5.3).

In February 1972, a dam broke in Buffalo Creek Valley, West Virginia, killing 125 people and leaving 4000 homeless. The wall of black water wiped away or severely damaged 14 mining towns. The stress of the destruction, escape from near death, and the death of friends and relatives had lasting effects. Titchner and Kapp (1976) studied 654 survivors of the disaster. They found that early symptoms included disorganization in thinking and decision making, and lack of emotional control, ranging from emotional outbursts to an inabil-

Figure 5.2 Percent of victims manifesting delayed symptomatology after Xenia, Ohio, Tornado.

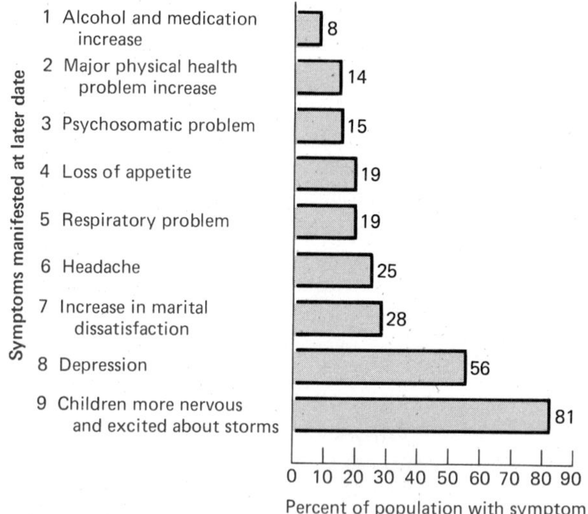

Based on Taylor (1976).

HIGHLIGHT 5.3
OBSERVATIONS ON THE SINKING OF THE ANDREA DORIA

Psychologically trained professionals have rarely been present at acute major disasters. They have usually arrived on the scene after the major events. However, on July 25, 1956, at 11:05 P.M., the liner *Stockholm* collided with the liner *Andrea Doria* off Nantucket Island, causing a major maritime disaster. Fifty-two people were killed, 1600 survived. Shortly after the crash, the liner *Ile de France* hove to at the scene to assist in the rescue of the *Doria's* passengers and crew. On board the *Ile de France* were two psychiatrists, Paul Friedman and Louis Linn (Friedman & Linn, 1957). They were able to interview, observe, and record the reactions of a large number of the survivors.

They noted that initially the survivors acted as if sedated. In other words, they appeared passive and compliant, their movements were slowed, they expressed little emotion (showed emotional numbness), and some showed mild amnesia. After this initial shock had worn off, the survivors could be interviewed, and many were willing to retell their experience almost compulsively, with identical details and emphasis. At this point, many of the survivors were angry that such an event should befall them, and blamed the crew of the *Andrea Doria* for carelessness and irresponsibility, even though the cause of the crash was unknown. Little panic had been apparent, possibly because of good leadership by some passengers who provided role models for others by taking charge and remaining calm (as did many of the crew).

Friedman and Linn noted that the "women and children first" principle had been followed, and caused serious dislocation and psychological trauma in many families. They also found that the lack of official lists of survivors promoted bewilderment: Several days passed before some families' members were reunited, with the subsequent escalation of fears that some had died.

ity to feel anything at all. Shortly afterward, almost all survivors experienced anxiety, grief, despair, severe sleep disturbances, and nightmares. Two years later, over 90 percent of the survivors still had significant symptoms of anxiety, depression, and character change. They were haunted by visions of the disaster and the related emotions of seeing blackened and torn bodies in the wreckage. Many had **survivor shame** about their behavior which had not met their own expectations during the crisis. Many attempted to "undo" the disaster through fantasy. They would relive the event in their minds with a more positive outcome, or fantasize heroic behavior.

How long may such reactions last? Leopold and Dillon (1963) studied 36 out of the 58 sailors who survived a sea collision involving a violent explosion and fire. They found that approximately four years later, only 12 of the men could bring themselves to return to shipboard work on a regular basis, and all who did felt anxious and fearful of a similar incident. All other survivors studied had major adjustment problems, some requiring hospitalization (see Table 5.1). Lifton (1969) found that 25 years after the atomic bombing of Hiroshima, the survivors still manifested major psychological disturbances. For many survivors, the disaster experience does not appear to be quickly forgotten; the emotional stress may be carried by them for years.

SUMMING UP

Whether an experience is stressful depends on two major factors: personal variables of the individual undergoing the experience and objective aspects of the environment. The more objectively stressful the environment, the less likely that personal vulnerabilities will be of major importance. Under extreme conditions of stress such as a concentration camp or major natural disaster virtually everyone experiences a stress reaction. However, even in these situations, personal vulnerabilities seem to influence the degree of disturbance.

Within the broad range of behavior called normal, there is a large variation in the degree

Table 5.1
Immediate and long-term psychological complaints of male survivors of a maritime disaster

	Percent with immediate symptoms (n = 36)	Percent with symptoms 3.5–4.5 years later (n = 34)
Mood and affect disturbance	72	96
Sleep disturbance	41	65
Somatic reactions		
Gastrointestinal	33	29
Other, mainly headache	30	30
Intellectual deficits	8	14
Sexual debility	0	17
Never returned to sea duty	N.A.	11
Returned to duty, but had to give it up because of symptoms	N.A.	45
Returned to sea duty sporadically or regularly, but had symptoms	N.A.	50
Psychiatric hospitalization		45

Based on Leopold and Dillon (1963).

of vulnerability to stress. Common events such as marriage, divorce, or leaving home are far less objectively stressful than armed combat, imprisonment, or the eruption of a volcano. Still, some individuals perceive these common crises as very stressful, and develop adjustment reactions. What characteristics do major stressors such as armed combat share with common events such as marriage or divorce?

From the perspective of the person experiencing stress, the event usually has at least these characteristics:

1. An important change in the environment.
2. Significant concerns about one's ability to handle the demands of the change.
3. The threat of psychological or physical pain or discomfort.
4. A sense of being unable to control important aspects of the change such as its duration or level of threat.

Some personal characteristics believed to result in defects in coping with the stress of common events have already been discussed. Once an individual develops a stress reaction, the immediate concern becomes one of resolving the behavioral disturbance. The next section discusses key treatments for stress reactions.

KEY TREATMENTS

The disturbed behaviors that occur as reactions to common stressors often disappear when the stress ceases to exist. When stresses are chronic or very severe, the disturbed behaviors may last for years. However, whether the stresses are chronic or short-term, the reactions to the stress may be subjectively so unpleasant that the individual seeks help in coping with either the stress or the reaction to the stress.

Crisis intervention

A typical treatment approach for adjustment reactions to common crises such as divorce, job loss, or school entry is **crisis intervention counseling.** The crisis counselor's role is to provide a setting where clients can ventilate feelings, discuss problems, examine their approaches to the problems, receive feedback, and obtain resources helpful in problem solution. At the very least, the goal of crisis intervention counseling is to return the individual to a level of adjustment equivalent to the person's functioning before the onset of the crisis. Effective crisis counseling may, however, allow the person to learn new ways of handling stress which result in an adjustment which is even stronger than the precrisis state (see Figure 5.1).

The pain of the crisis can act as a potent motivation for the individual to study him- or herself and to make changes in ongoing behavior. The crisis counseling setting provides the emotional support of the counselor for this difficult task. A major presumption of many crisis counseling theorists is that the presence of an understanding supportive listener is of major importance in the successful resolution of the crisis (Getz, Wiessen, Sue, & Ayers, 1974). Emotional support alone, however, probably is insufficient in enhancing the person's ability to deal with future crises. The crisis counselor must also directly teach the person (or assist in the learning of) new behaviors to facilitate dealing with future stresses.

Stress inoculation training

People who have difficulty coping with stress may engage in self-defeating thinking. They often think "It's too much to handle," "I'll never make it through this," "I'm falling apart," or "This is the worst thing that has ever happened to me." Donald Meichenbaum (1975) has developed an approach for training individuals to engage in cognitions (thoughts) which enhance their ability to deal with stress, called **stress inoculation training.** In this approach, the individual is trained to think positive cognitions which are "instructions" to cope in certain ways. For example, when preparing for a stressor the individual should think: "I can develop a plan to deal with it." A coping thought for confronting a stressor is "Don't think about fear, just about what I have to do"; "Stay relevant." A person who begins to feel overwhelmed may think, "Don't try to eliminate fear totally, just keep it manageable." Successful coping is followed by such self-reinforcing thoughts as "It worked, I was able to do it."

While practicing the self-instructional coping statements, the client also learns physical relaxation exercises which reduce many of the subjective experiences of anxiety. Once proficient at the relaxation exercises and the coping statements, the person practices the procedure under stress-provoking conditions with the supervision and guidance of the trainer. Stress inoculation training has been demonstrated to be an effective cognitive behavior modification technique, and is commonly used to enhance individuals' ability to cope with many types of stressful situations (Meichenbaum, 1977).

Treating combat reactions

Various treatment approaches have been utilized with men who have an adjustment reaction to combat. Among the best known is the use of hypnotism to treat combat stress–related amnesia, a technique frequently dramatized in Hollywood films. Treatment of combat adjustment reactions is usually much less dramatic than the use of hypnotism. Most cases respond to removal from battle for a short period of **supportive psychotherapy** which focuses on helping the person through the crisis, mild chemical sedation, food, and rest. A finding of major importance (Glass, 1955) is the impact of **expectancy.** If the expectation is maintained that the men will recover and return to their unit, the expectation will be fulfilled in approximately 65–75 percent of the cases. Most men will fulfil the expectation that they will get better. As Shatan (1978) has pointed out, however, others need long term psychotherapeutic assistance.

The Vietnam veteran. Estimates of the numbers of Vietnam veterans with delayed posttraumatic stress disorders vary, but a reasonable estimate is that 500,000 men in the United States are in this group. The treatment of Vietnam veterans is complicated by the fact that this war became very unpopular at home. Many veterans feel that a therapist who lacks firsthand experience of the conflict cannot really understand their dilemma. As a result, many therapy programs for these veterans use other veterans as therapists.

Williams (1980), a psychologist with Vietnam combat experience, describes four goals of psychotherapy with Vietnam veterans: 1. controlling anger, 2. reducing guilt, 3. expressing emotions, and 4. resocialization. Anger is a common problem. Many veterans are angry at society for rejecting them after they have "done their duty," angry at themselves for what they did in the war, and easily angered by day-to-day frustrations in civilian life. The men are often guilty about surviving when others have died, and may be guilty about their behavior in combat. The emotional numbing that occurred during combat must be broken in therapy by helping the veteran to become more aware of his feelings and more able to express them. A common problem is that veterans isolate themselves. In therapy they can begin to involve themselves in an emotional, verbal sharing process with another human being who knows from experience what the war was like. The therapist provides emotional support and can accept the client's feelings of guilt, anger, and isolation. In addition, the therapist provides a role model for new behavior, and may give homework assignments which involve the client trying out new forms of behavior.

Veterans are often treated in groups. In a group setting the veteran can share experiences and problems, and receive emotional support from group members in addition to the therapist. Often, the support of other members has more impact than the therapist alone. A therapist provides the following illustration of the impact of a group interchange on survivor guilt:

> Joe (who was a medic): I feel so bad about all the men that died in my chopper. I dream about them.
>
> Ted (an amputee with many other combat wounds): If it hadn't been for guys like you, I would have died. You must have saved a lot of guys' lives?
>
> Joe: Sure I did, but I haven't thought about that before.
>
> I [the therapist] had talked to Joe in individual counseling about looking at his experiences differently . . . but I simply did not have the impact on Joe that Ted had in group. [Joe] had been forgiven by a severely shot-up survivor. It was significant experience for both of them. That was the longest statement Ted had made in group in more than four months, and Joe cried, expressing immense relief. (Williams, 1980, pp. 38–39)

The clinical experience of therapists who work with veterans who have delayed or chronic posttraumatic stress reactions indicates that many problems can be resolved through these essentially verbal relationship therapies (Williams, 1980). However, these therapists are concerned that the posttraumatic stress syndrome is repetitive and cyclical. Many problems seem to resurface at a later date at a lower (but still uncomfortable) level of intensity. The resistant and chronic nature of delayed posttraumatic stress disorder is a phenomenon also seen in survivors of Nazi concentration camps.

Both Hoppe (1971) and Berger (1977) have attempted to treat the long-term results of Nazi persecution in death camp survivors. Berger has found a strong resistance in survivors to going back psychologically to work through the pain of these experiences. These investigators' work suggests that the reactions are very difficult to deal with because of the many years which have elapsed, and the magnitude of the trauma. Clinical experiences in the treatment of delayed combat stress reactions and the reactions to the stress of concentration camps suggest that early intervention is important for effective treatment of the disturbed behavior. The lessons learned from studying such experiences have led to an emphasis on rapid response to survivors of major stress experiences.

Treating survivors of major disasters

The treatment of survivors of major disasters such as earthquakes, floods, and major air crashes has many aspects. In natural disasters, many physical resources such as shelter and food must be provided immediately, and the immediate psychological shock experienced by individuals must be dealt with. Treatment must focus on reuniting families, encourage expression of feelings and experiences, encourage the reinstitution of routines, and involve the victims in the work of environmental reconstruction (Kafrissen, Heffron, & Zusman, 1975). The postdisaster symptoms require treatment focused on active recall and working through of painful memories primarily related to helplessness and loss (Titchner & Kapp, 1976). When a loved one has been killed in a disaster, a survivor may need psychotherapeutic assistance to work through the mourning process.

Like the combat veteran or concentration camp survivor, the survivors of a major disaster may be angry, guilty, or ashamed about their behavior during the disaster. Memories and emotions may be so painful that they are buried, pushed out of consciousness. A supportive psychotherapy setting is often necessary if the survivor is to regain awareness of these feelings and experience the relief of finally expressing them. The emotional support of a caring therapist may also aid individuals to return to the routine of making lives for themselves after working through the aftermath of the losses involved in the disaster.

Summary

1. Individuals with no obvious emotional disorder, who would be described as essentially normal, may develop behavioral disturbances under stress.

2. When stress is extreme and out of the ordinary, such as a major natural disaster or armed combat, a subsequent behavioral disturbance is called a posttraumatic stress disorder. When the stresses involve more common life situations such as marriage, death, or divorce, a subsequent behavioral disturbance is called an adjustment disorder.

3. The perception of an event as stressful depends both on the character of the event and on characteristics of the perceiver. Some people seem more vulnerable to perceiving common events as stressful than are others. Some events such as an earthquake or war are likely to be perceived as stressful by almost everyone.

4. People who cope well with stress usually are good problem solvers. They break the problem down into manageable pieces, anticipate the outcomes of their actions, practice their coping behaviors, and try to obtain as much information as possible. They engage in effective worrying. They avoid becoming preoccupied by things that they cannot control.

5. Individuals who are not effective at coping with stress may enter a crisis state; a short period of disequilibrium in a person who confronts a hazardous circumstance that for the moment cannot be escaped or solved. In the crisis state, behavior may become disorganized.

6. A number of common events may result in adjustment disorders if the individual perceives them as stressful and has insufficient coping skills. These events may include experiences which are often considered to be primarily positive such as marriage, vacations, and the birth of a child. Other events that may precipitate a stress reaction include job loss, divorce, ill health, retirement, and school transitions.

7. Armed combat has provided a laboratory for the study of posttraumatic stress disorders in three major wars. The reported incidence of immediate stress reactions decreased in the Vietnam war, but a high incidence of delayed reactions have appeared as Vietnam veterans have returned to civilian life.

8. The common symptoms seen in Vietnam veterans include depression, social isolation, rage, survival guilt, anxiety, sleep disturbances, intrusive thoughts, and the avoidance of feelings or emotional numbness.

9. Internment in POW or concentration camps has long lasting effects on survivors. The effects are generally negative, although some survivors of POW camps felt that they had grown stronger emotionally through the privation of the imprisonment. Survivors of concentration camps appear to have great difficulty putting their experiences behind them. Even those with a good superficial adjustment seem to have long-term negative effects from their wartime experiences.

10. Acute major disasters appear to have long-term effects on survivors. Most survivors will manifest a delayed reaction months after the experience. Common reactions include intrusive thoughts and vivid memories about the experience, depression, tension headaches, emotional numbness, sleep disturbances, and anxiety. Reactions to disaster experiences may last for years afterward.

11. Crisis intervention counseling consists of supportive verbal psychotherapy. Its goal is to assist individuals through stress-induced crises, and, at the least, help them regain a precrisis level of functioning.

12. Effective crisis counseling also focuses on teaching new stress coping skills. Within the emotionally supportive counseling session the client can focus on the problem, break it into manageable parts, and learn to deal with one part at a time.

13. Stress inoculation training is a procedure in which people are taught positive cognitions that prepare them to face stress. These cognitions are practiced in conjunction with a series of physical relaxation exercises, and are then implemented in stress-provoking settings under the guidance of the trainer.

14. Hypnotism is a dramatic treatment sometimes used with people who, when under combat stress, develop amnesia or psychologically caused paralysis.

15. Major stress reactions during combat are usually treated by removal from combat, short-term supportive psychotherapy, and mild chemical sedation. If it is expected that the individual will recover and return to combat, this outcome becomes more likely.

16. Veterans of Vietnam have a relatively high incidence of delayed stress reaction. Therapy with these veterans must take into account their feelings about having had to fight in an unpopular war. The goals of therapy with Vietnam veterans usually include: 1. controlling anger, 2. reducing guilt, 3. expressing emotions, and 4. resocialization.

17. Treatment of victims of major disasters focuses on dealing with feelings similar to those experienced by combat veterans and concentration camp survivors. Psychotherapy with survivors of disasters involves working through feelings of helplessness and loss, anger, and guilt. A caring therapist can facilitate the expression of buried painful feelings, and can help the survivor continue with the business of living.

KEY TERMS

Adjustment disorder. A disturbance of thinking, feeling, or behaving which is due to the effects of commonly encountered stressful events.

Autonomic nervous system. A section of the nervous system that influences the functions of visceral organs, endocrine glands, and cardiovascular activity. It is important in physiological reactions to stress.

Emotional numbness. A reaction to extremely stressful circumstances in which emotions are suppressed. The individual feels "wooden," as if there are no feelings.

Intrusive thoughts. Thoughts or memories that intrude into awareness despite the individual's attempts to avoid them.

Posttraumatic stress disorder. A disturbance in thinking, feeling, or behaving which is primarily due to the experience of an uncommon major stressor.

Psychosocial support system. A system composed of caring individuals, such as friends and family, who provide emotional support for an individual.

Ruminative thinking. Repetitious thoughts about an event or problem; "worrying."

Survival guilt, survivor syndrome, or survivor shame. These terms refer to a process in which survivors of a disaster or other major stress experience feel guilty or shameful about inappropriate behaviors which they manifested or about behaviors they feel they should have performed, but did not. This process is especially common when other people have died in the event. The survivors often feel they should have been the ones to die.

Uncomplicated bereavement. The normal expression of grief and mourning when a loved one dies. It is characterized by sadness and a sense of loss. Loss of self-esteem in the survivor is not part of this process.

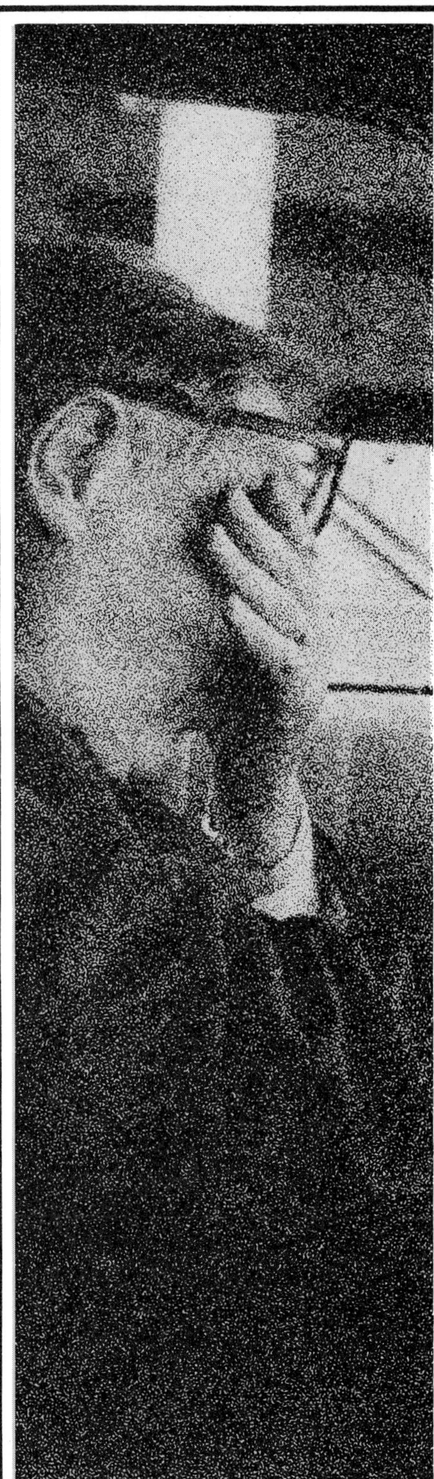

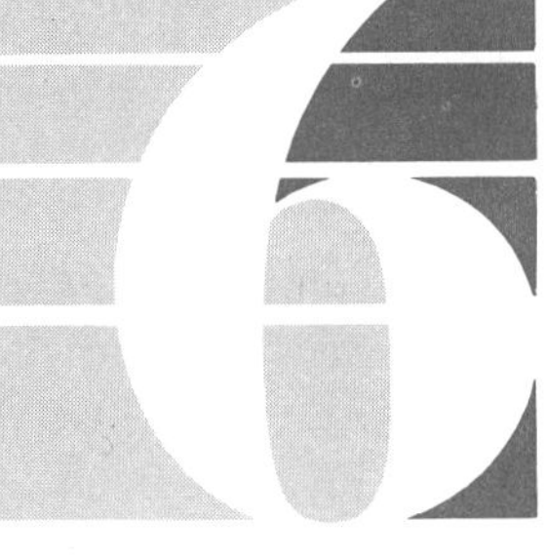

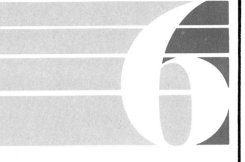

Disorders of psychophysiology

- Psychological factors affecting physical conditions
- Clinical patterns and DSM-III
- Common psychophysiological disorders
- Differential etiology: why he has ulcers and I have hypertension
- Key treatments
- Summary
- Key terms

In the previous chapter on reactions to major stressors, we saw that most individuals respond to extreme stress with psychological and behavioral disturbances. Emotions or stress can have a major impact on the physical as well as the psychological well-being of an individual. Most of us can identify some physical effects of intense emotion in our daily life—the churning feeling in our stomach when we are unprepared for a test, the heated flush of our cheeks when we are embarrassed, or the mild headache after a long and tension-filled day at work or home. Far beyond such commonplace emotional reactions are **psychophysiological disorders,** which are characterized by an actual physiological disturbance of an organ system, and direct or indirect involvement of psychological factors. In such disorders, physiological tissue damage occurs, as in peptic ulcer, or tissue change, as in the constriction of breathing passages in asthma. The symptoms of these disorders have traditionally been conceptualized as related to chronic autonomic nervous system arousal, and outside "conscious," or voluntary, control. In psychological reactions to major stress, the **autonomic nervous system** response is usually a factor in the fear or anxiety an individual experiences. In psychophysiological disorders, other types of emotions, such as anger, also seem to be important.

These disorders were called **psychosomatic disorders** by such early investigators as Helen Flanders Dunbar (1943) and Franz Alexander (1950). Unfortunately, this term came to be used incorrectly by most people to suggest that the symptoms or problems were "all in the head" and "not really a physical illness." This belief was particularly common in regard to disorders whose symptoms are not obviously physical, such as headaches, stomachaches, and muscular pain such as backaches. To avoid the negative meaning of "psychosomatic," the term "psychophysiological" was introduced. This term is quite popular among health care professionals, since more and more of them now believe that all physical illness has psychological components. Emotional and psychological factors appear to have pervasive effects on our general physical well-being.

PSYCHOLOGICAL FACTORS AFFECTING PHYSICAL CONDITIONS

The extreme extent to which psychological factors may affect one's physical condition is illustrated by documented cases of **voodoo death** (Cannon, 1957) and **sudden death** (Wendkos, 1979). Golden (1977) relates the following from his experience as a Peace Corps volunteer in West Africa:

> My landlady was fatally affected by such a curse. . . . For a year or so she had been suffering from severe and acute attacks of abdominal pains. She had had exploratory surgery performed by European doctors on three occasions with no positive result. Toward the end of my Peace Corps tour I noticed that she was losing weight and saw her less and less often in the marketplace. When she died, there was, uncharacteristically, no funeral celebration for her; she was buried on the outskirts of the cemetery. When I asked a friend of mine why, I was told that she had been cursed by the yehwe, one of the major cults in the village, because she had been an adulteress.
>
> For the curse to be successful, the victim has to be made aware that he or she has been cursed. Priests learn through divination ceremonies that gods or ancestors are angered due to the transgressions of a certain villager. It is not hard to imagine how in a small village the priests could obtain this knowledge in less than otherworldly ways. The priest's divination soon becomes common knowledge. The slightest suggestion is sufficient to cause tremendous fear in the victim. Tribal laws are rigid, and all members know them. The transgressor knows that there is nothing he or she can do to reverse or negate the curse. Death comes slowly but surely over a period of months.
>
> When the curse becomes known, the victim's family and friends as well as the entire community withdraw their support. The victim becomes an outsider to the few cohesive and organized activities of the village. He or she is thus no longer protected from the evil wishes of ancestors and witches.
>
> Feeling hopeless and helpless, the victim withdraws, thus furthering his or her isola-

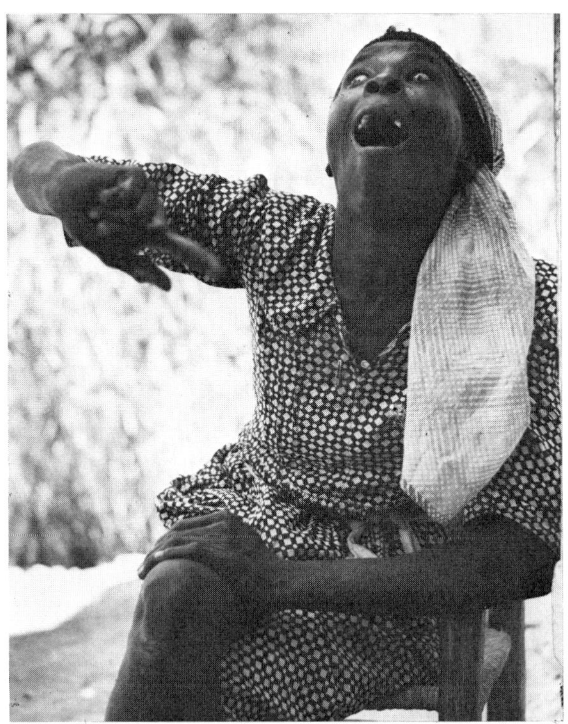

This Haitian woman believes she is possessed by a voodoo spirit. People who believe in curses may experience psychophysiological reactions and may even die, depending on the strength of their belief.

tion. Eating and drinking habits become irregular, and the victim settles into an increasingly lethargic state. Although the threat to life is not acute, the emotional strain of feeling hopeless is evident over an extended period of time. (p. 1426)

Although rare in countries such as the United States, voodoo death has many similarities to the phenomenon of sudden death. In sudden death, an individual dies suddenly, with no known prior fatal medical condition. For example, Engel (1971) describes the case of an apparently healthy 61-year-old woman who had accompanied her 71-year-old sister to an emergency room. The elder sister was pronounced dead on arrival. When given the news, the apparently healthy 61-year-old sister collapsed, developed irregular heart rhythms, and died.

Dimsdale (1977) has identified factors which may be implicated in such sudden deaths. In many cases there is overwhelming stress either from personal danger, or from situations of intense relief, triumph, or pleasure. This stress cannot be avoided, evokes intense emotions, and occurs in situations that the subject cannot control. Rahe and Romo (1974) studied 61 people in apparent good health who died suddenly. In the two years prior to death, the subjects had experienced a 250-percent increase in stressful life events and were found to have **coronary artery disease** (fatty deposits in the arteries). In other cases, hopelessness appears to be an important factor. Richter (1957) has demonstrated that a no-escape situation (being held in a human's hand) leads to death in some wild rats. He speculated that in these cases the heart slows down to such an extent that the beat becomes irregular, erratic, and finally stops because of disregulation by the **vagal nerve.** Wild animals and laboratory rats placed in extremely stressful circumstances often show destruction of heart muscle tissue (see Highlight 6.1).

Physiological processes may be disrupted by extreme stress and hopelessness. For example, cardiac rhythm and rate can be affected by even moderate emotional stress, with the rate often more than doubling under stress conditions (Moss & Wyner, 1970). A sudden death may be due to a stimulation of the vagal reflex and the release of adrenaline during an autonomic nervous system reaction. These events may result in death because the heart slows to the point of stopping, or speeds up dramatically to the point where the heartbeat becomes wildly irregular (Lown, 1980). Most cases of sudden death probably involve previous unknown heart disease or lowered physical resistance in the individual (a predisposition). It seems unlikely that a completely healthy individual would suffer sudden death; but sudden death does occur, and it may be a function of destabilization of a susceptible heart during an acute psychological disturbance (Wendkos, 1979).

The effects of the "mind" or emotion on the physical well-being of humans can be seen to be on a continuum from minor to major physiological impact (see Table 6.1). At one end are

HIGHLIGHT 6.1
COULD YOU BE SCARED TO DEATH?

The work of Dimsdale (1977), Engel (1971), and others on sudden death is reflected in the following *Reader's Digest* (News from the World of Medicine, 1980) note:

> Acute stress can provoke changes in the heart that may lead to death, say Drs. Marilyn S. Cebelin of Cleveland and Charles S. Hirsch of Cincinnati. The two doctors recently identified 15 cases in which people died after a physical assault, although the injuries alone would not have been enough to kill them. Eleven of the 15 cases showed a type of heart-cell death called myofibrillar degeneration, similar to a reaction in experimental animals who are helpless to anticipate or avoid danger. (p. 183)

the very dramatic examples of voodoo death and sudden death. Towards the center are the serious illnesses traditionally considered to be psychophysiological in origin. Still farther down the continuum are the other major "medical" disorders, which we now believe are affected by psychological processes. Toward the less extreme end of the continuum, we find "minor" illnesses and generalized physical states, such as feeling "lousy," "exhausted," or "tired," and the minor physical upsets that most humans have, such as minor aches and pains, occasional upset stomachs. Some investigators, such as Wright (1977), would go even further and include on this continuum the behavioral and psychological problems which occur subsequent to the development of a physical disorder. In effect, these would be "somatopsychic" disorders, such as the psychological reactions to diseases like cancer, cardiac disability, and paralysis. Such disorders can have devastating effects on an individual's psychological equilibrium, and can be a source of extreme stress in and of themselves. As D. T. Graham (1967) has aptly pointed out, psyche and soma cannot be treated in isolation from each other; each, alone, is incomplete.

In the classic formulation of psychophysiologic disorders, organ systems are considered to be adversely affected by the long-term physiologic response of the body to emotions or to the experience of stress. While some investigators have defined emotions as the *physiological* changes in the body (Lachman, 1972), it seems useful to include the individual's subjective perceptions in the definition. For example, since some of the physiological reactions of fear and anger are similar, the emotion experienced probably depends on the individual's evaluation of the circumstances in which the reaction of the autonomic nervous system occurs. Emotion may be considered an interpretation of both external and internal events.

Emotion and Autonomic Arousal

When an individual experiences an emotion, typical changes occur in the physiology of the body. Strong emotions are accompanied by autonomic nervous system arousal with far-reaching effects. Walter Cannon, a physiologist, regarded these changes as adaptive, since they are frequently seen during emergencies when the organism is threatened with injury or actually injured. In effect, the changes prepare the body for emergency action. This has been called the "fight-or-flight" response. The autonomic nervous system affects almost all of the body's internal functions. It is composed of

Table 6.1
A continuum of increasing physiological impact of psychological or emotional states

Generalized state of being: feeling lousy, tired, minor aches and pains	*Minor illness: colds, flu*	*Major "medical" disorders*	*Serious psychophysiological disorders: ulcers, asthma, etc.*	*Voodoo death and sudden death*
Minor physiological effects				Major physiological effects

two systems, the **sympathetic** and **parasympathetic,** which usually act in opposition to each other. The sympathetic acts to get the body ready for emergency. The parasympathetic acts to return the various systems to a balanced state.

Under conditions of stress or danger, the **sympathetic nervous system** is mobilized. A nervous impulse begins in the lower section of the **hypothalamus,** a part of the brain. The impulse descends the spinal cord and, about halfway down, leaves the cord at any of a number of junctions. The impulse then enters a bundle of nerve fibers called a sympathetic **ganglia,** which is connected to a whole series of these bundles. The impulse travels up and down this chain, exciting **neurons** (nerves) that connect with many organs. Several processes then occur (see Table 6.2 and Figure 6.1).

Epinephrine and norepinephrine, two **hormones,** are released from the adrenal glands into the bloodstream, resulting in a number of effects. Hormones are secreted by many different kinds of glands, and are biochemicals which have many effects on the body. Carbohydrates are released from the liver, providing immediate energy. Respiratory passages are dilated (increased in size), helping breathing. Red corpuscles increase in number, making more oxygen available to the muscles. A depression of the digestive processes occurs, and the blood is diverted to the **voluntary musculature,** muscles which control voluntary movement. Cardiac rate increases to enhance the blood flow, and blood clots more easily. The increased blood flow and perspiration enhances the body's release of heat generated by the increased use of energy. The body is now mobilized to fight or flee, and this arousal enhances the likelihood that all available energy reserves can be used to either combat the danger or get out of its way.

Once the danger has been resolved, the parasympathetic division reverses the emotional arousal and relaxes and calms the body. Parasympathetic impulses start from the upper part of the hypothalamus, travel down the spinal cord, and leave it either at the upper end or lower end. They, too, enter the chain of ganglia, travel up and down, and finally reach the same organs that the sympathetic impulses did (see Table 6.2 and Figure 6.1).

Table 6.2
Sympathetic and parasympathetic functions of the autonomic nervous system

Organ	*Sympathetic action*	*Parasympathetic action*
Eye pupils	Dilation	Constriction
Heart	Acceleration and dilation	Inhibition and constriction
Stomach and small intestine	Inhibition of secretion and of muscle action	Secretion and muscle action
Adrenal glands	Secretion	None
Colon	Inhibition	Increased tone
Rectum	Inhibition	Feces release
Bladder	Inhibition	Urine release
Genitals	Contraction of testicles (male) and vasoconstriction (female)	Erection (male) and vasodilation (female)
Liver	Sugar release	None
Sweat glands	Secretion	None
Hair	Erection	None
Blood vessels	Constriction (in skin and abdominal region)	Dilation
	Dilation (in heart and somewhat in voluntary muscles)	Constriction (in heart)

Adapted from Kleinmuntz (1974, p. 195).

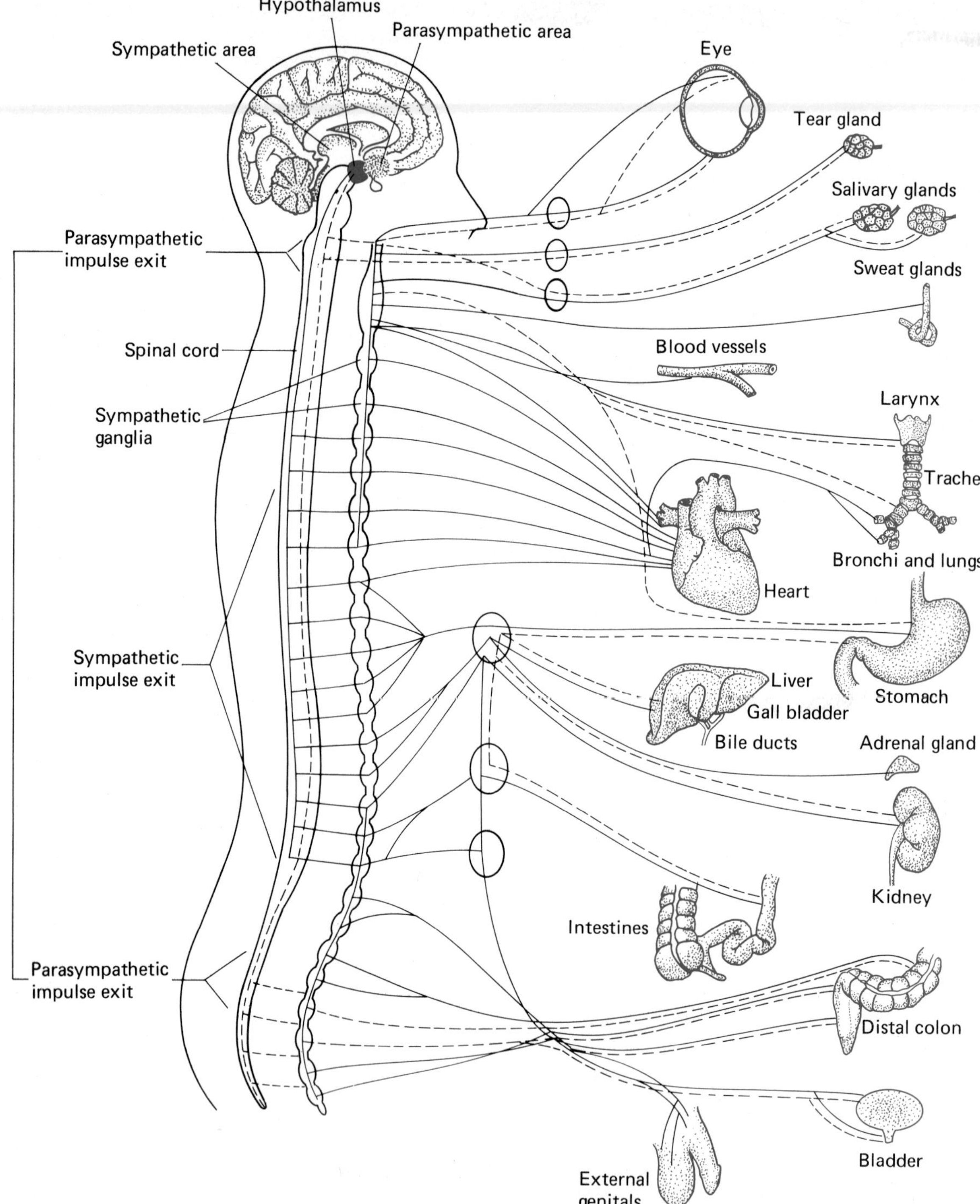

Figure 6.1. The autonomic nervous system and the organs it innervates.
Adapted from Krech, Crutchfield, Livson, and Krech (1976, p. 501).

The parasympathetic system acts to conserve and restore the resources of the body. For example, its action results in an increase in the diameter of skin and visceral (gut) blood vessels, and a lowering of heart rate. It promotes digestive action on food by an increase of salivary and gastric secretion; and the increased blood flow in the gut carries fuel to the other parts of the body, where it can be stored for later use. The parasympathetic system acts much more slowly than the sympathetic. That is why when one gets frightened, arousal occurs quickly, but it takes 20 to 30 minutes to become calm and relaxed after the danger has disappeared. Sometimes, however, the parasympathetic system may overreact during intense fear. (This overreaction may be the cause of fainting, and is also implicated in vagal, or sudden, deaths.) The organ systems affected by autonomic arousal are important in this chapter, since they all figure prominently in the classic psychophysiological disorders.

Stress and Life Events

As noted above, ANS (autonomic nervous system) reactions are prominent in situations of "stress." In Chapter 5 stress was defined in different ways. Selye (1976) defines stress as the psychophysiological response of the individual, mediated largely by the autonomic nervous system and a group of glands called the **endocrine system,** to any demand made upon him or her. Others have attempted to define stress in terms of the characteristics of events (Dohrenwend, 1973) and the individual's reactions to them (May & Sprague, 1976). The focus on stressful events has led to some highly interesting evidence and speculation on the impact of sociopsychological factors on physical health. Fontana et al. (1979) state in the boldest terms that "Extensive investigation has left little doubt that there is a significant relationship between the occurrence of a wide range of (stressful) events and a wide range of illnesses in people's lives."

Many studies have demonstrated that the greater the number of stressful events one experiences during a period of time, the more likely one is to develop a physical illness (Masuda, Lin, & Tazuma, 1980; Petrich & Holmes, 1977; Rahe, 1974). Such studies often define a stressful event as one that requires an energy expenditure—either psychological or physical—for adjustment. The relationship of life events to physical illness has led to an attempt to scale such events for level of stressfulness. Holmes and Rahe (1967) have developed one of the better known scales. They constructed a list of life change events and had a large number of subjects assign values to them, according to the intensity of stress and length of time needed for adjustment. Marriage was arbitrarily assigned a value of 500 by the researchers, and subjects rated other events in reference to this marker. The final scale was reduced numerically by a factor of 10, so that marriage was given 50 points and the scores for other events consist of the average of ratings given by subjects (see Table 6.3).

In a number of studies, Holmes and Rahe's scale and similar ones have demonstrated the relationship between life change events and a variety of illnesses. In a prospective study, for example, 2500 U.S. Navy officers and enlisted men were separated into high and low risk groups based on life change scores during the preceding six-month period (Rahe, Mahan, & Arthur, 1970). During the following six months at sea, the high risk group had almost 90 percent more illnesses than the low risk group. Obviously, such information could be quite important for use in illness prevention programs. If groups at high risk for medical disorders related to stress can be identified, then these individuals can be given special attention which may prevent or reduce the severity of illness.

The impressive evidence for the relationships between stress and disease has not gone unchallenged. Correlations between stressful events and disease in random populations are usually quite moderate, sometimes as low as .10 (Bowers & Kelly, 1979). The identification of events as intrinsically stressful is also problematic, since it tends to ignore the characteristics of the individual. Some individuals are psychologically better equipped than others to handle such events (Lazarus, 1974). In Chapter 5 we saw that psychosocial support systems are important in the degree of stress that is perceived (Cassel, 1976; Cobb, 1976). The presence of caring people, mutual relationships, a sense of self-esteem, and feeling loved, helps people deal with stress (Cassel, 1976; Cobb, 1976).

Table 6.3
Social readjustment scale

Rank	*Life event*	*Mean value*
1	Death of spouse	100
2	Divorce	73
3	Marital separation	65
4	Jail term	63
5	Death of close family member	63
6	Personal injury or illness	53
7	Marriage	50
8	Fired at work	47
9	Marital reconciliation	45
10	Retirement	45
11	Change in health of family member	44
12	Pregnancy	40
13	Sex difficulties	39
14	Gain of new family member	39
15	Business readjustment	39
16	Change in financial state	38
17	Death of close friend	37
18	Change to different line of work	36
19	Change in number of arguments with spouse	35
20	Mortgage over $10,000	31
21	Foreclosure of mortgage or loan	30
22	Change in responsibilities at work	29
23	Son or daughter leaving home	29
24	Trouble with in-laws	29
25	Outstanding personal achievement	28
26	Wife begins or stops work	26
27	Begin or end school	26
28	Change in living conditions	25
29	Revision of personal habits	24
30	Trouble with boss	23
31	Change in work hours or conditions	20
32	Change in residence	20
33	Change in schools	20
34	Change in recreation	19
35	Change in church activities	19
36	Change in social activities	18
37	Mortgage or loan less than $10,000	17
38	Change in sleeping habits	16
39	Change in number of family get-togethers	15
40	Change in eating habits	15
41	Vacation	13
42	Christmas	12
43	Minor violations of the law	11

From Holmes and Rahe (1967).

These psychosocial support systems are not measured by scales like the one in Table 6.3. Stress is not only a property of events but also includes the personal psychological and physiological characteristics of the individual experiencing the event: Individual differences in the perception of, and reaction to, stress are related to the development of the psychophysiological disorders.

In the section which follows, we will consider some distinct psychophysiological disorders and notions about their development. This will be followed by a consideration of the question of general etiology: Why do only some people react to stress by developing a major psychophysiological illness, and why that illness rather than another?

CLINICAL PATTERNS AND DSM-III

As pointed out, psychological and emotional factors and the perceived level of stressfulness impact on some individuals' physical well-being to the extent of being implicated in some types of sudden death, as well as colds, fevers, and general feelings of physical well-being. Evidence for this widespread impact is so convincing that DSM-III (1980) no longer lists the classic psychophysiological disorders. Some investigators believe that to list all of the psychophysiological illnesses would require a list of *all* physical illnesses! Rather than take such an unwieldy approach, DSM-III suggests that when psychological factors are suspected to be significant in the development or maintenance of a physical illness, a diagnosis of "Psychological Factors Affecting Physical Condition" should be made, and the relevant physical disorder then listed. However, the DSM-II (1968) classification approach to psychophysiological disorders remains useful as a focus for discussion. In this framework, psychophysiological disorders are characterized by physical symptoms in nine specific organ systems. The nine major organ systems are identified below, with examples of psychophysiological disorders:

1. Skin disorders: disorders such as neurodermatosis (inflammation), hyperhydrosis (dry skin), and eczema (severe flaking, scaling, and itching).

2. Musculoskeletal disorders: tension headaches, backaches, cramps, muscle spasms, and rheumatoid arthritis.
3. Respiratory disorders: bronchial asthma, sighing, hiccoughs, hyperventilation, sneezing, and coughing.
4. Cardiovascular disorders: tachycardia (rapid heart rate), hypertension (high blood pressure), migraine headaches, fainting, vagal depression of the heart rate.
5. Hemic and lymphatic disorders: disturbance in the blood or lymph system. Recent speculation suggests that leukemia, for example, may have a psychophysiological component.
6. Gastrointestinal disorder: peptic ulcer, chronic gastritis, ulcerative or mucous colitis, constipation, diarrhea, "heartburn," and hyperacidity.
7. Genito-urinary disorders: problems in menstruation (such as "cramps") or urination.
8. Endocrine disorders: malfunctions of the endocrine glands resulting in disorders such as hyperthyroidism and diabetes.
9. Disorders of special sense organs: glaucoma (increase in pressure within the eye) and disorders of the inner ear's semicircular canal (leading to problems in balance) are thought to be examples.

Here, a cautionary note must be inserted: While these disorders may be psychologically influenced in some or even a majority of individuals, it is possible that for others, psychological factors have only a small or nonexistent role in the genesis and development of the disorder. In some individuals, the cause of one of these diseases may be almost completely physical. We shall see that in most cases psychophysiological disorders are a result of an interaction between several factors, including **physiological predisposition,** psychological vulnerability, and environmental stressors.

COMMON PSYCHOPHYSIOLOGICAL DISORDERS

Ulcers, migraine and tension headaches, asthma, hypertension, and coronary heart disease are disorders which affect many people. With all these disorders, there is massive evidence for the impact of both nonorganic and organic etiological factors. These disorders are representative of the gastrointestinal (ulcers), cardiovascular (migraine, hypertension, and coronary heart disease), musculoskeletal (tension headache) and respiratory (asthma) systems.

Ulcer

Peptic ulcer is a syndrome characterized by the presence of an irritated area or actual hole in the lining of the stomach or the duodenum (the first 10 inches or so of the small intestine). This **lesion** is produced by the presence of an excess of hydrochloric acid (HCL). In the digestive process, HCL and enzymes (biochemical agents including pepsin and trypsin) break down food into components the body can use. Usually the inner wall of the digestive tract is protected from these **gastric acids** by a layer of mucus. The presence of excess gastric acids over long periods may lead to an erosion of areas of the protective mucus lining resulting in a crater-like wound of the intestinal wall. A primary symptom of such ulcers is abdominal pain. The pain has a uniform quality and location, tends to be rhythmical, disappears at times (especially after bland foods have been eaten), and tends to be chronic. Ulcers are often phasic in character, "flaring up" in times of stress.

In terms of overall incidence, it has been commonly reported that 1 out of 10 people will have an ulcer at some time. The relative incidence of ulcers in males and females has varied interestingly over time. Gove and Tudor (1973) report that 80 years ago, 12 women had ulcers for every ulcered male. Today men with ulcers outnumber women by approximately two or three to one, but the incidence of ulcers in women appears to be on the rise.

The following case described by Rosen, Fox, and Gregory (1972) illustrates the development of a peptic ulcer. It demonstrates how other behaviors in the life of an affected individual can complicate a psychophysiological disorder. In this case, the complicating behavior is the excessive use of alcohol, a particularly damaging habit for individuals who have a gastrointestinal disorder.

> The patient was the fourth of five boys. His father was an unsuccessful farmer whom the patient had disliked from an early age on and never respected. His mother, to whom he felt

much closer, was nervous, frail, and had numerous bodily complaints. . . . Nevertheless, she criticized and dominated her husband and nagged her sons into striving for the success that their father had never achieved.

Poverty and a small physical stature contributed to making the patient feel inferior to other children, but he compensated by striving for academic achievement. . . . He completed college and two years of law school in evening classes. In World War II he rose from private to captain. At the age of 24 he married and subsequently became the father of three children.

He was as ambitious and hard driving in his career as he had been in school and in the Army. He began to work for a large company at the age of 21 and over the ensuing 25 years rose to a senior executive position. He felt personally responsible for much of the company's growth and expansion. . . . For 15 years [he] never took a vacation with his family. But after reaching a high position he began to feel that his talents—which were considerable but which he undoubtedly overvalued—and his dedication were neither appreciated nor adequately rewarded. His future seemed bleak, with little opportunity for future advancement financially or in prestige. Every morning he felt sick over the prospect of another day's exhausting demands and inadequate rewards. However, he did not express his feelings of frustration and resentment while at work but became increasingly irritable at home. He also began to drink and smoke very heavily. At this point, he developed stomach ulcers. Sedative medication reduced his pain but he continued to drink and become increasingly depressed. . . . He became extremely unreliable on the job, often failing to keep business appointments, and finally was dropped by the company for alcoholism and unreliability.

Shortly thereafter he was referred to psychiatric treatment. He was angry, tense, tremulous, and depressed. As a consequence of losing his position, he was confronted with the necessity of reevaluating his goals and patterns of behavior. He was treated in psychotherapy and by minor tranquilizers and his tension and depression diminished. Being an intelligent man, he was able to acquire insight rapidly, his compulsive ambition decreased, he cut down on smoking and drinking, and his ulcer symptoms receded. He took a less demanding position with another company and during a two year follow-up period there was no recurrence of the ulcers. . . . (Rosen et al., 1972, pp. 176–177)

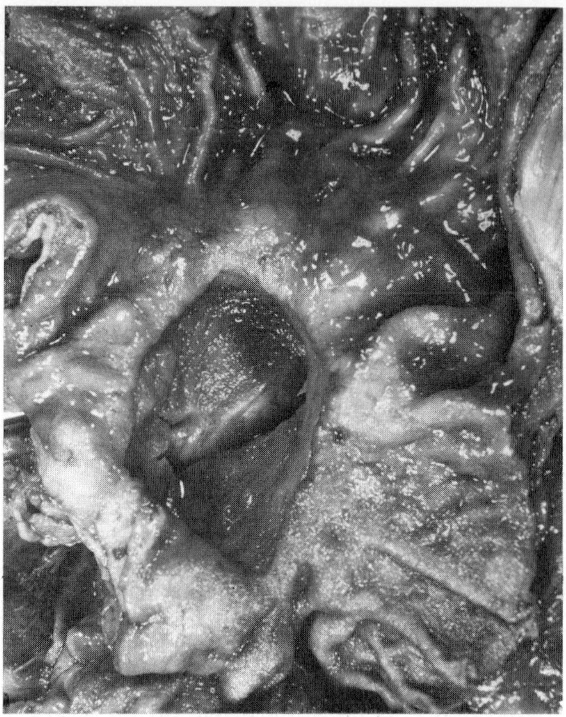
Human stomach with an ulcerated intestinal lining.

Causal Factors in Ulcers. Specific etiological factors have been identified for peptic ulcers. Individual physiological predispositions are clearly important. Mirsky (1958) has demonstrated that marked individual differences in **pepsinogen** levels exist even at birth (pepsinogen breaks down into the digestive enzyme pepsin). The importance of this finding is reinforced by a study of 2073 Army draftees (Weiner et al, 1957), which identified 63 men with the highest levels of pepsinogen and 57 with the lowest levels. All 2073 men had been given a complete physical, including intestinal X-rays, and were administered a series of projective personality tests. Four of the high-level pepsinogen men had ulcers at the start of the study, and by the end of Army basic training, 5 more men in this group were found to have developed ulcers. None of the low level secreters had ulcers at the beginning of the study, and none developed them during basic training. The data suggest that a biological predisposition towards high pepsinogen levels is an important factor in the development of ulcers under stress. Evaluation of the psychological data revealed that high level secreters who developed ulcers manifested major unresolved persistent conflicts about dependency, gratification, and hostility, which they could not express. The psychological profiles, when separated into two groups to predict high and low secreters, correlated highly (85 percent) with the physiological data.

The data from this study are fairly consistent with the psychoanalytic theory of Franz Alexander (1950), who proposed that frustration of dependency needs is important in the development of ulcers. Other factors also appear to be important. Conflict, for example, has been found to lead to the development of ulcers in some laboratory animals. When such animals are allowed to avoid an unpleasant situation, ulcers are less likely to develop than when the situation is unavoidable (Weiss, 1971). In general, the research suggests that individuals who develop peptic ulcers are likely to meet three criteria: 1. a biological predisposition towards high levels of pepsinogen secretion, which may be inherited; 2. the experience of a stressful life situation, and 3. the likelihood of unmet dependency needs or an anger-oriented reaction to stress. Although peptic ulcer is one of the best understood of the psychophysiological disorders, these conclusions remain tentative, especially those regarding the issue of dependency needs and unexpressed anger.

Asthma

Asthma is a disorder of the respiratory system which affects an estimated 2–5 percent of the population. Males are more frequently asthmatic than females by about two to one, and approximately 60 percent of asthmatics are under age 17. Bronchial asthmatic symptoms include shortness of breath, gasping, coughing, and wheezing caused by a narrowing of the airways of the lungs as a result of spasms of the bronchial muscles, swelling of the airway walls from an increase in cellular fluid, the secretion of excessive mucus; or collapse of the airway walls as a result of forced respiration. While inhalation and exhalation are both hampered, the primary restriction is during exhalation. Repeated attacks may result in reduced lung capacity and lung elasticity and, at times, chest deformity.

An asthma attack typically begins suddenly, with the subsequent symptoms lasting from less than an hour to several hours and, on rare occasion, days. The suddenness of the attack and the significant interference in the vital function of breathing often result in major subjective psychological reactions, especially in children. Significant panic or terror reactions, fatigue and exhaustion, and irritability are often associated with the attacks (Kinsman et al., 1974).

Causal Factors in Asthma. As in peptic ulcers, several factors are involved in the development of an asthmatic disorder, and at least one study indicates that psychological factors are unimportant in 30 percent of the cases. In this study, Rees (1964) examined 441 asthmatics and found psychological factors to be dominant in 37 percent of the cases, and secondary in 33 percent. Infective factors were the dominant cause in 38 percent of the cases, and allergic factors were dominant in 23 percent of the cases. These percentages cannot be considered exact representations, since they are based on only one study, but they do indicate that asthma has multiple causes. In a majority of cases, the initial precipitant of respiratory problems is apparently an infection or series of infections of the respiratory system, or the development of an allergic response. But even in most of these cases, psychological factors later become important. Thus, the data support a biological predisposition towards respiratory weakness (see Table 6.4).

Recent research in **immunology** has suggested that asthma may be due to a malfunction of the immunological system of the body (Frick, 1976; Hamburger, 1976). In this situation, strong emotions may act to block the sympathetic nervous system, ultimately leading to the release of biochemicals (histamines) that constrict the lung passages. The impact of emotions on asthma is well documented. Kleeman (1967) in a study of 26 asthmatics, found that almost 70 percent of their asthma attacks were

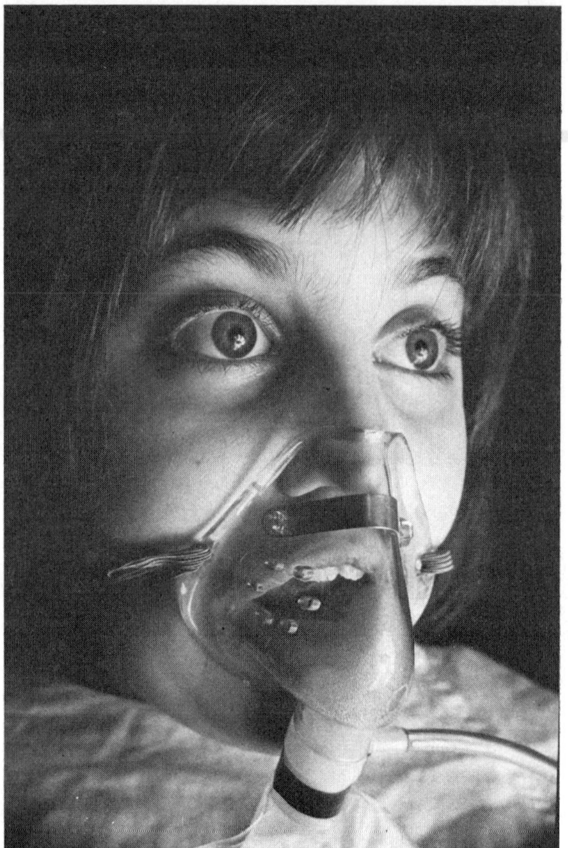

Some people with asthma need to use special devices to assist in respiration.

precipitated by a strong emotional reaction. Asthmatics' expectations also seem important. Philipps (1970) demonstrated that when asthmatics who were inhaling a neutral solution believed that this would cause breathing difficulties, they manifested asthmatic responses. When they believed they were inhaling a neutral solution (in fact, an airway spasm-inducing drug), they reacted with less intensity than they ordinarily would. The effects of suggestion and expectations were confirmed in a study by Luparello and colleagues (1971), in which 19 of 40 asthmatic patients responded with significant airway obstruction to a **placebo** (neutral) mist which they believed contained air pollutants. Of the 19, 12 had full asthma attacks. The airway obstruction decreased when the 19 thought they had received a drug that

Table 6.4
Percent contribution of allergic, infective, and psychological factors in asthma for 441 cases

Relative importance	*Factors*		
	Allergic	Infective	Psychological
Dominant	23	38	37
Subsidiary	13	30	33
Unimportant	64	32	30
Total	100	100	100

From Rees (1964).

would cause an increase in the airway. In fact, they had only received an inert substance. However, over 50 percent of the group of 40 asthmatics did not respond to the expectation effect. For these "nonreactors," asthma appeared to be exclusively a physiological problem.

The degree to which asthmatic responses may be learned, for example, through classical conditioning, remains unresolved. Some studies (Dekker & Groen, 1956; Turnbull, 1962) support such a conclusion. Other studies (Dekker, Pelser, & Groen, 1957) indicate that learning is a secondary factor. Recent work with biofeedback equipment suggests that autonomic reactions to stimuli do generalize (Stoyva, 1976) and, in this sense, one might learn to respond to certain stimuli with an asthmatic attack. For example, Lachman (1972) notes a case in which a patient who had asthmatic attacks regularly when exposed to roses also displayed an attack when confronted with an artificial rose. One simple way of viewing this example is to consider that the subject has learned through many repeated trials that rose pollen precipitates allergy attacks. The attacks are emotionally stressful. Confrontation with the artificial rose results in a strong emotional response—possibly fear or anxiety. The expectation of an attack and the reaction of fear or anxiety, then, may lead to the actual symptoms of asthma. However, in the absence of predisposing physiological factors and experience of previous asthmatic responses, it is unlikely that asthma attacks could be easily conditioned.

Studies have indicated that family interactions may be psychological causal factors in the development of asthma. They certainly contribute to the maintenance of asthmatic behavior in many cases, particularly in children. In a well-known study, Purcell et al. (1969) identified two groups of asthmatic children: group A, whose attacks were precipitated by emotional reactions; group B, whose attacks were not emotionally induced. After a four-week selection and preparation period, the parents and siblings were moved to a motel for two weeks, while the 26 asthmatic children stayed in their homes with mother substitutes. While the asthmatic children continued to be exposed to their normal physical environment, measures were taken of peak respiratory flow, degree of wheezing, daily medication, and frequency and intensity of asthmatic attacks. While separated from family, group A improved on all variables, while group B improved only on frequency of attack, and the improvement was not as great as for group A. When the families were reunited with their children, the asthmatic symptoms began to return to previous levels. The fact that symptoms improved in these children when family members were absent strongly suggests that the family members' behaviors precipitated asthmatic attacks or made the attacks worse once they had started. One factor which might account for this finding is the possibility that stressful relationships between parents (such as heated arguments) might emotionally upset the asthmatic child and induce an attack. Another possibility, which seems very probable, is the development of a situation in which the child receives unanticipated and subtle rewards for behaving asthmatically. Being sick (having asthma) may obtain "reinforcement" for the child, such as more parental attention, special privileges, avoidance of school, and special toys.

The recognition that the sick role can be reinforcing for a child (or for an adult) has led to the common treatment recommendation that asthmatic children be treated no different at home than healthy siblings. Parents are told to avoid overprotection and special consideration. A more positive approach is to react to the patient as having the potential to lead a normal existence. This does not imply the complete withdrawal of concern and support by family members. In fact, the absence of familial and social support appears to have an impact on the medication level required in the treatment of asthma. De Araujo et al., (1973) have found that under high stress, asthmatics with low familial/social support required over three times as much steroid medication to obtain equivalent levels of relief as those with high familial/social support. For asthmatics under low stress, the difference in required steroid medication was not significant between high support and low support groups (see Table 6.5).

Tension and Migraine Headaches

Although often lumped together in casual conversation, tension and migraine headaches are primarily disorders of two different organ systems. Tension headache is a disorder of the musculoskeletal system, while migraine is a disorder of the **cardiovascular system,** which is composed of the heart, arteries, and veins (see Figure 6.2).

The incidence of headache is astounding. There are an estimated 20 million migraine sufferers and 100 million tension headache sufferers in the United States (Budzynski, 1979). In the clinical headache population (those who seek treatment), Appenzeller (1973) found that migraines were the identified problem for 15–20 percent of the group. The most frequent type of headache is due to tension, and migraine is the second most common form, but other types of headaches also occur. These less frequent types of headache may be caused by tumors in the brain, increased **intracranial pressure** (pressure in the skull), intracranial infections; or the pain may be "referred" from other organic sites such as the eyes, teeth, ears, or neck. Treatment of these problems may be ignored if the headache is assumed to be from tension or migraine, and serious life-threatening consequences may ensue. Fortu-

Table 6.5

Relationship between stress (life change events), level of available social support, and steroid dosage (in milligrams) for asthmatic patients

		Stress (life change events)	
		HIGH	LOW
Level of social support	High	5.6	5.0
	Low	19.6	6.7

Based on de Araujo et al. (1973).

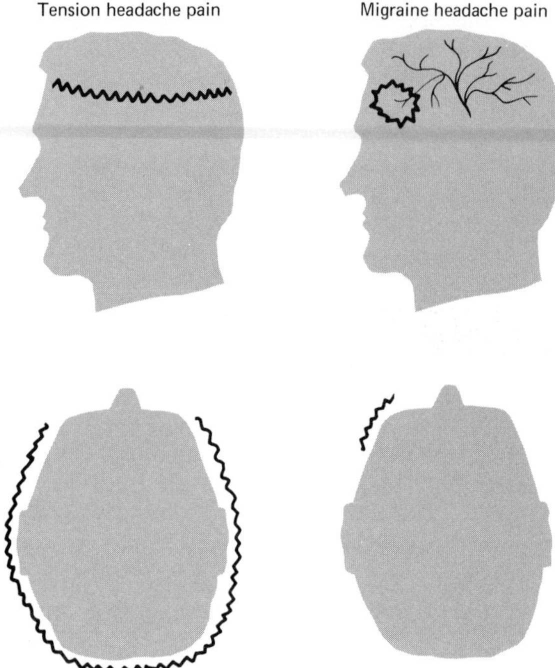

Figure 6.2. Tension and migraine pain. Tension headache pain is usually manifested as a painful band encircling the head, while migraine is often localized on one side in the area of the cranial arteries.

nately, as indicated, these other causes of headache are relatively infrequent.

Tension Headache. The common tension headache is a dull pain, usually encircling the head, although some sufferers report it to be localized on one side. It is commonly described as feeling that one's head is being compressed by a circular vise. Duration varies from a few hours to (rarely) a few months. Martin (1972), along with many others, has described the tension headache as a muscle contraction headache. This type of pain appears to be due to periodic intense contraction of face, scalp, neck, and shoulder muscles. Studies of neural action of the muscles of the head have provided strong support for this concept (Haynes et al., 1975). The chronic tension of the voluntary musculature which produces the pain symptoms is considered to be a function of emotional stress. The pain is due to vasoconstriction (constriction of the arteries, veins, and capillaries) caused by the contraction of the muscles surrounding the skull. Studies have indicated that during a tension headache there is a reduction in blood supply. Even when free of pain, tension headache patients are more vasoconstricted than normals; this indicates the possibility of a generalized higher resting tension level (a physiological predisposition), which can be accentuated by stress (Tunis & Wolff, 1954).

Tension headaches are typically untreated, with the sufferer self-prescribing a pain reducer such as aspirin. If the pain is serious enough, formal treatment is usually sought from a physician, who provides muscle relaxant drugs or pain-reducing sedatives. In recent years, however, psychological relaxation approaches and biofeedback treatment of tension headache, have gained popularity, to some extent because of their demonstrated effectiveness (Budzynski, 1979; Fuller, 1978).

Migraine. Migraine is an intensely painful headache usually localized on one side of the head over the region of the temple or to the rear of the eye. At times the migraine pain may generalize to involve an area similar to the tension headache. The "classic" migraine includes an **aura** which precedes the actual pain by a

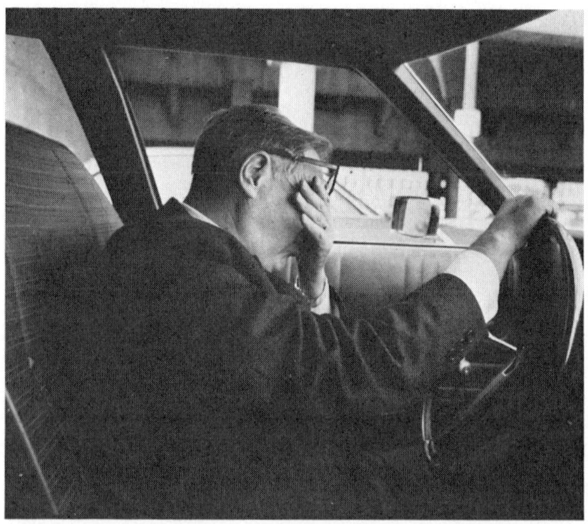

Headaches are a common psychophysiological disorder. Their pain can be incapacitating.

few minutes to three-quarters of an hour. The aura may consist of visual disturbances ("scotoma," such as bright flashes, geometric forms), tingling feelings, or numbness; these sometimes extend into the headache period. The term "common migraine" is used when the aura is not present. A third type of migraine is the "cluster migraine," characterized by sharp stabbing pains which occur in multiple episodes. Some individuals who have migraine have other symptoms besides pain. The pain often throbs in synchronization with the pulsing of the cranial arteries, nausea is often present, facial skin may be come tender and flushed or appear white and "drained" of blood, and the face and scalp tissue may swell. Some persons may suffer dizziness, fever or blurring of vision, excessive perspiration, and vomiting.

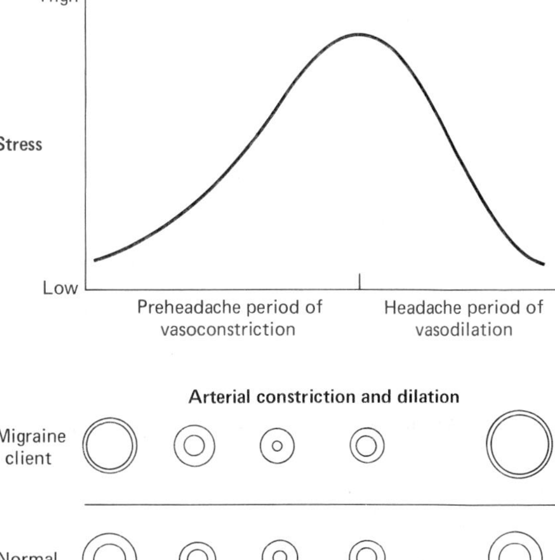

Figure 6.3. Stress and arterial constriction and dilation in migraine patients and normals.
Adapted from Budzynski, (1979).

Causal factors in migraine. Migraine headaches appear to be primarily due to the effects of changes in the vascular system, particularly in the cranial arteries. Budzynski (1979) describes a commonly accepted model which proposes that the experience of stress in migraine sufferers leads to vasoconstriction of the cranial arteries. The reduction of stress results in a relaxation of these arteries, which rebound into an excessively dilated state. At the point of excessive **vasodilation,** the intense migraine pain is experienced (see Figure 6.3). This explanation has received substantial support by investigators such as J. R. Graham and Wolff (1938) and Sokolov (1963).

There appears to be an inherited physiological predisposition in migraine (Refsum, 1968). Even when not in pain, migraine sufferers exhibit larger temporal artery pulsations than normals, have abnormal vasodilation responses, and show consistent differences in blood flow between the side of the head affected by pain and the side not affected (Bakal, 1975). A great deal of research evidence indicates that when individuals are unable to cope with perceived frustration and aggression, they develop temporarily increased blood pressure (Price, 1974). This fact may combine with a genetic predisposition to hypersensitive cranial blood vessels to produce a migraine sufferer. In addition, R. B. Williams (1977) has found typical migraine sufferers to be highly organized and perfectionists who need to be in control of events which affect them. For such individuals, life change events can be particularly frustrating.

The following case description (Vetter, 1972) illustrates the symptomatology and family history of migraine which are often seen.

> Severe headaches were a common occurrence in our family. Among my earliest memories are recollections of my sister and me tiptoeing around a darkened house while my mother lay moaning on the sofa with a damp cloth over her eyes. She had an inexhaustible supply of stories, which she told with grisly relish and a wealth of details, about others in her family who also suffered from migraine, including her mother, elder brother, and several cousins and aunts. . . .
>
> I have often been told that I take after my mother, although I strongly resented the suggestion and could never detect the resemblance. The only feature I ever felt we had in common was our inability to express our feelings—especially to one another. My sister, who is three years younger than me, is just the opposite. When she got upset as a child, the whole neighborhood knew it. . . .

> Although I had suffered from severe headaches since I was in high school, the first real migraine I can remember hit me while I was in college. It happened in the gym where several hundred of us were having an American history final. The pain was on the left side and it was incredibly violent, like nothing I had ever felt before. . . . I became nauseous and began to throw up. I had chills, perspired heavily, there was severe sinus pain, and I experienced scotomas for the first time, which scared me silly. This attack lasted for two days, including spasms of nausea and retching. Since that time, the attacks have occurred at intervals of about three weeks to a month. . . . (p. 153)

Essential Hypertension

Extensive evidence demonstrates that many normal individuals have significantly increased blood pressure when experiencing emotional responses (Benson, 1975). However, when a prolonged condition exists in which there is intermittent or chronically elevated blood pressure, which is not secondary to other disorders such as kidney disease, **renal** artery disease, obesity, or use of drugs, the disorder is called **essential hypertension.** An estimated 10–15 percent of the United States population has some degree of essential hypertension (Benson, 1975; Byassee, 1977). The problem may even be greater: Nelson (1973), in a survey of three middle-class Los Angeles neighborhoods, found that over 30 percent of the adults examined had high blood pressure. For reasons unknown, black Americans have twice the incidence of hypertension as whites (Kaplan, 1974). Suspected contributors to this difference include environmental stress (e.g., inner-city life), dietary differences, and possible genetic factors. Current evidence favors the conclusion that blacks inherit a genetic predisposition to the development of essential hypertension (Warren & O'Connor, 1980). The renal system of blacks seems to produce less of a vasodilator called kallikrein than do whites, and this may lead to an increased likelihood of hypertension in blacks.

Few symptoms of essential hypertension are apparent to the subject until the disorder is well established (Lyght, 1966). That is unfortunate, since if started in the early stages, appropriate treatment can have substantial impact on the disease. Subjective symptoms which sometimes occur include feelings of weakness, dizziness, nervousness, and fatigue. There also may be heart palpitations, insomnia, and headaches. If not treated or if unsuccessfully treated, chronic hypertension results in death, on the average, after 20 years. The actual cause of death is a stroke, heart attack, or other disease which is a function of the essential hypertension.

Causal Factors in Essential Hypertension. The reaction of the cardiovascular system to stress has been well established. In calm, the heartbeat is regular and slow, blood pressure is low. Under stress, the blood vessels of the **visceral organs** (like the stomach) constrict and divert blood to the skeletal muscles in the fight-or-flight response, which has been discussed before. The constriction of the visceral arteries forces the heart to work harder, as do other changes wrought by the sympathetic nervous system and the endocrine system, leading to an acute increase in blood pressure. This acute elevation of blood pressure subsides when the parasympathetic system is activated. Chronic elevation of blood pressure may be partly due to a predisposition to greater vascular reactivity when the autonomic nervous system is activated by stress, or to a generalized chronic hyperactivity of the sympathetic division of the ANS and a resulting increase in blood pressure.

The importance of stress in essential hypertension is well known. Many individuals who have hypertension seem to experience life as chronically stressful. The relationship of stress to hypertension has been shown in studies like that of Cobb and Rose (1973), who found that air traffic controllers (a notoriously high stress occupation) had six times the incidence of hypertension as a control group, and that the disease developed earlier in controllers working at high density (high stress) airports (such as New York's LaGuardia and Chicago's O'Hare airports) (see Table 6.6). In this study, the incidence of other psychophysiological disorders was also higher in the controllers' group. Life stresses other than occupation can also have effects on blood pressure; in fact, Kasl and Cobb

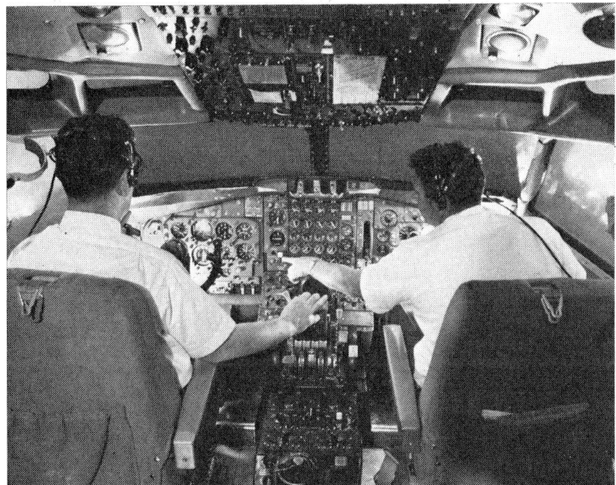

Some occupations involve tremendous pressures and responsibilities. Stress is virtually a built-in feature. Occupational stress, however, is only one possible factor in the development of a psychophysiological disorder.

(1970) found that job loss leads to increased levels of blood pressure. (One would presume that an air traffic controller who was fired would be particularly at risk!)

In addition to the factors of stress and a physiological predisposition to react hypertensively, investigators have considered personality variables in the development of this disorder. Franz Alexander (1950), for example, suggested that undischarged hostile impulses create a chronic emotional state leading to essential hypertension. The hostile impulses are due to unresolved unconscious conflicts. Little sound evidence supports the idea that unconscious conflicts are a primary factor in hypertension, but recent work provides some support for the importance of undischarged hostility or aggression in the development of essential hypertension.

David McClelland (1979) has suggested that the issue in hypertension is inhibited power motivation. In a major study, he found that individuals who have: 1. a strong need for power, 2. a tendency to inhibit expression of this need for power when it is manifested as aggression, and who 3. face strong situational challenges, are very likely to develop hypertension even when predisposing physiological factors are not present. In this study of 78 males, who were examined and followed up every 5 years for 20 years, the researchers were able to predict blood pressure at age 50 or 51 from an assessment of power needs on the TAT projective test given while the men were in college. McClelland's study is quite persuasive, in spite of the possibility that other uncontrolled factors have influenced his sample during the 20-year period.

Coronary Heart Disease

Coronary heart disease (CHD) is a major cause of death in the United States. One major form is called myocardial infarction (MI). In this disorder, oxygenation of heart muscle tissue is reduced below what is required, and portions of the heart muscle die. Myocardial infarction is commonly called a "heart attack." The reduction in oxygenation of the heart tissue is due to

Table 6.6

Annual incidence rates of hypertension per 1000 subjects in two samples: air traffic controllers and control group; air traffic controllers in high stress and low stress settings

Age group	*Controllers/control group*		*Controllers' stress*	
	CONTROLLERS (n = 4325)	CONTROLS (n = 8435)	HIGH (n = UNREPORTED)	LOW (n = UNREPORTED)
20–24	0	0	0	0
25–29	2	1	4	0
30–34	2	1	6	2
35–39	10	1	12	10
40–44	6	0	26	4
45–49	11	4	51	32
50+	15	4	0	36

a reduction in blood flow from blockage of the blood vessels to the heart muscle. The blockage is frequently due to deposits of fatty tissue or blood clots (coronary thrombosis). Another form of CHD is angina pectoris. In this disorder, the reduced blood supply is less serious than in MI, but people with angina pectoris have an obviously increased risk of an MI. In angina the pains are sharp and stabbing; they are located in the chest and may travel into the left shoulder and arm. In an MI, the pain is even more severe and long lasting.

Etiology of Coronary Heart Disease. A number of factors have been identified as increasing the risk of coronary heart disease: aging, sex (being male), elevated levels of fatty substances in the blood, hypertension, heavy cigarette smoking, family history of heart disease, obesity, and physical inactivity (Glass, Contrada, & Snow, 1980). Obviously, many of these factors are behavioral: eating foods high in fatty substances, smoking heavily, overeating, and living a sedentary existence. In addition, clinicians and researchers have discovered that coronary heart disease is often associated with a particular life-style, now labeled **Type A behavior** (see Highlight 6.2).

Type A behavior is described as an action-emotion complex in which people struggle to achieve more and more in less and less time (Friedman & Rosenman, 1974). Type A people are achievement oriented, competitive, time urgent, and hostile, but they keep feelings of hostility deeply under cover. Type As are re-

HIGHLIGHT 6.2
TYPE A BEHAVIOR AND SELF-CHANGE

The difficulty of changing one's health-threatening behavior is well known. Even though smoking, drinking, and overeating can cause health problems, these habits are very difficult to modify. Most physicians report that it is often quite difficult to get their patients to complete the treatment regime prescribed. Even people well aware of the dangers of certain behaviors may find them hard to change.

> Stan Crawford was a well-known psychologist, professor, and author. Like many successful professionals, he had personal characteristics which met the criteria of a Type A personality. He was an energetic, dynamic man. In his forties he was the picture of a "man on the go." He was chairperson of a psychology department, an active member of his church, coauthor or author of a half-dozen journal articles and two books, and organizer of a psychological assessment and treatment center. He smoked a pack and a half of cigarettes a day, ate and drank more heavily than he should, but by age 50 still seemed tireless. At that time he was warned by his physician that both his blood pressure and his blood cholesterol were approaching dangerously high levels.
>
> In his early fifties Stan suffered a massive coronary occlusion (blockage) and nearly died. After recovery he quit smoking, watched his diet, and exercised regularly. However, he could not slow down his hectic professional life. He was still directing graduate student research, organizing workshops, editing and writing, going on lecture tours, and working in a busy consulting practice. In spite of repeated warnings from his physician, family, and friends, he was as overcommitted as ever. Stan seemed determined to live his life in the fashion he had grown used to, even if it killed him. A few weeks after returning from a national convention he suffered a fatal cardiac seizure. (based on McCall, 1975, pp. 496–497).

Stan Crawford found it impossible to significantly change his life-style, even though he was well aware of the danger of coronary heart disease. Changing Type A behavior appears to be a difficult task. Clinicians and researchers are, however, beginning to look for ways to modify this behavior (Glass et al., 1980). The National Heart, Lung and Blood Institute is currently engaged in a five-year study of 600 Type A individuals with coronary heart disease. The approach being used to treat this group involves small group sessions, role playing, and behavioral practice in which individuals are learning behaviors which should reduce their overinvestment in hectic work schedules, their impatience, and their emotional overarousal in uncontrollable stress situations.

ported to be twice as likely to develop heart disease as Type Bs (those who do not have the identified behavior pattern of Type A). In one study, 3000 men were followed up for 8½ years. The group was split into 1500 Type As and 1500 Type Bs. The study provided strong support for a relationship between Type A behavior and heart disease. It also found that other factors such as smoking rate and elevated **serum cholesterol** (fatty compounds in the blood) could not account for the differential in disease rate (Rosenman, Friedman, & Strauss, 1964). The Type A individuals had *twice* the incidence of CHD as those who did not manifest Type A behavior (Rosenman et al., 1964). A second MI was five times as likely in Type As as in Type Bs when both had had one previous heart attack.

What mechanisms might connect Type A behavior with coronary heart disease? Recent research indicates that when under stress (especially stress that the individual perceives is outside of his or her control) Type As have higher levels of epinephrine and norepinephrine in their blood than do Type Bs. (High levels of norepinephrine and epinephrine indicate ANS arousal). Some investigators believe that these high levels of norepinephrine and epinephrine can result in damage to arterial walls and an increased likelihood of blood clots and fatty tissue deposits. The high levels of these substances are also associated with increased blood pressure. Glass (1977) suggests that the cumulative negative effects of an excessive rise and subsequent fall of epinephrine and norepinephrine in Type As, who must contend with what they perceive to be uncontrollable stress, lead to an increased risk of CHD. His hypothesis makes sense and is currently being tested (Glass et al., 1980).

The evidence for the association of Type A behavior with CHD is impressive. We need to remember, however, that most Type A individuals do not develop CHD, and that some Type Bs do. An individual's development of coronary heart disease is most likely the result of a combination of many factors including genetic physiological predisposition, type of behavior (A or B), presence or absence of high risk behaviors such as smoking or overeating, and the degree of stress encountered.

DIFFERENTIAL ETIOLOGY: WHY HE HAS ULCERS AND I HAVE HYPERTENSION

Organic Concepts

So far, we have noted the likelihood of physiological predispositions in the etiology of the psychophysiological disorders. Such predispositions may be a result of a variety of factors. As Lacey (1967) has pointed out, there are early differences in autonomic reactivity in newborn infants. We have seen that differences in physiology exist between, for example, ulcer victims and normals, and hypertensives and normals. These differences could conceivably be the result of genetic influences. The sensitivity of specific organ systems to stress may also be a result of prior damage, as in the development of ulcers in a heavy drinker. In asthma, for example, many sufferers have had previous respiratory diseases, which may damage lung tissue and make it more susceptibile to irritants. The possibility that individuals develop a particular type of disorder depending upon which organ system is most responsive to ANS activity is now quite widely accepted (Claridge, 1973).

Organ system specificity may also be related to the concept of the **general adaptation syndrome** (GAS) in the development of specific psychophysiological disorders. The GAS refers to a three-stage response to stress first identified by Hans Selye (1976), a Canadian physiologist. He noted that the initial symptoms of almost any disease appear very similar; after studying these symptoms, he concluded that the body reacts in three stages to any prolonged stress: 1. alarm, 2. resistance, and 3. exhaustion. In the alarm reaction, the body mobilizes its resources (the autonomic nervous system's sympathetic action) to cope with the stress. After the body becomes stabilized (possibly by the action of the parasympathetic system), the alarm reaction disappears; but this adjustment is costly in terms of energy reserves. If the stress continues, a stage of exhaustion is reached, when stress hormones are depleted and the body may develop a psychophysiological disorder, organ failure, or a collapse of an organ system that is physiologically predisposed to weakness.

Recent work has implicated the body's immunological system in the development of a number of disorders (Weiner, 1977). This system acts to defend the body against infectious and other foreign bodies. When functioning adequately, it will attack and destroy foreign invaders. However, when it malfunctions, several errors are possible: it can be hyperreactive, underreactive, or misguided (Bowers & Kelly, 1979). Examples of each of these errors in order are bronchial asthma (the body overreacts to respiratory irritants), cancer (the body does not react to kill cancer cells), and **rheumatoid arthritis** (the body attacks itself). The immunological system has been shown to be sensitive to the activity of the autonomic nervous system. For example, in stress-provoked allergic responses, the body produces immunological substances which result in the inflammation of body tissue (Frick, 1976). People who are depressed show lowered efficiency of the cells (T-cells) that usually destroy cancerous cells (Bartop et al., 1977). Some hormones released in the ANS response to stress are believed to upset the general functioning of the autoimmune system, which could lead to an increased risk of disease (Reiser, 1975). The relationship of the immunological system to psychophysiological diseases remains speculative. Further research in this area may discover specific individual immunological reactions to stress which lead to specific diseases.

Psychological Factors

The work of Alexander (1950) and Dunbar (1943) has been influential for many years. In the psychoanalytic framework, the specific disorder is seen as a symbolic manifestation of underlying unconscious conflicts. Alexander, for example, proposed that an underlying frustration of dependency needs during the oral stage of development was the issue in ulcer development. An ulcer results from the individual's constant preparedness to take in and digest food, which is a symbol of the need for satisfaction of the dependency. This preparedness leads to a constant flow of digestive juices, which digest the intestinal wall. Little empirical support for Alexander's theories exists. While unconscious conflicts and neurotic personality styles do not have sufficient research support, enduring personality traits may influence the development of specific psychophysiological disorders.

Earlier, we saw that McClelland (1979) has demonstrated a relationship between power needs and hypertension. The idea that specific personality factors are related to certain diseases is valuable, particularly when one considers traits rather than personality per se. Since Grace and Graham (1952) first focused on the relationship of attitudes and emotions to type of illness, many researchers have been studying this concept. D. T. Graham (1972) suggests that *specific attitudes* are related to certain psychophysiological changes which result in specific diseases. In interviews of 128 patients, Grace and Graham (1952) found clearly defined enduring attitudes (traits) that apparently did relate to particular changes in physiology:

1. Asthma: When facing a difficult situation, the individual wants to make it go away, blot it out, ignore it.
2. Duodenal ulcer: The individual is revenge seeking.
3. Arterial hypertension: The individual feels he must be constantly prepared to meet all possible threats.
4. Cold, moist hands: The individual feels she should undertake some sort of activity, even though she does not know what to do. In Raynaud's disease, in which lowered blood circulation in the hands leads to painful coldness, the attitude is one of a desire for hostile action, which is not acted upon.

Some experimental studies have provided support for the specific attitude theory, while others have not (D. T. Graham, Stern, & Winoker, 1958; Peters & Stern, 1971). Although these specific attitudes (Grace & Graham, 1952) may not be supportable, the issue of personality trait variables is still an open one, as McClelland's (1979) study has demonstrated. For example, recent research has suggested that in Raynaud's disease the trait of alienation is a significant factor (Surwit et al., 1979). Perhaps further research will provide more conclusive data.

Behavioral Theories

Can a specific psychophysiological disorder be learned? Sheldon Lachman thinks so. He does not deny the importance of physiological predisposition or of stress. In addition to the concept that autonomic responsivity can be modified through learning, Lachman (1972) proposes five learning processes which can lead to the development of specific symptomatology:

1. The role of stimulus-substitution learning. . . . Stimuli originally incapable of eliciting a response but closely associated in time with effective emotion-provoking stimuli may themselves, sooner or later, come to be effective in producing emotional reactions. For example, [while it is raining a child is frightened by several lightning bolts and loud thunder. On subsequent occasions, even gentle rain may lead to a reaction of fear, in the absence of thunder and lightning. The stimulus of rain has substituted for the original stimuli of lightning and thunder, and can now elicit the emotion of fear and its associated autonomic reactions.]
2. The role of emotional reintegration. A single component in the stimulus-situation earlier associated with a complex pattern of emotional reactions (i.e., physiological responses) may itself be effective in producing the total complex pattern of emotional reactions. A boy, while fishing on a bridge [fell] 30 feet into the ice cold water, was swept down a rocky rapids, and almost was drowned. Now the sight of that bridge or river or of people fishing or of the rocky rapids serves to revive vividly all of the complex stimulus situation and emotional reactions associated with the earlier event.
3. The role of stimulus generalization. An internal response that has been associated with a particular stimulus may come to be elicited by a variety of somewhat similar stimuli, that is, stimuli somewhat like the originally learned stimulus but varying along one continuum or another. Such stimuli become capable of eliciting an internal response—an emotional reaction or aspect thereof—that they did not elicit prior to learning. [Swimming may evoke the emotional reaction that the boy felt after falling in the icy water, in item 2 above.]
4. The role of symbolic stimuli. Stimuli that in the personal history of the individual represent effective emotion-provoking stimuli, may themselves become emotion-provoking. At the human level, such symbolic stimuli (or stimulus symbols) are frequently but not always language stimuli. [The word "rape" may provoke strong emotional reactions in a woman who has been sexually assaulted.]
5. The role of ideation. Organismic effects of stimuli, probably largely in terms of central nervous system manifestations, may persist in the form of "central percepts," "thoughts," or "ideas" (i.e., neural images or cognitive symbols) that can be revived in the absence of the originally relevant external stimulus situation, to produce a characteristic implicit emotional-reaction constellation. [An individual may think about an emotional event (being criticized by an employer) and may feel the associated emotion (anxiety).] (pp. 66–67)

Lachman suggests processes through which one may learn to manifest chronic ANS arousal. However, the issue of the specificity of a person's disorder (e.g., hypertension vs. migraine) is left by his theory to physiological predisposing factors such as genetic inheritance. Evidence that one differentially learns to be hypertensive rather than migrainous is lacking.

Diathesis/Stress

The theories proposed to explain both the general and specific etiology of psychophysiological disorders enable us to draw some conclusions. Obviously, there is a great deal of agreement on the necessity for some physiological predisposition towards an organ system weakness. The weakness may be due either to genetic transmission or to organ damage over time. Secondly, stress is clearly implicated as a serious contributing factor to the ongoing physical condition of the human body in disorders ranging from simply "feeling bad" to major illness.

The issue of personality variables is less clear. Evidence both supports and denies their impact. Perhaps we have not yet asked the right questions in this regard, but the work of McClelland and others seems promising. Finally, the impact of learning on symptom formation has some support, but needs further research. The specificity of psychophysiological disease appears to be a function of the organism operating as an interactive system—with physiological predispositions, levels of perceived threat, and psychological factors all impacting on the individual's life adjustment. A specific psychophysiological disorder is due to a **diathesis** (a physiological or psychological predisposition) which is influenced by the level of stress that the individual encounters. Given enough stress and a strong enough diathesis, the individual is likely to develop a psychophysiological disorder. We will see that the approaches to treatment of the psychophysiological disorders reflect these concepts of the development of the disorders.

KEY TREATMENTS

Varied approaches are used to treat the psychophysiological disorders, either alone or conjointly. Some focus on changing the psychosocial environment to reduce stress, some on changing the stress reaction or building coping abilities, and others on intervening in the sequence of events leading to disease (Warnes, 1979). However, the medical approach remains the most commonly utilized. Most individuals who suffer from a psychophysiological disorder receive medical treatment, but rarely seek out or are referred to individuals trained to deal with the nonphysiological aspects of the disorder. Many reasons exist for this state of affairs.

Medical approaches

A major reason why medical approaches are so common is that many psychophysiologically disordered patients have difficulty accepting that their disease is causally related to psychological processes. They reject the notion that the disorder is "all (or even partly) in the head." Some appear to focus almost exclusively on the physicalness of their symptoms in an attempt to defend against psychological insight (O'Connor, 1970). Sifneos (1973) in a study of 25 psychophysiologically disordered patients and 25 normal controls found that the patients' characteristics would not tend to make them interested in psychological approaches: little fantasy life, constricted emotional functioning, inability to verbalize feelings, and a lack of interest and ability in self-examination. A compounding problem is that many medical practitioners feel they can handle the disorder without the collaboration of psychologists or psychiatrists (Wolff, 1965). Many physicians, in fact, feel that such collaboration is useless. Since the obvious symptoms of the psychophysiological disorders are physical, the patient rarely gets beyond symptomatic alleviation through **pharmacological treatment** or surgical techniques, and encouragement by the physician to "take it easy," "avoid stress," or "find a hobby." The common somatic treatments for several psychophysiological disorders are given below (based on Lachman, 1972, pp. 173–174):

> **1.** Peptic ulcer: Rest. Typically bland diet involving milk as the basis and several daily feedings of easily digested, palatable, nonirritating foods. Multivitamin capsules. Medication to minimize stomach acids and intestinal spasms. Blood transfusion for bleeding ulcers. . . .
> **2.** Essential hypertension: Administration of drugs which lower blood pressure. If obese, weight reduction may be desirable. Short-term periods of rest advised. Multivitamin tablets. Diet with restriction of salt; rice emphasized in a special diet that restricts elements which raise blood pressure. . . .
> **3.** Bronchial asthma: Many drugs may relieve asthma symptoms—ephedrine and epinephrine are two examples.

While criticism of the medical approach as being psychologically naive is well founded, some progress has occurred in recent years with the advent and popularization of behavioral medicine. Particularly in the major medical centers, one is more likely to find an approach to the treatment of specific psychophysiological disorders, and to the treatment of "physical" disease in general, which takes into account human physiology *and* psychology.

Psychodynamic approaches

Psychotherapy of the psychoanalytic or supportive type has had mixed results with people suffering from psychophysiological disorders. Kellner (1975), in a survey of controlled studies, concluded that psychotherapeutic approaches are effective for some patients with some disorders. For example, peptic ulcer, asthma, and migraine appear to be more amenable to such treatment than do hypertension and ulcerative colitis. However, he points out that few of these studies have been replicated, and the evidence remains tentative. Karasu (1979) confirms that many studies have demonstrated the difficulty of applying psychotherapeutic approaches to these disorders, and suggests that the success of the approach may be enhanced if the patients are properly prepared for psychotherapy. He proposes as the first phase of this preparation the *health alliance,* in which the therapist becomes an extension of the physician in the medical treatment of the disorder, and builds trust in the patient by being supportive. The second phase is the *life alliance,* in which the prospective therapist becomes a "trustworthy, reliable, benign 'friend-parent.'" In this stage the early phases of therapy begin. These phases, says Karasu, may take a year or two before formal analytical therapy begins. Obviously, one major disadvantage of this approach is its length. Since analytic therapy may take 3–5 years, this approach from beginning to end may involve 4–7 years of treatment.

Hypnosis has been reported to be an effective treatment technique for some individuals. Bowers and Kelly (1979) have examined some disorders and the impact of hypnotic treatment on them. A major point which they make is that the characteristics of the person, rather than the type of disease, are important in determining the usefulness of the techniques. They indicate that high hypnotic ability in the subject is predictive of successful use of hypnosis in the treatment of psychophysiological disorder, while low hypnotic ability is not. A review of the application of hypnosis to the treatment of skin disorder, headache, and asthma, however, indicates that the evidence that hypnosis can directly influence autonomic nervous systems functioning, even in people who can be deeply hypnotized, remains equivocal (de Piano & Saltzberg, 1979).

Behavioral approaches

Since the early 1960s behavior therapy has frequently been applied to psychophysiological disorders. In a survey of treatment approaches, Price (1974) reports that a wide variety of specific behavioral techniques have been used to change behavior which influences the course of psychophysiological disorders. The techniques have been used to modify the environmental contingencies which seem to maintain symptoms, to directly inhibit a supposedly pathological autonomic nervous system, and to modify behaviors that increase the risk of illness (e.g., smoking cigarettes). The successful application of behavioral techniques to physical illness has led to the development of a new specialty called **behavioral medicine.**

The impact of a behavioral approach on a psychophysiological disorder is illustrated in the following case study in which the therapists used an *operant behavioral* technique to reduce the degree of symptomatology in an asthmatic child.

> Patient was a seven-year-old boy who had suffered from asthma from the age of six months. Prior to treatment he suffered from frequent attacks which did not appear to be managed well by medication and dieting restrictions. His most intense coughing and wheezing occurred at bedtime, when attacks would often last over an hour (as measured during baseline). Nighttime responding was therefore chosen as the target behavior for therapy.
>
> The parents were requested to discontinue all attention and medication during bedtime asthmatic attacks. Once the bedroom door was closed, no parent-child interaction was to occur until morning. Additionally, the parents were to give the boy lunch money—as he preferred, (rather than having him take his lunch to school) if he coughed less frequently on a given night than the night before. . . . Neisworth and Moore (the therapists) found that the combined extinction and reinforcement treatment program dramatically reduced bedtime attacks to about five minutes [per night]. An eleven month followup indicated that bedtime attacks had been reduced to 2–7 minutes and that daytime coughing had also declined sharply. (Price, 1974, pp. 139–140)

The pure operant approach makes no assumptions about any impact on the physiological functioning of the body. In contrast, **biofeedback** is a technique which assumes a direct impact on the autonomic nervous system. The use of biofeedback with psychophysiological disorders has grown tremendously in recent years. Fuller (1978) defines biofeedback as the "use of instrumentation to mirror psychophysiological processes of which the individual is not normally aware and which may [then] be brought under voluntary control." Commonly instrumented feedback includes muscle tension levels, skin temperature, brain-wave activity, heart rate, and blood pressure. Fuller describes biofeedback as an established major new therapeutic approach. Others are not so optimistic about the degree of confidence to be placed in biofeedback as an established approach (Budzynski, 1979; Engel, 1979; Turk, Meichenbaum, & Berman, 1979), although they believe it has great promise. Schwartz (1973) has pointed out that the basic research in biofeedback is well controlled and methodologically sound. However, much of the clinical research focused primarily on the single case design without control groups. Since Schwartz's article some progress in clinical research has occurred, although further work must be done before we can really accept biofeedback as a well-documented clinical technique (Basmajian, 1979).

A hypothetical but prototypal example of the use of biofeedback (in this case, electromyographic, or muscle tension, feedback) is provided by Astor (1977):

> Let us consider a typical patient who comes to the therapist with a classical complaint of simple tension headache. This is usually a bilateral, dull-aching frontal headache. These headaches may start gradually in the morning and sometimes last all day. Assuming proper diagnosis is made, the treatment plan for this symptom would be electromyograph (EMG) biofeedback. In the first few sessions, electrode attachments might be placed on the forearm extensor muscle for beginning training in relaxation. In later sessions, the patient will train with electrode placements on the frontalis muscle of the forehead. The subject will be instructed to keep a low tone on the EMG by relaxing the "hooked-up" muscle. As he gets better at doing this, the feedback system is gradually turned up so as to require small increments of increased muscle relaxation. Feedback success is conveyed to the patient by a lowering of light, sound, or meter intensity, depending on the type of display his equipment provides. This particular training system may be likened to a form of operant conditioning, in that it helps to change and shape behavior by providing immediate positive reinforcement to each successful muscle relaxation response.
>
> Should the patient be unable to lower his muscle tension on EMG, he is given some form of relaxation training. . . . Once he demonstrates successful ability to relax, he is put back onto biofeedback treatment. Patients usually receive two or three thirty-minute treatment sessions per week for a period of four to eight weeks. Silent trial sessions without feedback may be interspersed, to enable the patient to transfer his training. Patients are encouraged to practice at home at least once or twice a day, and are often given tape recordings with relaxation suggestions as an aid. If inexpensive biofeedback devices are available, they are loaned to patients to assist them in home practice. Patients are usually required to maintain logs on treatment progress, recording the intensity, frequency, time and duration of headaches. As patients progress through tension headache biofeedback therapy, they report increased awareness of tension and greater ability to reduce it. (p. 619)

In clinical applications, biofeedback techniques are often used in conjunction with other approaches such as medical treatment, psychotherapy, and **relaxation training.** Recent studies have begun to examine the relative merits of the techniques alone and in conjunction with other approaches (e.g., Andrasik & Holroyd, 1980; Jacobson, Manschreck, & Silverberg, 1979). The relationship of human individual differences to the effectiveness of these techniques is also being explored (e.g., Acosta, Yamamoto, & Wilcox, 1978; Surwit et al., 1979). Blanchard and Young's (1974) comments remain relevant; it would be premature to hail biofeedback as a panacea for psychophysiological disorders.

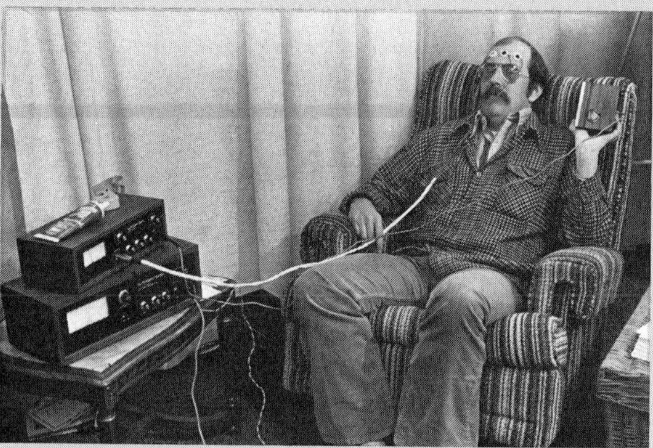

Electromyographic (EMG) feedback of muscle tension in the forehead (frontalis muscles) is used to treat tension headache.

Application of treatment approaches to some specific psychophysiological disorders

Asthma. Medical treatment of asthma is usually symptomatically oriented. When emotional factors appear significant, psychotherapy or hypnosis is often tried (Collison, 1975; Karasu, 1979). More recently, biofeedback techniques, which focus on dealing with stress through procedures such as relaxation (Stoyva, 1976), have been used. In the following case, Lerro, Hurnyak, and Patterson (1980) used **thermal biofeedback** to treat a woman with acute severe bronchial asthma in which psychological factors appeared to be particularly important.

> Ms. A, a 58-year-old woman, had suffered from asthma attacks for one year before seeking . . . consultation. At that time her admitting physician noted that she had been hospitalized on nine occasions during the past several months for acute bronchial asthma attacks. Prolonged treatment

with substantial doses of intravenous [medication was] usually required to relieve the attacks . . . Ms. A noted that during the past two years she had suffered three major traumas in her life: her brother's serious cardiac illness and the deaths of her sister and mother. According to her, she did not experience much emotional change after these incidents, but she said that she "shook for days" following her mother's death. . . .

We believed that her three family traumas that preceded her asthmatic disorder were significant in contributing to the asthma, and we recommended continued psychiatric contact with supportive psychotherapy. Two psychiatric office visits during the next few weeks appeared to lessen her anxiety and interrupt her pattern of recurrent asthma attacks and hospitalizations. Nonetheless, two months later she was hospitalized again with chest pain and [breathing difficulty.] Following her discharge, Ms. A discontinued psychiatric contact. She began experiencing asthmatic episodes with even greater severity, and shortly thereafter she was hospitalized. During the next four months she was in the hospital on three occasions for a total of 3½ months. . . .

During her last hospitalization we discussed biofeedback with Ms. A, and she agreed to try it. . . . The biofeedback therapist noted Ms. A's extreme breathing difficulty: her breathing was erratic, she often gasped for breath, her face was red and puffed, her eyes were glassy, she appeared extremely anxious, her hands shook, and her gait was unsteady. However, she appeared to be motivated and cooperative. We taught Ms. A how to use a heat-sensitive biofeedback apparatus . . . that displayed a digital readout of her skin temperature as measured through a sensor attached to her right index finger. She was directed to elevate her skin temperature, and we suggested that she might accomplish this by increased relaxation. We emphasized the importance of her active participation in the process, and we taught her deep muscle relaxation by asking her to concentrate on feelings of warmth and heaviness in her limbs. Ms. A performed these exercises twice daily. She had five weekly sessions while still hospitalized. By the third session, her physicians noted marked clinical improvement in her breathing pattern, anxiety level, and general appearance. By the fifth session she showed no tremor and was moving around on her own. At this point she was able to raise her [finger] skin temperature (4°–5° F. in less than 10 minutes) and maintain the increase for 10–15 minutes. One week after she was discharged from the hospital she was driving her car and going places alone. She maintained normal breathing and after two outpatient biofeedback sessions, her biweekly visits were reduced from one to one-half hour. Her . . . medication was tapered off. Within 2½ months her biofeedback visits were reduced to once a month. Six months after discharge, she had required no further hospitalizations, although during the following six months, she was hospitalized briefly twice for acute bronchitis. No severe breathing difficulty was observed on either occasion. (pp. 735–736)

Migraine. Symptomatic medical treatment of migraine involves the use of strong **analgesic** (pain-killing) drugs, such as Demerol, since aspirin is relatively powerless in relieving the pain of this condition. Vasoconstrictive drugs, such as ergotamine tartrate, are also prescribed and are of some benefit (as are the tranquilizers Valium and Librium) for the reduction of generalized anxiety levels. Psychotherapeutic approaches to migraine have had varying success, with Wolff (1972) reporting about a 65-percent success rate. Unfortunately, the criteria for success in many of these psychotherapeutically focused studies involve subjective clinical impressions. In an interesting study, Cedercreutz (1978) reported excellent success using hypnosis with 23 migraine sufferers who were capable of moderate to deep hypnotic trance. At an 11-month follow-up, all 23 deep-to-moderate trance subjects had no migraine symptoms. However, most migraine sufferers of the 100 treated in the study were only able to obtain lighter trances, and were not symptom free.

A major new focus in treatment of migraine headache has been on relaxation training and the use of biofeedback techniques to gain control of the vascular response system (Budzynski, 1979). One migraine biofeedback approach is very similar to the one described in the treatment of asthma, where the temperature of the extremities is lowered. However, recent evidence suggests that a different form of biofeedback is more effective with migraines. In this treatment, the subject is provided with feedback on pulse pressure in the cranial arteries. Subjects are trained to lower the temporal pulse, which is an indication of constriction of the artery. Since migraines are due to a dilation of cranial arteries, this constriction should reduce the migraine. In a controlled study (Elmore, 1979), subjects who used this procedure had less than 50 percent of the number of headaches than before treatment. In the same study, subjects who used thermal biofeedback of the extremities reduced their headaches to a lesser degree. In addition, the latter approach took longer, and headaches during treatment were experienced as more painful, than in the temporal pulse group. The use of temporal pulse (or cephalic blood volume pulse, as it is sometimes called) has been confirmed as effective in a later study by Bild and Adams (1980).

Most biofeedback approaches have been at least somewhat effective with many migraine patients (Friar & Beatty, 1976; Russ, Hammer, & Adderton, 1977). In a study by Pearse et al. (1975), a biofeedback treatment program led to considerable improvement in 73 percent of the patients and significant medication reduction in 55 percent of those treated. Many questions remain about which biofeedback approach is most effective with migraines, though the evidence currently favors temporal, or cephalic blood volume, pulse feedback.

Essential hypertension. Essential hypertension is another disorder with multiple causes: a possible predisposition towards physiological vascular reactivity, an impact of stress on the autonomic nervous system, and a likelihood of a complicating personality style. The treatment of the disorder has focused on all three areas: medical treatment to deal with the physiological factors, psychological approaches to deal with the ANS stress response, and psychotherapy to deal with personality variables. Medical treatment has primarily used drugs to reduce blood pressure. However, drugs often have unpleasant and sometimes dangerous side effects. While some controlled studies have indicated that verbal psychotherapy is effective in the treatment of many psychophysiological disorders, hypertension appears to be very difficult to treat in this manner (Kellner, 1975). In fact, one of the few controlled studies on psychotherapy with hypertensive patients found that during the course of therapy, patients' hypertension became worse (Titchner, Sheldon, & Ross, 1959).

Recent research on biofeedback and relaxation therapy has indicated promise for the treatment of hypertension (Price, 1974). Both approaches can be used to train subjects to significantly lower their blood pressure. Patel and North (1975) have demonstrated that the combined use of yoga meditation and biofeedback led to a significant average reduction of 26.1 points in blood pressure for hypertensive patients. Simply providing direct feedback of blood pressure levels without training in meditation also can lead to a 10–15 percent reduction in pressure (Kristt & Engel, 1975). But studies of the clinical application of these techniques are not completely positive. Although Agras, Taylor, Kraemer, Allen, and Schneider (1980) found that relaxation treatment significantly reduced hypertensives' blood pressure, Taylor et al. (1977) found that relaxation therapy had no greater impact than other therapy or medical treatment when evaluated one year after the treatment period. In this study, the immediate positive effects of relaxation therapy were lost due to the absence of what the authors concluded was an essential requirement: periodic maintenance training in the relaxation techniques. Surwit, Shapiro, and Good (1978) found that relaxation treatment, muscle tension reduction, and cardiovascular feedback were of little value with borderline hypertensives, and suggested that these approaches are useful when the initial values of the clients' blood pressures are very high. The current status of biofeedback and relaxation approaches warrants further study and clinical trials. They do not have enough support to justify calling them established treatments (Engel, 1979).

A concluding comment

The effective treatment of psychophysiological disorders is difficult. Many procedures have been tried and continue to be tried. Medical approaches are primarily symptomatic. They reduce symptoms, but do not resolve issues related to stress and personality or life-style factors. Traditional psycho-

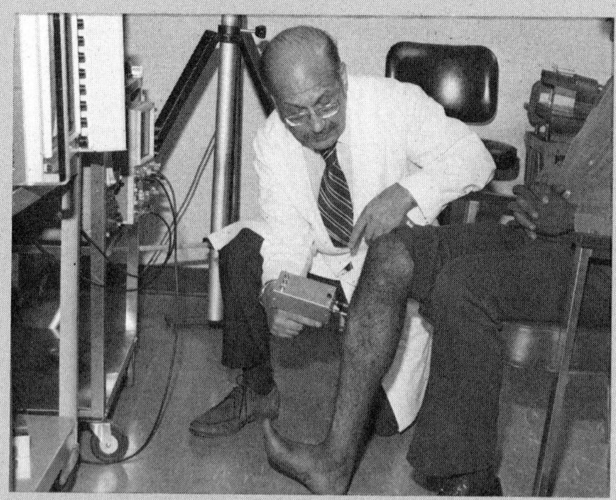

John Basmajian, a noted clinician and researcher, uses a biofeedback device to test a patient's improved muscular control.

therapeutic approaches are either ineffective or too time consuming. During the years that psychotherapy takes, the physical organism is at risk of continuing deterioration. The preliminary evidence for the relatively rapid positive effects of the behavioral approaches, especially the anxiety reduction techniques of relaxation training and biofeedback, has led to tremendous enthusiasm for these techniques. They have virtually exploded onto the scene in the past decade. Still, we have many questions about them. Which techniques are most effective with which disorders? What exactly makes these techniques work? Are the effects specific or nonspecific? We cannot answer these questions; we must wait to see what current research will tell us.

Summary

1. The experience of stress can have a broad range of effects on the physical condition of humans, from minor feelings of fatigue and "lousiness" to the development of a major physical illness.

2. Significant correlations have been found between many life events (not all of which are negative) and physical health. A critical factor appears to be how the individual perceives the event, and the degree of social support available.

3. The classic formulation of psychophysiological disorders focuses on the concept of various organ systems being adversely affected by long-term physiological responses to emotions or stress, as manifested in the sympathetic activity of the autonomic nervous system. This response has significant effects on the major organ systems, particularly if stress is prolonged or chronic.

4. Nine major organ systems have traditionally been identified with psychophysiological disorders.

1. The Skin
2. The Musculoskeletal System
3. The Respiratory System
4. The Cardiovascular System
5. The Hemic (Blood) and Lymphatic System
6. The Gastrointestinal System
7. The Genito-urinary System
8. The Endocrine System
9. The Sense Organs

5. This chapter has focused on six common disorders: ulcers, tension and migraine headaches, asthma, hypertension, and coronary heart disease.

6. Ulcers are most likely in individuals who: 1. have a biological predisposition towards high levels of pepsinogen secretion, 2. are experiencing a chronically stressful life, and 3. have unmet dependency needs or react to stress with anger.

7. Asthma is a respiratory disorder which most likely begins with a biological predisposition to respiratory infection or allergy. In many cases the predisposition is influenced by emotional factors, stress, and learning. The degree of importance of these factors in the etiology and maintenance of asthma varies from individual to individual.

8. Tension headaches appear to be due primarily to emotional stress, although some evidence suggests a physiological predisposition.

9. Migraine headaches are the result of a disorder of the vascular system. Substantial evidence exists for a biological predisposition towards hypersensitivity of the cranial blood vessels, which may be inherited.

10. Essential hypertension is a silent killer. The chronic high blood pressure of essential hypertension is most likely due to a combination of a physiological predisposition, the perception of a chronic stress situation, and personality variables which may result in a reaction to stress which involves undischarged hostility or aggression.

11. Coronary heart disease is related to many factors. Risk of heart disease is increased by aging, obesity, high cholesterol levels, lack of physical activity, smoking, and a familial history of the disorder. Type A behavior, which is characterized by a hectic overcommitted life-style, has been correlated with coronary problems. Most individuals who fit the Type A category do not have coronary heart disease. Research is currently being conducted in an attempt to identify specific aspects of Type A behavior which may be particularly associated with CHD. One factor being investigated is people's reaction to uncontrollable stress.

12. The issue of differential etiology (e.g., why one individual develops ulcers, but another develops hypertension) has been presented in terms of several concepts: physiological predisposition, response sensitivity of specific organ systems, the general adaptation syndrome, immunological reactions, psychoanalytic concepts, personality traits and specific attitudes, and learning theory.

13. The best conclusion that we can draw regarding the development of a specific disorder in a specific individual is that a physiological predisposition towards an organ system weakness must be present. Second, it appears very likely that some psychological vulnerability is present. This vulnerability may consist of a personality trait or a learned behavior; the evidence is not clear. Third, the physiological and psychological vulnerability interacts with the individual's perception of life stresses, and results in the development of a psychophysiological disorder. This is a diathesis-stress formulation of psychophysiological disorders.

14. The treatment of psychophysiological disorders has been mainly medical and symptomatic. In recent years there has been a greater emphasis on behavioral medicine: the utilization of a broad variety of psychologically oriented techniques to treat classic psychophysiological disorders and, not so incidentally, "ordinary" physical disorders.

15. Psychodynamic psychotherapy has not been shown to be efficient with psychophysiological disorders. Although some studies have demonstrated that psychotherapy is effective with some disorders, others have indicated that it is not. Even in cases where it might be effective, psychotherapy is not efficient. It is so time consuming that serious physical damage is likely to result from the psychophysiological disorder while treatment continues for years.

16. Reports of the successful application of behavioral techniques to health-related behaviors and to specific psychophysiological disorders have led to the development of a field called behavioral medicine.

17. The reduction of stress-related anxiety and tension has been a focus for behaviorists who treat psychophysiological disorders. Two predominant techniques, which may be used alone or in conjunction, are relaxation training and biofeedback.

18. Dramatic successes have been reported in the literature using behavioral techniques with psychophysiological disorders. However, many studies have been reports of success with individual patients. Negative results are rarely submitted for publication. Controlled studies contrasting the relative effectiveness of various behavioral approaches are now being done, but to hail any behavioral technique as a clearly established treatment of choice for a psychophysiological disorder would be premature.

19. The application of behavioral techniques to the treatment of psychophysiological disorders, and more generally to all physical disorders, is an exciting new area in clinical psychology. However, many important questions remain about the effectiveness of behavioral medicine.

KEY TERMS

Immunology. The study of the systems of the body which protect the individual against disease. The autoimmune systems of the body fight against foreign bodies which might cause disease.

Pharmacological treatment. Medical treatment that utilizes various chemical substances (drugs) to deal with the symptoms or organic causes of disorders.

Physiological predisposition. Some organic factor that predisposes the physical organism to react in a particular way.

Placebo. A neutral or inactive substance which the individual believes is effective as a treatment. Using a placebo control group is one way to control for the effects of subjects' expectations when studying the effectiveness of a particular treatment.

Renal. Pertaining to the kidneys.

Rheumatoid arthritis. A form of arthritis characterized by inflammation of connective tissue such as skeletal joints, muscles, and heart valves.

Thermal biofeedback. A treatment in which information about the temperature of the extremities (usually a finger) is provided to the individual. The goal of the treatment is to raise the finger's temperature, which is considered to be a sign of increased blood flow and thus of relaxation of the vascular system.

Vagal nerve. Also called the *vagus nerve,* or *tenth cranial nerve.* The vagus nerve is important in regulating the rate and regularity of the heartbeat.

Vasodilation. A relaxed or dilated state of the blood vessels. A dilated vessel is one in which the cross-section has increased in size, allowing a higher rate of flow with less pressure.

Visceral. Pertaining to the viscera, or internal organs, especially those in the abdomen.

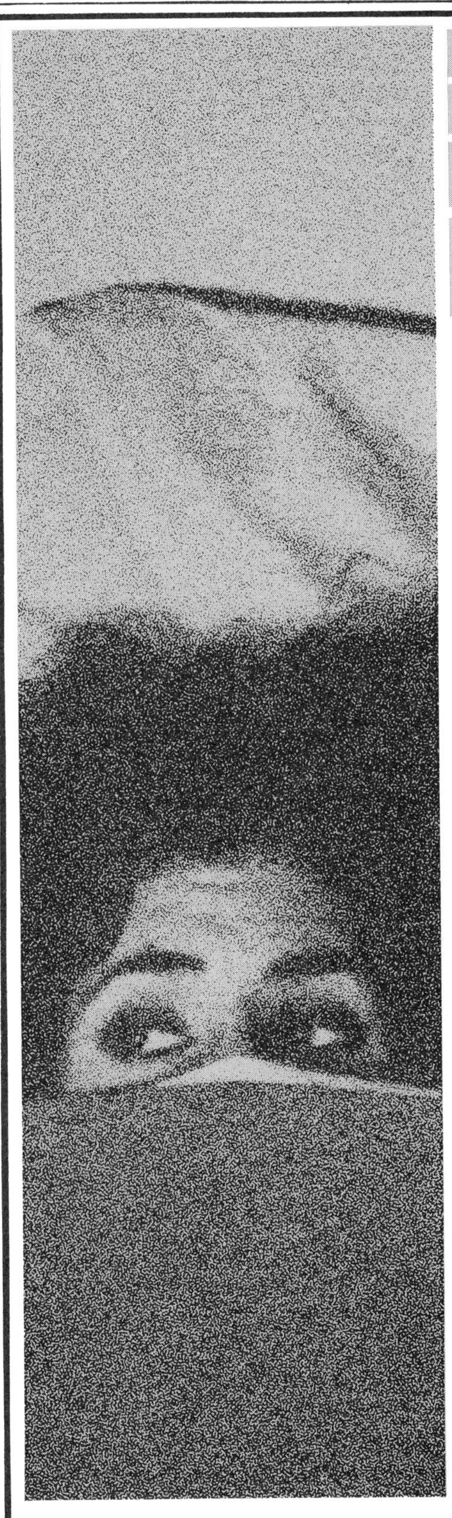

7

Anxiety and related disorders

- Anxiety
- Specific disorders associated with anxiety
- Final comments on etiology
- Key treatments
- Summary
- Key terms

Anxiety is so commonplace that the modern era is often called the "age of anxiety." We have already seen that during times of major stress many people react with **anxiety.** Depending upon the level of stress perceived, some people are unable to cope and they develop an adjustment reaction, as discussed in Chapter 5. In Chapter 6, we saw that under some circumstances, stress may lead to major physiological reactions, including sudden death. In this chapter, we will explore another possibility. Certain disorders are characterized by the subjective experience of unpleasant levels of anxiety or by behaviors that appear to have the function of avoiding situations that provoke anxiety. Anxiety or anxiety-avoiding behaviors are considered abnormal when they disrupt functioning to such an extent that the individual becomes incapacitated. The anxiety is so unpleasant that it interferes with human relationships, with life goals (such as study or work), or is simply extremely painful and disconcerting. The experience of intense anxiety or behaviors designed to avoid anxiety often end up being self-defeating. Anxiety *disorders* differ from normal anxiety primarily because of the intensity of the anxiety experienced and its repetitive nature.

The subjective experience of the condition we call anxiety can range from mild to severe. For example, some one taking an exam or meeting a "blind date" or having a job interview might feel mild "concern." This might consist, among other things, of worry ("Will I do well?"), "butterflies" in the stomach, slight sweating of the palms of the hands, and a sense that the heart is beating more quickly. But the subjective experience can also be much more unpleasant. Some people might react to the same situations with an extreme sense of dread and panic, including difficulty in catching their breath, irregular heart rhythm, chest pain, a choking sensation, dizziness, and severe trembling. Although similar, this reaction has sometimes been differentiated from fear. The word "fear" has usually been applied to these types of symptoms when the individual faces an objective, real danger, such as a burglar holding a gun, while "anxiety" is the label for such symptoms when the danger is "irrational." Such a distinction is not particularly helpful; the responses which we call fear or anxiety are very similar.

Most of us have experienced mild levels of anxiety, and some may have experienced the disabling reaction of panic. The following first-person account may provide some understanding of just how unpleasant severe anxiety can be.

> I don't think I'll ever forget it! It was just before I took the Graduate Record Exam before applying for graduate school. For a couple of days I'd been worrying about it. You know. Like—what if I don't get a good enough score to be accepted. All the time I knew it was silly, 'cause I'd always done well in college, and shouldn't have any trouble. But that morning, wow—it was a bummer. I overslept, and thought I'd be late, and maybe I couldn't get in. While I was driving over there, I could feel my stomach grinding away, my throat tasted sour, and I drove faster and faster, my heart pounding louder and louder in my ears! I made it, about 10 minutes late, and just got in. I thought the world was going to end! I was shaking, my stomach was upset, and everything closed in on me. I was really upset! At the desk, I was dizzy and sweating like a pig, my chest hurt, and my hands were shaking so hard I could hardly hold a pencil. I've never been so scared in all my life! I tried to take deep breaths to calm down, but it didn't help, and I was afraid I'd throw up so I had to get out of there. I told the proctor I was going to be ill, so he told me to leave, and guess what, I went to the john and threw up! The next time I took the GRE, I was anxious but not like the first time!

It is obvious from the above self-report that anxiety is not only a subjective experience but also has objective behavioral and physiological components, some of which are not directly perceptible to the individual.

ANXIETY

Physiological Aspects of Anxiety

In Chapter 6, we studied the physiological actions of the autonomic nervous system (ANS). We saw that when an individual is threatened by some real danger, such as an impending automobile accident, the ANS is activated. We have also seen that the experience of chronic stress or threat may activate this physiological system. A third aspect of this system is important in human behavior: its relationship to the experience of anxiety.

People experiencing anxiety, as we have pointed out, typically feel that their heart is pounding. In anxiety-provoking situations, heart rate increases. In addition, depth and rate of respiration escalate, palms tend to perspire, a generalized increase in tension of the voluntary musculature occurs. These events are relatively available to the subject's awareness. Also possible are other physiological changes that the subject is less likely to be aware of, such as changes in stomach activity (Katkin, 1975). People are likely to be completely unaware of some of these changes unless assisted by special equipment; these changes include increased electrical resistance of the skin due to perspiration (Katkin, 1975; Lehrer, 1972), increased blood pressure (Lader & Mathews, 1970), and increased diameters of the pupils of the eyes (Janisse, 1976). The measurement of these physiological effects has played an important part in the experimental study of anxiety and in its treatment through relaxation therapies (see Figure 7.1).

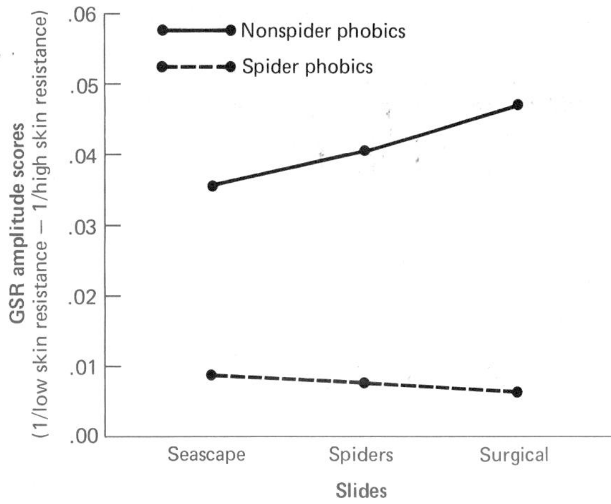

Figure 7.1.
Measurement of physiological changes has been used to determine autonomic reactivity in anxiety-provoking situations. The graph demonstrates the change in electrical skin resistance (GSR, or galvanic skin response) in phobic individuals when viewing slide photos of their feared insect (spiders), and compares their GSR responses to nonphobic controls.
From Prigatano and Johnson (1974, p. 174).

The physiological signs of anxiety are signs of autonomic arousal, and have often been characterized as the **fight-or-flight response.** This arousal presumably prepares the person to either fight against or flee from danger or stress. As we saw in Chapter 6, on psychophysiological disorders, when the autonomic nervous system is aroused, it activates the smooth muscles of the blood vessels, stomach, intestines, kidneys, endocrine glands, and other organs, including the heart. The two parts of the autonomic nervous system, the sympathetic and the parasympathetic, work in unison at times, and at other times oppose each other's effects. The sympathetic system dilates the pupils (pupils increase in size), accelerates the heart, inhibits digestion, and stimulates the other smooth muscles and glands—changes which prepare the individual for rapid strenuous activity. The parasympathetic system acts more as a **homeostatic mechanism** (a system which acts to keep bodily processes in balance) which shuts down the systems activated by the sympathetic branch. This division is not always clear-cut (e.g., the parasympathetic system also has some stimulating actions), but for our purposes, the above description is adequate. (See Figure 6.1 and Table 6.2 to review this system.)

Autonomic arousal, as we have seen in Chapter 6, is not unique to the experience of anxiety. The physiological changes seen during anxiety are often precipitated by *other* stimuli (e.g., sexual arousal, anger, or novel experiences) which do not involve a subjective sense of anxiety (Masters & Johnson, 1966; Rule & Nesdale, 1976). Another complicating factor is that the intercorrelations among these physiological events are generally not high (Hodges, 1976). In other words, not all individuals manifest all the effects each time they experience anxiety, and some of these physiological effects are experienced with differing emotions.

Behavioral Aspects of Anxiety

Frequently, **behavioral observation** is used to determine if a subject is anxious; the observer watches for signs commonly construed to indicate anxiety. These signs may include trembling, nail biting, changes in voice pitch, visible perspiration, and more global behaviors such as physical attack (indicating anger or rage rather than anxiety) or avoidance of stimuli, which would be construed as indicating fear. Obviously, these behaviors may occur for reasons other than anxiety. One may tremble because of cold or anger. One may perspire from exertion, and one may avoid stimuli because they are boring. Since there may be many reasons why the autonomic nervous system becomes activated, and many reasons why behaviors associated with anxiety can occur, we often rely on individuals' verbal reports to determine if they are anxious.

Subjective Experience

The subjective experience of anxiety is often, but not always, correlated with the physiological events described above. When someone is threatened, physiological changes occur and the subject's assessment of these changes may result in the subjective awareness of anxiety. For example, if on your way to take an exam you feel your stomach churning and your heart pounding, you might report that you are anxious. However, if you had this same physiological experience just after being rudely insulted, your subjective report might be one of anger. The subjective experience may vary with situational factors, even when the behavioral and physiological signs or symptoms are the same or similar.

Self-reports of subjective experience can be quite informal (such as the one presented earlier in this chapter) or they can be very structured and standardized. One commonly used standardized measure is the Taylor Manifest Anxiety Scale (TMAS). Many of this scale's items were taken from the Minnesota Multiphasic Personality Inventory (MMPI), which was discussed in Chapter 4. The subject answers true or false to a series of statements such as "I am usually calm and not easily upset." Instruments such as the TMAS appear to measure what we call **trait anxiety,** anxiety considered to be a characteristic, enduring trait of the individual. Individuals appear to have differing generalized levels of anxiety, so that some people appear to be typically more "nervous" than others. (Notice in Figure 7.1 that phobic individuals had a higher level of arousal when viewing photos of a neutral seascape than did nonphobics.) Their level of nervousness is an enduring factor in their personality makeup. Some researchers are more concerned with **state anxiety,** or the degree to which the experience of anxiety is due to variables within a particular situation or experience. Bowers (1973) has concluded that any individual's experience of anxiety is due both to situation variables and to trait variables.

SPECIFIC DISORDERS ASSOCIATED WITH ANXIETY

While most of us have experienced anxiety to some degree, for some individuals anxiety becomes an overwhelming aspect of their daily life. Traditionally, the disorders associated with anxiety either directly or indirectly have included free-floating forms of anxiety, an experience of generalized irrational fear not attached to a specific object or situation; **phobias,** or unrealistic fears of specific objects or situations; obsessions and compulsions; the hysterical conversion and dissociative disorders; depression; and some sexual disorders. These disorders were previously called "neurotic disorders," (see Highlight 7.1). In DSM-III (1980) these disorders are categorized into anxiety disorders, somatoform disorders, and dissociative disorders. Somatoform and dissociative disorders will be covered in Chapter 8. Depression and psychosexual disorders are covered in later chapters, and are no longer grouped with anxiety disorders and somatoform and dissociative disorders in DSM-III.

The experience of anxiety is central to some disorders; for example, in **panic disorder, generalized anxiety disorder,** and **phobic disorder.** The relationship, as we will see, is somewhat less obvious in the **obsessive-compulsive disorder.** The anxiety disorders are estimated to occur in 2–5 percent of the population (Marks & Lader, 1973).

HIGHLIGHT 7.1
"NEUROTIC" DISORDERS

Individuals with anxiety disorders were described, in the past, as "neurotic." Although this term is still occasionally used, current professional practice avoids it as much as possible. The concept of a neurosis is primarily associated with one particular theoretical persuasion: psychoanalysis. The term can be used descriptively to differentiate an individual who is maladjusted but not psychotic (i.e., disturbed, but not out of touch with reality). However, it most accurately designates an etiological process which involves an unconscious conflict that leads to anxiety. The anxiety is supposedly handled through a defense mechanism—a behavior that results in a symptom.

We will see that the evidence for the psychoanalytic theory of the etiology of anxiety disorder is not more convincing than the evidence for other theoretical formulations. Rather than imply acceptance of the psychoanalytic formulation by using the term "neurosis," many clinicians now prefer to use the more descriptive terminology "anxiety disorder."

Panic Disorder and Generalized Anxiety Disorder

Both panic disorder and generalized anxiety disorder are primarily manifestations of severe anxiety. Symptoms include apprehension, a sense of impending doom, worry, and fear of losing control; motor tension, such as shakiness, twitches, trembling, and jerky movements; and autonomic manifestations, such as sweating, pounding heart, hot and cold spells, flushing, and rapid breathing (see Table 7.1). In addition, the sense of apprehension may lead to increased vigilance and distractability, and the individual may have difficulty sleeping. Frequently, people experiencing these disorders also feel depressed.

The primary differentiation between panic disorder and generalized anxiety disorder is in intensity and duration. In panic disorder (or anxiety attacks) the subject experiences *recurrent* short-term episodes of intensified severe anxiety which are not usually associated with specific situations or objects, and therefore are relatively unpredictable. The individual rarely knows in advance when the panic will occur.

The generalized anxiety disorder is usually characterized by a lesser level of intensity of symptoms, which are relatively durable or chronic. The intense fear or terror of the panic attack is absent, and the individual instead feels a relatively constant mood which ranges from uneasiness to a clear subjective feeling of anxiety. In clinical settings, the differentiation between disorders is often not precise, as the following case illustrates. The individual exhibited the symptoms of generalized anxiety disorder, but later developed a panic disorder (episodes of acute anxiety).

> The patient, an American oil geologist for many years resident abroad, aged thirty-two and unmarried, was referred by his company for diag-

Table 7.1

Symptoms shown by 50 percent or more of patients with anxiety disorder, compared with controls

Sympton	*Patients*	*Controls*
Palpitation of heart	97	9
Tires easily	95	19
Breathlessness	90	13
Nervousness	88	27
Chest pain	85	10
Sighing	79	16
Dizziness	78	16
Faintness	70	12
Apprehension	61	3
Headache	58	26
Paresthesia (unpleasant sensations such as tingling or burning)	58	7
Weakness	56	3
Trembling	54	17
Insomnia	53	4
Unhappiness	50	2

Based on Marks and Lader (1973).

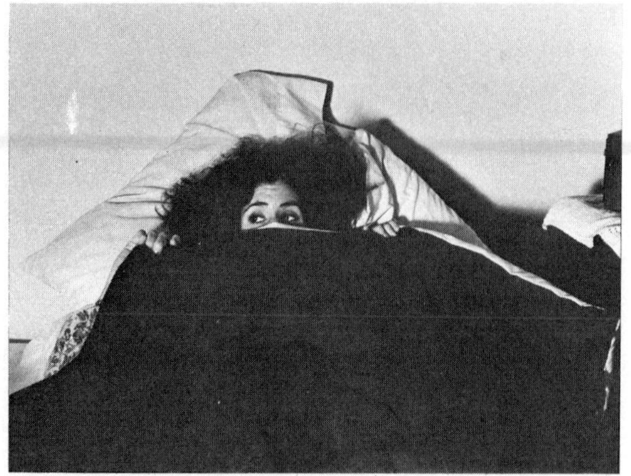

Panic attacks may occur at any time.

nosis because of numerous complaints which he believed meant that he must be insane. For five or six years he had been suffering from intermittent attacks of dizziness, blurred vision, weakness, and unsteady gait, for which no satisfactory explanation had been found by his medical examiners. For three years the patient had been bothered by almost constant "nervous tension," irritability, increased sex pace with incomplete satisfaction, inability to relax, poor sleep, and frequent troubled or terrifying dreams. His neck seemed always strained and he frequently rubbed it and made rotatory head movements to relieve the pull. For about a year the patient had been so restless he could scarcely sit still and stand still in the daytime or lie still at night. He walked so vigorously that he tired everyone else out and himself too. As long as he kept on the move he felt in reasonably good spirits, but he was intolerant of delay and opposition no matter from what or whom it came. The moment he let up in overt activity his symptoms increased, his legs ached, he felt "jumpy" and he could get no satisfaction unless he drove himself on to further activity, even though he felt worn out. He began to rely more and more on whiskey to steady him during the day and on barbiturates to get him to sleep at night.

One day, about eight months before his referral for diagnosis, while the patient was dressing to go out for an evening's entertainment, he felt something in his head suddenly snap, everything around him looked unnatural, and he seemed to be about to faint. He lay down on his bed for a long time, his heart pounding and his breathing labored, while the thought kept recurring, "I'm dying, I'm dying." Eventually he managed to sit up, weak and shaky, to drink about a pint of whiskey and take a double dose of sedative, after which he slept through the evening and night. Following this, the patient had frequent recurrences of anxiety attacks which consisted of "queer head sensations," weakness, sweating, coarse tremor, palpitation, and the conviction that something terrible was happening to him. He had only one repetition of the snapping in his head, but he dreaded its return more than anything else. He stated that, from the time of the first snapping to the present, he had never regained his previous ability to think clearly, concentrate, or remember. (Cameron, 1947, pp. 251–254)

Biophysiological Issues. There is good evidence that innate differences exist in the ease with which individuals are aroused and in the magnitude of peoples' autonomic reactivity (Hare, 1975; Lacey, 1967). It seems that the more labile (easily aroused) the autonomic nervous system, the more likely an anxiety disorder is to develop. People with easily aroused autonomic nervous systems seem more likely to experience a subjective sense of extreme anxiety. They would, therefore, encounter more situations that they would attempt to avoid. If the situation is unavoidable, their discomfort can interfere with their ability to function in the setting.

Is this difference in autonomic reactivity inherited? Slater and Shields (1969) studied 17 identical and 28 fraternal same-sex twins to try to find out. One twin of each pair was known to have an anxiety disorder; 41 percent of the identical co-twins also had anxiety disorders, but only 4 percent of the fraternal co-twins shared the disorder. Such differences suggest a genetic influence in the predisposition to develop anxiety disorders. However, little evidence exists that specific anxiety disorders are inherited. For example, in Slater and Shields's study, one twin was likely to have one type of anxiety disorder (e.g., panic disorder) and the co-twin was likely to have a different anxiety disorder (e.g., a phobia). This evidence supports the possibility of an inherited predisposition towards ease of anxiety arousal. It does not provide evidence for the genetic transmission of specific anxiety disorders. Cohen (1974), after evaluating the available evidence, concluded that the concept of genetic transmission in this broad range of disorders has not yet been adequately supported. However, the disorders may well be related to an inherited physiological mechanism (a highly reactive autonomic nervous system) that allows psychological factors to impact on the physiology of the body (Blanchard & Young, 1974).

Panic and Generalized Anxiety as Learned Behavior. Learning theorists have made interesting contributions to the conceptualization of anxiety. Most theorists view the basic physiological response as being innate and present at birth in the form of the **startle response.** In young infants, the presentation of a sudden stimulus, such as a loud noise, results in this response, which consists of a startled jerking of the arms and legs. Hans Eysenck (1961; Eysenck & Eysenck, 1968) suggests that ease of emotional arousal is, to some degree, inherited; this concept has received considerable experimental support. However, the general level of chronic autonomic arousal, the situation in which an increase in anxiety will be experienced, and the specific symptomatic manifestations of anxiety may be strongly influenced by learned behavior. For example, Mowrer (1947) demonstrated that laboratory rats could learn to avoid a previously neutral event to which they had developed a conditioned fear.

One way of thinking about the anxiety in panic and generalized anxiety disorder is that the anxiety response is learned because it is reinforced. If a stimulus (an object or situation) is associated with anxiety (e.g., with autonomic arousal) and the person escapes from the stimulus, the reduction in anxiety is reinforcing. The person learns to avoid the stimulus, so that we have **avoidance learning.** A different possibility is direct reinforcement of anxiety. For example, if a child becomes anxious and its mother comforts it and cuddles it, these are positive reinforcers. Do we train people to be anxious in this manner? Most research has indicated that the complete anxiety response is very difficult to train in this manner, although some aspects of physiological arousal can be changed using direct reinforcement procedures (Blanchard & Young, 1974).

Could other factors be involved? In Chapter 3, the social learning approach was presented, with its core notion of internal mediating responses. Some theorists have focused on this process in regard to anxiety. In a very interesting study, Geer, Davison, and Gatchel (1970) demonstrated that human subjects who believed they could control the amount of **aversive stimulation** (painful or unpleasant experiences) they would receive were less anxious than subjects who believed they were helpless, regardless of the subjects' actual ability to control the variables. In this study, subjects were given painful electrical shocks lasting six seconds to determine their autonomic responses as measured by the **electrodermal response,** or the degree of electrical conductivity of the skin. As each shock occurred, subjects were to press a switch as quickly as possible so that their reaction time could be measured. Once this baseline was established, the subjects were split into two groups. One group was told that the duration of the shocks would be cut by 50 percent if the subjects could achieve a particular speed in throwing a special switch. This group's members believed that by changing their own behavior, they could control the amount of aversive stimulation they would receive. The other half of the subjects were simply informed that each of the next 10 shocks would be shorter. In fact, in the second phase of the experiment, both groups received three-second shocks rather than six-second shocks, regardless of the speed of their reactions. The subjects who incorrectly believed they were in control of the duration of the shocks manifested significantly less autonomic arousal than those who were helpless (see Figure 7.2).

The evidence that a belief that one is in control of the environment reduces anxiety supports the importance of internal mediators in anxiety. The way we think (how we perceive) or what we think (what we perceive) can be important influences in how we react. These mediators may be important even when they do not accurately reflect reality, when they are irrational.

Some clinicians believe that the influence of learned irrational beliefs or expectations on

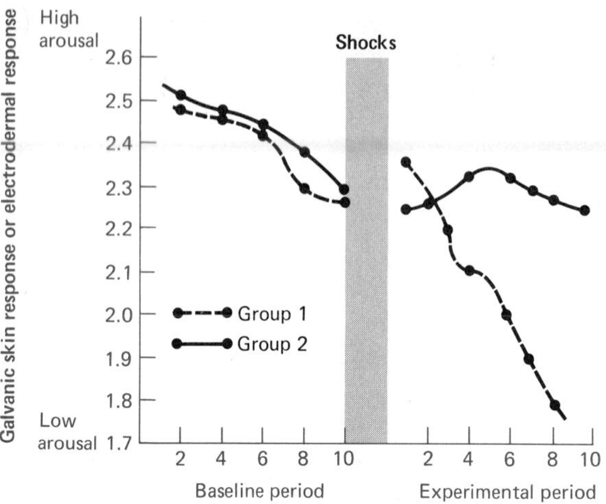

Figure 7.2. Change in anxiety level due to a perception (belief) that the individual can control the environment.

In the baseline period, all subjects were treated the same. In the experimental period, group 1 subjects falsely believed that they could reduce shock duration through their own behavior, while group 2 subjects believed that their behavior had no effect on shock duration. Adapted from Geer et al., 1970.

anxiety is extremely important. For example, a person who believes that "I always make a fool of myself" might become anxious in a public setting because of the perceived danger that foolish behavior might occur. Ellis (1973) and Beck, Laude, and Bohnert (1974) have pointed out that people with anxiety disorders tend to have irrational beliefs about how people should behave and about their own likelihood of experiencing "catastrophic" events (e.g., "looking foolish"). In addition, a strong relationship has been found between the level of anxiety and the severity and likelihood of the anticipated event (Beck et al., 1974). Beck and Rush (1975) have found that in 50 cases suffering from severe anxiety experiences, the subjects experienced thoughts consisting of an anticipation or visualization of physical or psychological danger such as criticism, rejection, or interpersonal failure. The thoughts exaggerated both the degree and likelihood of harm; and such thoughts or cognitions were highly resistant to reason. The individuals resisted logical arguments against these beliefs.

The behavioral approaches suggest that individual differences in anxiety may be partly due to a combination of: 1. innate factors that influence autonomic arousal, 2. conditioned learning, and 3. learned cognitive beliefs. In addition, social learning theorists suggest that a person may learn to manifest generalized anxiety through "modeling" or "imitative learning." Some studies have indicated that parents of people with these disorders are likely to manifest more symptoms of anxiety than the general population. Perhaps individuals who have a biological predisposition to be easily aroused autonomically learn to be generally anxious through an interaction of this predisposition with conditioned fear responses, avoidance learning, and the modeling of parents' behavior and beliefs.

Psychoanalytic Concepts. An alternative formulation of anxiety disorders comes from psychoanalytic theory, which uses anxiety as a central concept for almost all disorders. (The psychoanalytic theory of anxiety has been discussed in Chapter 3.) To review briefly, Freud conceptualized anxiety as based on the flooding of excitation during the birth trauma, and subsequently as a signal of a threatened overstimulation by id impulses. Wachtel (1977) has described anxiety as a fear of our deep-seated desires. The function of anxiety is to signal the need for repression and/or the activation of the defense mechanisms, such as projection or regression. The irrationality of anxiety (experiencing fear when no objective threat is present) is a function of the repression of the actual danger, the id impulse. This impulse is either sexual or aggressive, and may subsequently be linked to some symbolic object or situation in the environment. An individual manifests a disablingly high level of generalized anxiety or has panic experiences which are not related to objective threats because the repression of id impulses and the other defense mechanisms are ineffective. The individual is in danger of having the id impulses break through into consciousness or behavior. The person, in fact, experiences conflict between the instinctual impulsive pressure to act on the id impulse and gratify it, and, on the other side, the necessity to keep the impulse under control. The need for control results from the need to avoid guilt or to avoid the punishment by society which would occur if the impulse broke through.

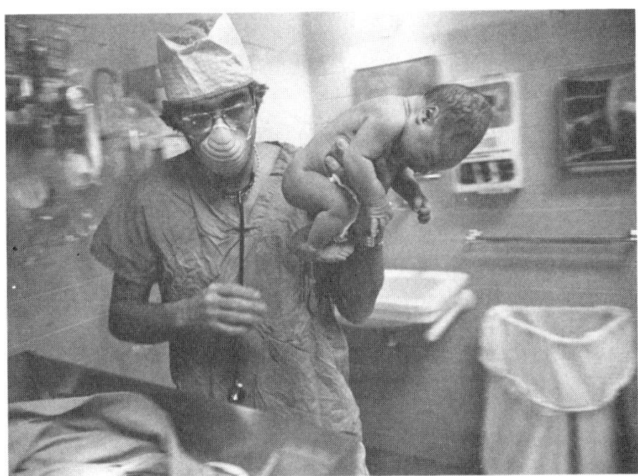

Freud believed that sensory overstimulation due to being introduced suddenly to the bright lights, loud sounds, and possible painful stimuli at birth was the prototype for anxiety.

Later psychodynamic theorists have proposed alternative notions about anxiety. Alfred Adler saw anxiety as being due to a sense of inferiority. Karen Horney felt that "basic anxiety" was a result of a lack of satisfaction of the child's need for the security provided by parents. She proposed that the "basic anxiety" leads to feelings of isolation and helplessness, and the individual develops "strategies" to cope with these feelings by developing **neurotic needs,** needs that are due to unconscious impulses such as the need to "exploit" others. Harry Stack Sullivan also conceptualized anxiety as a response to frustration of the need for security. The more secure one is, the less anxious one will be. In his formulation, generalized anxiety and panic are due to deepseated insecurities which develop when parents do not provide the security needed by a child. Like Freud's psychoanalytic approach, these theories are extremely difficult to prove or disprove, since they do not yield to an experimental approach designed to establish cause and effect.

Phobic Disorder

When an individual goes to great lengths to avoid a harmless object or situation because of irrational fear, or to avoid intense anxiety, the behavior is called phobic. When confronted with the phobic stimulus, an individual with a phobic disorder experiences anxiety symptoms, often to the extent of panic. For some persons, even thinking about the phobic stimulus results in extremely uncomfortable sensations of anxiety.

Many individuals have irrational fears of objects such as spiders, snakes, and worms, but these fears do not interrupt their daily activities. For example, a strong aversion or fear of touching a worm would be unlikely to have great impact on an urban apartment dweller. However, it could be quite distressing to a professional gardener. In the former case a clinical phobia would not exist, but in the latter it would. In a clinical phobia, the irrational fear must be persistent, must be a source of significant distress, and the fears are usually recognized by the subject as unwarranted.

Many types of phobias have been identified according to the object or situation feared. Some examples are acrophobia—a fear of high places; nyctophobia—a fear of darkness; claustrophobia—a fear of enclosed places; hematophobia—fear of blood; mysophobia—fear of germs; and even phobophobia—fear of irrational fear! Current practice, however, uses three categories: **agoraphobia, social phobia,** and **simple phobia.** Of these, agoraphobia is the most commonly seen in clinical practice (Leitenberg, 1976).

The individual with *agoraphobia* has a significant fear of either being alone or being in public places. A significant aspect of this fear is the concern that should something happen to the individual, either no one will be available to help, or those available will be strangers and will provide no assistance. Agoraphobia frequently develops after a series of panic attacks, and the individual often feels that the anxiety attack is the threatened event which may occur when alone or in crowds. As with other anxiety disorders, agoraphobics are often mildly depressed and manifest mild obsessive-compulsive behavior, perhaps in an attempt to deal with the anxiety (Marks, 1978). Such individuals tend to be passive, shy and dependent, anxious, and are more often female than male. In extreme cases, the individual may be limited to the home environment and require constant companionship—a very restrictive existence:

Donna, at the age of 37, had recently returned from visiting distant relatives who lived abroad. The visit was stormy, with many old family quarrels being resurrected. After her return to the United States she experienced several panic attacks which were inexplicable to her and her husband. Neither could make sense of her odd experiences. The attacks consisted of a subjective sense of anxiety, sweating, shakiness in her legs, and a pounding in her chest.

As time passed, Donna became frightened of being alone, lest the attacks reoccur. Her husband had to work, however, and one day while Donna was driving to a store, she had another attack. After this experience Donna would feel intense anxiety when she tried to leave the house. She accommodated to this by staying indoors, near a phone, so that she could call her husband if she had an emergency. Donna soon became "housebound." She began calling her husband at work frequently during the day, in order to receive reassuring contact. If he was unavailable, she would begin to feel anxious. Donna's "disability" required many adjustments by her husband. He had to take over all her outdoor chores and errands, including all the shopping for the family. Only when Donna's frequent phone calls at work caused problems with his supervisor did her husband demand that she seek treatment. At this point Donna had not been out of the house (except for a few minutes in the yard) for 17 months.

The *social phobia* involves an irrational fear and avoidance of situations in which one must interact with others. The fear usually involves the possibility of humiliation or embarrassment by others. A common example is disabling anxiety over public speaking. One can see how incapacitating such a phobia would be in, for example, a college instructor! The following case example illustrates agoraphobia and social phobia in the same individual:

A man of thirty-nine complained that he had fear of open spaces, of large rooms, and of meeting people. The reason he gave was that such situations produced "panics" in which he felt giddy, trembled, had curious sensations in his legs, and saw everything as if through a mist. The panic lasted sometimes for many minutes, and in the intervals he was always more or less apprehensive of them. He had been subject to occasional panics in open spaces or large buildings since later childhood, but this had not interfered with his work until four months before he came for advice. They had increased in frequency until he was entirely disabled. The first panic of any kind had occurred in a schoolroom when he was eleven years of age, when there was an epidemic of mumps in the school and the patient feared he might be infected. Suddenly he felt a lump in his throat, and wondered if it meant mumps. A schoolmate said, "You look pale—are you ill?" and the patient promptly became very much afraid and had a panic similar in all respects to those from which he suffered in later life. The patient was married with one child . . . and his wife in the last eighteen months had seemed very cold towards him. He had a

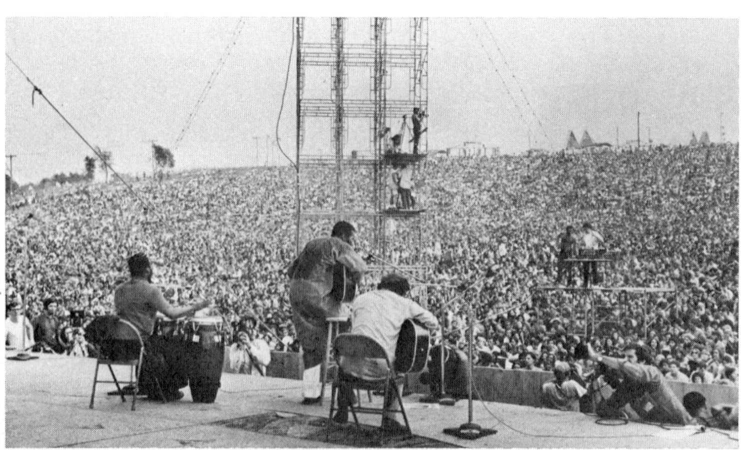

For some people, being part of a vast and packed crowd like the one shown in this photo of a rock concert would create intolerable anxiety.

feeling of guilt with regard to her, because he had flirted a good deal about a year ago. . . . In addition to this, he gave in response to inquiry the information that he was in business or partnership with his father-in-law. Business had not been going well for the past two years. He was in some awe of his father-in-law, feeling that he was inferior to him, and was afraid to discuss business with him. Another relative was in the same business and the patient did not get on well with her. His financial affairs were in a serious muddle. . . . (Henderson & Gillespie, 1969, p. 242)

When individuals' irrational fears compel them to avoid contact with objects or situations other than those described above, the disorder is classified as a *simple phobia*. This classification includes the many phobias of objects, which most frequently involve animals. If the object is avoidable, little impairment may occur; but if confronted by the phobic object or situation, the individual may suffer an extreme panic attack. The simple phobia appears to often begin in childhood, a time when many unrealistic fears are not uncommon. Mussen, Conger, and Kagen (1974) have found that about 20 percent of childhood fears are unrealistic, and these unrealistic fears seem stronger than realistic ones. However, most such fears are outgrown. Direct confrontation with the phobic object is not necessary for the individual to experience turmoil. The phobia may cause difficulty when the individual thinks about the phobic object. Some simple phobias also decline with age. For example, notice in Figure 7.3 that the incidence of fear of injections peaks at age 10, remains constant until age 20, and then declines. A similar decline is seen in regard to snake phobia after the age of 20. In contrast, fear of crowds (social phobia) is most prevalent between the ages 50 to 65. The case that follows illustrates a simple phobia:

Mrs. R. M., a housewife in her thirties, has had an irrational fear of sharks for years. Although she has no contact with sharks, the fear prevents her from viewing movies or television programs with such creatures involved, and even reading about them leads to unpleasant anxiety experiences. She has always been aware of the irrational character of the fear, but this was recently emphasized when she felt forced to reject a free three-week cruise on a ship captained by her brother, because the ship would travel out of the Great Lakes and St. Lawrence Seaway into the Atlantic Ocean. The decision evoked anxiety reactions until she resolved to reject the offer. She currently prefers to live with the phobia, as treatment sounds "painful" to her (in terms of facing the anxiety) and she believes that such a major interference in her life is unlikely to occur again.

In discussing the development of anxiety, we

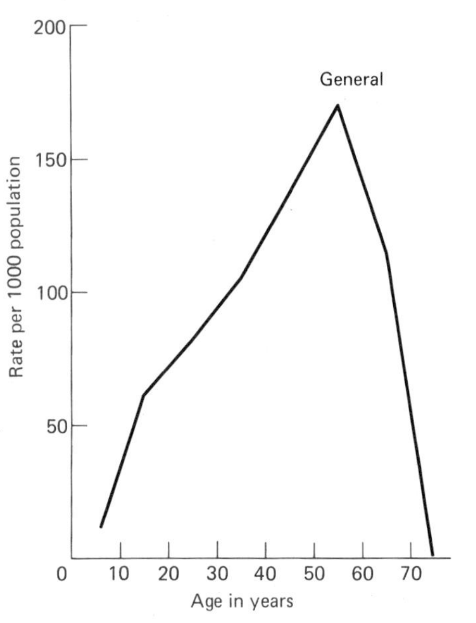

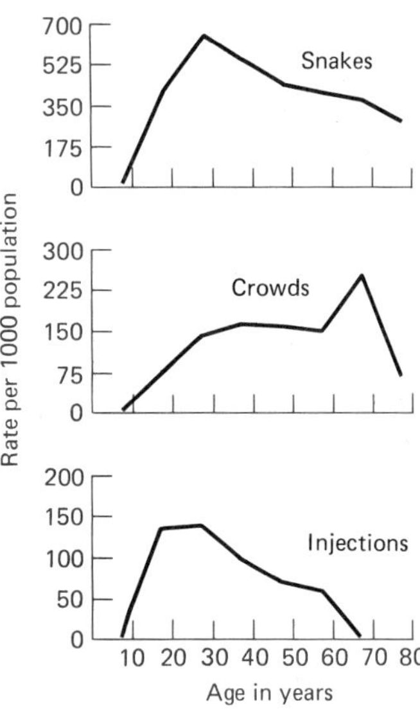

Figure 7.3.
Prevalence rates for phobias vary with age in the general population, and appear to peak at different ages for various phobias.
Adapted from Agras, Sylvester, and Oliveau (1969, p. 153).

saw that many researchers have studied the possibility of innate physiological differences in autonomic reactivity, and some have found evidence that these differences may be inherited. In a study of basically normal twins, Torgersen (1979) found greater concordances for identical twins than for fraternal twins on some types of fears. Torgersen was studying fears which, if exaggerated, would be considered phobias. However, we must remember that identical twins are more likely to have more similar environments than fraternal twins. We have already seen that evidence for the direct inheritance of specific anxiety disorders is inconclusive. What might account for one person being phobic and another not, and why would one person develop a phobia and another develop a generalized anxiety reaction?

Phobia as a Learned Disorder. The conditioned fear hypothesis of phobia has been a classic one since Watson and Rayner's (1920) experiment on Little Albert (see Chapter 2). In this experiment a neutral stimulus (a white rat) was paired with a stimulus that evoked an unconditioned fear response (a steel bar was loudly banged to frighten the child). After several pairings of these stimuli, presentation of the white rat alone frightened Albert and he attempted to get away. (He would huddle in a far corner of his crib when the rat was introduced.) This conditioned fear appeared to generalize to other objects similar to the furry rat, such as a rabbit, a fur coat, and a Santa Claus mask. Many investigators suggest that phobias develop like Albert's fear of the white rat. A traumatic event is associated with a stimulus, and the stimulus later results in phobic behavior. For example, a child who is attacked by a snarling dog may generalize this fear to all dogs, and end up as an adult with a simple phobia toward dogs, even those that appear friendly. Thus, the adult's fear of all dogs or big dogs or brown dogs depends on the circumstances of a traumatic event years before, and indeed appears irrational. The following case history illustrates the development of an irrational fear apparently precipitated by a classic conditioning experience.

> Sally was hospitalized at age 20 months and underwent major chest surgery, with no preparation for or subsequent explanation of the experience and the resulting scar. After her hospitalization, Sally changed from a happy, outgoing, affectionate, apparently well-adjusted toddler to a withdrawn child, excessively fearful of doctors, strangers, and of noise and faces on the television.
>
> In spite of improved physical health, nurturance by the family, and patience on the part of medical personnel, exposure to doctors continued to cause Sally to cry hysterically and shake visibly. Because frequent medical visits were salient reality factors, Sally was referred for treatment 4 months after surgery to reduce doctor- and hospital-related fear reactions. [Her phobia had also generalized to elevators, as became apparent when she had to visit a dentist for a routine screening.] Sally entered the dental school in high spirits, but once she was in the elevator her exuberance turned almost immediately to debilitating dread. She sobbed and started to shake perceptibly. Sensing her panic, I held Sally to comfort her and cut short our visit to the building. Later information that Sally's only prior experience with elevators had been during her hospitalization made her dramatically labile emotions more understandable. (Wallick, 1979, pp. 1325–1326)

If this child had not been successfully treated, she might have grown into an adult with an apparently irrational fear of doctors and elevators. In Sally's case we can see that a traumatic event is associated with the phobic stimuli. However, Rachman (1977) has noted that many situations or objects associated with traumatic experiences do not become phobic stimuli. For example, despite several million auto accidents every year, the frequency of automobile phobias is not high.

The recognition that certain situations or objects have an unusually high frequency as phobic stimuli has led to the suggestion that humans have a predisposition to be easily conditioned to some stimuli, but not others (Seligman, 1971). This **preparedness theory** also involves the notion that certain unpleasant experiences may be more easily associated with certain types of neutral stimuli. For example, nausea is an unpleasant experience that is more likely to be associated with recently eaten food (even though the nausea is a result of the flu) than is the unpleasant experience of a headache (even though the headache may be due to a food allergy). The idea of preparedness has been examined in a study of conditioning using pictures of two stimuli that are uncommon phobic objects (a house and faces) and one stimulus of a common phobic object (snakes) (Öhman, Erixon, & Löfberg, 1975). All the subjects in the study were presented with all three sets of pictures, but half were given an electric shock (an unconditioned stimulus) immediately after seeing each of the pictures of a snake (a conditioned stimulus). The other half were shocked only after viewing either each picture of a house or after viewing each picture of a face. All three conditioned stimuli elicited about the same degree of autonomic arousal (measured by change in the electrodermal response) in the subjects. That is, each type of object (face, house, or snake) elicited the same degree of conditioned fear at the end of this phase of the experiment. Although these data seem to suggest that preparedness was not a factor, the conditioned fear (or autonomic arousal) elicited by the pictures of snakes was more resistant to extinction than the fear elicited by photos of faces or houses (results convincingly replicated by Hugdahl & Karker, 1981, using different phobic and nonphobic stimuli). These findings have also been amplified by the demonstration that fears are more easily conditioned in individuals who have high levels of initial physiological arousal (Hugdahl, Fredrikson, & Öhman, 1977). People who have low levels of autonomic responsivity are less easily conditioned to have fear responses to neutral stimuli.

Does the combination of high levels of autonomic reactivity and preparedness and classical conditioning make sense as an overall explanation for the development of phobias? One problem has consistently been noted: Most phobics do not seem to have had a specific traumatic experience with the feared object or situation (e.g., Eysenck, 1976). Something more must be involved.

May modeling be important in the development of phobic disorder? Social learning theorists, such as Albert Bandura, think so. Many laboratory experiments have demonstrated that fear responses can be learned by modeling or imitative learning. It is not difficult to imagine a child attending to increased tension levels of a parent who is in the presence of something the parent is afraid of. Nor is it difficult to imagine a parent directly communicating to a child that something is to be feared. (An interesting way of looking at these types of modeling behaviors is to consider that they may constitute the process in which preparedness develops.) In the case of Sally, we have no information about the parents' reaction to her initial hospitalization. Did they communicate to her their own fears about her surgery? either overtly or subtly? Perhaps they were so solicitous after her surgery that Sally found she received rewarding attention if she behaved fearfully when she had to visit a doctor (operant learning). If her parents responded by removing her from the situation (the doctor's office), Sally would soon feel better, and would realize that she could avoid unpleasant consequences by behaving fearfully.

Phobias seem to be due to the interaction of multiple factors. Weekes (1978), for example, approaches phobias as a problem of multiple causation. She has found that persons with phobic disorders, particularly agoraphobia, first experience heightened autonomic arousal. Then they have a panic experience during a time of major stress, and are indecisive about coping procedures. They experience bewilderment, constant anxious introspection, and discover that avoidance of some object or situation provides relief. In her formulation, deep-rooted psychodynamic conflicts may well be operative in the development of the phobic behavior.

Psychodynamic Factors. The psychodynamic perspective conceptualizes phobic behavior as a defense against the recognition of threatening sexual or aggressive impulses. Anxiety, which is experienced when the impulses threaten to break through into consciousness, is displaced onto the phobic object. By avoiding the phobic object or situation, the individual avoids recognition of the impulses and reduces the danger that they will break through. Another psychodynamic concept of phobia is the displacement of anxiety to defend the self-concept. Feeling threatened by some situation which they feel expected to cope with, individuals displace the anxiety and fear onto an object or situation of secondary importance which can be more easily defended against, such as snakes. The defense, of course, is ineffective, since the original anxiety producer remains active, in effect, "feeding" the phobia.

For example, an individual on the way to a supervisory conference with an employer is angry about being called in. The anger may arouse deep-seated aggressive impulses. However, such impulses cannot be expressed because of the threat of losing the job. The danger that the impulses present result in anxiety, yet the individual cannot admit to being anxious about such feelings because he or she "knows" that one should "be able to handle meetings with bosses." The anxiety is then displaced onto the elevator which one must ride in order to get to the boss's office. By avoiding the elevator, the individual avoids recognizing the aggressive impulses, and may even be able to avoid confrontation with the employer. However, this behavior is self-defeating in the long run. The individual avoids the expression of forbidden impulses for the moment, but has a phobia which will cause future difficulty. Such a formulation involves a great deal of inference about what is "really" going on inside the person's unconscious processes, and is difficult to demonstrate experimentally.

Obsessive-Compulsive Disorder

Individuals may have only obsessive thoughts, they may have only compulsive behaviors, or they may have both **obsessions** and **compulsions.** In one study of 150 obsessional patients, for example, 69 percent had obsessions and compulsions, 25 percent had only obsessions, and 6 percent had only compulsions (Wilner et al., 1976). *Obsessions* are unshakable, recurrent thoughts. Obsessive thoughts are occasionally experienced by most of us, at least in the minor way that a word or song lyric runs through our thoughts for a few minutes or hours. Normal examples of compulsive behavior include "magical" thinking, as manifested in superstitions such as knocking on wood to prevent unlucky occurrences, throwing spilled salt over one's shoulder to prevent bad luck, and avoiding walking under ladders for the same reason. However, for the true obsessive, the thought, idea, impulse, or image is extremely persistent, seems involuntary, and is usually unpleasant or threatening. *Compulsions* are behaviors (such as cleaning, washing hands, manipulating objects) repeated with a ritualistic pattern, often at a very high frequency. They actually have no functional end (the hands are already clean), but may be momentarily tension reducing. The individuals see themselves as compelled to engage in what they perceive as irrational behavior. They cannot resist the compulsion without experiencing a discomforting escalating sense of tension, which is reduced when they "give in" (Carr, 1971). Some individuals' recognition that the behavior is irrational may lead to an increase in overall anxiety. Though the disorder is relatively rare, Akhter et al. (1975) studied a group of 82 obsessive-compulsive subjects and found several categories of obsessions and compulsions.

Obsessions

1. Obsessive Doubts: Recurrent thoughts that a previously completed task had not been appropriately finished were found in 75 percent of the subjects.
2. Obsessive Thinking: Interminable chains of thought about future events that might affect them were experienced by 34 percent of the subjects.
3. Obsessive Fears: Fears about loss of self-control and doing something embarrassing plagued 26 percent of the subjects.
4. Obsessive Impulses: Of those interviewed, 17 percent had strong impulses to engage in behaviors ranging from silly acts, such as drinking ink, to assaultive behavior.
5. Obsessive Images: A small proportion (7 percent) were bothered by cognitive images of imagined events or by images of events recently seen. These images were most often unpleasant; for example, a woman imagined her infant being flushed down a toilet.

Compulsions

1. Yielding Compulsions: Of the subjects, 61 percent yielded to an obsessive urge and were compelled to engage in the act.
2. Controlling Compulsions: Of the subjects, 6 percent were able to avoid acting on an obsession by repetitively engaging in an alternative behavior. In effect, the alternative ritual gave control over the threatened urge; for example, counting to 10 to avoid an obsessive sexual impulse.

The compulsions and obsessions are characteristically **ego alien**, that is, foreign to individuals' perception of themselves, and thus distressing. In contrast, behaviors such as "compulsive" gambling or "compulsive" drinking are usually considered enjoyable by the individual who engages in them and are not categorized as obsessive-compulsive disorders. When true compulsive behavior is interrupted, the individual may experience a flood of anxiety. For these reasons, obsessive-compulsive behavior has often been conceptualized as a defense (although an ineffective one) against anxiety-provoking impulses. In some cases, situational anxiety or stress appear to be important precursors to the development of the obsession or compulsion. In the developmental sequence of the behaviors, most individuals find that the problem escalates and gradually involves more and more of their daily life and activity. Individuals with this disorder are often described as bright, with a tendency to intellectualize (focus on thinking rather than emotions), and to have been orderly and rigid throughout their lives. In addition, they are often described as relatively emotionally cold, controlling, stubborn, and insensitive to others. The obsessive-compulsive disorder can be extremely disabling, and frequently has associated symptoms of anxiety and depression. The following case excerpt illustrates obsessional fears, compulsive behavior, and the widespread impact they have on a person's life-style (Rachman & Hodgson, 1980).

> [A] severely disturbed woman, was . . . dominated by her obsessional fears and washing compulsions. Practically every action of every day was planned and assessed in terms of the probability of contracting cancerous contamination. It determined where she lived, and when she moved (frequently), it determined what clothing she was free to wear (very few items indeed). It determined whom she could speak to and whom she could touch (practically no one). It determined the homes and public places that she could visit (very few). It determined the type of work she could undertake (very limited and always unsatisfactory). The risk of contamination precluded any form of sexual activity. She was unable to pick up any reading material except and unless she wore protective clothing. Her conversation was confined mainly to a discussion of her fears and the actions she was obliged to take in order to avoid or escape from them. Ultimately, after thirty years of this form of existence, the obsessions and compulsions had become the core and substance of her entire life. (p. 59)

Physiological Factors. As with the other anxiety disorders discussed in this chapter, a common hypothesis about individuals who develop obsessive-compulsive disorders is that they are especially prone to states of pathological physiological arousal (e.g., Beech & Perigault, 1974). The evidence supporting this type of predisposition in anxiety disorders as a group is, of course, applicable to obsessive-compulsive disorder. Rachman and Hodgson (1980) have summarized the tentative research findings specifically related to obsessive-compulsive disorder. When obsessive-compulsive individuals are exposed to real or imagined stimulation of the obsessive thought or compulsion, autonomic arousal increases. Execution of the ritualistic behavior is followed by a prompt decline in arousal and a decline in subjective discomfort. Since most studies are of individuals who already have the disorder, we do not know if this physiological overreactivity is present before the disorder develops. However, many researchers and clinicians suspect that it is, and we can expect further research on this issue.

Another area of study that is relevant to the physiology of obsessive-compulsives is the **habituation** of the arousal response. Habituation is a common phenomenon of autonomic arousal in most individuals. If a stimulus that arouses an autonomic response is presented to a subject repeatedly, the magnitude of the autonomic response diminishes. The individual becomes habituated to the stimulus. If obsessive-compulsives do not experience physiological habituation, or experience less or slower habituation than normal, their irrational thoughts and behaviors continue to first arouse a physiological reaction and then decrease it. For example, obsessive thoughts about contamination would arouse an autonomic response, cleaning would decrease the response, and a repetitive cycle would ensue. If the individual is prevented from doing the cleaning, the arousal associated with the obsessive thoughts will not habituate (decrease in level) or will do so more slowly. Once the individual is free to engage in the response, the compulsive cleaning is likely to occur in order to reduce subjective discomfort. This deficit in habituation, if present, could explain why obsessive-compulsive disorders last for so many years and why they are so resistant to treatment. Rachman and Hodgson (1980) have pointed out the lack of studies of habituation with obsessive-compulsives, but such research is likely to occur in the near future. The existence of a physiological overreactivity (either genetically transmitted or otherwise developed) could be very important in the development and maintenance of the obsessive-compulsive disorder.

Learning and Obsessive-Compulsive Disorder. The discussion of factors relating to the development of generalized anxiety disorder and panic presented some evidence that subjects' ability to control and predict aversive stimulation is important in determining whether they feel anxious. In addition, studies have found that anxious individuals have more irrational beliefs than people who do not have anxiety disorders. The way people think about the world and their place in it may interact with other factors in the development of obsessive-compulsive behavior. Carr (1974) suggests that obsessive-compulsives adopt a cognitive view of life that overestimates the probability of potentially harmful events. All of us, for example, encounter daily situations where we are exposed to bacteria that might cause disease. The obsessive-compulsive overestimates the likelihood and potential danger of these encounters and, thus, according to Carr, is more likely to engage in certain behaviors to ward off the threat.

This particular cognitive set (and other relevant cognitions) could be learned from a lifetime of consistent experiences within the family. The families of persons who develop obsessive-compulsive behavior tend to share certain characteristics (Adams, 1973). The parents generally are very concerned with correct behavior and in believing "the right thing." The families are generally formal in their relationships with each other, and seem to lack warmth in their interactions. They emphasize "good" behavior and "good" thoughts and are critical of "bad" thoughts and behaviors.

A social learning perspective would consider obsessive-compulsive behavior to be learned partly through modeling. The rigid behaviors of the compulsive are modeled from the parents. The child who deviates from the rules experiences anxiety, and this unpleasant emotion is reduced by "being good"; the compulsively correct behavior then is reinforced by anxiety reduction (Meyer & Chesser, 1970). However, most studies have indicated that the children of obsessive-compulsive parents (from whom these behaviors could most easily be modeled) are not likely to have an obsessive-compulsive disorder (Rachman & Hodgson, 1980). Rather, the studies indicate that obsessive parental behavior may lead to a generalized anxious behavior pattern in the child, which is fertile soil for the development of a obsessive-compulsive disorder.

Could obsessive-compulsive behavior be due to direct operant reinforcement? Skinner (1948) demonstrated that pigeons could be taught what he called "superstitious" behavior ("purposeless" ritualistic behavior) through shaping and reinforcement. This discovery has been used to support the notion that obsessive or compulsive behavior may develop from chance reinforcement of human behavior. If parents are extremely involved in teaching their children to have the "right" thoughts, and children model such behavior, and if compulsiveness is an important life-style in the household, it would not be surprising that the child who has "wrong" thoughts experiences shame, guilt, and anxiety. It would be quite likely for the child (or adult) to experience anxiety relief by engaging in a compulsive behavior, particularly when the behavior is associated with "bad" thoughts. For example, individuals who are having "dirty" (sexual) thoughts might feel that these make them dirty (an irrational belief). They might then discover that washing their hands helps them feel clean and reduces their anxiety. Soon they might be washing their hands frequently to avoid feeling dirty in the first place.

If the contributions of behavioral social learning theory are viewed in the context of what we know about the physiological responses of obsessive-compulsive individuals, the development of these disorders seems more understandable. An individual with a predisposition to overreactivity of the autonomic nervous system learns through modeling that one should have good, clean, correct thoughts. The likelihood of anyone having a bad thought is probably fairly high, and the potential obsessive-compulsive would be very discomforted by such ideas. When the thought leaves (as all thoughts eventually do), the discomfort would be relieved. As an alternative, the individual might find discomfort reduced by certain cleaning behaviors or other rituals. Thus, the person would be intensly reinforced by trying to avoid certain thoughts (a difficult task) and by engaging in ritualistic behaviors. Although the formulation is very simplified here, the combination of physiological predisposition, childhood modeling, and operant reinforcement provides the underlying structure for many clinicians' views of obsessive-compulsive disorder.

Psychoanalytic Concepts. Psychoanalytic concepts are a major alternative to behavioral or social learning views of obsessive-compulsive disorder. The psychoanalytic concept of the development of the obsessive-compulsive disorder again involves the notion of instinctual processes breaking through into behavior, and a resulting defense reaction. The impulses are seen as mainly aggressive (sometimes sexual) and due to a fixation at the anal level of development. The fixation is presumed to result from rigid and harsh toilet training by the parents. The obsessive-compulsive symptoms usually represent an unsuccessful attempt to defend against the id impulse and against the anxiety resulting from threatened punishment of the impulse. At times the defenses do not work, and the id impulses break through in symbolic form (the obsessive thoughts). When the **ego defenses** or defense mechanisms are marshaled, the thoughts can be pushed away, or ritualized behavior can be used to symbolically banish them.

The defenses used by obsessive-compulsives include **intellectualization:** They isolate their feelings from their thinking. They use reaction formation: They become concerned, for example, with cleanliness or morality to avoid impulses to be dirty (which symbolize "dirty sex"), or they become orderly to defend against chaotic aggression. They may use "undoing" to defend against aggressive behavior. In the play *Macbeth,* using undoing Lady Macbeth ritualistically washes her hands to remove imaginary blood which symbolizes her involvement in a murder. The obsessive-compulsive may engage in ritualized behaviors to undo the harm of even "feeling like" hurting someone. A parent might be compulsively careful about preparing meals in order to avoid an **unconscious impulse** to poison a spouse or children.

Whether or not their impulses are instinctual, many obsessive-compulsives have thoughts or impulses to act which they see as unacceptable to others, and they seem to defend against these impulses or thoughts by engaging in other behaviors which may become ritualistic. In addition, they often feel they have engaged in behavior or thoughts which they themselves feel are wrong or bad. Many of their actions seem to be an attempt to undo the action symbolically, and to remove the guilt they feel about the bad behavior. As has been noted, psychoanalytic views about human behavior have not been subjected to rigorous research. They are based on theoretical speculation about clinical cases using retrospective data.

FINAL COMMENTS ON ETIOLOGY

Many theories have been proposed to account for the anxiety disorders. Some theories have research support; others are supported by the experience of clinicians and tentative experimental findings. Still other theories are predominantly supported by retrospective clinical data and theorists' speculation. The data and theories presented in this chapter allow some tentative conclusions to be drawn.

1. Individuals with anxiety disorders appear to be more autonomically reactive than normal individuals. This overreactivity may be genetically transmitted, but we are not sure. This reactivity seems to be a predisposition in the development of anxiety disorder.

2. Learning, both in the form of reinforcement through reduction in anxiety and in the form of modeling, seems very important in the development of anxiety disorders.

3. Cognitions are important in the development of anxiety disorders in the form of mediating thoughts and self-perceptions.

4. Childhood experiences are important either in terms of what one is directly or indirectly taught, and possibly in terms of more obscure factors like those dealt with from a psychodynamic perspective. Research evidence in support of psychoanalytic concepts such as psychosexual stages of development, unconscious processes, fixation, and defense mechanisms is unsatisfactory, yet psychoanalytic and psychodynamic explanations remain persuasive for many clinicians.

KEY TREATMENTS

The prevalence of anxiety disorders is such that most people suffering from these disorders "grimace and bear it" and do not seek treatment. For those who do, several possibilities are available. Many people seek help from their family physician, and are prescribed **tranquilizing medication** (such as Valium or Librium), which supresses the symptoms of their disorder and allows about 70 percent to function at a higher level. This may be the most common treatment approach, as more tranquilizers are sold in the United States than all other medications combined. This approach, however, does nothing to resolve the central issue of self-defeating behavior.

Psychotherapy

Individuals who suffer extremely from recurrent panic attacks, generalized anxiety, phobic behavior, or compulsions and obsessions may seek psychotherapy. This is more likely if they recognize that these behaviors are extremely self-defeating. If the therapist is psychoanalytically oriented, the therapy will focus on uncovering buried childhood experiences and repressed wishes. This uncovering occurs in a procedure called free association. In traditional analysis, the patient lies on a couch and engages in an unrestrained monologue. The analyst pays special attention not only to what the patient says, but also to what he avoids saying. The patient is likely to avoid talking about thoughts or feelings associated with the repressed conflict or impulses. Dreams which the patient relates are analyzed in terms of symbolic meanings, since they are presumed to be a window into the unconscious. As the repressed impulses or conflicts are uncovered, the patient "works through" them. This **working through** process involves reliving old experiences in the context of an intense emotional relationship with the analyst, called **transference.**

In transference, the patient transfers irrational feelings onto the analyst. The analyst, in effect, is experienced and treated by the patient in much the same way that the patient related to the parents. The therapist interprets these reactions to the patient, who, over a long period, gains a deep insight into his or her behavior. The insight, which is both emotional and intellectual, strengthens the ego, so that instinctual drives can be expressed appropriately, realistically, and in a socially acceptable manner. The anxiety is no longer necessary as a danger signal, and the defense mechanisms are no longer needed, since the instinctual impulses can now be expressed in acceptable ways. This form of psychotherapy is complicated and time consuming. Critics argue that it focuses too much on insight and not enough on behavior. Psychoanalytic therapy is more extensively presented and evaluated in Chapter 20, with other forms of treatment.

If the individual seeks treatment from a Rogerian client-centered counselor, the focus will in contrast be on the here and now. The counselor will attempt to create a therapeutic situation in which the client feels unconditionally accepted. This acceptance allows the client to examine her self-defeating behavior, see the problems involved, and try out new behavior which will help her cope with the anxiety-provoking situation or with the anxiety itself.

In this humanistic approach, the important factors in treatment are the clients' recognition that the therapist values the client unconditionally, that the therapist understands the client's dilemma, and has empathy for her. A therapist who is "genuine," that is, who behaves honestly and is caring, enables the client to get "in touch" with "real" feelings; then behavior can become congruent with these feelings, and the anxiety will no longer be overwhelming.

Behavioral approaches to anxiety disorders

Behavioral approaches have been remarkably successful with the anxiety disorders (Barlow & Wolfe, 1981). While the behavior therapies tend to focus on specific behaviors or symptoms, they appear to have broad positive effects on the individual's overall functioning (Marks, 1978). The basic presumption of these approaches is that the individual has learned to manifest anxiety to a particular situation (as in phobias); or if the anxiety is not situation specific, the anxiety has generalized to many situations. Generalized anxiety is often treated through biofeedback and/or relaxation therapy. In biofeedback, manifestations of autonomic arousal such as muscle tension are monitored, and feedback is provided to the subject. In another example, the temperature of a finger might be measured. A low finger temperature implies cardiovascular constriction that is due to autonomic nervous system arousal; an increase in temperature implies dilation of the blood vessels from relaxation. The subject is taught to relax, gaining some control over the ANS. This learning is generalized through practice under a variety of conditions, and is used to abort the experience of anxiety.

Systematic densensitization is an anxiety reduction procedure based on a classical conditioning model. In this procedure, conditioned anxiety is counterconditioned utilizing the concept of **reciprocal inhibition,** the idea that anxiety is inhibited (cannot be present) when an antagonistic response is manifested. One response considered antagonistic to anxiety is relaxation. If a phobia is being treated with this procedure, the therapist and client first identify the phobic object or situation. They then develop a **hierarchy** (graded series) of events or situations which arouse the phobic anxiety. For example, in the case of a fear of enclosed spaces, the hierarchy might begin as follows: "1. being in a fenced in yard, 2. being in a house, 3. being in my living room, 4. being in a bathroom, 5. thinking about being in a narrow corridor."

The hierarchy would continue in graded steps to the most anxiety-provoking settings: "17. walking down a hallway, 18. knowing I have to get my coat from a closet, 19. standing in a closet with the door open, 20. being locked in a small, dark closet."

In the next step the therapist would teach the client a procedure that leads to relaxation. The therapist might teach the client a series of exercises involving alternate tensing and relaxation of voluntary muscles, might use relaxing imagery (lying on a sun-dappled beach), or a combination of both. After several sessions of instruction and practice, when the client can effectively use the relaxation exercise, the therapist and client return to the developed hierarchy. The client is instructed to visualize the first anxiety item on this hierarchy. If the patient can remain relaxed during the presentation, the procedure continues and a next higher stimulus on the hierarchy is presented. The task of the patient and therapist is to move through the hierarchy to even more potentially threatening stimuli, with the patient consistently remaining relaxed. If the patient becomes anxious (as is likely), the therapist "desensitizes" the patient (reduces the level of anxiety using the previously taught relaxation procedure during several presentations of the stimulus) and gradually moves on to stimuli higher in the hierarchy.

When the client is able to vividly imagine the most anxiety-provoking item on the hierarchy and consistently remain relaxed, the procedure is complete. Some therapists try to go a step further and may accompany the client into a real life setting where the phobic object or situation is present, in order to continue the desensitization. However, even when this is not done, therapists have consistently reported successful anxiety reduction in 8 or more out of 10 people treated with this procedure (Kazdin & Wilcoxon, 1976; Wolpe, 1981).

Another technique used with anxiety is **cognitive rehearsal.** This can be used when the individual becomes anxious about doing something because of expected failure. Suppose an individual becomes anxious when confronted with the need to talk to

In systematic desensitization, the therapist uses a relaxation technique to prepare the client for confronting anxiety-provoking experiences. Photo shows Dr. Lazarus of Princeton, N.J. conducting a relaxation session with several clients.

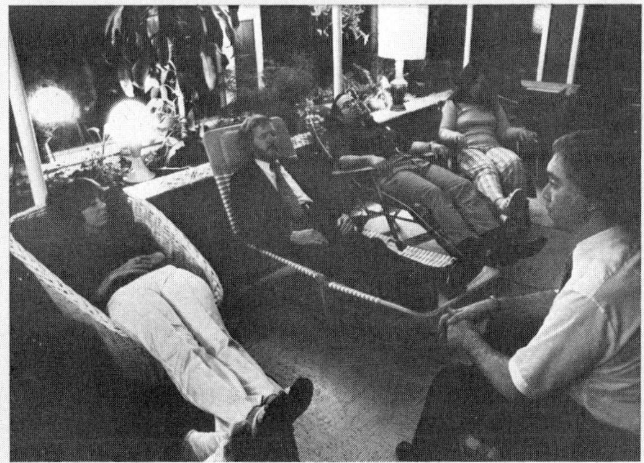

strangers or slight acquaintances because "I won't know what to say." The therapist works with the client to develop strategies so that the client will know what to say; for example, developing a "script" of what to say when introducing oneself, or topics for conversation. The client then rehearses the conversations or behaviors mentally, perhaps even practicing them with the therapist. These behavioral techniques may be used in conjunction with other behavioral approaches, such as direct positive reinforcement of coping skills.

In the obsessive-compulsive disorder, the cognitions or thoughts that the individual has are important. Cognitive therapists have developed several techniques which focus on changing such irrational, intrusive thoughts and beliefs in an attempt to treat these disorders (Mahoney, 1974). We have already seen how cognitions may be significant aspects of the anxiety disorders: the recurrent thought that one's hands are dirty, for example, or that some danger exists in a particular setting or event, when none does. Cognitive therapists may use **thought stopping** to deal with some of these problems. In this procedure, a client has an obsessional thought, the therapist presents a distracting stimulus (yelling "Stop!") when the patient indicates that the thought is present. The distraction often terminates the obsessive thought. The process is repeated several times and the client begins to say "Stop" rather than the therapist. Finally, the client silently says "Stop." When successful, the client has a mental technique which can be used anywhere to stop obsessive ruminations.

In many obsessive-compulsive disorders, the individual's prime concern is the compulsive ritualistic behavior. Rather than focus on the cognitions or thoughts, some therapists simply try to stop the ritualistic behavior. Foa, Steketee, and Milby (1980) studied the relative effectiveness of two techniques for this purpose. In one technique, "exposure," the subject is repeatedly exposed to the discomfort-evoking stimuli (in this case, dirt), with the underlying assumption that eventually the stimuli will no longer evoke discomfort. The other technique is "response prevention"; the subjects are simply prevented from engaging in the ritualistic response (washing). Foa et al. studied two groups of four patients each. Group A was first treated with exposure, then with exposure and response prevention combined. Group B was treated first with response prevention alone, and then with response prevention and exposure both. The results are shown in Figure 7.4. In this study, response prevention was a highly effective rapid technique for the reduction of ritualistic washing behavior, more effective and rapid than exposure to the discomfort-evoking stimuli. However, response prevention did not reduce the subjective sense of anxiety, while exposure did. When the treatments were combined, during the period from phase 1 to posttreatment, ritualistic behavior and subjective anxiety were reduced about the same degree in both groups. The combination of response prevention and exposure has been reported to be effective, and to yield positive long-term results (at least two years) in other controlled studies (see Rachman & Hodgson, 1980).

Treatments of anxiety disorders consist primarily of either tranquilizing medication, psychotherapy, or behavior therapy. Unfortunately, most persons who could benefit from such treatments probably do not take the opportunity to use them. Furthermore, the treatments do not help every individual who attempts them. It would simplify matters tremendously if we could say that one of these treatments was clearly superior to the others, or that a specific treatment was the best one for a specific disorder. At this point such claims cannot be made. In Chapter 20, the various treatment approaches will be evaluated more fully, and the reasons that categorical statements cannot be made will become clearer.

Figure 7.4. Mean washing times for group A and group B.

In phase 1, group A was treated with exposure only and group B with response prevention only. In phase 2, both groups received exposure and response prevention treatments. From Foa et al. (1980, p. 73).

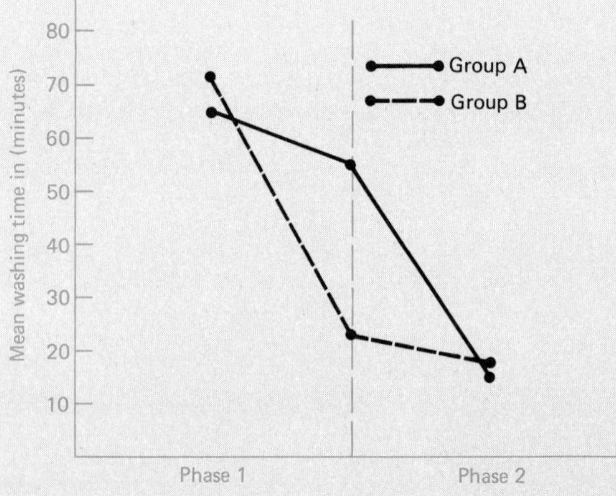

Summary

1. Anxiety may be one of the more universal human phenomena, ranging from mild to severe from individual to individual. The term is used to conceptualize the subjective experience, behaviors, and objective physiological manifestations we sometimes call fear. Although there is not universal agreement on its definition, anxiety remains a useful concept, and attempts at reliable measurement and refinement of its identification continue.

2. For some individuals, anxiety apparently becomes such a serious problem that it, or the person's reaction to it, significantly interferes with adaptive functioning. Their behavior becomes disordered. The disorders which have been theoretically related to anxiety have been presented. The chapter covers the anxiety disorders of panic and generalized anxiety states, the phobic disorders, and the obsessive-compulsive disorder.

3. Panic disorder consists of recurrent short-term episodes of intense anxiety. Generalized anxiety disorder consists of chronic, somewhat less intense anxiety, which is subjectively discomforting.

4. Consistent evidence exists supporting innate differences in ease and magnitude of arousal of the autonomic nervous system. Autonomic overreactivity may be a predisposing factor in the development of the anxiety disorders; however, little evidence supports the idea that a specific anxiety disorder, such as phobia, is inherited.

5. Some learning theorists accept the notion that the degree of generalized autonomic reactivity acts as a predisposition in anxiety disorders; however, they see this reactivity as influenced by learning. Thus, the development of an anxiety disorder may be due to factors such as classical conditioning, avoidance learning, modeling, mediating cognitions, or some combination of them.

6. Psychoanalytic theory proposes that panic and generalized anxiety disorder are due to threatened overstimulation by id impulses. Anxiety is seen as a signal of danger. The individual's discomfort and disturbed behavior is due to the ineffectiveness of the defense mechanisms.

7. Phobic disorder involves the experience of intense anxiety or fear which is associated with a specific object or situation. Common phobias include agoraphobia—fear of being alone or of being in public places; social phobia—fear of situations in which one must interact with others; and simple phobia—fear of any of a number of specific objects, animals, or special situations.

8. A predisposition to autonomic reactivity is considered an important possibility in the development of phobias. Classical conditioning has been considered an important factor in the development of phobias. However, the high frequency of certain objects or situations as phobic stimuli (e.g., snakes, crowds) suggests that people are more prepared to fear some objects than others. Furthermore, modeling of others' fears is considered an important factor, as is the direct reinforcement of avoiding a feared situation.

9. The psychoanalytic formulation of phobias is similar to that of panic and generalized anxiety disorders. It differs in that the anxiety is seen as focused on an object or situation that symbolically represents the unconscious conflict between the impulsive desire and the threat of punishment.

10. Obsessive-compulsive disorder consists of persistent intrusive ego-alien thoughts, compulsive ritualistic behaviors, or a combination of both. The thoughts provoke anxiety, which can be relieved by avoiding the thoughts or by engaging in the compulsive behavior. However, these actions can lead to a resurgence of anxiety, since they are ego alien.

11. Obsessive-compulsive disorder is associated with a suspected predisposition to autonomic overreactivity and a possible deficit in habituation (decline in reactivity upon repeated presentations of a stimulus). Obsessive-compulsives seem to overestimate the likelihood of environmental danger. This and other cognitive factors may be due to childhood experiences in a rigid, overorganized family environment. Physiological reactivity, cognitions, and modeling may combine with direct reinforcement through anxiety relief to produce the obsessions and compulsions.

12. From a psychoanalytic perspective, obsessive-compulsive behavior is believed to be due to a fixation at the anal psychosexual stage of development. The fixation is thought to occur because of overly rigid and harsh toilet training. Obsessions are seen as symbols of id impulses, and compulsions as rituals used to banish the impulse. As is the case for psychoanalytic formulations of the other anxiety disorders, the research evidence in support of this viewpoint is very limited.

13. Psychotherapeutic approaches to the anxiety disorders focus on developing a relationship with the patient. In psychoanalysis the focus is on uncovering buried wishes, impulses, or conflicts through free association or dream analysis. The uncovered material is then worked through in a transference relationship with the therapist. This is an intense, emotionally significant relationship in which the patient is believed to transfer buried irrational feelings onto the therapist. The goal of therapy is intellectual and emotional insight, which strengthens the ego so that id impulses can be accepted and expressed in socially acceptable ways.

14. Client-centered counseling is another common form of psychotherapy for people who have anxiety disorders. It focuses on here-and-now relationships. The patient's history is relatively unimportant. The therapist creates an accepting atmosphere, in which the client feels understood, so that the client can achieve congruence between real feelings and behavior.

15. Behavioral treatment approaches focus on the direct reduction of anxiety. Biofeedback has been used to train individuals to gain control over indirect manifestations of autonomic arousal, such as muscle tension or the temperature of the extremities. Relaxation training is often used in association with the feedback on the autonomic processes. In systematic desensitization, relaxation training is used to develop a relaxed state considered to inhibit anxiety. This state is then used to desensitize the client to a series of progressively more anxiety-provoking stimuli. The stimuli are specific to the anxiety reactions of the client, who has ranked them in a hierarchy.

16. Cognitive therapy has been applied to anxiety disorders in different formats. If an individual is anxious because he expects to fail at some task, a therapist may help him practice cognitions which will prevent anxiety and help him act effectively. This procedure is called cognitive rehearsal. Thought stopping is a technique that can be used with obsessive-compulsives. Obsessive thoughts are interrupted by the therapist who yells "Stop" when the client indicates their occurrence. The client then learns to use the same procedure and to do it silently (mentally yells "Stop").

17. Obsessive-compulsive disorder has consistently been described as extremely resistant to traditional treatment approaches. Recent evidence indicates the effectiveness of a behavioral approach in which the repeated exposure to obsessive or compulsive stimuli (e.g., dirt) is combined with response prevention (the individual is not allowed to engage in the compulsive ritual). The technique is described as effective, relatively rapid, and having effects which last for periods up to several years in individuals who benefit from it.

KEY TERMS

Birth trauma. The inferred subjective experience an infant has at the moment of birth. The transition from the quiet, warm, dark, comfortable womb into a cold, noisy, bright world is speculated to be an important trauma for the infant by many psychodynamically oriented theorists.

Ego alien. Refers to a thought or behavior which an individual feels is out of character or unacceptable. It is experienced as foreign to the concept of self.

Ego defenses. Behaviors identified by psychoanalytically oriented theorists which serve to defend against recognition of unacceptable impulses and anxiety.

Empathy. A deep understanding of another person. Being able to "walk in another's shoes."

State anxiety. A condition of subjective anxiety that is due primarily to external factors.

Trait anxiety. A subjective sense of anxiety that is due to enduring, internal factors of the individual.

Unconscious impulse. An impulse, usually believed to be innate, that the individual has no conscious awareness of.

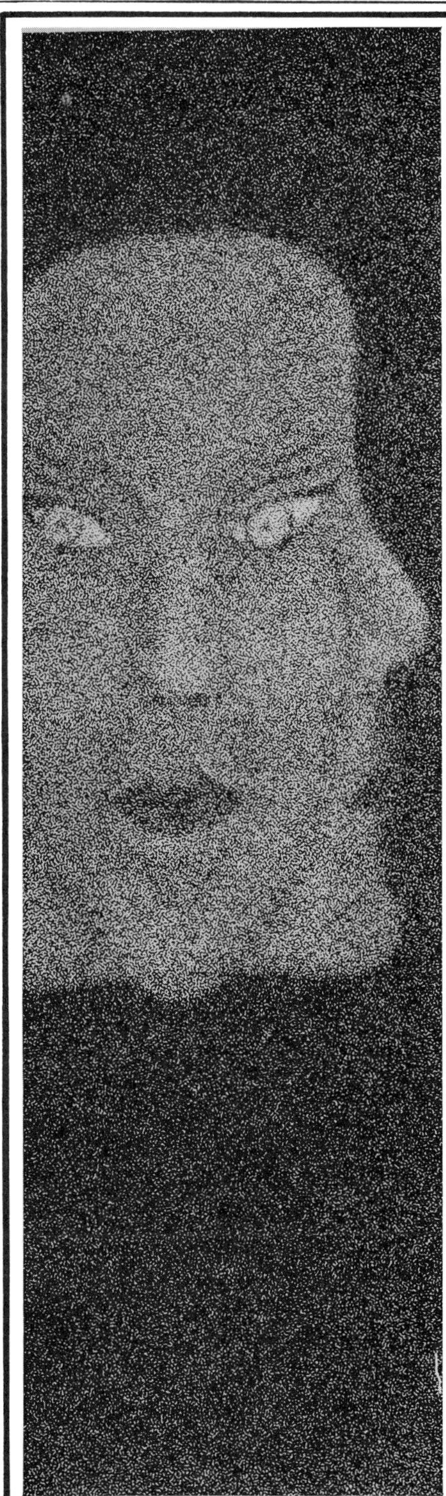

8

Somatoform and dissociative disorders

- Somatoform disorders
- Dissociative disorders
- Summing up
- Key treatments
- Summary
- Key terms

The somatoform and dissociative disorders have traditionally been associated with avoidance of anxiety-provoking situations. Now the evidence is less clear. **"Somatic"** means "pertaining to the body." **Somatoform disorders** have the form of a physical disorder, but do not have a demonstrable physical cause or underlying physiological mechanism. The **dissociative disorders** are named from the phenomenon of **dissociation.** The individuals dissociate themselves from certain behaviors. That is, they seem not to be consciously aware of what they are doing or what they have done in the past. In extreme cases of dissociation, the individual has more than one distinct personality. Dissociative disorders have often been called disorders of consciousness.

SOMATOFORM DISORDERS

The somatoform disorders include **somatization disorder, hypochondriasis, psychogenic pain disorder,** and **conversion disorder.** The extent to which these disorders are clinically distinct remains unclear. Because conversion disorder has the most dramatic symptomatology of the somatoform disorders and has been studied most extensively, it will receive special attention in this section.

Somatization Disorder

Beginning before the age of 30, most frequently in adolescence, somatization disorder is characterized by recurring multiple physical complaints which have no physical cause. Physical symptoms may be **pseudoneurological** (double vision, muscle weakness), gastrointestinal (stomachache, gas, diarrhea), reproductive (painful menstruation, nausea in pregnancy, sexual indifference), or cardiopulmonary (palpitations, chest pain). Pain or a feeling of "sickliness" may be felt for a large part of the subject's life. The complaints are often presented in a dramatic or exaggerated manner. People with this disorder seek medical treatment more frequently than most of us. They apparently interpret their symptoms as having a greater severity than most of us would if we had them. The physical symptoms are commonly experienced by most people at some time in their lives, but most people interpret them as relatively minor and do not seek treatment.

Hypochondriasis

Hypochondriasis is similar to somatization disorder, but it occurs after age 30, and it is characterized by the individual's unrealistic interpretation that relatively common physical sensations are abnormal. This misinterpretation is associated with another major feature, the development of an irrational preoccupation with or fear of having a major disease. The individual cannot be reassured by a medical examination which finds normal physical functioning, and tends to move from physician to physician until one treats the nonexistent disorder. Such individuals often end up being "treated" with **placebos.** Placebos are medically inert substances (such as sugar pills) which have no physical or physiological effect upon the body.

Life for people with hypochondriasis revolves around health and illness. They are almost constantly preoccupied with the functioning of their bodies. They may keep charts of bodily functions such as excretion, digestion, flatulence, and body temperature. They often make special efforts to keep abreast of medical news, in order to be aware of possible treatments for the disease they fear, and to keep informed of new diseases which could threaten them.

Psychogenic Pain Disorder

The individual with psychogenic pain disorder either experiences pain in the absence of physical causes, or experiences much more pain than is normal for the physical cause that is present. Such individuals seem to flirt with being an invalid. The pain may be sensed as excruciating, and may interfere greatly with a functional life-style. Much like the person with somatization disorder and hypochondriasis, these individuals move from doctor to doctor, and at times become addicted to pain-relieving medication.

These three disorders share many similarities, and in the past were often lumped together under the term "hypochondria," an abnormal concern about one's state of health. Some individuals manifest little anxiety about their disorder, and almost seem to enjoy ill health. For them, the disorder may be a way of avoiding demands that might lead to anxiety. Others do manifest significant anxiety. They are often complaining, demanding people who are extremely frustrating to live with. The following case is representative.

> Mrs. Agnes S. was referred by an internist for psychiatric evaluation. She was a forty-eight-year-old, childless married woman whose major center of interest had gradually come to be her physical self, her functions, and sensations. Her doctor had described her as having "numerous psychosomatic symptoms and a great deal of concern over her health."
>
> Mrs. S. complained of frequent indigestion, "neuritis," and aching in her abdomen. She was very heart-conscious, and she suffered from frequent headaches. . . . Her symptoms had become much worse following the death of her mother seven years previously from cancer of the throat. . . .
>
> Her medical history was extensive. She had had thorough studies by several very competent physicians. In addition, she had been through the diagnostic clinics of two university medical centers. Two of her doctors had tentatively talked of the possible value of a psychiatric consultation. A new set of symptoms always arose to interfere and to send her into a new round of tests, studies, and observations. Her present physician had made a most exhaustive study. . . . It took him fifteen minutes alone just to list the many tests she had received. . . . It was as though he was trying to prove to her and to himself an absence of organic dysfunction.
>
> Not only did each new possibility that occurred to him for exploration absorb the patient's attention in neurotic fashion, but it strengthened her conviction of a physical etiology, renewed her interest in further studies, and reinforced her secondary defenses. The physician had hoped to eventually logically disprove her belief in a physical basis. Instead, she had taken his interest and each new test as evidence of uncertainty on his part and his lack of security, or of his being not at all convinced about the emotional basis which he had intermittently suggested. (Laughlin, 1956, pp. 501–502)

Factors in the Development of Somatization, Hypochondriasis, and Psychogenic Pain Disorder

Somatization, hypochondriasis, and psychogenic pain disorders may have several causal factors. Some individuals with these disorders have reported being raised in homes in which parents apparently overemphasized bodily concerns; this raises the question whether the behavior may have been learned through modeling. In addition, these individuals often have had an actual physical injury or illness early in life, with subsequent "secondary gain" as a result. By secondary gain, we mean that avoiding school and personal responsibilities, or gaining increased attention and concern from others, because of illness is reinforcing. For many individuals, illness (or complaints of illness) can have gratifying consequences. In a disturbed marital or work situation, expectations for performance are often reduced for an "ill" partner. The "pressure" is off. Being ill also allows one to gain control over others, making it more likely that one can obtain one's own way.

These less than admirable achievements are difficult to recognize in one's own behavior, and individuals who have the somatoform disorders engage in **denial.** That is, they are extremely resistant to accepting that their behavior may have these secondary gains. The need to avoid seeing oneself in an unfavorable light may explain why such persons cannot accept reasonable medical evidence that no physical cause exists for their symptoms. It may also explain their rejection of proof that their fear of developing some serious ailment is irrational because they are in good physical condition.

Perhaps these disorders develop as a result of modeling a parental behavior or parental overconcern with bodily functions, and the reinforcement of the sick role from secondary gains. The effectiveness of these behaviors in gaining reinforcement and in the avoidance of life's demands may partly explain their resistance to change.

Conversion Disorder

The characteristic symptoms of conversion disorder were described at least as early as Hippocrates who called the disorder **hysteria.** Freud used the term "conversion hysteria," and in DSM-II (1968), the disorder is called a "hysterical neurosis, conversion type," and linked to the dissociative disorders. In DSM-III (1980) it is simply listed as a somatoform disorder. The frequency of the conversion disorder was once reported to be high. (In World War I, it was the most frequently diagnosed psychiatric disorder among soldiers.) Many authorities feel that its incidence has declined over the years with the increasing medical and psychological sophistication of the general populace. Some estimates have placed its incidence at 5 percent of disorders currently treated by general physicians. Some investigators, however, have reported that as many as 20 percent of patients going to see an **internist** or **neurologist** (physicians who specialize respectively in diseases of internal organs and nerve function) have a conversion disorder rather than a physical illness (Ziegler, 1970).

The major characteristic of conversion disorder is the manifestation of a significant physical symptom in the absence of physical or organic pathology. Its similarity to the somatization disorder is obvious, the primary difference being that in conversion disorder, the symptom is circumscribed, such as blindness or deafness. In the somatization disorder, various somatic symptoms are present. Conversion disorder can occur in the sensory area, motor area, or visceral area.

Specific sensory symptoms may involve any of the senses, but commonly include numbness, excessive sensitivity, loss of sensitivity to pain, and tingling or prickling in the limbs. Less common but more dramatic are deafness and blindness. Motor symptoms may include limb paralysis, **mutism** (inability to talk), and convulsive movements of the limbs. Visceral symptoms may involve choking, coughing, hiccoughing, and **pseudopregnancy.** Watson and Buranen (1979) studied 40 male conversion disorder subjects and found that the most frequent symptoms were pain (58 percent), paralysis or partial paralysis, (42 percent), anesthesia (numbness) (38 percent), headache (32 percent), mock heart attack (25 percent), and dizziness and fainting (22 percent). The classic symptoms of blindness, deafness, tunnel vision, and full limb paralysis were absent or rare in this study. Similar results had been found in a study by Woodruff, Goodwin, and Guze (1974) (see Table 8.1).

The symptoms of conversion disorder are reported more frequently in women than men. Such individuals have been described as highly suggestible and dramatic, prone to exaggerate, manipulative, and demanding. In addition, they often have shallow emotional relationships. Traditionally, individuals with a conversion disorder have been described as manifesting **la belle indifference,** in which they seem remarkably unconcerned over their symptoms. They may be indifferent about suddenly becoming blind, but willing to discuss the problem at length. The few studies on this aspect of conversion disorder have found conflicting evidence of its presence. Stephens and Kamp (1962) found indifference in only one-third of the case histories of 100 hysteric conversion reactions they reviewed. Their sample was primarily composed of females. Mucha and Reinhardt (1970), on the other hand, found la belle

Table 8.1

Percent of patients manifesting conversion disorder symptoms in two studies[1]

Symptom	*Watson and Buranen*	*Woodruff et al.*
Pain	58	88
Paralysis or partial paralysis	42	84
Anesthesia	38	32
Headache	32	80
Mock heart attack/chest pain	25	72
Dizziness	22	84
Fainting	22	56
Blindness	0	20
Deafness	0	4
Tunnel vision	0	0
Full limb paralysis	8	12

[1]The percent of individuals with various symptoms in these two studies differs, probably because of the samples studied. C. G. Watson and Buranen (1979) studied 40 males hospitalized for the disorder. Woodruff, Goodwin, and Guze studied about the same number of females being treated on an outpatient basis. But blindness, deafness, tunnel vision, and full limb paralysis were very rare in both samples.

indifference in all 56 male aviation students with conversion disorders whom they studied.

Since the symptoms of conversion disorder may appear quite real, they must be differentiated from the true physical disorder. This is a difficult task, although the disorder often does not make anatomical sense, as in "stocking" or "glove" anesthesia. In this condition, **tactile insensitivity** (lack of sensation of touch) follows the pattern of a glove on the wrist and hand, with a sharp demarcation line, or the outline of a stocking on the ankle and foot. Such a distribution of tactile anesthesia is not possible anatomically (see Figure 8.1). The differential diagnosis is extremely important, as demonstrated by Slater and Glithero's (1965) finding that some patients diagnosed as conversion reactions later developed clear symptoms of organic diseases of the central nervous system. A characteristic sometimes helpful in differentiation is the selectivity of the symptoms (Weintraub, 1977). For example, a paralysis may not be consistent, so that a person cannot walk, but can move the legs while in bed. Theodor and Mandelcorn (1973) have also demonstrated that some people with conversion disorders are more disabled (i.e., perform more poorly) than persons with a true physical disorder. They reported that a girl who was psychogenically blind in her peripheral vision made more errors than an organically blind person would when identifying a peripheral visual target.

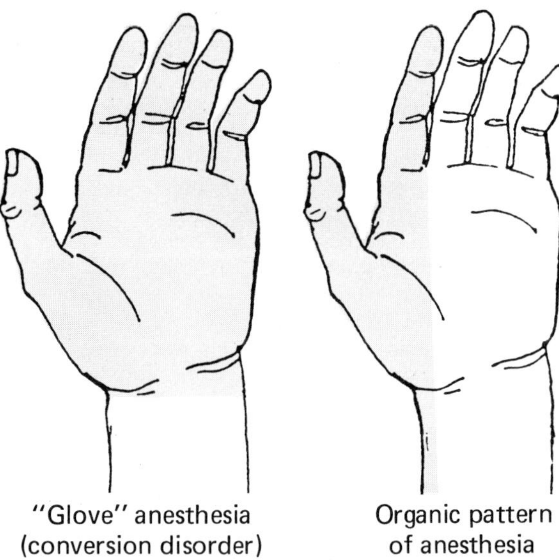

Figure 8.1.
The sharp demarcation line at the wrist in "glove" anesthesia is typical of conversion disorder, and is not found in true organic sensory loss.
From Bourne/Ekstrand (1982, p. 417).

Was this girl faking? Perhaps. The issue of **malingering** (intentional faking) is important in conversion disorder, since a true conversion disorder requires that the behavior be out of conscious or voluntary control. Most authorities agree that the malingerer does not show la belle indifference, is usually not defensive if the inconsistencies in symptoms are pointed out, and rarely objects to being intensively examined.

The following case illustrates a conversion disorder with motor symptoms (Cameron, 1947):

> The patient, daughter of a ranchman whose means and education were both very limited, was in early adolescence when her [conversion] disorder had its onset. While she was alone in the ranch house one afternoon, according to her story, a relative entered and threatened her with rape. She screamed for help, her legs gave way and she slipped to the floor, where she was found unharmed a few moments later by her mother. She was carried to her bed and waited upon there with unaccustomed devotion for several days. When, however, attempts were made to get her up, it was discovered that her legs buckled under her and she could not stand. The family physician attributed this reaction to fright, in which he was probably right, and advised keeping her in bed until her legs grew strong again, in which he was unquestionably wrong. The family added confusion to the situation by relating her illness to an epidemic of paralysis among ranch animals which had appeared in the neighborhood.
>
> As it became evident that the girl was not recovering, she was allowed to displace her father in the parental bedroom, which opened into the living room. Her mother slept with her at night. Neighbors paid frequent visits, brought her homemade things to eat and to wear, and discussed her disability over and over. As an invalid and a victim she received the best of food and attention. Her mother

massaged the paralyzed legs morning and evening. . . . She did not lose the ability to move her legs around in bed, and she could reach for things with her toes and pull them toward her.

The patient would probably never have come to the attention of neurologists and psychiatrists but for the intervention of a newcomer in the neighborhood ten years later. The newcomer recognized the possibility that the paralysis might be hysterical in character, but made the mistake of arousing hopes of a medical miracle among relatives and friends of the patient. Upon the patient's admission to the hospital, it was obvious that her relatives expected something to be done immediately which would make her well. It was equally obvious that the patient herself resented the whole move and regarded the physician's questions and examinations as covert accusations against her honesty. She, her family, and the neighbors appeared to believe completely in her illness as [an organic] "paralysis."

[At the hospital whenever] she was supported in a standing position, her legs became limp, whereas when she lay in bed they were not. She leaned with her entire weight upon the nurses supporting her and let her feet drag when the nurses tried to help her to walk. Both she and her relatives expressed frank disbelief when it was suggested to them that their interpretation of the disorder might be mistaken. The mother said, "It's you and not her that's supposed to do the curing." At the end of a month the patient was removed against advice, even though her stay cost the family nothing, and returned to her home to resume her life-role as the community's invalid girl. (pp. 328–330)

Psychoanalytic Formulations. How might a conversion disorder develop? A common psychodynamic view of its development in women is that sexual impulses towards the father are repressed during the Electra conflict. Later in life the impulses threaten to break through, and anxiety is *converted* into a physical symptom which keeps the impulse from being acted upon.

More recent modifications of psychoanalytic theory have tried to account for conversion disorder in both males and females, giving less importance to the Electra conflict and Oedipus conflict (Sperling, 1973). In general, these theories focus on strong emotions such as sexual desire or aggression, which cannot be expressed because of fear of the consequences. Consider the individual who experiences a rage impulse against a loved one, and feels extreme guilt and fear for having this "evil" feeling. The act may be defended against unconsciously by having one's arm become paralyzed, so that the person cannot strike out. Or someone who wishes to see a forbidden sexual act may become blind because such desires are "bad." Or the person with strong impulses to say "dirty" things may become mute to defend against this unacceptable behavior.

In the case cited above, a psychoanalytic explanation might propose that the girl's unconscious sexual impulses were aroused by the threatened rape. To defend against acting on the impulse, she collapsed (her legs gave way). Continued paralysis created a situation which defended against future unacceptable impulses (sexual behavior with a relative). An alternative psychoanalytic explanation might be that the paralysis was a result of her not meeting her own expectation that she should have run away from the threatening rapist.

In wartime, conversion disorders frequently follow extreme battle stress experiences during which the subject did not perform up to his own expectations. In cases of paralysis, the individual often ran from the scene or felt like running, and suffered extreme guilt because others had died during his "act of cowardice." In these cases, the primary issue seems to be guilt and self-punishment. Hypnosis had to be used to help many subjects remember what had occurred on the battlefield. They seemed to forget or repress the traumatic situation. Since the time of Charcot and Bernheim—before the turn of the twentieth century—hypnosis has figured prominently in the study of conversion disorder.

Hypnotic Behavior and Formulations about Conversion Disorder. People manifesting somatoform disorders have been described as highly suggestible, dramatic, and emotional. Hypnotic states have often been characterized as states of heightened suggestibility (see Highlight 8.1). There seems to be a similarity between conversion disorder and a hypnotic experience. Many investigators have shown that

HIGHLIGHT 8.1
HYPNOSIS

Hypnosis has already been mentioned in the regard to the studies of hysteria before the turn of the century, and in regard to mesmerism and animal magnetism. Its relevance to the study of somatoform and dissociative disorders requires that we define it. Unfortunately, the nature of hypnosis is the subject of some controversy. Hilgard (1965) suggests that the hypnotic state has the following characteristics:

1. Increased suggestibility. The subject is more accepting of suggestions from the hypnotist than when in the waking state.
2. Attention is redistributed. Subject intensely attends to what the hypnotist is saying, and becomes less aware of other surrounding stimuli.
3. Increased ability to engage in fantasy. Visual images appear to be more vivid in this state.
4. Increased acceptance of persistent distortions of reality. The subject seems willing to accept perceptual distortions which would be rejected in the waking state. For example, smelling the odor of a nonexistent rose when the hypnotist suggests that it is present.
5. A heightened ability to assume a role. In the hypnotic state, it is easier for the subject to behave "as if." The subject can behave "as if" deaf, or drunk, and so on.

Is hypnosis a dissociative "state"? Theodore Barber (1969) says "No." He makes the same criticism of a hypnotic state that other experimental psychologists have made of the concept of dissociation. Barber proposes that hypnotism is not a state of altered consciousness, but simply a set of behaviors which requires no inferences about mental states. He says that the behaviors of hypnotized subjects can be duplicated by nonhypnotized subjects who are simply *simulating* the behavior of being hypnotized. Barber's critics claim that simulators can do this because they have "slipped into" a hypnotic state. Arguments continue to be leveled and refuted by both sides of the debate. However, the evidence produced by Hilgard and associates (see Figure 8.2) is convincing that hypnosis is more than simple simulation of a role.

hypnotic induction and suggestion can cause "normals" to develop conversion disorders that are hard to distinguish from "naturally" occurring cases. Perhaps the same mechanisms are operative in both instances.

Hypnosis seems to involve a restriction of attention. Through the induction procedure, the subject "tunes out" all but a few stimuli such as the hypnotist's voice. You may have experienced mild hypnotic states yourself while, studying or reading a novel; you may have been so attentive to your reading that you "tuned out" most other stimuli without being aware of it. Hypnotism also requires that the subject be willing to cooperate with the hypnotist, and to take the roles suggested.

Under these circumstances, subjects who have been given the suggestion that they will not feel pain have, when tested under hypnosis, reported less pain from aversive stimuli than when not under hypnotic induction (Hilgard, 1969; Hilgard et al., 1978). Hilgard and colleagues' (1978) experiment is depicted in Figure 8.2. Such studies suggest that conversion disorders may be a function of the restriction of attention or of high levels of concentration, combined with a strongly motivated desire to escape from a situation that makes stressful demands.

Sackheim, Nordlic, and Gur (1979) have sug-

This therapist is testing the depth of the subject's hypnotic state by using an arm levitation suggestion.

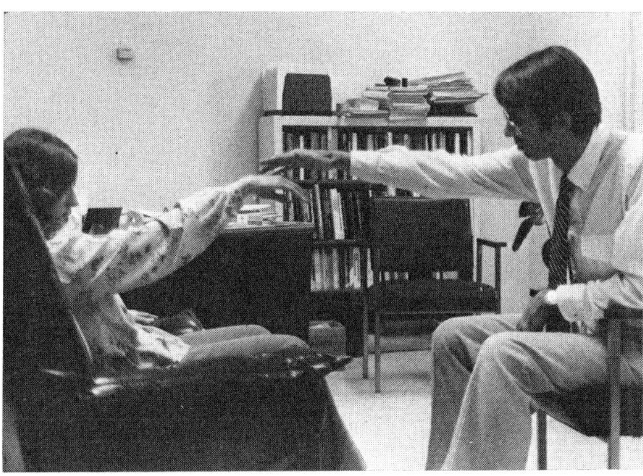

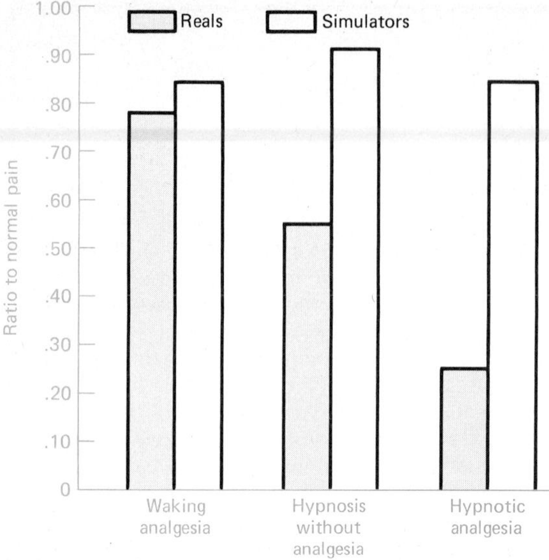

Figure 8.2. Hypnotic pain reduction: Real or fake?

Is the pain reduction of hypnotism real or are subjects faking? Hilgard and his colleagues used an "honesty interrogation" to find out. The procedure was designed to maximize truthfulness. Their study indicates that highly hypnotizable subjects experienced less pain when it was suggested they would feel no pain while hypnotized. Simulators felt virtually the same level of pain when awake, when simulating a hypnotic state without analgesia, and when simulating a hypnotic state with analgesia. Hypnotized subjects reported less pain when hypnotized than when awake, and even less pain when hypnotized and given an analgesic suggestion.

From Hilgard et al. (1978, p. 243).

gested a process by which this may occur. They believe that the sensory neural impulses reach the brain, but the person has learned to block the central process involved in bringing the information to awareness. The individual is able to deny the information to consciousness, so that the information remains outside awareness. Exactly how the individual learns to do this is not clear. Nor do we fully understand why some people have and use this ability, while others do not.

Conversion Disorder as Learned Behavior. Conversion disorder and hypnosis are both extraordinary forms of behavior. Are they simply learned? As yet, there is no convincing evidence that simple learning results in conversion disorders, although learning may well contribute to their development. Conversion disorders often allow the individual to avoid unpleasant consequences and anxiety, and to gain attention and solicitude. The typical person who develops conversion disorder has been described as suggestible, dramatic, manipulative, demanding, and inclined to exaggeration. Such a person's behavior might well be shaped by the environment into a conversion symptom, which is maintained by secondary gains. In the ranch girl's case, the secondary gains from her "paralysis" are obvious. They appeared so significant that the girl left treatment and returned home to be taken care of, as she had been for the previous 10 years.

Interestingly, many people who have a conversion disorder have had some acquaintance with the symptoms they manifest from a relative who "modeled" the behavior (i.e., the relative was actually blind, deaf, or paralyzed; Mucha & Reinhardt, 1970). This type of learning need not be conscious or under voluntary control. Investigators such as Schwartz (1973) have convincingly demonstrated that humans can learn to modify physiological activity previously thought to be outside voluntary control and awareness.

A very interesting model of the somatoform behaviors has been proposed by Ullmann and Krasner (1975). They suggest that these behaviors are a manifestation of a learned **role enactment.** In conversion disorder, they suggest, the subject has not really "lost" any voluntary function, but engages in behavior that matches his or her *concept* of the social role a person with the true physical disorder would enact. (Remember that glove anesthesia does not match an anatomical anesthesia.) This framework conceptualizes the behaviors of hypnosis in the same way—as role enactment rather than as a distinct form of altered consciousness—and the similarities between a hypnotic state and conversion disorder therefore supports the theory.

Ullmann and Krasner go on to suggest that once the person has adopted the role (e.g., being blind) and has acted in this manner, a return to the healthy role is unlikely. The "sick" role is maintained by the immediate benefits of avoidance of unpleasant situations and the positive secondary gains already discussed.

In addition, to give up the role behavior would subject the person to the unpleasantness and embarrassment of admitting that the disorder was not real. Keep in mind that this type of role enactment goes far beyond play acting. This formulation focuses on the behavior emitted, and does not deal with the conscious or unconscious dimensions of the subject's awareness of the behaviors being manifested.

DISSOCIATIVE DISORDERS

The dissociative disorders are described in DSM-III (1980) as sudden temporary alterations in the normally integrative functions of consciousness, identity, or motor behavior. DSM-III includes **psychogenic amnesia, psychogenic fugue, depersonalization disorder,** and **multiple personality** in this category. Other types of behavior may also be a type of dissociation (see Highlight 8.2). In the past these states were considered to be a category of the hysterical neurosis, along with conversion disorder. From clinical observation, many practitioners had noticed that individuals from both groups of disorders appeared to share similar personality variables, labeled the **hysterical personality.** These characteristics included **egocentricity** (self-centeredness), poor self-awareness, childlike emotionality, and a high degree of suggestibility and dependency on others.

Clinicians such as Chodoff (1974) have suggested that the concept of hysterical personality is used so loosely that it is almost without value. Because of disagreement on the validity of the concept of the hysterical personality, the DSM-III has moved in the direction of treating the dissociative disorders as conceptually separate from conversion disorders, even though the personality characteristics noted above are often seen in persons with either of these disorders.

Psychogenic Amnesia

Amnesia, the partial or total inability to recall past events or periods of one's life, has many causes, including organic factors such as a blow to the head. *Psychogenic amnesia* occurs in the absence of physical causes. Faced with an unbearable situation or experience, the individual uses massive repression or perhaps avoidance learning to keep thoughts about the experience out of awareness. The amnesia usually occurs in situations that the person cannot realistically escape. The "forgetting" may involve a few hours or days or, more rarely, a whole lifetime of memories. While mem-

HIGHLIGHT 8.2
SOMNAMBULISM: A DISSOCIATIVE DISORDER?

Sleepwalking, or **somnambulism,** is quite common in children, probably occurring at some time at least once in most persons' childhood (Jacobson, Kales, & Kales, 1969). It is unusual in adults, however, and often appears to be a dissociative state for them (Kales et al., 1979). Somnambulism (the formal term for sleepwalking) usually occurs in the early hours of sleep. The individual moves with open eyes, is apparently able to see obstacles, has a bland expression, and may engage in purposeless but complicated behaviors with varying degrees of effectiveness. The sleeper is very difficult to awaken and usually returns to bed, but sometimes lies down elsewhere and wakes in the morning wondering how she or he got there. There is no memory of the events of the episode, although at times the walker may remember dream fragments. The notion that it is dangerous to awaken a sleepwalker is myth, as is the idea that the sleepwalker is in no danger while sleepwalking. The individual can fall down stairs and so on when in such a trance.

Somnambulism seems to occur in some adults under stress from environmental or personal conflict. It remains a poorly understood disorder, with few reports of successful treatment. The primary response may be to ensure that the sleep locale (bedroom or house) is securely locked and dangerous objects removed during the period the behavior occurs. Some sleepwalkers have been successfully treated with psychotherapy that focused on uncovering and resolving conflicts, and reducing stress.

ories of places, people, and one's own name and experiences may be forgotten, the person's basic behaviors and personality structure remain intact. The following case illustrates a severe case of psychogenic amnesia which was successfully treated by hypnotism, the technique most commonly used with such individuals:

> Miss B.Q., aged seventeen years, was brought to the clinic in a complete state of amnesia. She was found at a church in a disheveled state and could not tell who she was. She spoke coherently but did not know her name, her address, who her relatives were, how old she was, where she went to school, or any other fact about her past life. Her mental processes were otherwise intact, and she could read, write, and discuss specific problems intelligently.
>
> Under hypnosis the essential history of her past was brought to light. She and her sister lived with their widowed father. He was a domineering, sadistic person who demanded implicit obedience and exact accounting of the household budget. On the day the amnesia developed, the patient was given the money for rent, and when she arrived at the agency discovered the money had been lost. The fear and panic that seized her was so great that rather than go back and face certain and severe punishment—she "forgot" all about herself. (Kraines, 1957, p. 80)

Psychogenic Fugue

Fugue is quite similar to amnesia, but has one notable difference. Individuals in a fugue state not only lose their memory but also travel away from their usual environment. They develop a new identity, which may range from vague memories of a different past life to a complex identity with a complicated, vividly remembered, nonexistent past. Psychogenic fugue is such a rare disorder that virtually no controlled research has been completed on it. It may simply be one type of amnesia. Some individuals in a fugue state have started totally new lives with new identities far from home and family, and have successfully lived their new lives until either being accidentally discovered or suddenly regaining their memories of their true past. As in psychogenic amnesia, fugues can be of a duration as short as hours or days, but fugues sometimes last for years, unlike the simpler psychogenic amnesia. The psychiatrist Jules Masserman (1961) cites such a case:

> Bernice L., a forty-two-year-old housewife, was brought to the Clinics by her family, who stated that the patient had disappeared from her home four years previously, and had recently been identified and returned from R. . . ., a small town over a thousand miles away. On rejoining her parents, husband and [child, she] had begun to insist that she really had never seen them before, that her name was not Bernice L. but Rose P., and that it was all a case of mistaken identity. . . .
>
> The patient was raised by fanatically religious parents, who, despite their evangelical church work and moralistic pretenses, accused each other of infidelity so frequently that the patient often questioned her own legitimacy. . . . [In] the troubled loneliness of her early years the patient became deeply attached to her older sister, and together they found some security and comfort; unfortunately, this sister died when the patient was seventeen and left her depressed and unconsolable for over a year.
>
> However, during her second semester at the University, [while studying to be a missionary] she was assigned to room with an attractive, warm-hearted and gifted girl, Rose P., who gradually guided the patient to new interests, introduced her to various friendships, and encouraged her to develop her neglected talent as a pianist. The patient became as devoted to her companion as she had formerly been to her sister, and was for a time relatively happy . . . the patient . . . fell "madly in love" with her friend's fiance, and spent days of doubt and remorse over her incompatible loves and jealousies. The young man, however, paid little attention to his fiancee's shy, awkward, and emotionally intense friend, married Rose P. and took her to live with him in Canada. The patient reacted with a severe depression. . . .
>
> On completion of her [school]work she entered into a loveless marriage with a man designated by her parents and spent six unhappy years in missionary outposts in Burma and China. The couple, with their two children, then returned to the United States and settled in the parsonage of a small midwest town. Her life as a minister's wife, however, gradually became less and less bearable as her husband became increasingly preoccupied with the af-

> fairs of his church, and as the many prohibitions of the village (e.g., against movies, recreations, liberal opinions and even against secular music) began to stifle her with greater weight from year to year. During this time the patient became increasingly prone to quiet, hazy reminiscences about the only relatively happy period she had known—her first two years in college with her friend, Rose P.—and these years, in her daydreaming, gradually came to represent all possible contentment. Finally, when the patient was thirty-seven, the culmination of her disappointments came with the sickness and death of her younger and favorite child. The next day the patient disappeared from home without explanation or trace, and her whereabouts, despite frantic search, remained unknown to her family for the next four years.
>
> Under treatment in the Clinics, the patient recollected that, after a dimly remembered journey by a devious route, she finally reached A . . ., the college town of her youth. However, she had lost all conscious knowledge of her true identity and previous life, except that she thought her name was Rose P. Under this name, she had begun to earn a living playing and teaching the piano, and was so rapidly successful that within two years she was the assistant director of a conservatory of music. Intuitively, she chose friends who would not be curious about her past, which to her remained a mysterious blank, and thereby eventually established a new social identity which soon removed the need for introspections and ruminations. Thus, the patient lived for four years as though she were another person until the almost inevitable happened. She was finally identified by a girlhood acquaintance who had known both her and the true Rose P. in their college years. (pp. 35–37)

As in amnesia and the other dissociative disorders, the individual who develops a fugue is often egocentric, immature, suggestible, and faces an intolerable situation from which escape is often impossible.

Depersonalization Disorder

The most frequent dissociative disorder may be *depersonalization disorder*. Fleiss, Gurland, and Goldberg (1975) found that 23 of 57 normal students had experienced it. Depersonalization involves a sense of things or experiences as being "unreal" and a feeling of estrangement from oneself or one's surroundings; both feelings have an unpleasant quality and are experienced as a distinct change from one's usual mode of functioning.

The depersonalization experience can be quite frightening, and the individual often experiences panicky anxiety and a feeling of losing control. One of the more disturbing symptoms is the sense that one's body is distorted, often to the point of grotesqueness. The "astral projection" or "out-of-body" experiences that some persons report seem quite likely to be episodes of depersonalization disorder. The same may be true of the experiences reported by some people who have "died" for a few minutes and been brought back to life by emergency measures. A few of these individuals report glimpses of "heaven" or "limbo." They sometimes report floating above their bodies, looking down to see the doctors working to bring their bodies back to life, and then feeling "pulled" back into their bodies as the doctors succeed in reviving them.

Like the other dissociative disorders, the depersonalization disorder is often episodic, with periods of normal functioning in between. Episodes of depersonalization tend to be short, lasting minutes or hours rather than long periods such as years, as do some fugues. The presumed greater frequency of this disorder than the other dissociative disorders suggests that it may be a milder form of dissociation and possibly more amenable to treatment. However, more research is necessary before such issues can be clarified. Its etiology is probably similar to that of the other dissociative disorders—an escape or avoidance of some psychological stressor in the environment that cannot be avoided through other coping mechanisms.

Multiple Personality

Multiple personality is one of the most dramatic dissociative disorders, and has received a large share of attention in the popular media. The movies *The Three Faces of Eve* and more recently *Sybil* have dramatized the situation in which one individual has two or more unique personalities or identities coexisting in one body. This disorder has been infrequently seen, but the incidence of reports is now increasing (Bliss, 1980).

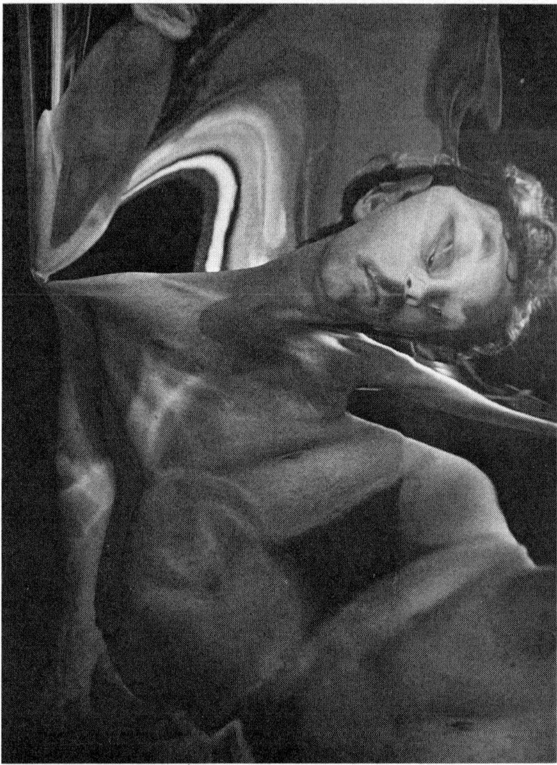

Depersonalization may result in the sense that body parts are distorted.

Some authorities have suggested that the typical multiple personality appears in sets of threes, consisting of a moralistic character, a character who acts out behaviorally, and a relatively well-balanced character (Thigpen & Cleckley, 1957); others have found that any variety of personalities is possible (Luria & Osgood, 1976). Each personality has a relatively unique and stable identity with its own emotional structure and thought process, but usually one appears to be the primary personality from which the others have "split" or dissociated (Jeans, 1976). The individual may switch from personality to personality in a matter of minutes or hours, with the primary personality holding sway most of the time. The separate personalities usually have no awareness of each other, so that the primary personality blanks out for periods, then "comes to," only to find evidence of having done something in the lost interval. The primary personality often is told by other people what "he" or "she" has been doing; frequently, the behaviors are very foreign to the primary personality (e.g., sexual promiscuity, excessive drinking). Here we are not talking about role playing. As Luria and Osgood (1976) point out, "All of us have somewhat different personalities in different social situations, but for most of us there is no dissociation (which Jeans emphasizes is the 'hallmark' of multiple personalities)—when we are at home with the family we do not forget [everything that] we said and did at the office."

The existence of truly different personalities in one person has received validating support from the work of Osgood, Luria, Jeans, and Smith (1976) in their study of Evelyn. In this study, Osgood, Luria, and Smith did a blind analysis of double testings of the three personalities of Jeans's patient "Evelyn," using the semantic differential (see Figure 8.3). The three personalities were: 1. Gina, an efficient businesslike moralistic person, unhappy in her relationships with others, the "presenting personality"; 2. Mary, childlike, feminine, emotional, and seductive; and 3. Evelyn, more mature but still shallow. With no direct knowledge of the patient or her background, Osgood et al. were able to describe the personalities of Jeans's patient based on the data from the semantic differential, to an extent that is impressive in its agreement with Jean's clinical data. Osgood et al. were even able to specify actual features from the patient's early life history.

The causal development of the multiple personality remains unclear, although many theories have been advanced. In general, theorists have focused on the existence in the individual of major conflicting desires which are repressed, but are so strong that they break through. However, the desires are so unacceptable to the original personality that, in breaking through to behavior, a new personality is formed to allow their expression. Howland (1975) has emphasized that the initial dissociation occurs during a period of extreme stress, and is an effort to maintain psychological survival. In the individual who manifests the features of the hysterical personality, who is threatened by unacceptable feelings, and who feels parentally rejected (Osgood et al., 1976),

Father

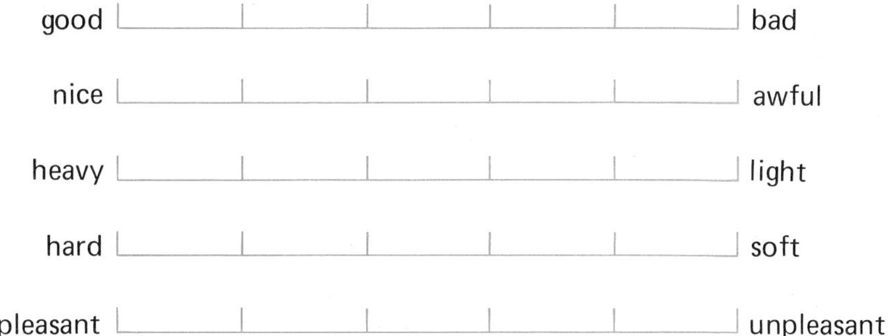

Figure 8.3. Sample item from Osgood's semantic differential measure. Osgood has developed this rating scale to assess the meaning of concepts to individuals. In the example shown, the subject would rate the concept "father" on the qualities listed, determining where father would fall between good and bad, and so on. In the study of "Evelyn," reliable and obvious differences appeared in ratings made by her different personalities.

the development of alternative personalities may be the only available coping mechanism. One case which fits this concept—in which anger/rage was the impulse which required dissociation before it could be expressed, and which was *so* intense it had to be expressed—is adapted from Winer (1978).

By the age of 24, Nancy had been hospitalized twice for depression, anxiety, and multiple personality. Her life had been a turmoil of unhappy times. As child she had been isolated from other children by her mother who was a brutalizing, aggressive woman. Mother and father fought constantly and violently. Nancy had been sexually abused at the age of 5, by her mother's grandfather, and raped at age 13 by her mother's boyfriend. Nancy had married and divorced three men who shared the characteristics of heavy drinking, unfaithfulness, and abusiveness. She finally remarried her first husband, the father of her two children. He had supposedly reformed his "habits."

Nancy's personalities appeared following a sense of "pressure" in her head. At first, she was only aware of "blacking out" for a period of time, but friends and relatives described the behavior during "blackouts" and she finally realized that she had more than one identity in her. "Nancy" (the most frequent personality) was insecure, dependent, anxious, and usually depressed. "Kitty" was present as a 14-year-old, childlike and frightened of men. "Lillian" was sly, seductive, sophisticated, and knew everything that Nancy did, and some of what Kitty did. Kitty did not know about Nancy or Lillian, and when not present spent her time in a "dark place."

During treatment sessions, Nancy was hypnotized so that the other personalities could be "drawn out." Interactions between the therapist and the various personalities revealed the apparent reasons for the dissociation of the two additional personalities. Kitty was a splitting off of part of Nancy's personality when she was 14. Kitty remembered an incident at age 14 in which she "killed" her mother with a butcher knife. The event had actually not taken place; Nancy had felt like killing the mother when Nancy saw her mother having sexual intercourse with Nancy's boyfriend. These intense homicidal feelings could not be tolerated and split into Kitty, who in fantasy did the murder. "Lillian" split off when Nancy was having her second child. While she was in the hospital, Nancy's parents told her that they had seen her husband kissing another woman in the hallway. Nancy was so hurt it "almost killed her." However, Lillian split off, and was "furious." Apparently, Nancy could not allow herself to experience extreme rage or anger. Perhaps she was frightened of losing control and killing someone, so that the other personalities had to split off to handle these feelings.

This case illustrates several common characteristics of multiple personalities. If the primary personality (in this case, Nancy) seeks help, it is usually for ancillary issues such as depression, low self-esteem, insomnia, and lack of energy. The early family relationships are extremely troubled, and an abusive (either psychologically or physically) parent is often present. However, the subject in adulthood often seems more involved with one or both parents than most people are, in spite of the abuse received as a child. Each additional personality develops when the subject is under extreme stress and is experiencing an intense emotion such as rage. This emotion cannot be expressed, and the new personality splits off to protect the original personality from the consequences of feeling the intense affect.

Factors in the Development of Dissociative Disorders

Psychoanalytic Concepts. Psychoanalytic views regarding dissociative states are similar to psychoanalytic views of somatization disorders, since both were once believed to be very similar reactions. According to these formulations, dissociation occurs to control an unacceptable impulse. The immediate stress that is usually present at the time of dissociation is considered to have activated some deeply repressed or extremely unacceptable impulse which relates to the Oedipal conflict (see Chapter 3). The dissociation defends against the anxiety due to the threatened breakthrough of the impulse, which is then unconsciously expressed, for example, in the fugue state or in a new personality.

Let's examine part of Nancy's case from this perspective. We can speculate that in the violent household in which she grew up, she was unable to resolve her earlier Oedipal conflict. She continued to have unresolved feelings of rage and hostility towards her abusing mother, yet she needed her mother to care for her. Upon finding her mother engaging in a sexual act with Nancy's boyfriend, Nancy becomes enraged and has an impulse to kill, but must repress this unacceptable, evil thought. The only way she can do this is to dissociate into Kitty, who in *fantasy* kills the mother with a knife. Nancy is able to be hurt and disappointed about mother, and in fantasy, as Kitty, is able to express the violent feelings that she must repress. Such a formulation of dissociation requires many inferences about the subject's past history.

Dissociation as Learned Behavior. In the discussion of conversion disorder, we have seen that hypnosis can result in a "tuning out" of stimuli, and that there may be a central brain processing mechanism which can be blocked to keep information out of individual awareness. Perhaps people can learn to use this process to develop a "not thinking about it" response. Bliss (1980) reports that people who have multiple personalities seem to be able to enter hypnotic like states easily, even as children (see Table 8.2). If so, they could engage in various behaviors while in a fugue state while "not thinking about" their previous life. Or they could experience a traumatic event and later have amnesia of the unpleasant event because of this massive "not thinking about it" response. This speculative idea has been entertained by some learning theorists as an explanation of dissociation. It suggests the assumption that hypnotizability (or hypnotic suggestibility) is a trait or predisposition, as has been proposed by some investigators.

Social learning theorists have proposed that dissociation may be due to an individual modeling the behaviors of others. Ullmann and Krasner (1975) would describe dissociation as an elaborate role enactment. In the case of multiple personality, persons act "as if" they contain different personalities. The information the person needs to do this may have come from popular media account of multiple personalities such as *The Three Faces of Eve.* The role enactment model can also be applied to amnesia or fugue. Some investigators have suggested that the role enactment of a multiple personality may be unintentionally suggested by psychotherapists during the course of therapy for other problems.

Consider Masserman's (1961) case of Bernice

Table 8.2
Multiple personality and hypnotic suggestibility

Subject	Reports of patients: History of hypnosis during early years
1	I feel as though I have always been able to hypnotize myself. I don't honestly remember a time when I couldn't. I could always get inside myself and I always thought everyone could and did.
2	I think perhaps half my life has been lived in another realm of time.
3	I began even before the age of eight when my dying mother and I shared a room. Her screams of pain came to be unbearable for me as a child. I curled up in a ball and concentrated all my efforts on being nonexistent. I blocked out all noise and imagined myself as being a part of the atmosphere, just floating and nonexistent. I could feel nothing. This would happen every night.
4	Every year my teacher wrote on my report card that I sat in class and daydreamed. I never understood until we did hypnosis what it was.
5	I spent an awful lot of time in hypnosis when I was young. I would wish for music and then hear it. I've always lived in a dream world. Now that I know what hypnosis is, I can say that I was in a trance often. There was a little place where I could sit, close my eyes and imagine, until I felt very relaxed just like hypnosis—and it could be very deep. . . . I know I was in hypnosis when I eloped. During my first marriage I was in and out of it all the time.
6	As far back as junior high school my teachers always commented. "You always seem to be in a world of your own." Since I was a little girl there was this hideaway—a retreat.

From Bliss (1980, p. 1392).

L., who was able to escape from a very unpleasant life by becoming Rose P., a girl she had many opportunities to model while in college. Becoming another person is probably the most intense modeling or role enactment situation conceivable. We can think of it as acting a role which has been learned, but it has the added aspect of avoiding thinking about one's real past because that past is too painful to think about. Bernice had hostile moralistic parents and a cold unloving husband who also was very condemning of "good times." In contrast, Rose P.'s life seemed ideal to Bernice. Finally, Bernice received a crushing blow: the death of a favored, loved child. These events were so unpleasant that Bernice seems to have become Rose P., and never again allowed herself to think of her real past. Her new life was extremely reinforcing, and to think about the past would have been very aversive. Bernice would have to admit that she had run away, left her husband, abandoned her family—behaviors which she could not accept as part of herself, which she could not "own."

SUMMING UP

Theories of the development of somatoform and dissociative disorders share many similarities. This is not surprising, since for many years these disorders were considered subtypes of the same category of diagnosis. Much about these disorders remains speculative. However, some factors are striking.

1. The phenomenon of hypnotism has striking similarities to many behaviors seen in somatization disorder and dissociative disorder. Individuals with both disorders appear particularly suggestible, and degree of suggestibility is very important in hypnotizability.
2. Learning, especially modeling and role enactment, may be important in the development of somatization disorder. Reinforcements (e.g., avoidance learning) clearly seem to be important in the maintenance of the behavior. However, research findings regarding hypnotism, suggest that, at least in conversion disorder, more is going on than *acting* "as if sick."
3. Dissociation appears to be an escape from extremely uncomfortable feelings or impulses. In clinical cases, it is a convincing demonstration of the psychoanalytic concept of repression and unconscious processes. The extent to which this finding can be used to develop a general theory based on psychoanalytic formulations is limited. However, the learning theory concepts used to explain these phenomena (such as role enactment, a learned "not thinking about it" response) are also very limited.

Although there are some useful ideas about these types of behaviors, the superiority of one theory over another has yet to be demonstrated.

KEY TREATMENTS

Somatoform disorders

Treatment of somatoform disorders has been extremely difficult. Although psychotherapy has been used, it has been relatively ineffective. Behavior therapy seems to hold some promise for treating somatoform disorders. Fordyce (1979) has used behavior therapy successfully with pain disorders; and the modification of environmental contingencies has often been used with hypochondriacal and somatization disorders. Once established, these behaviors tend to be reinforced by the environment. The individual receives sympathy and attention from friends and relatives. Unpleasant tasks such as household duties and occupational demands can be avoided. A great deal of attention is offered by medical personnel. Behavioral approaches which restructure the environment to eliminate such reinforcers as sympathy and attention, to make avoidance of unpleasant life tasks impossible, and to provide for positive reinforcement of behaving "as if not sick" have had moderate effectiveness in the treatment of these behaviors.

These disorders remain very resistent to treatment, since it is often extremely difficult to convince subjects that their problem is behavioral or psychological, not organic. Most individuals with somatization and hypochondriacal disorders who are in treatment have usually looked for help for other problems, such as depression, rather than for the primary symptoms. Most people with somatoform disorders avoid entering psychological treatment for what they perceive to be purely physical disorders.

The treatment of conversion disorder has often centered on a psychodynamic psychotherapeutic approach using hypnotism, particularly when the disorder is suspected to originate from some traumatic guilt experience. Under hypnosis, the subject relives the experience and ventilates the feelings, with a subsequent reduction in physical symptomatology. This procedure is often combined with an attempt to reduce the secondary gains or reinforcers in the environment which may work to maintain the symptom (such as giving sympathy and attention; treating the person as poor, sick, helpless). These short-term approaches are usually augmented by a long-term effort to modify the individual's coping styles and even the basic personality structure in an attempt to avoid recurrence of the conversion disorder symptomatology.

The use of fairly strict behavioral approaches with conversion disorder has not been frequently reported. However, Hersen et al. (1972) report an example which indicates that the operant approach may have some utility. In this case, a young man was admitted to a hospital with complaints of lower back pain; pain in the legs and hips; and difficulty in walking, sitting, and standing. No physical cause could be found. A female therapist began a behavioral approach by visiting his hospital room three times a day. For three days she chatted with him and encouraged him to walk, but provided no reinforcement. During this baseline period, there was no change in his behavior. For the next three days she told him to walk and reinforced his attempts by giving him attention, smiles, and encouraging comments. During the next three days he was instructed to walk, but no reinforcement was given. During the next (and final) three days the instructions to walk were again paired with reinforcement. His baseline consisted of a total absence of walking; twelve days later he was walking approximately 1000 yards per day.

Dissociative disorders

Dissociative disorders have been most commonly treated by psychodynamic psychotherapy. Many therapists see dissociation as an avoidance of anxiety-provoking or very unpleasant stressful experiences. Thus, psychotherapy focuses on the development of skills which will assist the individual in dealing with the anxiety-provoking material or the traumatic stress in such a way that psychological retreat is not necessary.

Hypnotism is a psychotherapeutic technique often used to uncover the precipitating factors in dissociative disorders. In a hypnotic state, individuals appear to be able to recall traumatic events and the emotions associated with these events, which they have pushed out of awareness. The recall is often marked by ventilation (expression of the feelings), which leads to a sense of relief. Through suggestions of the therapist the dissociated material (the repressed material or the various identities) can be more easily remembered when the patient is no longer hypnotized, although this may take many sessions. The formerly repressed memories or identities may then be integrated into the conscious personality with the assistance of the psychotherapist.

The application of psychodynamic psychotherapy to multiple personality has been the subject of popular books and films. These popularized versions of cases suggest that this approach is time consuming but extremely effective when used by talented therapists. It may be, but hard evidence is not available to document this viewpoint. In one of the most publicized cases (which was turned into a book and the movie *The Three Faces of Eve*), the impression is given that the three personalities were integrated into one. In fact, the real patient (Chris Sizemore) had to return for many more years of therapy, and ultimately manifested over 20 different personalities. Since multiple personalities often do not even appear until after psychotherapy has begun for some other disorder, some authorities have proposed that the use of hypnosis with highly suggestible patients may elicit personalities which otherwise would not have developed (see Howland, 1975). The psychotherapist also provides a relationship in which the client can learn new, more functional ways of dealing with the types of emotions which surrounded the trauma, and which are likely to occur again. Behavioral techniques have rarely been used with dissociative disorders, probably in part because of the low frequency of manifestation of the classic dissociations of amnesia, fugue, and multiple personalities. However, since these disorders seem to function to avoid stress, anxiety, or emotional trauma, we can speculate that behavioral anxiety reduction techniques (such as systematic desensitization) or cognitive techniques (such as thought stopping or cognitive rehearsal, discussed in Chapter 7) might well work once the stress had been uncovered. Perhaps we will soon see reports of the successful application of these techniques to the dissociative disorders.

Treatment of the somatoform and dissociative disorders remains an area in which little controlled research has been done. The disorders (especially conversion disorder and the dissociative disorders) are relatively low in incidence, compared to anxiety disorders, and have not been studied to the same extent. Much of the information that we have about treating these disorders is based on anecdotal case material. Perhaps because of these cases' rarity, few treatment approaches other than psychodynamic psychotherapy and hypnotherapy have been used. These disorders remain among the least studied of all abnormal behavior.

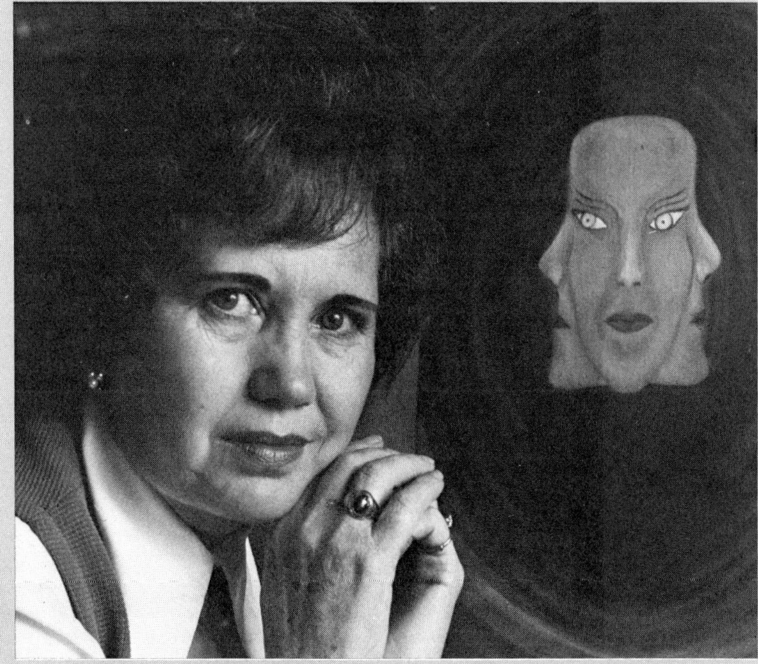

Chris Sizemore, shown with her self portrait, was the famous "Eve" of the book and film *Three Faces of Eve*. At last count, she had in fact manifested twenty-two different and distinct personalities.

Summary

1. The somatoform disorders are characterized by behaviors that have physical manifestations, but no known physical cause or underlying physiological mechanism.
2. Somatization disorder includes recurrent and vague or ill-defined physical complaints such as muscle weakness, stomachache, nausea, or chest pain.
3. Hypochondriasis is characterized by unrealistic interpretation of relatively common physical sensations, and irrational preoccupation with or fear of having a major disease.
4. In psychogenic pain disorder, the individual experiences more pain than would be expected during an illness or injury, or experiences pain in the apparent absence of physical causes.
5. Conversion disorder is characterized by physical symptoms such as paralysis or partial paralysis, anesthesia (numbness), or dizziness in the absence of physical causes. Better known but less common symptoms include blindness, deafness, and full limb paralysis.
6. The psychoanalytic view of somatoform disorders is that the symptoms are symbolic representations of repressed impulses. In conversion disorder, for example, unacceptable sexual or aggressive impulses are repressed, and the individual unconsciously defends against their expression through the formation of a physical symptom. Blindness may guard against the impulse to see a sexual act. A limb paralysis may prevent acting upon an impulse of aggression.
7. A more general psychodynamic view is that conversion disorder is one type of symptom of repression which occurs when very upsetting emotions are experienced. The individual feels guilt over unacceptable behavior or impulses, and to punish the self, develops a conversion disorder symbolic of the conflict. A soldier who runs away from battle, or feels like running, may become paralyzed.
8. Conversion disorder can be induced and removed through hypnosis. Many investigators believe that both hypnosis and conversion disorder may be similar phenomena that occur in suggestible individuals through a restriction of attention to limited sensory input.
9. Many theorists suggest that conversion disorder is at least partly due to the modeling of behavior and/or role enactment of the "sick" role. Such modeling or role enactment may not occur with the individual's full awareness. A conversion disorder may be reinforced by the benefits of being "sick."
10. The dissociative disorders are sudden temporary alterations in the normally integrative functions of consciousness, identity, or motor behavior. They include psychogenic amnesia, psychogenic fugue, depersonalization disorder, and multiple personality.
11. Psychogenic amnesia consists of the partial or total inability to recall significant past events or periods of one's life. Fugue is similar to amnesia, but also involves physical flight from the usual environment and the development of a new identity.
12. Depersonalization disorder involves a sense of things or experiences as being unreal and a feeling of estrangement from one's self or one's surroundings.
13. Multiple personality is an infrequent disorder in which an individual has two or more discrete personalities which switch back and forth. Some of the personalities may have some knowledge about the others. Usually the personality which is present most often experiences "blackouts" when other personalities emerge.
14. The splitting off of additional personalities seems to occur at times of extreme trauma and stress. Some have proposed that this splitting off is a way of coping with otherwise totally unacceptable conflicts.
15. Psychoanalytic theory about the dissociative states is similar to psychoanalytic theory about somatoform disorders. Analysts view dissociation as a massive repression of parts or all of the personality. Immediate stress or trauma reactivates unconscious impulses. The dissociation is an extreme defense against major conflict and the associated anxiety.
16. Dissociation may be due to a "tuning out" of stimuli similar to what occurs during hypnosis. If the process is reinforced, people may learn to use this process to avoid unpleasant experiences.
17. Dissociative behavior may be a form of elaborate role enactment. Highly suggestible people may learn about amnesia, fugue, and especially multiple personality from the popular media of books, television, and movies.
18. The somatoform disorders are resistant to treatment. Individuals with these disorders have difficulty accepting that their physical symptoms have no organic cause; thus, these persons are not motivated for psychological treatment.
19. Conversion disorder is one somatoform disorder that has apparently had considerable treatment success. Many clinical case reports have demonstrated that a psychodynamic approach using hypnotism can be successful in alleviating conversion symptoms. Behavioral approaches have not been frequently used with conversion disorder, although a few successful treatment cases have been reported.
20. Dissociative disorders have also been treated

primarily with psychodynamic therapy and hypnotism. Hypnotism facilitates the integration into consciousness of the split material (either repressed memories or personalities which have split off). The goal of psychotherapy is the development of new strategies for dealing with the types of impulses or intense feelings which led to the dissociative process.

21. The dissociative disorders are so rare that almost no reports exist of the use of behavior therapy with amnesia, fugue, depersonalization, and multiple personality. However, behavioral techniques might be useful in dealing with the stress that leads to dissociation.

22. The reports of treatment of somatoform and especially dissociative disorders are mainly single case clinical studies. These reports tend to be inferential and subjective, and it is difficult to evaluate the effectiveness of treatment. The rarity of these disorders makes research difficult, and they still are not well understood.

KEY TERMS

Denial. Refers to a process by which the individual does not allow the self to be aware of unpleasant aspects of reality.

Dissociation. The separation of aspects of thought, emotion, or behavior from awareness. They are "split off" from consciousness.

Hysteric. Manifesting hysteria.

Hysterical personality. A personality type believed to be subject to hysteria or what we now call somatoform and dissociation disorders. This personality is characterized as suggestible, demanding, and dependent, with a tendency towards exaggerated emotional reactions. This designation has been criticized as a subtle form of chauvinistic labeling, since it is most often applied to females by male mental health workers.

Malingering. The conscious, intentional faking of an illness in order to gain something or to avoid unpleasant events.

Mutism. The inability or refusal to speak.

Pseudoneurological. Having the form of a neurological disorder, but without an organic neurological cause.

Pseudopregnancy. Manifesting the symptoms of pregnancy, but in fact not being pregnant. In some cases, this includes a swollen abdomen.

Psychogenic. Due to psychological causes.

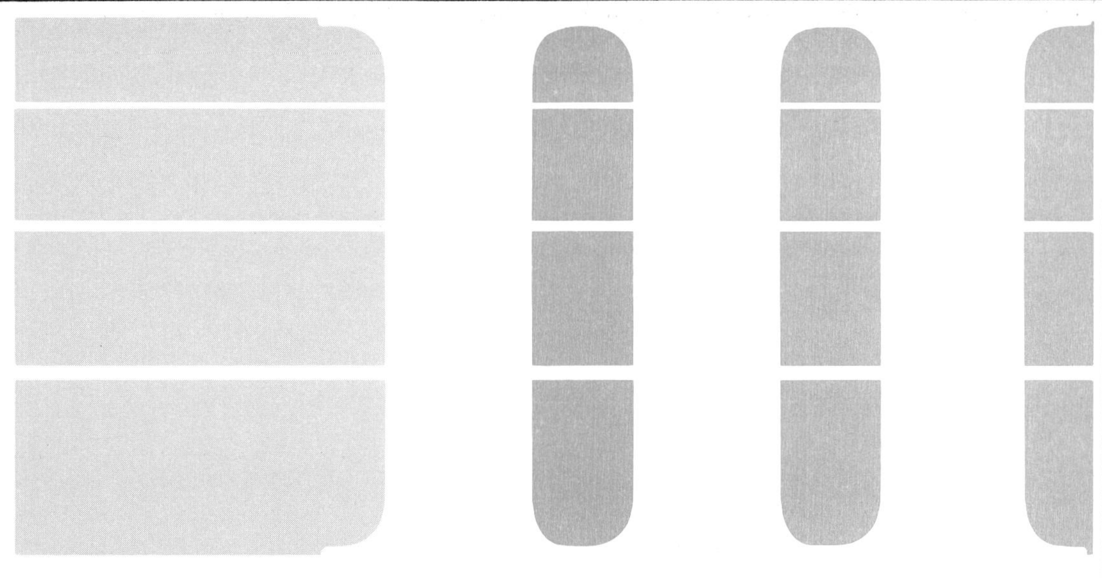

INDIVIDUAL PROBLEMS OF SOCIAL CONCERN

Many behaviors are as much as or more of a problem for society than they are for the individual. Some disturbed behaviors are *mostly* a problem for society, since the individual would not identify the behavior as something to be particularly concerned about. In this section, many of these types of behaviors are covered.

Sexual behavior may be of concern to an individual when it does not meet his or her expectations for fulfillment. Sexual functioning is also an area of many social prohibitions. Chapter 9 begins with coverage of normal sexual functioning and sexual dysfunction. Some sexual behaviors present serious problems from the viewpoint of society. In this chapter, the less accepted behaviors of sexual deviations, incest, and rape are considered, and the controversies about homosexuality are presented.

In Chapter 10, the problem of drug abuse is presented. Most individuals abuse drugs for long periods before they identify their behavior as a problem. Although society has legalized the recreational use of some drugs (such as alcohol), the use of many other drugs is against the law. Laws prohibiting drug abuse have been relatively ineffective, but they demonstrate social concern about the consequences which people believe are a result of the use of illegal substances.

Chapter 11 covers the personality disorders, enduring patterns of behavior which some people consider to be exaggerations of normal traits. The personality disorders include a wide range of behaviors which individuals often accept as "ego syntonic." The behaviors objective observers describe as problems are often seen by the individual manifesting them as "just the way I am." One of the most studied personality disorders is the antisocial personality. These individuals are usually content with their behavior, even though it often violates the rights of others. Society has identified such individuals as problems.

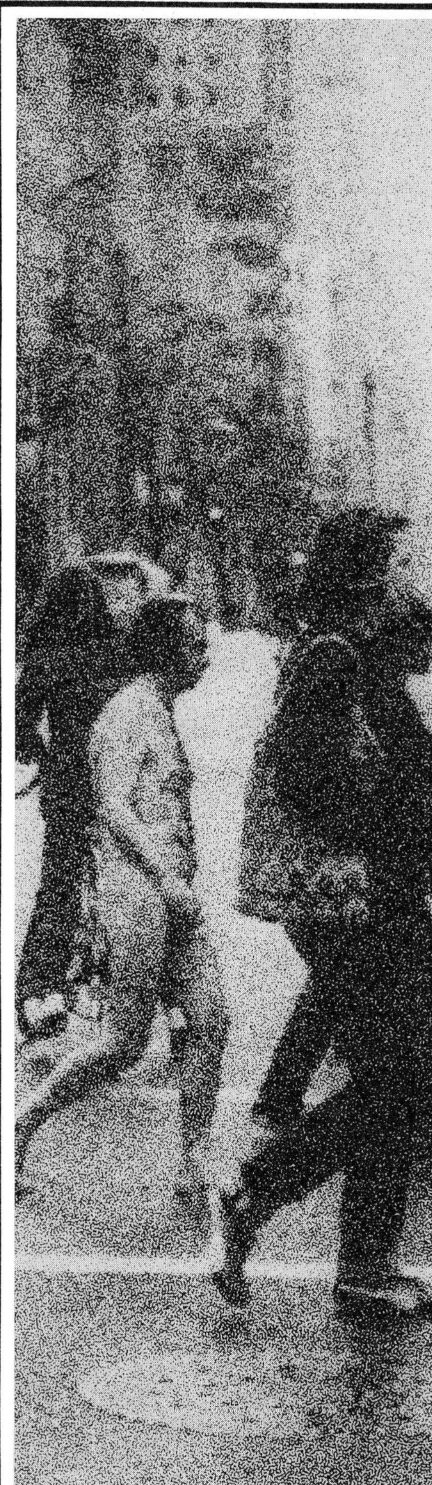

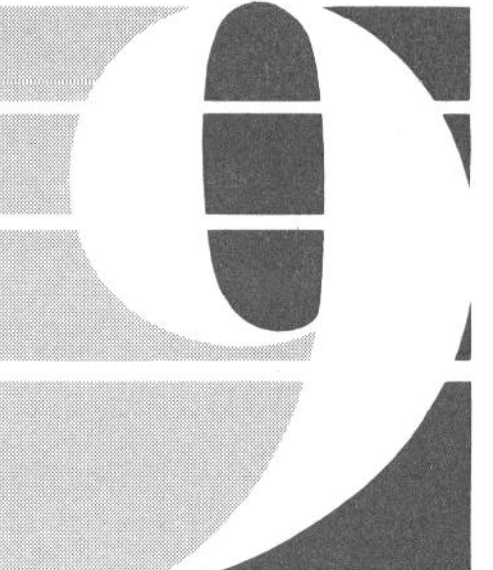

The human sexual response and abnormal behavior

- Sexual behaviors: normal or abnormal?
- The human sexual response
- Psychosexual dysfunction/sexual inadequacy
- Etiology of psychosexual dysfunction/sexual inadequacy
- Gender identity disorder (transsexualism)
- The paraphilias
- Sexual behavior of special significance
- Key treatments
- Summary
- Key terms

The nature of the human sexual response has only recently become a respectable area of scientific study. Until the Kinsey studies in the late 1940s and early 1950s, and the work of Masters and Johnson in the 1960s and 1970s, human sexuality was a topic characterized more by myth than by reality—in spite of the overwhelming importance of sexual behavior in our lives.

In childhood, sexual behavior is important because it is prohibited. Adults apparently prefer that children be uninterested in sex. In adolescence, sexuality is important as an area of exploration, adjustment, and possible trauma. Adults, married or single, tend to be concerned with the questions "Do I?" "Don't I?" "How often?" "With whom?" and "How well?" Whatever our opinions are, sexuality exists. It is in movies, books, magazines, and advertising. We find it in *Playboy* and *Cosmopolitan*, *Time* magazine, and the Bible. But mostly, we find it in our minds (see Highlight 9.1).

Attitudes about sexuality have varied dramatically through the ages, and from culture to culture. In recent years, there has supposedly been a "sexual revolution." Prohibitions have lessened, laws have been liberalized, attitudes have become more flexible. At least so it appears. More couples live together before marriage in a consenting sexual relationship than in the past; and both women and men seem more liberated, less constricted, about sexual behavior. Yet sexual inadequacy remains a concern of many, and others feel that the increased emphasis on sexual pleasure dehumanizes relationships. Perhaps the changes are not great.

As recently as the 1920s, devices for the prevention of **masturbation** which look more suited to the torture chamber than the home were available across the counter in drug stores throughout the country (G. S. Schwartz, 1973). Today, many people consider masturbation as a relatively harmless and acceptable sexual outlet. Some would say that it is abnormal, a sin against "nature" (see Highlight 9.2). Would most people perceive the following sexual behavior as abnormal? At a wedding, the bride engages in sexual intercourse with all the men present, one after another. As she satisfies each man, she becomes prouder and prouder; so does her husband, since she is showing his friends and relatives that she will be a good wife. Abnormal? No, this is culturally sanc-

HIGHLIGHT 9.1
FANTASY AND SEXUAL EXCITEMENT

Fantasies often give us the opportunity to engage in behaviors which in real life we would avoid for a variety of reasons. As Stoller (1976) has pointed out, in fantasy, frustration and trauma are often converted to triumph. Friday (1973) surveyed a large number of women to determine their types of sexual fantasy. The results demonstrate that sexual fantasy is common and often centers on being irresistible to others. Perhaps sexual fantasy is so common because we are in total control of what happens. A typical woman's fantasy from Friday's book follows:

> I imagine a variety of things when I masturbate. Sometimes it's that a man has come to the door selling something, and I invite him in. While he stands there displaying his Fuller brushes or whatever, I begin to caress myself. He watches, obviously aroused, and finds it harder and harder to continue his sales spiel. I remove my clothes and begin to masturbate, all the while watching his efforts to control himself. He's in a real state, and of course I'm very cool—in one sense, but I'm also getting very worked up. . . . (pp. 88–92)

Stoller (1976) indicates that men's fantasies are usually more assertive than women's, but in both cases, the fantasizer remains in control. A typical man's fantasy follows:

> I'm at work in my office and my secretary is behaving very flirtatiously, you know, giving me the "come on." I ignore her, but she persists. Finally in exasperation, I grab her and push her onto the couch. I pull off her clothes and fondle her breasts and thighs. She can hardly stand it,' cause she wants me so much. We have a really wild sexual experience, and she's exhausted, but tells me I'm the best she ever had.

HIGHLIGHT 9.2
MASTURBATION

Many individuals who masturbate (and surveys have indicated that a large majority of both men and women masturbate) feel guilty or are concerned that it will damage them in some way. The overwhelming evidence indicates that masturbation has no negative physical effects on the human body; in fact, in terms of overall sexual responsivity, this activity can be beneficial. Exclusive masturbatory activity when sexual intercourse is possible, however, may be a sign or symptom of **psychosexual** dysfunction.

Many myths about masturbation still linger on from the era when masturbation was thought to lead to a variety of physically dangerous consequences. In the 1800s and early 1900s, this belief was so strong that tortuous devices were invented to prevent what was called "self-abuse."

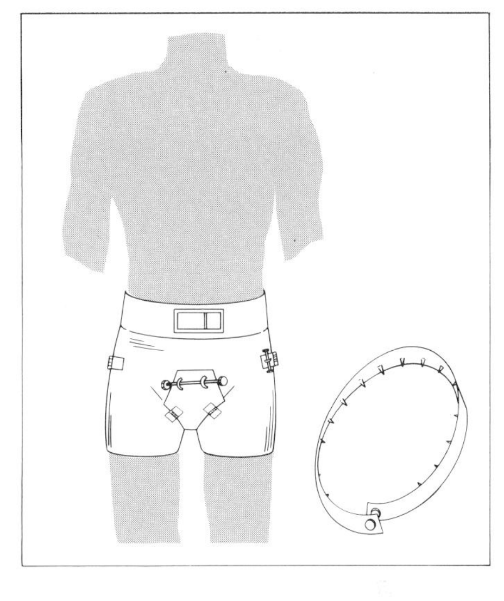

tioned behavior in the Marquesas Islands (Wincze, 1977).

SEXUAL BEHAVIORS: NORMAL OR ABNORMAL?

The discrimination of normal and abnormal sexual behavior remains difficult. It is an area of opinion, myth, morality, and cultural value that still needs to be explored. Some behaviors are consistently viewed as abnormal or pathological, such as sexual activity between adults and young children; other behaviors such as **homosexuality** remain the center of controversy.

In distinguishing normal or "healthy" from abnormal or "sick" sexual behavior, the comments of several experts may be helpful (Marmor et al., 1977). Healthy normal sexual behavior: 1. is motivated by feelings of affection and tenderness; 2. is not used to discharge anxiety, hostility, or guilt, nor does it lead to these feelings; 3. does not inflict pain or harm on oneself or one's partner; 4. is not performed using force on a nonconsenting person.

While experts disagree to some extent with each other, their opinions are more similar than different. They all raise the issues of motivation, the infliction of pain or exploitation, involvement of human partners rather than nonhuman objects, internal distress, and consent in their definitions of healthy sexuality. Sexual health or sexual sickness is not generally found in the specific behavior, but in its effect on the participants.

We will consider several normal and abnormal behaviors in this chapter, beginning with the typical human sexual response, as described in the pivotal work of the researchers Masters and Johnson (1966). Since as many as 50 percent of all married couples may experience at least some transient sexual dysfunction, the **psychosexual dysfunctions** will also be examined. The much less frequent psychosexual behaviors which are more popularly seen as abnormal or deviant will then be covered. The label of abnormality is applied to these behaviors primarily because they are either socially unacceptable, do not involve affection or tenderness, use unconventional objects, or result in harm. These include **gender identity disorder** or **transsexualism,** and the **paraphilias** (unconventional sex objects or modes of behavior). In addition, sections on incest, rape (due to its exceptionally intrusive nature), and on homosexuality are included. The chapter ends with a section on treatment approaches to sexual disorders.

HIGHLIGHT 9.3
THE SEXUAL GENITAL RESPONSE IN MEN

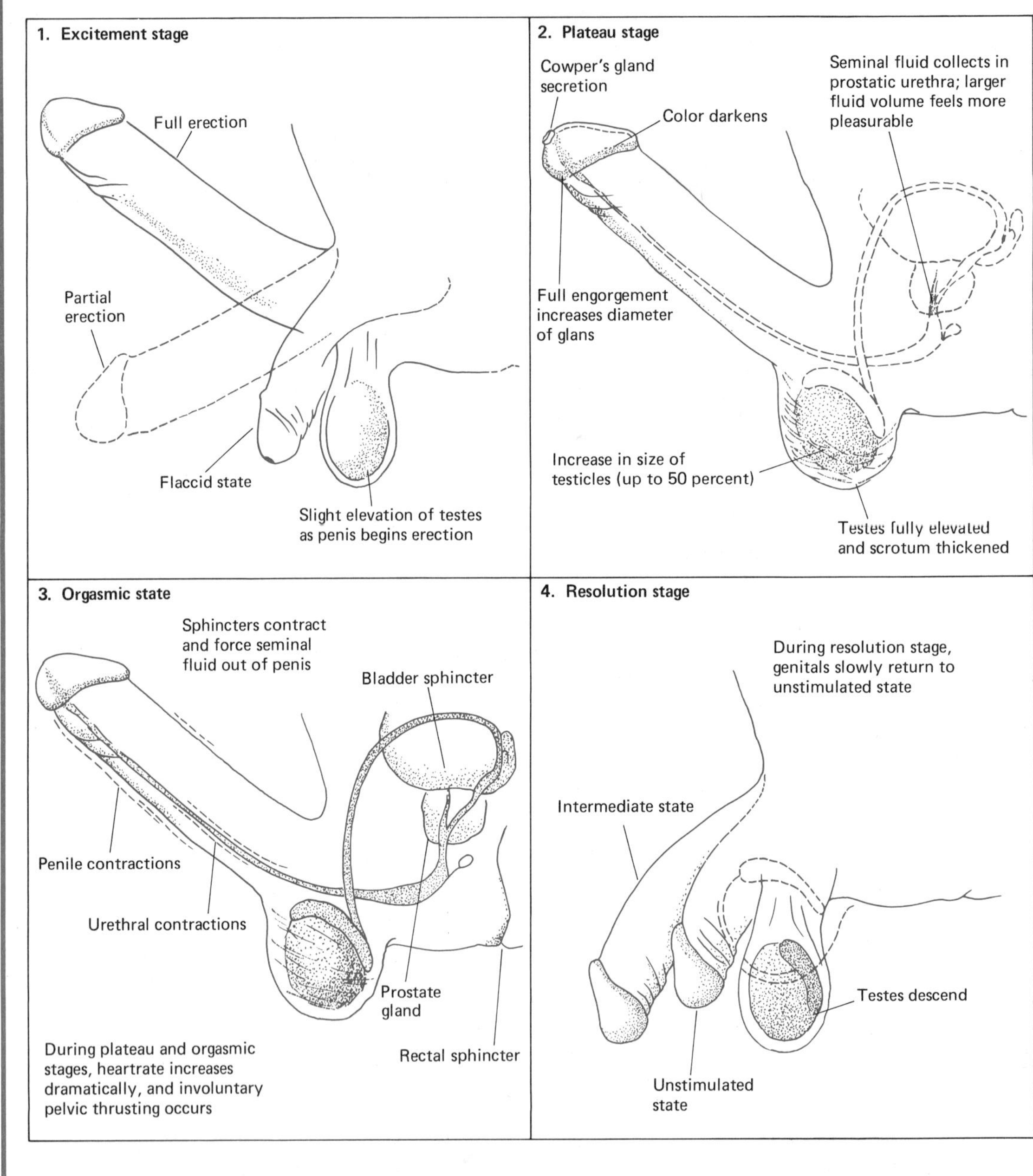

1. Excitement stage
Full erection
Partial erection
Flaccid state
Slight elevation of testes as penis begins erection
2. Plateau stage
Cowper's gland secretion
Color darkens
Seminal fluid collects in prostatic urethra; larger fluid volume feels more pleasurable
Full engorgement increases diameter of glans
Increase in size of testicles (up to 50 percent)
Testes fully elevated and scrotum thickened
3. Orgasmic state
Sphincters contract and force seminal fluid out of penis
Bladder sphincter
Penile contractions
Urethral contractions
Prostate gland
Rectal sphincter
During plateau and orgasmic stages, heartrate increases dramatically, and involuntary pelvic thrusting occurs
4. Resolution stage
During resolution stage, genitals slowly return to unstimulated state
Intermediate state
Testes descend
Unstimulated state

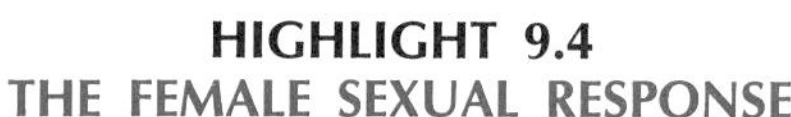

HIGHLIGHT 9.4
THE FEMALE SEXUAL RESPONSE

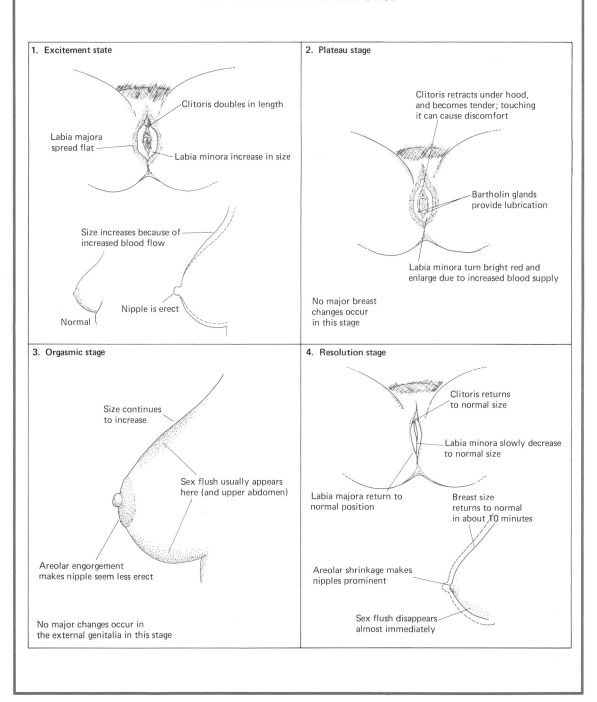

1. Excitement state

Clitoris doubles in length
Labia majora spread flat
Labia minora increase in size
Size increases because of increased blood flow
Normal
Nipple is erect

2. Plateau stage

Clitoris retracts under hood, and becomes tender; touching it can cause discomfort
Bartholin glands provide lubrication
Labia minora turn bright red and enlarge due to increased blood supply
No major breast changes occur in this stage

3. Orgasmic stage

Size continues to increase
Sex flush usually appears here (and upper abdomen)
Areolar engorgement makes nipple seem less erect
No major changes occur in the external genitalia in this stage

4. Resolution stage

Clitoris returns to normal size
Labia minora slowly decrease to normal size
Labia majora return to normal position
Breast size returns to normal in about 10 minutes
Areolar shrinkage makes nipples prominent
Sex flush disappears almost immediately

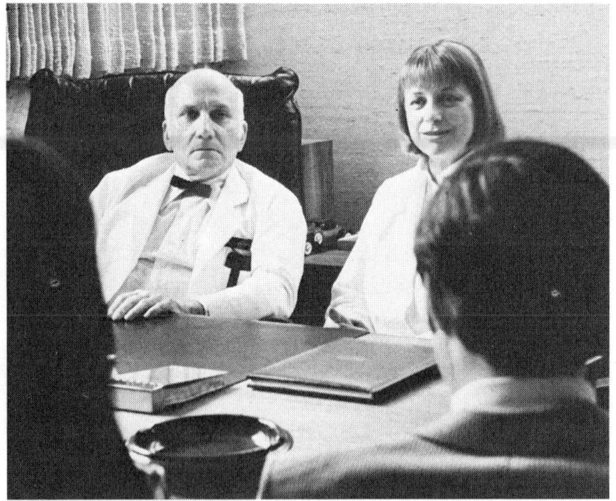

William Masters, physician, and Virginia Johnson, psychologist, who opened many closed doors in the study of human sexuality.

THE HUMAN SEXUAL RESPONSE

The physiology of the human sexual response was studied intensively by Masters and Johnson (1966) in their pioneering efforts in the 1950s and 1960s. William Masters and Virginia Johnson risked their professional reputations to study this area, which had long been considered an area lacking scientific respectability. They based their conclusions on the observations of 312 men, ranging in age from 21 to 89, during 2,500 cycles of sexual response, and 382 women during more than 10,000 cycles of sexual response (Masters & Johnson, 1966, 1970).

They found a surprising similarity between males' and females' physiological reactions to sexual stimulation. Generally, there is widespread vasocongestion (increase in blood supply) and an increase in muscular tension. The physiological response in both males and females can be divided arbitrarily into four stages (see Highlights 9.3 and 9.4).

1. Excitement (the early stage of sexual arousal). If excitement is strong enough and uninterrupted, increased levels of sexual tension lead to the next stage, the plateau.
2. Plateau (a stage of high sexual arousal). If orgasm does not occur to lower sexual drive, or if stimulation ceases to be effective, a long period of slowly decreasing sexual tension occurs. If drive and stimulation continue to be effective, however, the next stage, orgasm, is achieved.
3. Orgasm. An involuntary response consisting of the few seconds when the bodily changes resulting from stimulation reach maximum intensity. This is followed by the final stage, resolution.
4. Resolution (a return to the unstimulated state). In this stage, women are capable of achieving another orgasm. Men enter a refractory period during which they cannot be restimulated; its length depends on both physiological and psychological factors.

It must be remembered that these four stages are a formulation of convenience. They should not be used as a standard to measure individual sexual responsiveness. In addition to the observation of the human sexual response, Masters and Johnson found evidence to contradict some commonly held misconceptions about human sexual behavior. For example, they found that the size of a man's penis has little to do with his sexual enjoyment and his ability to sexually satisfy his partner (except possibly in the situation when his partner psychologically invests in the size of his penis) (see Highlight 9.5). They also found that most females' **clitoral orgasms** are just as intense and satisfying as those from vaginal stimulation, demonstrating that Freud's assertions of the superiority of **vaginal orgasm** were based on ignorance and speculation. A final example of their myth-dispelling data is their discovery that having the goal of achieving simultaneous orgasm can be so distracting that couples often experience less pleasure in the sexual act.

Masters and Johnson courageously opened the door for others to engage in this type of research, broke ground in the development of instrumentation for the study of the human sexual response, and provided baseline data for the study of human sexual inadequacy. However, a note of caution is due. The data from their early work are not based on a random sample of the population. Initially, they studied prostitutes, then turned to volunteers from their local university community. Their volunteers were screened to reject persons who were emotionally disturbed and who were not capable of having an orgasm; yet one must suspect a self-screening process in an era when such research was quite controversial. The "average person" in the late 1950s and early 1960s would not be likely to volunteer to be instrumented and observed during sexual intercourse and masturbation under laboratory conditions—nor would the average person even now.

PSYCHOSEXUAL DYSFUNCTION/ SEXUAL INADEQUACY

Masters and Johnson's early work on the human sexual response led to the study of sexual inadequacy. Their work at the Reproductive Biology Research Foundation in St. Louis, Missouri, resulted in a greater understanding of the development of sexual inadequacy and its treatment (Masters & Johnson, 1970b). This knowledge has grown considerably through their work and the work of others. For convenience, sexual inadequacy can be discussed under the general categories **arousal dysfunction, erectile dysfunction, ejaculatory dysfunction, dyspareunia, vaginismus,** and **orgasmic dysfunction** (see Highlight 9.6).

Arousal Dysfunction

Some individuals experience an inhibition of desire or loss of sexual interest. For males, this may result from fatigue, stress, or a defensive maneuver to avoid performance anxiety. In some cases, it may be due to depression (Wise, 1976). In women, this lack of sexual responsivity was called "frigidity," but has more recently been termed "general sexual dysfunction" (H. S. Kaplan, 1974). S. H. Rosenthal and Rosenthal (1975) cite the following case:

> [Mrs. A] described a strict upbringing with a great emphasis on guilt with regard to premarital sex and a very strong home emphasis on not being seen even partially unclothed by other family members. In six years of marriage, Mr. A had never seen his wife undressed in the light. Their infrequent sexual relations were stereotyped, performed in the dark. . . . There was little or no foreplay. Mrs. A's chief complaint was that she did not enjoy sex, that she would not care if she never had sex, that she would rather not be bothered, and that during sexual relations, she wishes that she were someplace else. She gets very little if any feeling of sexual arousal, usually does not become lubricated, and finds penetrations somewhat painful. She tries to avoid sexual relations whenever possible. (p. 145)

In both sexes, arousal dysfunction may be a resultant of many factors, perhaps even sexual dysfunction in the partner (Derogatis & Meyer, 1979); or the condition may lead to sexual dysfunction in the partner. H. S. Kaplan (1979) suggests that inadequate desire or arousal may be the most prevalent sexual dysfunction.

Erectile Dysfunction

Erectile dysfunction has in the past been called **impotence.** Masters and Johnson distinguished between primary impotence, in which the male

HIGHLIGHT 9.5
"MICROPHALLNEUROSIS"

The male's concern about the size of his penis has been called microphallneurosis by Glenn (1972). Such concerns are quite common. Many researchers have studied the common ranges of flaccid and erect penis size, and their combined results yield the following data:

> The flaccid penis has an average length of about 4 inches, with a common range of 2.3 inches to 4.5 inches. Erect penis length averages about 6 inches, with a common range of about 4.5 inches to slightly over 8 inches. The circumference averages 4.2 inches. These measurements vary somewhat from study to study and do not include the unusually small or large penis. An interesting finding (Masters & Johnson, 1966) was that the smaller flaccid penis increased to a greater degree when erect than the larger flaccid penis, and that penis size bears almost no relationship to the male's overall body size.

HIGHLIGHT 9.6
SEXUAL BEHAVIOR AND DSM-III

The categories of sexual disorder or behavior in DSM-III (1980) include the following:

A. Psychosexual Dysfunctions
   1. Inhibited Sexual Desire
   2. Inhibited Sexual Excitement
   3. Inhibited Female Orgasm
   4. Inhibited Male Orgasm
   5. Premature Ejaculation
   6. Functional Dyspareunia
   7. Functional Vaginismus
   8. Atypical Psychosexual Dysfunction.

These disorders are equivalent to the psychosexual dysfunctions described by most researchers such as Masters and Johnson, and avoid the somewhat perjorative terms "frigidity" and "impotence."

B. Gender Identity Disorders
   1. Transsexualism
   2. Gender Identity Disorder of Childhood
   3. Atypical Gender Identity Disorder.

C. Paraphilias
   Includes disorders such as transvestism, pedophilia, voyeurism, etc. These disorders were previously called "sexual deviations," and the individuals who manifested them were called "sexual deviates." "Paraphilia" avoids the negative connotations of these terms.

D. Other Psychosexual Disorders
   1. Ego-dystonic Homosexuality
   2. Psychosexual Disorders Not Elsewhere Classified

"Psychosexual Disorders Not Elsewhere Classified" is a residual, wastebasket term. The use of **Ego-dystonic Homosexuality** reflects a belief that homosexuality is a disorder only when it causes the homosexual significant psychological difficulty (is not accepted by the ego), not when the individual is accepting and adjusted to his or her sexual orientation.

has never been able to achieve an erection sufficient for intercourse (a relatively rare condition), and secondary impotence, in which the inability to attain an erection sufficient for intercourse is current, but the individual has been potent at least once in his life. Serious long-standing erectile dysfunction may be due to physical causes such as diabetes or the use of certain medications, but most investigators agree that the most frequent causes are psychological. Reports of erectile dysfunction are increasing, most likely because of the increased acceptance of seeking help for sexual problems. However, some researches (e.g., Ginsberg, Frosch, & Shapiro, 1972) suggest that the increase is due to males' perceived threat of having to live up to the sexual performance expectations of "liberated" women. Wise (1976) gives the following example of erectile dysfunction related to complex psychosocial aspects in the home situation:

> . . . A 37-year-old married male sought psychiatric consultation due to the recent onset of impotence. The patient noted that for the past few months he had had increasingly frequent episodes of loss of erection upon penetration. At the time of consultation, his wife refused to attempt any sexual relations with him since his impotence made her feel like a failure. The couple was able to have fully satisfactory sexual relationships whenever they went away for the weekend or on a short vacation. At home their sexual dysfunction returned. (p. 151)

We can see from this example that sexual dysfunction has an impact on the partner, whose reaction to the impotence may complicate the problem. In addition, the problem seems to be sensitive to the setting. Away from home, the couple's sexual performance was satisfactory.

Ejaculatory Dysfunction

Masters and Johnson identify premature ejaculation and ejaculatory incompetence as problem behaviors, the latter being quite rare or at least underreported. In ejaculatory incompetence, the male cannot **ejaculate** in the vagina, although erection and entry may not be a problem. Premature ejaculation refers to the male's inability to delay ejaculation for a sufficient time to allow entry and satisfaction of an adequately functioning partner. LoPiccolo (1978) suggests that a male who cannot delay ejaculation for up to four minutes of stimulation may suffer from this problem. Such definitions are quite arbitrary, since many factors, most notably age, affect the male's ability to voluntarily control ejaculation (H. S. Kaplan, 1974). Younger, inexperienced males tend to be less likely to be able to delay than older, more experienced males.

Ejaculatory dysfunction may result from hostility and guilt (Offit, 1977), or may be learned in early sexual experiences where there was a fear of being "caught" and a need to rush the sexual act. For example, a young married couple had to live in a small apartment with the husband's grandparents for economic reasons. Their "bedroom" was an alcove with a curtained doorway. The grandparents were restless sleepers, often awakening and walking by the curtained alcove during the night. The young couple feared that the grandparents would walk by, a few feet from their bed, while they were in the middle of sexual relations; and the young husband soon developed premature ejaculation in his rush to complete the act. They soon became complete abstainers until they could find their own apartment to ensure privacy, then their sexual behavior became satisfactory.

Dyspareunia

Dyspareunia means "painful intercourse," a disorder rare in women and even rarer in men. Painful intercourse is most frequently caused by organic factors such as lesions, infections, cysts, or other structural abnormalities (Bunge, 1970; H. S. Kaplan, 1974) and it frequently causes other sexual dysfunctions when it is present. Temporary dyspareunia (e.g., from an infection) can result in vaginismus in some cases.

Vaginismus

Folklore has commonly described a sexual scene in which a man's penis is trapped within a woman's vagina by an involuntary muscle contraction of the vaginal walls. Unfortunately, the folklore is true, although this disorder, called vaginismus, is rare. In this disorder, an involuntary contraction of the muscles in the lower third of the vagina makes penetration difficult or impossible; in rare cases where entry has occurred, the penis may be trapped temporarily. Though frightening for both partners, withdrawal is usually possible shortly after the man's erection subsides. Only in the rarest and most unusual circumstance is medical intervention (administration of a muscle relaxant to the female) necessary. Vaginismus is frequently associated with inexperience, fear of sexual intercourse, anxiety, and tension. H. S. Kaplan (1975) describes the experience of a 21-year-old wife and her 21-year-old husband, an Air Force enlisted man:

> When they first came for therapy they had been married for ten months and had not been able to achieve entrance. She had had a strict upbringing and "strong morals," and before they were married, only gradually consented to genital petting which, however, she seemed to enjoy very much. On their honeymoon she had [a thickened **hymen**], and his attempts at penetration were painful and frustrating for them both. She became frightened and puzzled throughout their honeymoon, and he became fed up, disgusted, irritated, and resentful. . . . By the time they had come to see us four or five months later, they had almost ceased trying to have intercourse and were ready to give up on the marriage. They responded well to treatment. (pp. 122–125)

Orgasmic Dysfunction

For years, women with orgasmic dysfunction have been labeled frigid, implying that they lack warmth, are anti-erotic, and unresponsive to males. While some women are like this, others with orgasmic dysfunction are not. Masters and Johnson identified primary orgasmic dysfunction as existing in women who have never had an orgasm by either masturbation or intercourse. Situational orgasmic dysfunction exists in women who have had at least one orgasm, but are nonorgasmic in one or more specific situations. For example, someone might be nonorgasmic with one individual but not another, or nonorgasmic in intercourse but not in masturbation.

There appears to be a decrease in reported cases of orgasmic dysfunction (Hunt, 1974). About 1 out of 10 women seems to have some degree of orgasmic deficiency (H. S. Kaplan, 1974). However, Singer and Singer (1978) have pointed out that the subjective experience of female orgasm varies so widely that the accuracy of assessments of incidence are questionable. The following case history from Ince (1973) is typical of situational, or secondary, orgasmic dysfunction:

> W. L. was a twenty-one year old woman who experienced a change in her sexual desires approximately one month prior to her marriage. She and her husband had engaged in sexual intercourse for more than one year before they were married, frequently three or four times per week. Her only fear was of becoming pregnant and she did not experience any feelings of guilt during this time.
>
> About one month prior to her marriage, the patient lost all desire for sexual relations and only engaged in intercourse to please her fiance. She did not enjoy the activity, and, in fact, "could hardly wait for it to be over." On her honeymoon she did not want to be sexually intimate with her husband. Since then she had not enjoyed sexual relations at all and her desires for sexual intercourse had progressively decreased. When her husband approached her in bed she "tensed up all over" and remained tense during foreplay and intercourse, which had recently become painful because of vaginal constriction.
>
> The patient was extremely unhappy about her feelings and reported that her marriage was suffering as a consequence. She had been married for nine months prior to entering psychotherapy. (pp. 447–448)

ETIOLOGY OF PSYCHOSEXUAL DYSFUNCTION/SEXUAL INADEQUACY

Several factors may result in the development and maintenance of psychosexual dysfunction. Masters and Johnson (1970b) have identified two types: historical and maintenance. Historical factors originate before the onset of the dysfunction.

Historical Factors

Sexual Trauma. Early unpleasant, painful, or terrorizing sexual experiences may lead to later sexual dysfunction. Rape, incest, discovery, and punishment are examples. Ridicule of early sexual behavior may also be an issue. Anxiety over the size of one's penis, or "microphallneurosis," (Glenn, 1972) may lead to impotence in males. Such anxiety about one's physical acceptability appears widespread in our culture.

Sociocultural Factors. As Masters and Johnson (1970) have pointed out, many cultures subtly influence sexual behavior, particularly in women. Women often are to be the Madonna, the Virgin, pure, with no sexual thoughts or desires. As noted, these sociocultural factors are changing in favor of seeing women as naturally sexual, but this change may be leading to problems for males (Burros, 1974). Some men appear to feel pressure to perform, to completely, totally satisfy the "new" sexual woman, and this pressure and performance anxiety may lead to male sexual dysfunction.

Religious or Moral Restrictions. Rigid religious or moral teachings may dwell on the evil or sinfulness of human sexuality. The transition from such attitudes to a free sexual relationship in or out of marriage is difficult. Such attitudes can be buried deeply, and affect behavior even when rational sexual behavior is acceptable.

Ignorance and Bad Advice. As Masters and Johnson (1966, 1970) found out, many people are extremely naive about the sexual functioning of the body, expecting perhaps that sexual behavior will "just happen," that it is instinctual, and that one will "naturally" do the right thing. Quite the opposite, effective sexual behavior requires knowledge, practice, and feedback from one's partner. This pervasive ignorance is compounded by bad advice from both amateurs and professionals (H. S. Kaplan, 1974, 1977). People with sexual problems may be told to "forget about it, and it will go away," or they may be advised to "sleep around and put some spice in your sex life." Such advice is unlikely to be followed, and if it is, is more likely to compound the problem than solve it.

Homosexuality. Some individuals enter into heterosexual relationships knowing or suspecting that they are homosexual (Masters & Johnson, 1970). The homosexual who attempts such a relationship often finds it a difficult task, leading to sexual dysfunction. Bieber and Bieber (1975) raise the interesting problem of the heterosexual who has fleeting homosexual ideas, fantasies, or attractions. Such thoughts may be quite anxiety provoking and lead to heterosexual dysfunction, which compounds the anxieties and may lead to more severe dysfunction. Masters and Johnson found underlying homosexuality to be a cause of heterosexual dysfunction in about 20 percent of their dysfunctional subjects. Current work, however, indicates that homosexuality is one of the less common historial factors in psychosexual dysfunction.

Physical Causes. Some sexual dysfunctions are the result of physical trauma, illness, or abnormality. Scars, infections, or other physical problems may lead to sexual dysfunction, as may drugs used to treat certain physical illnesses. A major drug often implicated in male dysfunction is alcohol. The central nervous system depressant effect of alcohol may lead to a lowering of inhibitions and an increase in sexual interest, but the same nervous system depressant effect makes the attainment of an erection more difficult. Secondary impotence often begins when an intoxicated man attempts sexual behavior and fails to attain an erection. The anxiety resulting from such failure may begin a vicious cycle.

Maintenance Factors

Fears about Performance. Once sexual dysfunction occurs, individuals usually react with anxiety and fears about future performances. These fears and anxieties may be present before the first sexual experience, or occur during a functional initial experience, growing as time passes until dysfunction occurs. In either event, as the likelihood of a sexual encounter nears, the fears and anxiety level probably increase. Frequently, this overconcern grows into what Masters and Johnson (1970, 1975) call the "spectator role."

Spectator Role Adoption. The **spectator role** may be a defensive maneuver and a manifestation of anxiety. The individual distances him/herself from the sexual act in progress. One becomes a spectator observing the performance, looking for flaws which prevent adequate functioning. Spectator role adoption may also be due to interpersonal problems between the sexual partners. As Lobitz and Lobitz (1978) have noted, interpersonal problems can lead to sexual behavior loaded with insecurity or resentment. The adoption of the spectator role prevents the passive, uncritical acceptance of sexual stimulation necessary for adequate function. The individual is unable to "get into" sexual enjoyment.

Sexual dysfunction rarely occurs in a vacuum. Derogatis and Meyer (1979) have studied the *invested* partner, who they describe as "an individual whose partner in a couple or maritial unit is suffering from a diagnosed sexual dysfunction but who is himself or herself free from any sexual disorder. In addition, the sexually functional individual must indicate a substantial personal investment in the relationship and accept a degree of responsibility for the shared disorder." They studied 51 such subjects (33 men and 18 women) and compared them with 200 controls. In general, they found the invested partners to be lower in self-esteem than controls, with the difference more pronounced for males. Males and females were both constricted in their range of sexual experience, females more than males, and female invested partners had a lowered sexual drive. Derogatis and Meyer ask whether these differences are due to the experience of living with a sexually dysfunctional partner, or perhaps are a contributory cause to the development of a sexual dysfunction in the partner. Their research could not answer this question.

GENDER IDENTITY DISORDER (TRANSSEXUALISM)

The term "gender identity disorder" is used to refer to a disturbance of the relationship between anatomic sex and one's subjective experience of sexual identity. In this disorder, an anatomical male has the subjective experience of being a female trapped in the body of a man; an anatomical female has the subjective experience of being a male who has the body of a woman through a "quirk" of nature. This disorder in adults is called *transsexualism.* In children, it is termed gender identity disturbance of childhood. Not all children with a gender identity disturbance develop transsexualism.

Transsexuals may engage in "homosexual" behavior, but from their perspective, such behavior is "heterosexual." In addition, while transsexuals do **cross-dress** (i.e., wear clothing consistent with their subjective rather than their anatomic sex), they are not **transvestites.** A true transvestite's self-perception is consistent with anatomical sex, and the transvestite is usually physically heterosexual, but gains sexual excitement from cross-dressing.

Transsexualism is rare, and is less common in women than in men. Onset of the gender disturbance can usually be traced to early childhood (R. Green, 1974). Children who later become transsexual usually assume, at least partially, the role of the opposite gender in their play and cross-dressing. Such behavior is often accepted and even promoted by the child's parents. Many adult transsexuals can recollect early childhood events which supported their gender confusion and cannot remember a time when they were secure in their anatomical sex role. Male transsexuals often report early recollections of hating their penises and wishing the "ugly growth away." It appears that basic gender identity becomes established in both normals and transsexuals very early, probably by 18 months of age, and is quite resistant to later attempts at change. By adulthood, transsexuals consider themselves to be of the opposite sex, and they dress accordingly and behave accordingly when possible.

Transsexuals move from homosexual to heterosexual behavior, and back agan, having difficulty being accepted by others and often finding social life excruciating. The conflict is constant: "Should I behave as I feel myself to be, or should I behave as my anatomical endowment demands?" Some transsexuals attempt heterosexual marriage, usually with disastrous results. When an anatomically appropriate relationship is established by a transsexual (anatomical male with an anatomical female), the transsexual subjectively experiences the relationship as *homosexual.*

Many experts believe that the development of transsexualism is most likely due to early childhood learning and, in males, to an overattachment to a binding mother (Pauly, 1974; Stoller, 1975). Recent research though has implicated hormonal factors. In order for testicles to develop in the male embryo, hormones called the **H-Y Antigen** must be present. Male transsexuals develop testicles, so this H-Y Antigen must have been present while the embryo was developing. Hoenig (1981) found that in 88 percent of the adult male and female transsexuals he studied, the H-Y Antigen levels were abnormally low in males and abnormally high in females. Hoenig suggests that through some unknown biological mechanism, the H-Y Antigen levels change after the embryo's physical sexual characteristics have developed. The change in levels may lead to changes in the individual's perception of sexual identity. Hoenig's findings are tentative, but will certainly lead to further research.

THE PARAPHILIAS

The group of disorders presented in this section were once called sexual deviations, a label that many still use. The term "paraphilia" is used in DSM-III (1980). This label comes from the latin words *para* (meaning roughly "deviation") and *philia* ("attraction for"). The change is intended to avoid the loaded connotation of the terms "sexual deviation" and "sexual deviate" (see Highlight 9.7).

The paraphilias are sexual behaviors that require unusual, bizarre imagery or acts for sexual excitement and satisfaction. The behaviors tend to have an "involuntary" character and involve either: 1. repetitive sexual activity with nonconsenting partners; 2. repetitive human sexual activity that includes real or simulated suffering or humiliation; or 3. preference for the use of a socially unacceptable or nonhuman object for sexual arousal. Individuals who manifest a paraphilia rarely seek therapeutic help. They are often satisfied with their sexual behavior, or they are ashamed to admit their acts. Treatment is often sought at the insistence of a spouse or other relative; and frequently the

HIGHLIGHT 9.7
SEXUAL BEHAVIOR AND LABELING

Although we try to avoid using terminology that has unintended meaning, this is not always possible. Ideally, paraphilia or other sexual behavior should be discussed using terms that do not imply that these forms of behavior are limited to one extreme of the population. For example, to say "The *voyeur* attains sexual excitement from the act of viewing others who are nude or engaged in a sexual act, without their consent" implies that only one distinct group finds sexual excitement in this behavior. The phrase "individuals who engage in voyeuristic behavior" does not suggest that the behavior is seen only in "sexual deviates." Unfortunately, the latter terminology becomes awkward and stilted if used constantly. In the section on paraphilias, terms such as "voyeur," "transvestite," and "pedophile" are used for conciseness. We must remember that these labels apply to only one part of a person's behavior, and less extreme forms of these behaviors may not be considered disordered.

treatment is court ordered, since some of these behaviors are illegal in most states.

Transvestism

As noted in the discussion of transsexuals, **transvestites** cross-dress for sexual excitement. This appears to be an exclusively male disorder. The male transvestite may masturbate when wearing women's clothing, or may wear women's clothing when engaged in sexual acts with a partner. Most transvestites are heterosexual, and many are married (Bentler & Prince, 1969). Their cross-dressing behavior is usually known only to immediate family and intimates, if to anyone. Stoller (1967, 1974) has indicated that some transvestites report parental support of their cross-dressing during childhood.

Fetishism

The individual with a **fetish** needs a certain object to be present in order to attain sexual arousal and gratification. Sometimes a fetish is represented by an exaggerated interest in a particular part of a partner's body, such as the foot. Fetishists appear to be primarily males. Fetishistic objects may include a wide range of objects such as female underclothing, baby buggies, and rubber boots.

Often, the fetish object must have been used. That is, a newly purchased pair of panties will not suffice; they must have been worn. The acquisition of such objects may lead a fetishist into difficulty with the police, since he may resort to theft to obtain the object. The following first-person account is typical of fetishistic behavior (A. W. Epstein, 1965):

> I always seem to have been fascinated by rubber boots. I cannot say exactly when the fascination first started, but I must have been very young. Their spell is almost hypnotic and should I see someone walking along with rubber boots, I become very excited and may follow the person for a great distance. I quickly get an erection under such circumstances and I might easily ejaculate. I am most excited by boots that are black and shiny and hip length. Whenever I see a picture of boots in a magazine, I become excited.
>
> I frequently dream of boots and when I do, I have a seminal emission. Sometimes I just

The male transvestite often practices his behavior in private but, on occasion, may go public.

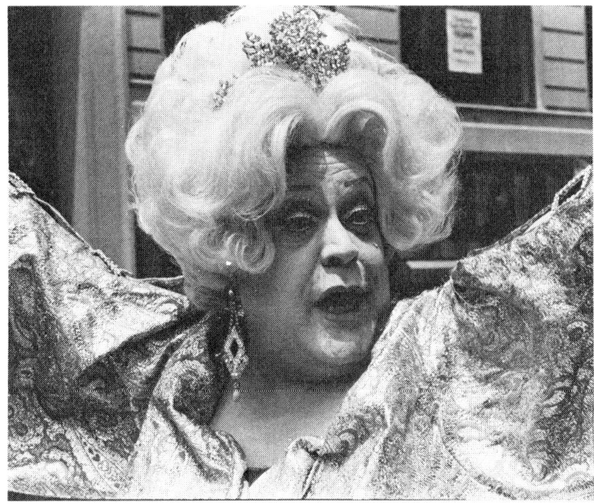

see a pair of boots in the dream—and I quickly have an emission. I self-stimulate myself (masturbate) frequently—I either look at a pair of boots, then, or simply allow the image of boots to come to my mind. When I am sitting alone, the thought and the sight of the boots makes me tense—it becomes painful, although usually the thought of the boots brings on a very pleasant feeling. I often put the boots on and look at myself in the mirror—this makes me stimulate myself. I often will take the boots to bed with me, caress them, kiss them, and ejaculate into them. (pp. 515–516)

Pedophilia

In 1912, Krafft-Ebing coined the term **pedophilia erotica** to label an adult's sexual desire for children. Such individuals are often called child molesters, and their behavior is illegal throughout the United States. The pedophile is often perceived as very dangerous, or often imagined to be an "old lecher" who waits outside schoolyards to lure children into a car for immoral purposes. In fact, most child molesters are neither dangerous nor old, and some are friends or members of the child's family. Two-thirds of pedophiles are quite harmless physically to children, although some of the remaining one-third can be quite dangerous. The typical sexual behavior of the pedophile consists of genital fondling and petting of the child. At times it includes having the child handle the genitals of the molester.

Several types of pedophiles have been identified. M. Cohen, Seghorn, and Calmas (1969) have identified the fixated molester, the regressive molester, and the aggressive molester.

The fixated pedophile is psychologically and psychosexually immature; the term "fixated" implies a psychological fixation at an earlier level of development. Such an individual is unable to develop an adequate adult hetero- or homosexual relationship and is only comfortable with children. The regressive pedophile has apparently adequate psychological and psychosexual relationships with adults, but this adjustment is tenuous. Under stress, the individual feels inadequate both sexually and otherwise; and when the sexual adequacy is threatened, turns to children for sexual and emotional satisfaction. The aggressive pedophile may not only be inadequate in adult psychological and psychosexual adjustment but may also vent rage and hostility through sexual acts on defenseless victims. Aggressive pedophiles are obviously the most physically dangerous type, although in a panic, some of the other types of pedophiles may inflict injury on a child. Most pedophiles will not injure the child, but some do (Kozol, 1971). It is tragic when the injury or death of a child results from such an act.

Exhibitionism

Sexual **exhibitionism** refers to the exposure of one's genitals to a nonconsenting individual, usually with the intent to achieve sexual self-stimulation or autoerotic (masturbatory) satisfaction. Many exhibitionists masturbate soon after exposing themselves, and some during the exposure; however, most male exhibitionists' penises are flaccid during the act of exposure. Sexual exhibitionism under conditions of sexual arousal is rare in women, and when seen it is usually in very seriously disturbed psychotic women. Women who exhibit their body for money (strippers, nude models) are primarily motivated by financial gain and attention, and their behavior rarely results in their own sexual arousal.

Male sexual exhibitionism is one of the most frequently reported "sexual offenses" (M. P. Feldman, 1977). Exhibitionists are almost never physically dangerous. Like pedophiles, exhibitionists are usually psychologically immature men who have difficulty approaching adult females on a mature level. Many are married, but have inadequate sexual relationships with their wives, and grave doubts about their own sexual adequacy (Witzig, 1968). They frequently exhibit when under increased levels of stress. Macdonald (1973) has described them as inhibited, puritanical, and fearful.

Commonalities in the developmental period of many exhibitionists have been noted (Zechnick, 1971). A striking lack of privacy often existed in their childhood homes. This may have been perceived as meaning that the penis "doesn't make any difference" to the women of the household. The later exposures might serve to prove that the penis does make a difference. It has been suggested that when the victim reacts with revulsion, shock, and escape, the exhibitionist feels gratified: His penis has been impressive. If the victim responds matter-of-factly, "M-m-m, that's very interesting, but what can it do?" the exhibitionist receives no sexual gratification and flees. Psychoanalysts view these behaviors as evidence that exhibitionism results from an unconscious fear of being castrated, a concept elaborated later in the discussion of the etiology of the paraphilias. In a sense, the behavior is a psychologically hostile act of defiance towards "castrating" women. Defiance and anger are illustrated in the following case, cited by Bond and Hutchinson (1965):

> His first exposure occurred at 13 following sex play with a 10-year-old neighbor girl. He had felt a desire to perform coitus, but the girl appeared indifferent to his suggestion and had refused. Her indifference hurt him; this was followed by rage, then by the exposing of his erect penis to her. During an exploratory hypnotic interview he recalled having seen this same girl urinate some five years before this episode, and his experience of astonishment at the appearance of her genitals. (p. 246)

Voyeurism

A person who engages in **voyeurism** obtains sexual excitement from the act of viewing others (usually strangers) without their consent or knowledge when they are undressing, nude, or engaged in a sexual act. The nonconsensual aspect is primary to this behavior. Becoming sexually excited from viewing another naked person who has consented is not voyeurism, nor is the viewing of pornographic materials. While secretly viewing someone, the voyeur becomes sexually excited and often masturbates. The elements of danger of discovery and secrecy apparently contribute to the sexual excitement, while the solitary nature of the act protects the voyeur from the shame of others' awareness of his inadequacy and sexual failure (McCary, 1973).

Many voyeurs are lonely, submissive, and dependent; if they are married, their marital sexual life is usually unsatisfactory. The basic voyeur is not dangerous, although some rapists may have elements of voyeurism, and may observe their intended victim prior to the rape, sometimes over a long period.

The following excerpt is from a fairly typical case (Hamilton, 1972) and illustrates the sense of power and "taking" that voyeurism may provide to the voyeur.

> Each voyeuristic expedition, he felt, was "unique," allowing him "the possibility of exclusive possession of the woman and of penetrating her secrets. It is like trespassing on someone's privacy. I am uninvited but not participating. I want warmth and intimacy, but feel as if I am stealing it. I steal it because I can't afford it." (p. 284)

Sexual Sadism and Sexual Masochism

The infliction of pain on another person to obtain or enhance sexual gratification is called **sexual sadism.** The need to have pain inflicted upon oneself to enhance sexual pleasure or to attain gratification is called **masochism.** Each behavior is named after a historical figure: sadism after the Marquis de Sade (1740–1814), who wrote extensively about the joy of his sexual gratification through the infliction of pain on others; and masochism after the novelist Leopold Sacher-Masoch (1836–1895), whose protagonists usually experienced sexual pleasure from pain. In addition to the sadist and masochist, some **sado-masochists** experience pleasure from both giving and receiving pain. When psychological pain such as frustration and humiliation are the primary behaviors, we refer to sexual dominance-submission syndromes, which may be either heterosexual or homosexual (Tripp, 1975). Since these behaviors are often consensual, their incidence is not known.

Very mild infliction of pain (e.g., love bites) may be fairly common in many sexual relationships, since the experience of mild pain seems to be stimulating. However, the sexual sadist and masochist go far beyond this. Cleckley (1957) cites a case with elements of fetishism and cross-dressing which illustrates a sexual sado-masochistic relationship:

> [The subject,] though somewhat indifferent, customarily treated his wife with respect and politeness. Apparently he felt, most of the time, a measure of personal affection for the attractive woman he had married. Ordinary intercourse was practiced usually and both partners enjoyed physiologic satisfaction.

At intervals of five or six weeks the husband insisted upon carrying out a different and rather remarkable procedure. The routine varied little. Forcing his wife to take a servile role and address him as "sir," and in every conceivable way to humiliate herself, he got her to cooperate with him in choosing instruments for her [punishment]. Agreement being reached on a hairbrush, he would then send her out to cut a stick from the limb of a nearby tree. The two together picked what dress she would wear for the beginning of the ceremonies planned.

He himself meanwhile discarded his own clothes, put on the wife's girdle, her stockings, and sometimes other lingerie. Not being able to get his feet into her shoes, he had bought himself a pair of high-heeled evening slippers which fitted. . . . Before the actual beating began, and also during its progress, he insisted that she prostrate herself in various indignities, that she grovel while describing herself in obscene terms, calling herself a dirty slut, and so forth. Kissing his feet while he expressed loathing and made gestures of contempt and derision, she tried to cooperate despite her extreme distaste. Often he tied her to a chair while she was completely dressed and beat her until she bled and screamed. Later, tearing off her clothes, he continued the blows, using now the hairbrush, now the rough stick she had cut for him. Sometimes her wounds and bruises remained visible for a week or more. (pp. 285–286)

Etiology of the Paraphilias

The paraphilias involve a wide range of behaviors. Some of the less well known are noted in Highlight 9.8. What general factors could account for this diversity of sexual behaviors which most people consider unacceptable?

Psychoanalytic theory suggests that paraphilias develop because of unconscious fears associated with the more socially acceptable forms of sexual relationships. Sexual impulses are then displaced from socially acceptable outlets onto objects or behaviors which are less intrapsychically threatening. An important factor in the psychoanalytic view is the belief that the disturbed individual has not resolved the Oedipal conflict; he (most people with paraphilias are men) associates adult women with his mother and finds them unapproachable like mother: powerful and forbidden. One reason why this might happen is because at an unconscious level he associates normal sexual behavior with an adult woman, to the danger of castration. Psychoanalysts believe that a young boy's sexual feelings towards his mother are repressed because of castration anxiety, a supposed fear of the son's castration by the father. This threat is resolved by the son's identification with the aggressor (father). If this identification is successful, normal adult sexual behavior is likely; if not, a paraphilia may develop. The application of psychoanalytic speculation to specific paraphilias could lead to ideas such as the following:

1. The transvestite has identified with a mother who encouraged his cross-dressing. The sexual excitement of cross-dressing is due to his symbolic possession of his mother, in the form of his *own* body dressed in women's clothes.
2. An object becomes a fetish because it is unconsciously associated with mother. For example, as a child, the man saw mother's panties and later panties become the fetishistic object.
3. Exhibitionism reduces castration anxiety and proves to "mom" (symbolized by the woman who sees the penis) that the man *is* a sexual creature.
4. A child becomes the preferred sexual object because sexual behavior with children does not lead to castration anxiety.
5. The voyeur is symbolically "peeping" at mother, or mother and father. The secret act gives him power over his parents.
6. Sadism is a demonstration of power over mother, and a demonstration that the man is as powerful as his father.
7. The need to be punished to obtain sexual satisfaction that exists in masochism is a symbolic reenactment of the dangers of sexual desire for a parent. The actual punishment symbolizes the punishment of the parent, and it satisfies the guilt over sexual behavior, which can then occur.

Although psychoanalytic speculation about the etiology of paraphilias is intriguing, there is virtually no direct evidence to support these ideas.

Are the behaviors learned? We have already seen that some transvestites have reported that their cross-dressing was reinforced by parents (usually the mother). Sexual arousal is reinforc-

HIGHLIGHT 9.8
AN ARRAY OF STRANGE SEXUAL BEHAVIORS

At the extreme range of low frequency sexual behavior, there is a broad variety of sexual objects and modes of function which have been described and named. Some are listed and described below:

1. Zoophilia. Sexual use of animals through masturbation or intercourse. This disorder is more frequently seen in rural areas, but cases have been described in which household pets have been trained to engage in sexual acts with humans.
2. Coprophilia. The need to have feces present either visually or tactiley to enhance sexual satisfaction. An example from Cleckley (1957) follows: "He would go to places where he was not known and there he would visit the public men's rooms of the railroad station in search for pieces of feces. Then he collected them, wrapped them up carefully and carried them around with him, thus experiencing sexual-orgastic relief."
3. Necrophilia. Sexual activity with a dead body.
4. Frottage. Rubbing against other persons' bodies (typically strangers) to obtain sexual satisfaction; most frequently occurs in public places such as crowded elevators and subways.
5. Saliromania. Dirtying or mutilating female bodies or clothing to obtain sexual satisfaction.
6. Piquer. Obtaining sexual satisfaction from stabbing another in the breast or buttock with a sharp pointed instrument such as a needle or ice pick. The intent is not usually to kill. Fortunately, this is an extremely rare behavior.
7. Klismaphilia. Sexual gratification obtained from giving or receiving an enema.
8. Obscene Telephone Calls. Only about 25 percent of the estimated 3 million "obscene" telephone calls received each year have a sexual content. The other 75 percent are harassing or threatening. Most such calls are made by males. The sexually oriented calls appear to be made exclusively by males, who are usually lonely, under stress, feel inadequate, and obtain a sense of strength and pleasure from the shocked reaction of the female who answers the call—especially if the reaction involves outrage. The most functional reaction is simply to hang up and report the call to the police.
9. Satyriasis and Nymphomania. Compulsive promiscuity, often called "satyriasis" in males and "nymphomania" in women, involves high frequency sexual behavior of a "driven" quality, which is rarely satisfactory to the individual. While orgasm can occur (and usually does in males), shortly after the sexual experience the individual is dominated by the need to engage in a sexual act again. In the classic case, the individual is searching for love, but feels unlovable, and must go from sexual liaison to sexual liaison in an attempt to prove to the self that he or she really is worth loving.

ing, and early childhood events may result in an individual associating unusual behaviors with sexual stimulation. In one case report of a masochistic individual, this seems to be how the paraphilia developed (Hirschfield, 1948):

> One evening they were surprised in the act [of masturbation] by the governess. She locked the door behind her and said: "You're now going to get a good hiding, and every evening for eight days, before bedtime, you're going to get the same." She fetched a stick, laid each of the boys across the arm of the sofa and raising his shirt—all that he was wearing—she laid on with the cane until his buttocks changed colour. Both boys submitted. "It burned my behind like fire, but at the same time it prickled so pleasantly, so delightfully. And it was the blows that did it, it had never been so nice when we masturbated, which we did again. And later I noticed that the governess's hands, during the now regular chastisements, frequently strayed between my legs and stayed there. So we were glad of the blows and when the happy days were over we longed for them."

In this example, the boy was physically punished, but the governess's behavior led not only to pain but also to a subjective experience of pleasure. The young man learned to associate pain with sexual pleasure.

A learning process has been suggested as the etiology for fetishistic behavior. The frequent experience of sexual gratification in the presence of an object may lead to classical conditioning. Even in the absence of the object, the fetish could be learned through fantasy association (Abel & Blanchard, 1974; Rachman, 1966; Stoller, 1976). However, if association with sexual arousal were the only thing necessary, we would expect more fetishisms to sheets, pillows, and ceilings than anything else (Baron & Byrne, 1977). In fact, these items are not common fetish objects.

In discussions of the etiology of other types of behavior disorders, the role of modeling has often been implicated. Could the paraphilias be modeled? It may be difficult to imagine a direct modeling experience as being an important etiological factor in these disorders. However, Krueger (1978) has reported on a multigeneration family in which voyeurism was passed from grandparent to parent, and transvestism was passed from parent to son:

> Mr. A [the parent] remembered that his father [the grandparent] loved and collected pornographic magazines and encouraged Mr. A. to engage in voyeuristic acts. He was arrested at age 17 while window peeping at a house of prostitution. His father told tales of Mr. A's grandfather going to the park "to sit around and have girls in the bushes with him." Mr. A believed his family had a history of sexually oriented men and was proud of this history.
>
> Mr. A reported that he was first introduced to the idea of cross-dressing when, as a young teenager, he went to the movies and bars "to learn how to be a man," since he did not see much of his father due to the latter's long work hours. At the bars he heard stories about men who wore women's clothes. He said he tried it himself for the first time at about age 16. Mr. A's wife reported first being aware of his cross-dressing after about a year of marriage, when he cross-dressed after times his father was especially critical of him.
>
> Mr. A would cross-dress, donning women's underwear, after some kind of stress, e.g., a fight with his wife or children, an occasion when his boss was critical of his work, a sexual problem (impotence or loss of erection), his wife's refusal to have sex, or when he was especially depressed. He described a domino effect. Typically, when his boss or wife would "come down on me," he would cross-dress. He would subsequently belittle and criticize his *sons*, who would then cross-dress. (p. 739)

Here we have three generations of paraphilias in one family line. Mr. A had three sons, and two had observed the cross-dressing. They engaged in transvestite behavior, the other did not. One case study does not prove that modeling is important in *all* transvestism, but indicates that it is a possible etiological factor.

Simple concepts of learning are probably too limited to adequately explain the paraphilias. However, if we include a few additional notions, the probable etiology becomes clearer.

1. Experiences in childhood and adolescence may create predisposing situations; for example, reinforcement of cross-dressing, or parental attitudes towards privacy as in the case of an exhibitionist.
2. Some individuals may have conditioned learning experiences that lead directly to the paraphilia. Later the association of relevant sexual fantasies with sexual arousal and gratification may reinforce the unconventional sexual activity. Cognitions (fantasy) are important in normal sexual arousal, and it would not be surprising if they are important in the paraphilias.
3. Even when conditioned learning does not precede a fantasy, fantasies about unusual sexual practices may be associated with sexual arousal and reinforcing gratification.
4. Some males who manifest paraphilias are often described as inadequate in their masculine roles. It is not certain, but seems likely that this inadequacy is present prior to the development of the paraphilia. This inadequacy, and anxiety about relating to mature females may be an important factor in predisposing the individual to engage in unusual sexual behaviors.

When these factors are considered, the paraphilias appear to develop in several possible ways: 1. They may be learned in a complex process that involves either: a. direct reinforcement of the behavior, or b. fantasies associated with masturbation and later experiences and sexual gratification. 2. Some individuals are predisposed to alternative forms of sexual behavior because of personal inadequacies in heterosexual behavior. They are likely to find that unusual forms of sexual activity avoid the anxieties about these inadequacies, and also that the behavior is reinforcing because of sexual stimulation and gratification. Although these are neat explanations of how paraphilias might be learned and maintained, they, like the psychoanalytic view, are based primarily on generalizations from case reports. Much more research must be done before the etiology of the paraphilias is clear.

SEXUAL BEHAVIOR OF SPECIAL SIGNIFICANCE

In this section three types of sexual behavior are treated separately because of their special significance. Incest is an old problem which is receiving increasing attention. Rape will be discussed here because of its relatively high frequency, the nonsexual aspects of this behavior, and the significant trauma experienced by the rape victim. In addition, homosexuality is presented here because of the controversy over whether it is, in fact, abnormal, "sick," or deviant.

Incest

Under some circumstance, incestuous behavior fits the parameters of pedophilia, for example, when the pedophile is a parent or sibling and the "victim" is a child under 12. **Incest** is usually considered to be the occurrence of sexual relations between parent and child, or between sibs of any age. In some cultures, the incest prohibition extends beyond immediate family members; only a few sociocultural settings have condoned incest, the most notable being the pharaohs of ancient Egypt.

The **incest "taboo"** as it was called by Freud, appears to have a meaning beyond simple morality or attitude. Adams and Neel (1967) studied infants born from 18 incestuous relationships and found that only 7 of the 18 could be considered normal. By the age of 6 months, 5 of the 18 had died, 3 had borderline intelligence, 2 were severely mentally retarded, and 1 had a cleft palate. In a control group of 18 infants, only 2 were abnormal. Although small in sample size, the study suggests that children of incestuous relationships may have a substantial risk of genetic defect. Even when an infant is not born from such a relationship, the effects of the experience can be quite damaging psychologically to the participants, since the behavior is far outside the bounds of what most people find acceptable.

Recent studies have indicated that the frequency of incest and pedophilia is much higher than suspected. Summit and Kryso (1978) estimate that there are 200,000–300,000 cases of sexual abuse of children each year (36,000 are father-daughter incest). The frequency of incest may be much higher than Summit and Kryso estimate. The shame and embarrassment about incestuous behavior may lead to the underreporting of such experiences.

By far the greatest percentage of reported incest occurs between fathers and daughters; and in the rare cases between mothers and sons (about 4 percent of reported cases; Maisch, 1972), the mothers appear to be even more psychologically disturbed prior to the initiation of the act than do incestuous fathers. When father-daughter incest occurs, the father often initiates the original act while his judgment is impaired by alcoholic intoxication. The behavior often begins when these fathers are under a strain which threatens their masculinity, commonly when the wife is rejecting the husband's sexual interest towards her. The husband then turns to a sexually developing child for sexual and usually emotional gratification. In families where the prohibitions against incest break down, the family is often disorganized. Family members do not communicate and, in fact, tend to deny sexuality. The wife-mother frequently denies the possibility of the act, and fails to protect the daughter even when she hears the daughter complain about it. Instead, she often attacks the daughter as a "liar" or as a seductress (Bernstein, 1979). To outsiders, these families appear quite normal and respectable and come from all social classes.

Often the child is only vaguely aware that something is "wrong" with the incestuous behavior, that it is unusual. Once this understanding grows, the adolescent female may try to terminate the behavior, and may feel ashamed, guilty, and angry. The subsequent perception of one's father as doing this "bad" thing may distort the daughter's later psychological and psychosexual adjustment, particularly if the father used intimidation and coercion (James, 1977). The primary treatment of such reactions to incest has been psychotherapy, but family therapy programs developed in recent years seem to have been successful in preventing a recurrence of the behavior and in dealing with the incest victims' reactions to the victimization (Giaretto, 1978).

Rape

Rape consists of forcible sexual intercourse, which is against the will of the individual who is coerced. Hilberman (1976) has described it as the "ultimate violation of the self short of homicide." Approximately 60,000 rapes are reported to police each year, but estimates place the actual incidence at 250,000 cases per year, perhaps more. Of the 60,000 reported cases, as much as 18 percent may be false accusations (Macdonald, 1973); however, this percentage must be balanced by the awareness that there is a strong tendency for males to disbelieve a woman's report of rape (Brownmiller, 1975; Hilberman, 1976). Rape occurs primarily with men as the perpetrator and women as the victims, although this is not always the case. Storaska (1975) has reported cases in other cultures of rape by women against men, although this is exceedingly rare in the United States, with only a few known cases. Rape by men of other men is more common. Groth and Burgess (1980) studied 22 cases of such male-male rapes occurring in the community; they suggest that it is much more common than believed, and almost never reported due to the male victim's shame and humiliation.

A demonstration sponsored by the National Organization of Women's Rape Prevention Committee. Public protests against rape have helped to generate media coverage of this serious issue.

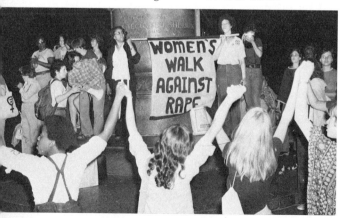

The Rapist. Is the rapist engaging in a sexual act? Many authorities say "no." Some say that sexual gratification is at most a secondary factor in rape (Groth, Burgess, & Holmstrom, 1977). Others claim that rape is a ritualized process for the subjugation of women which has little to do with sexual behavior (Brownmiller, 1975).

Most rapists are young, adult males, and about half are married. Most who rape once will rape again. Abel et al. (1977) have found that rapists are as strongly stimulated by rape scenes (or even scenes of pure aggression; Abel, 1979) as they are by scenes of consenting intercourse, unlike normal males. Could biological factors, such as increased levels of male hormones, be a contributing factor? Perhaps, but the evidence to date suggests not. A lifestyle that supports the development of aggressive behavior towards weaker victims, and feelings of anger, rage, and contempt for women appears to be a significant factor. Groth et al. (1977) have intensively studied rapists and have found that in all cases of forcible rape, the needs to express power, anger, and sexuality are present, with the expression of power and anger being dominant factors. They consider sexuality as simply the vehicle for the expression of these motivations. Groth et al. have found broad variations in personalities of rapists, but have developed several typologies which assist in the description of rapists:

1. Power-Assertive Rapist. For him, rape is an expression of virility, mastery, and dominance. During the rape, his inadequacy as manifested in his identity and life effectiveness can be denied through an act of power over another person.
2. Power-Reassurance Rapist. He commits the rape to reassure himself of his own sexual adequacy and masculinity. His need is to place women in a helpless position to eliminate his doubts and bolster his weakened self-perception.
3. Anger-Retaliation Rapist. Rape for him is an expression of anger and rage. The motive is revenge and his aim is degradation and humiliation. These men often have histories of abandonment or rejection by important female figures in their lives.

4. Anger-Excitation Rapist. This rapist is a sexual sadist who is excited by and finds pleasure in the suffering of his victim. His aim is to punish, hurt, and torture the victim. These rapists are likely to have histories of assaultive behaviors which in many instances are not associated with sexual activity. Fortunately, only 5 percent of rapists apparently fall into this category.

In their study of male rapes of male victims, Groth and Burgess (1980) found very similar dynamics. The motivation of the rapist was to express power over others, retaliate for perceived injury or slights, and assert strength and manhood. In this study, only 12 percent of the rapists were homosexuals, 38 percent had bisexual experiences (they had sexual activities with both men and women), and 50 percent were exclusively heterosexual, even though all had raped a man. The self-perception of these rapists supports the contention that the act is one of power and anger, rather than sexuality.

The Victim. Not only does the rape victim suffer the trauma of the event but also the trauma of reporting the assault. Most apparently avoid this additional trauma by suffering in silence. Hilberman (1976) points out that often the victim (who is only rarely male) is blamed for the attack: She was seductive, a flirt, dressed provocatively. The accusations against the victim are rarely true. Bryant and Cirel (1977) have estimated that only 4 percent of rape victims have contributed to the situation in *any* way.

Women cope with rape in a variety of ways. They use cognitive strategies (think through alternatives to prevent or defuse the event), verbal strategies (try to talk their way out), physical action (flee or fight); and some become psychologically paralyzed and numb (Burgess & Holmstrom, 1976). Burgess and Holmstrom report that during the physical attack, many victims mentally disengage and try to stay calm, others scream; some try to reason with the rapist; some struggle; and some experience involuntary gagging, choking, nausea, and even loss of consciousness. Once free of the rapist and safe, a series of reactions may occur (Notman & Nadelson, 1976). Victims are anxious and fearful, but often not immediately angry. Anger, when it appears, comes later. Guilt and shame are universal, and supported by the rejecting attitudes of friends, family, and strangers. Very commonly, the victims go through a period of lack of trust in men. Many women are so distraught they try to start life over; they find new places of residence, new jobs, new friends. The victims' reactions can be considered a posttraumatic stress disorder, like those discussed in Chapter 5.

Homosexuality

Within abnormal psychology and the other mental health professions, a major debate involves the normality or abnormality of homosexual behavior. This controversy will not be settled soon.

Until the work of Alfred Kinsey (Kinsey, Pomeroy, & Martin, 1948; Kinsey et al., 1953) most knowledge about homosexuality came from clinical studies of homosexuals who had entered therapy because of psychological difficulties. The data from these relatively unrepresentative samples led most clinicians to believe that homosexuality was not only a deviation from the norm in frequency but also was abnormal in a pathological sense, so that homosexuals were "sick." The Kinsey studies, however, indicated that the incidence of homosexual behavior or attraction was much more common than previously thought. In these surveys of 5300 men and 5940 women, who were randomly selected, interesting discoveries about homosexuality were made. These early surveys indicated that about 4 percent of the adult white male population was exclusively homosexual, and that about 37 percent of males had at some time experienced a homosexual orgasm. About 28 percent of the women surveyed had at least one homosexual experience.

While the Kinsey research has become dated since its publication more than 30 years ago, Bell and Weinberg (1978) have recently confirmed many of the Kinsey findings. They studied 979 homosexually oriented males and females from a sample of 5000 homosexuals in the San Francisco area and compared them to 500 heterosexual control subjects. Each subject was intensively interviewed for 1.5 hours, and each was asked the same series of structured questions. Although the sample may not be representative of homosexuals across the United States, some interesting findings stand out. There were no differences in occupational choice (the supposed predominance of homosexuality in the arts is a myth), and less than 10 percent of the homosexuals were in "feminine" occupations, (such as hairdressing or home decoration). Approximately 25 percent of the homosexuals regretted their homosexuality, less than is commonly thought. There was no significant difference in level of psychological distress between most of the homosexual group and the heterosexual control group. Most homosexuals could not be distinguished from heterosexuals in terms of "pathological" thought processes. However, about 28 percent of the homosexual men and 16 percent of the homosexual women were either psychologically disturbed (depressed) or isolated—problems which may have been due to the social unacceptability of homosexuality. In addition, at least 50 percent of the homosexual males reported having at least 500 different sexual partners during their sexual careers. Bieber (1978), a proponent of the view that homosexuality is a symptom of emotional disorder, regards this average of 20 new relationships per year for 25 years as a level of promiscuity that indicates significant "pathology."

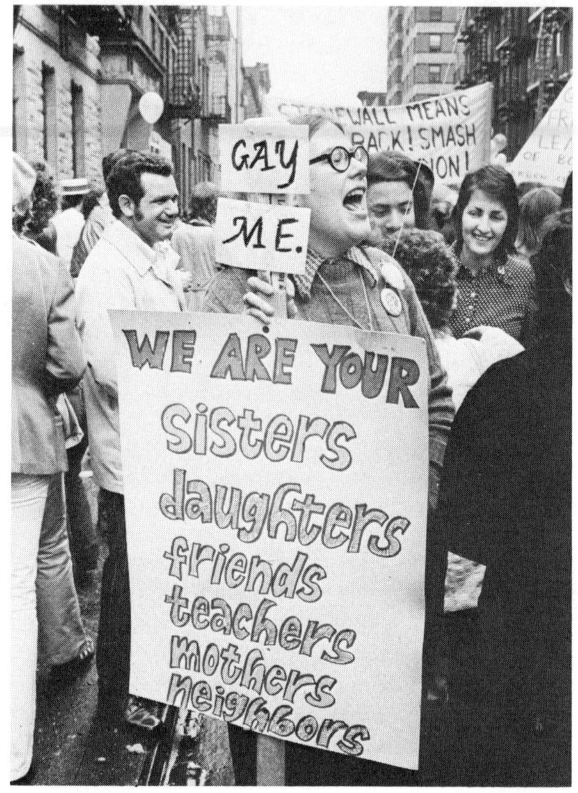

Homosexuals have become much more militant in expressing their desire for freedom from social discrimination.

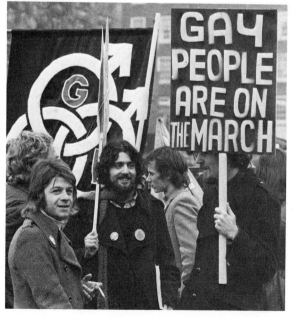

Homosexual Life-Styles. Misconceptions exist about the life-style of homosexuals; for example, homosexuals are supposedly obvious because they walk oddly, are "limp wristed," and lisping if males, and masculine appearing if females. These notions have been disproven by studies such as Bell and Weinberg's (1978). The following typology (one of several available) is useful in describing homosexual life-styles:

1. The situational homosexual. An individual who engages in homosexuality when no heterosexual partner is available; common in prisons. This individual does not usually consider him/herself to actually be a homosexual. The behavior is a matter of sexual necessity.
2. The hidden homosexual. Often known as a "closet" homosexual; one who hides the fact of the sexual preference; may be married or feign marriage. Only very close friends know of the homosexuality, perhaps no one knows but his or her lover. Bell and Weinberg (1978) found that

most of the individuals they studied kept the homosexuality a secret from all but a few. The subjects' mothers were most likely to be the member of their family who had been told.

3. The adjusted homosexual. Those who have close relationships with another homosexual partner or partners, handle their occupational status vis-à-vis their sexual preference well, and who are linked with the gay community. Some hidden homosexuals may overlap into this category. They manifest few of the stereotyped mannerisms of the behaviorally obvious homosexual.
4. The behaviorally obvious homosexual. These individuals fit the stereotyped limp-wristed, swishing femininity of the flagrantly flaunting male homosexual or the masculine, gruff, "butch" or "dyke" lesbian. Also included here are the male effeminate cross-dressers. This category is a minority. Most homosexuals are definitely not recognizable through mannerism or appearance.
5. The "tearoom" homosexual. An apparent minority, these individuals (perhaps exclusively males) engage in furtive "one-night stands." Approximately half are married, and it is likely that all are "hidden" in addition. Bell and Weinberg (1978) would consider them "dysfunctional." The term "tearoom trade" refers to homosexual behavior in public washrooms.

Possible Factors in the Development of Homosexuality. Humans are not simply heterosexual or homosexual. A great deal of research suggests that sexual behavior falls on a continuum for each of us. Homosexual thoughts are not uncommon in behaviorally heterosexual individuals (Bieber & Bieber, 1975) and heterosexual fantasies are common in behaviorally homosexual persons (Bell & Weinberg, 1978). As Mosher and O'Grady (1979) have demonstrated, in spite of a prevailing cultural rejection of homosexual behavior, a random sample of the heterosexual male population can be sexually aroused by homosexual stimuli, even though most heterosexual males experience disgust and anger in conjunction with the arousal. But why are a majority of adults behaviorally and subjectively heterosexual, and why do some become homosexual?

Physiological factors. Some investigators have implicated genetic and hormonal factors in homosexuality. However, Money (1970); D. Rosenthal (1970); Brodie et al. (1974); and Tourney, Petrilli, and Hatfield (1975) have found no consistent support for these etiological theories. Some studies have found low levels of male hormones in the blood of male homosexuals, others have found high levels. Similar contradictory results have been found for female homosexuals (Meyer-Bahlburg, 1979). This area of research remains so filled with discrepant findings that no conclusions can be effectively drawn.

Psychoanalytic theories. Psychoanalytic theories have also been proposed to account for homosexual behavior. One major view is that the individual turns to sexual behavior with a member of the same sex because of unconscious fears about heterosexual behavior. The fears are traced back to an unresolved Oedipal or Electra conflict. The adult avoids heterosexual behavior because it stimulates unacceptable incestuous feelings which were never resolved in childhood. Some studies of homosexuals in psychoanalysis seemed to indirectly support this theory. For example, Bieber et al. (1962) compared 106 male homosexuals in treatment with 100 heterosexuals in treatment. The homosexual subjects reported that their mothers were more domineering and demanded more intense emotional relationships with them than was reported for the mothers of the heterosexual males. These characteristics of the mother are called **close binding.** In addition, male homosexuals reported that their fathers were distant or hostile, and were poor figures for role identification. Because Bieber et al.'s findings were derived from homosexuals in treatment, they cannot be generalized to all homosexuals.

A later study (Evans, 1969) of homosexuals who were not in treatment found that some homosexuals (but not all) remembered their mothers as being close binding and their fathers as being distant and unacceptable. The members of the heterosexual control group in this study were less likely to describe their parents this way. Obviously, some homosexuals remember their parents as being of a particular type. However, it is a major leap to infer from this type of recollection that all (or most) homosexuals suffer from castration anxiety. Many experts (e.g., Bieber, 1978) still retain this view, in spite of criticisms leveled by other researchers (e.g., Siegelman, 1974).

Learning and homosexuality. Can homosexuality be learned? Perhaps. It has certainly been unlearned in some cases (Barlow, 1973; McCulloch & Feldman, 1967). An example of how homosexual behavior might be learned might include the following scenario: A shy boy finds acceptance with male peers less stressful than encounters with females, since he believes he cannot meet girls' expectations. By late adolescence, he has learned that he becomes anxious and inept when he tries to socially interact. Several unpleasant rejections by females lead him to become socially isolated from women *except* when he removes the threat by not considering them as sexual objects, and relates as a "brother" or platonic friend. His self-doubts about his heterosexuality (common in many adolescent males) crystalize during a relationship with a warm and open male friend, and the two enter a caring homosexual experience. His questions about his sexuality are eased by the positive reinforcement of the sharing relationship, and he begins to think of himself as a homosexual. Obviously, not all homosexuals develop this way, but the possibilities of homosexuality as a learned sexual preference require exploration.

KEY TREATMENTS

Psychosexual dysfunction

Various traditional treatment approaches have been tried with individuals who have psychosexual dysfunctions, generally with poor results. An exception has been the application of behavioral techniques to these disorders.

Systematic desensitization, a technique described in Chapter 7, has often been used to decrease the anxiety associated with sexual behavior. Ince (1973) describes the successful treatment of a woman who was so anxious about sexual intercourse that she had developed orgasmic dysfunction.

> The patient was asked to describe the sexual relationship between her and her husband, that is, the lovemaking, in precise detail, and to relate which aspects of it made her anxious. An outline of the sequence of acts, in order of occurrence and also in order of anxiety arousal is as follows:
>
> 1. Her husband moves toward her in bed
> 2. Her husband kisses her
> 3. Her husband embraces her and she returns the embrace
> 4. Her husband caresses her breasts and she caresses his penis
> 5. Her husband stimulates her vagina while she continues to caress him
> 6. Intercourse, occasionally preceded by oral-genital stimulation.
>
> Systematic desensitization was the treatment method employed. The patient was trained in relaxation by means of suggestion. Within two sessions she was able to completely relax. Then, under conditions of relaxation, the lovemaking sequence was described to her in detail by the therapist. The patient was first directed to indicate to him when she clearly visualized each scene, and also to indicate when she felt anxious by raising her hand. Each time anxiety occurred she was relaxed again prior to continuation of therapy. The patient was also given the task of relaxing herself at home in bed, prior to engaging in sexual relations, and her husband was instructed to postpone his advances until she had done so.
>
> Following the initial desensitization session, the patient had intercourse with her husband and was able to remain relaxed and enjoy the activity. She did not, however, experience orgasm. The following night she came the nearest to having an orgasm that she had since she had been married. One week later she had her first strong desire for sexual intercourse.
>
> Two days later she awakened in the night with a desire for intercourse, awakened her husband and enjoyed the sexual act immensely but did not have an orgasm. One week after that she began to feel as affectionate toward her husband as she had felt prior to her marriage and her sexual desires were "as they had been before."
>
> Within five more days she experienced her first orgasm and from then on reported no more difficulty in reaching an orgasm during her now frequent lovemaking sessions. The entire duration of therapy was one month. (pp. 448–449)

The treatment of sexual dysfunction is often based on the pioneering work of Masters and Johnson (1970) and their continuing research. Therapists such as Masters and Johnson, H. S. Kaplan (1975), and LoPiccolo (1978) tend to approach treatment of these dysfunctions very similarly. The major features of such approaches involve: 1. physical examination to rule out organic problems; 2. **sensate focus**—teaching the client and partner how to experience pleasure from touching and caressing each other's bodies while not engaging in intercourse; 3. programmed sexual experiences in the privacy of the client's residence; 4. ongoing counseling to resolve misconceptions, anxieties, and interpersonal difficulties. This approach does not use **sexual surrogates** (paid professionals who engage in sexual activities with the client and partner). Helen S. Kaplan (1977) has strongly presented her view, also the view of many other reputable sexual dysfunction therapists, that the use of sexual surrogates is unnecessary and even damaging to the therapeutic process; that therapists who use this approach are engaging in quackery, even subtle prostitution.

In the Masters and Johnson approach, physical problems that exist (they occur only in a small percent of cases) are dealt with, if possible. Assuming that they have been treated, or if no physical problems exist, the therapy is primarily psychological and educative. The counseling setting allows the therapists to work with the clients in a situation of relatively low anxiety. Clients' concerns and preconceptions about "appropriate" sexual behavior can be explored, and *educative* feedback can be given. As sexual misconceptions are resolved, homework is given. The clients (the plural is used, since sexual dysfunction therapy usually involves a couple) are instructed in sensate focusing. They are taught how to give and experience pleasure from touching each other. At home, they practice these behaviors with the injunction that no matter how much they may wish to, they are not to engage in intercourse. This prohibition takes away the pressure to perform and, hence, reduces anxiety. Finally, after much sensate focusing practice, the couple is instructed to begin to practice sexual intercourse in the privacy of their own home. Again the therapists caution the couple to avoid demanding or expecting too much. Problems encountered are resolved in open communication during counseling sessions, and successful activity is reinforced. This slow step-by-step process seems to be quite successful.

Both Masters and Johnson (1970) and H. S. Kaplan (1975) have reported success rates approaching 100 percent for the disorders of premature ejaculation and vaginismus. The success rates for other dysfunctions are lower, but Masters and Johnson's overall success rate is reported as 80 percent. Other equally competent therapists using the Masters and Johnson approach have not been quite as successful. This discrepancy has led to serious criticisms of Masters and Johnson's data collection and success criteria by other therapists and researchers (Zilbergeld & Evans, 1980). Masters and Johnson may have screened out the more difficult cases, and their success criteria may have been too subjective. Their high percentage of positive results may also have been due to positive rater biases.

Behavioral approaches have also proven effective with a variety of psychosexual dysfunctions. For example Nemetz, Craig, and Reich (1978), worked with 22 women suffering debilitating sexual anxiety; 7 of the 22 women manifested primary orgasmic dysfunction and 15 had secondary or situational orgasmic dysfunction. The women were provided with individual and group relaxation training. They then viewed 45 videotaped vignettes of graduated explicit sexual behavior. The tapes demonstrated various sexual behaviors such as masturbation and different types of intercourse. If the women became anxious while viewing the tapes, they were to use a relaxation exercise to decrease the anxiety. A waiting list control group showed no improvement, while the treatment group manifested positive changes in sexual attitude, behavior, and pleasure and a decrease in anxiety level. Although orgasmic frequency did not increase, the other positive changes were stable at a one-year follow-up.

The successful behavioral treatment approaches all utilize anxiety reduction and behavioral practice. H. S. Kaplan (1975) feels that therapy for sexual dysfunction must go beyond these two factors. Sexual dysfunction occurs in human relationships, most of which have been in existence for many years. Kaplan's approach emphasizes psychotherapy in addition to direct sexual training and anxiety reduction. She feels that if the interpersonal difficulties of the sexual partners are not resolved, the gains of strict behavioral sexual therapy may be undone.

Transsexualism

Transsexualism has attained a great degree of notoriety from popular media reports on the use of **sex reassignment surgery.** Beginning with George Jorgensen, who became Christine Jorgensen in 1953, and more recently with Renee Richards, an

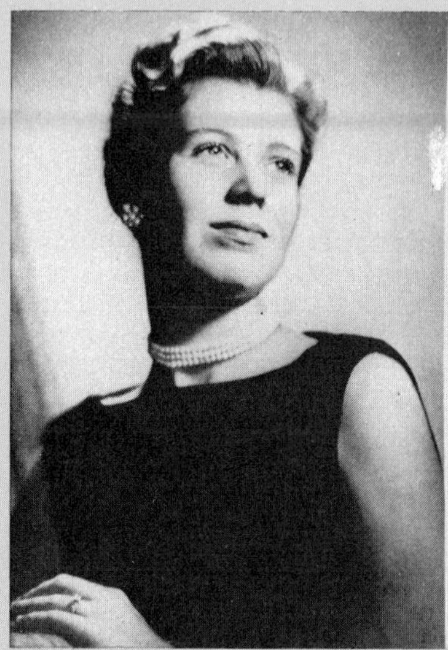

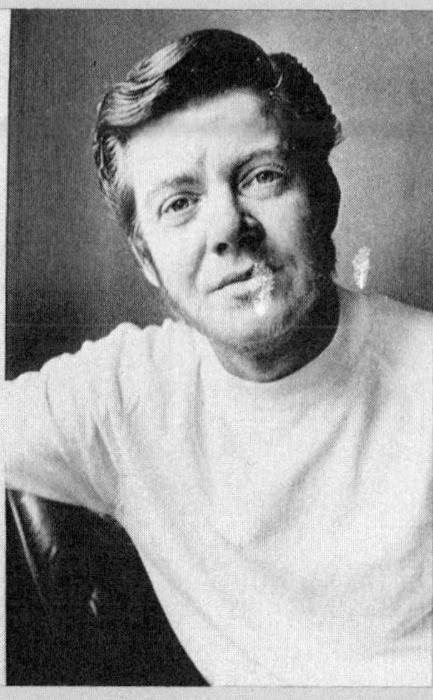

This individual was born with the anatomy of a woman **(left).** After entering a heterosexual marriage, she underwent sex reassignment surgery to become a man **(right)** and subsequently filed for a marriage annulment.

anatomically female professional tennis player who before surgery was a male, sex reassignment surgery has been a controversial but common treatment of transsexualism. Sex reassignment surgery for a male involves castration, the creation of a vaginal opening, and surgical augmentation of breasts. For a female, it involves surgical removal of the breasts, uterus, and ovaries, and the creation of a penis. The surgery for females is usually less satisfactory than for males, since the created penis cannot become erect. For men, the newly created vaginal opening is functional for intercourse, and some surgically altered transsexuals, who after surgery are females, can attain orgasm through the stimulation of their new vagina.

Prior to sex reassignment surgery, applicants are intensively screened. R. Green (1971) and Newman and Stoller (1974) have identified types of people who may seek sex change surgery, but for whom it is contraindicated. These include transvestites, effeminate homosexuals, and grossly psychotic persons. The screening is designed to weed out these individuals. Surgery is limited to those who are sincerely committed to the visible gender change because of their transsexual identity, and who are psychologically sound enough to have a good chance of postsurgical adjustment. Prior to surgery, applicants receive hormone treatment to begin the anatomical change. This treatment is reversible. The individual is then required to live totally in the role of the preferred gender from one to two years to demonstrate ability to adjust fully to such a life. If they are successful, sex reassignment surgery is possible. Individuals who are screened from surgery often have a very difficult time adjusting to the loss of this possibility and may experience a great deal of psychological turmoil. Some transsexuals have attempted the surgery on themselves, with mutilatory results (Greilsheimer & Groves, 1979). However, a screening technique is necessary because the surgery is irreversible.

When the subject is accepted, and the procedure performed, the subsequent results have been reported to be good in most cases. D. D. Hunt and Hampson (1980) conducted a long term follow-up (average of 8.2 years after surgery) on 17 biologic male transsexuals. They found that none of the 17 regretted the surgery, and all would choose it again if necessary, in spite of the pain and expense. D. D. Hunt and Hampson found gains in sexual adjustment and family acceptance, but little change in personality. A "high level" of functioning was reported for 60–70 percent of the sample. However, the surgery was not a panacea. The subjects continued (as many of us do) to struggle with the problems of intimacy and economics, and 24 percent still felt "driven" to have additional surgery. Earlier follow-up research on sex reassignment surgery has also been fairly positive.

The apparent effectiveness of this surgical approach and the apparent ineffectiveness of other approaches to gender identity change has led many to propose it as the primary treatment (R. Green, 1974; Hastings, 1971; Money, 1971; Pauly, 1971). Sagarin (1971), however, believes that the literature on this approach is filled with contradiction and distortion; and although the surgery may be effective, it is much too drastic.

In fact, other approaches short of surgery appear to be somewhat effective in the treatment of transsexualism. For example, Barlow, Reynolds, and Agras (1973) utilized a behaviorally oriented approach with a 17-year-old male transsexual. They used modeling and videotape feedback to train masculine styles of behavior. Social reinforcement was used to modify the way the subject sat, stood, and walked. In addition, his sexual urges and arousal patterns were modified in the direction of greater heterosexuality through social reinforcement and punishment of homosexual arousal. A one-year follow-up revealed that the masculine behavior remained dominant. The subject was dating, and his sexual responsiveness was to females rather than males. Five years later, his gender identity continued to be masculine and his sexual behavior was heterosexual (Barlow, Abel, & Blanchard, 1979). R. Green, Newman, and Stoller (1972) have reported five successful cases of treatment of boyhood transsexualism using family therapy, the development of a therapeutic relationship with each boy, and direct intervention to change family dynamics. In these reports, the transsexuals were young, suggesting perhaps that early psychotherapeutic intervention may be a feasible alternative to later sex reassignment surgery.

The paraphilias

Many individuals with a paraphilia never seek treatment. Some seek help under pressure from a spouse (DeBetz, 1975). Although many of the cases of paraphilia which have been reported have been treated with traditional psychotherapy, these techniques have not been particularly successful in changing the problem behavior. In the few successful cases, the treatment has taken many years (e.g., Bemporad, Dunton, & Spady, 1976).

Aversion therapy is one technique that has shown some promise in changing these behaviors. For example, the use of **aversive treatment** has been reported by Marks and Gelder (1967), in which electric shock was paired with the fantasy of the fetishistic object. They successfully treated several individuals in this manner, and Marshall (1974) successfully treated a trouser fetish with a similarly aversive conditioning procedure. The application of an aversive stimulus such as an electric shock to an individual in order to change sexual fantasys or behaviors is less common today than is the use of imagined noxious events. Barlow, Leitenberg, and Agras (1969) have demonstrated that the use of an imagined noxious scene (throwing up) could reduce pedophiliac attraction when paired with the presentation of an attractive child in a fantasy situation. This presentation of aversive stimuli in fantasy is called **covert sensitization.** It has been applied successfully to a range of behaviors. An exhibitionist, for example, is instructed to vividly imagine an unpleasant scene and associate it with the process of exhibiting himself (Matelzky, 1974; Wickramsera, 1976). One such scene might involve the following:

> You are standing in a doorway and, as an unsuspecting woman walks past, you open your pants. Suddenly, a blinding light sears your eyes. It is the police! The sirens are wailing and a crowd gathers. People are jeering and pointing. You feel ashamed and embarrassed, frightened about what will happen to you. The police have you by the arms and handcuff you. Reporters are taking pictures for the newspaper. Sick to your stomach, you know the whole town will discover your secret. They'll call you "perverted and sick." You'll lose your job and your wife will divorce you. Your minister will use you as an example of a sinner in his sermon. You will have ruined your life.

Covert sensitization has shown consistently impressive results in decreasing the behaviors associated with most paraphilias (Little & Curran, 1978). However, it is also desirable to increase the frequency of more acceptable behavior. One early behavioral attempt in this direction was tried by Stevenson and Wolpe (1960), who treated a pedophile by desensitizing his anxiety to normal heterosexual situations. A more intensive approach involves **orgasmic reconditioning.** In this procedure the subject masturbates and over a period of time substitutes socially acceptable sexual fantasy stimuli for the undesirable fantasy. The goal is to increase the individual's arousal by more desirable stimuli. In one report, a young man with a shoe fetish was treated by a combination of covert desensitization, anxiety reduction, orgasmic reconditioning, and psychotherapy (Anonymous), Chambers, & Janzen, (1976). At the end of treatment, he no longer collected shoes, did not need their presence to enhance his sexual behavior, and had been functional in a heterosexual relationship.

Reports of behavioral therapy with paraphilias are

promising. However, most reports are single case studies, and many clinicians still feel that these disorders are extremely resistant to treatment. Treatment is especially difficult when the subject is in treatment at the request or demand of someone else (a spouse or the courts).

Treating the rapist and the victim

Rada (1978) indicates that few treatments are effective with rapists, although many have been tried. In spite of some reported success of psychotherapy, others find this approach to be limited (M. Cohen et al., 1975). Perhaps the most promising work is by Abel and colleagues (Abel, Blanchard, & Becker, 1978), who use a combination of psychotherapeutic approaches and behavioral conditioning techniques with consenting rapists. There are no studies of the long-term effectiveness of their approach, however. Programs for imprisoned rapists have yet to be shown to be more effective than simple imprisonment, and imprisonment seems to have little effect on reducing the likelihood of a rapist again engaging in rape once released.

A major development in recent years has been the creation of rape victim crisis counseling centers in most major cities to help victims work through the trauma of the experience. The rape experience may haunt some victims for years. Rape crisis centers provide immediate emotional support and assistance for a woman who must face police, spouse, and relatives after a very brutalizing experience. The long-term effects of rape on the victim may require ongoing treatment. The victim may need help in dealing with shame, guilt, and the reactions of those with whom she lives and works (Burgess & Holmstrom, 1976). The treatment required is often very similar to that described in Chapter 5 for posttraumatic disorders.

Homosexuality: treatment or acceptance?

Sexual reorientation of the homosexual has been attempted through approaches ranging from the psychoanalytic to the behavioral. Bieber et al. (1962) reported a success rate of 27 percent using psychoanalysis, a rate higher than many have reported for this approach. Among the more effective sexual reorientation approaches, therapists have used aversive conditioning, covert sensitization, and positive reinforcement of heterosexual behaviors (Barlow, 1973; Callahan & Leitenberg, 1973; Ince, 1973). Recently, Masters and Johnson (1979) have reported successful treatment of 65 percent of homosexuals motivated for sexual reorientation therapy, a quite impressive figure.

A major debate rages, however, over whether homosexuality per se ought to be treated. If homosexuality is simply a sexual life-style, one point on a continuum of normal sexuality, its "treatment" makes little sense. The confusion over this issue is illustrated by the fact that homosexuality was included in DSM-II (1968) as a mental disorder. In 1973 a majority of the membership of the American Psychiatric Association voted to have homosexuality dropped from the manual. Many other members were incensed at this action. In DSM-III (1980) homosexuality is considered a disorder *if* it is *ego dystonic,* that is, if the individual is upset by this form of behavior and wishes to be heterosexual. In this case, it is implied, the individual should be treated for sexual reorientation. Many experts (e.g., Bieber, 1976; Halleck, 1976; Sturgis & Adams, 1978) would agree with this position, and perhaps even go so far as to contend that all homosexuals need treatment.

Gerald Davison (1976, 1978) is a psychologist who is a major opponent of the belief that all homosexuals (or even those who wish treatment) should be sexually reoriented. Davison believes that our culture is so prejudiced towards homosexuality that the ego dystonic homosexual regrets the behavior and has problems not because it is pathological, but because our society makes homosexual adjustment so difficult. Davison (1978) says that homosexuals seeking treatment ought to be treated, but the focus of treatment should be to treat the psychological and behavioral difficulties that are a consequence of the difficulty of adjustment. The aim should be to help the individual be more secure in the homosexuality, not to attempt sexual reorientation. He would say that even when a homosexual *requests* sexual reorientation, the therapist should not acquiesce.

Davison's position would be the one endorsed by the "Gay Liberation Movement." This group of homosexuals has banded together in the spirit of politicalization to fight against society's obvious and subtle discrimination against homosexuals. Their interest has been to publicize their plight, assert their normality, and to change laws which discriminate against individuals because of their sexual preference. Their open and often successful challenge to these laws and attitudes has led to a backlash, and the organization of community activists to fight the liberalization of these laws. The long-range effects of these sociopolitical activities remain to be seen.

Summary

1. Human sexuality encompasses an at times confusingly diverse group of behaviors. During the past quarter-century, data have been found which dispel many myths about human sexual functioning, and raise additional questions. Probably at no other time has more factual knowedge about this area been available.

2. The typical physiological sexual response is much more clearly understood through the efforts of Masters and Johnson and others, and has been described in the convenient model of: 1. excitement, 2. plateau, 3. orgasm, and 4. resolution. The major psychosexual dysfunctions appear to be much more common than previously thought.

3. Psychosexual dysfunctions may take several forms: arousal dysfunction, erectile dysfunction, ejaculatory dysfunction, dyspareunia, vaginismus, and orgasmic dysfunction.

4. Masters and Johnson identified two types of factors in the etiology of psychosexual dysfunction: historical and maintenance. Historical factors include sexual trauma, sociocultural attitudes, rigid religious or moral restrictions, poor sexual education, homosexual concerns, and physical causes. Maintenance factors involve performance fear (anxiety) and the adoption of a spectator role.

5. Gender identity disorder (transsexualism) involves a sense of being trapped in a body that is the incorrect biological sex. This is a rare disorder which tentative evidence suggests may be due to abnormal levels of sexual hormones. Many experts, however, believe that transsexualism is due to early learning experiences.

6. The paraphilias are sexual behaviors that involve: 1. nonconsenting partners; 2. suffering, pain, or humiliation; or 3. preference for socially unacceptable or nonhuman objects of sexual arousal. The paraphilias discussed in this chapter include transvestism, fetishism, pedophilia, exhibitionism, voyeurism, and sexual sadism and masochism.

7. Psychoanalytic views of paraphilias theorize that adult heterosexual relationships stimulate high levels of anxiety. The individual turns away from these relationships and develops the paraphilia to avoid castration anxiety, which is the result of incestuous feelings for the mother. No direct evidence supports this view. Paraphilias have also been conceptualized as being the result of learning. The behaviors may have been directly reinforced, reinforced in fantasy, or learned through modeling and subsequently found to be reinforcing. The association of fantasies with sexual arousal and gratification seems to be an important factor.

8. Incest has recently been recognized as a problem of increasing significance. It may have effects which last into adulthood for children who experience it.

9. Rape is a sexual behavior motivated by aggression, not simple sexual desire. The rapist is expressing power, retaliation, and rage.

10. Rape victims suffer the trauma of the violent act and must face a culture that often blames the victim for "stimulating" the rapist. Victims of rape are likely to develop a posttraumatic stress disorder.

11. Homosexual behavior, like rape, has a special significance in that many experts assert that it is not a sexual disorder. Instead, homosexuality is considered to be one end of a continuum of normal sexual behavior. Several studies have demonstrated that most homosexuals have no more pathology than heterosexuals. Still many clinicians, especially those of a psychoanalytic orientation, believe that homosexuality is a pathological sexual adjustment. Homosexuality has been attributed to several etiological factors including castration anxiety, abnormal levels of sex hormones, and learning.

12. Treatment for psychosexual dysfunction has become more common in the past 25 years. The behavioral approaches have made major contributions to the treatment of these dysfunctions. Behavioral approaches such as systematic desensitization focus on the reduction of anxiety related to sexual activity. Many therapists use an approach similar to that developed by Masters and Johnson which involves: 1. treating the rare physical problem if present, 2. teaching clients how to give and receive physical pleasure, 3. reducing performance fear through programmed sexual practice without the demand for orgasm, and 4. sex education counseling.

13. Transsexualism has been treated with sex reassignment surgery. The drastic nature of this surgery has stimulated attempts to treat transsexuals with psychological techniques. Several published reports have demonstrated the success of treatments based on the social reinforcement and rehearsal of gender-appropriate behavior. Family therapy has also been reported effective in some cases of childhood gender identity disorder. Perhaps these approaches will be useful as early intervention approaches.

14. The paraphilias have not been treated very successfully with psychotherapy. Successful behavioral approaches have included aversive stimulation with electric shock or other noxious stimuli. Covert sensitization involves presenting an unpleasant imagined scene, which is integrated into a fantasy about the unacceptable sexual behavior. These techniques, which are designed to reduce the paraphilia behaviors, can be used in conjunction with orgasmic reconditioning, in which sexual arousal is reconditioned to more acceptable sexual stimuli (e.g., arousal is reconditioned from children to adults).

15. Treatment of rapists has not been very effective. Rapists are generally not treated until they are arrested; many do not consent to treatment; and treatment is unavailable in many prisons. Some rape victims may have access to rape counseling centers, which provide emotional support and counseling services.

16. Homosexuality has been treated using behavioral techniques similar to those used with people who have paraphilias, and by psychotherapy. The treatment of homosexuality is very controversial. Many experts believe that homosexuality is a sexual preference, not a disorder, and that it is unethical to try to change a person's sexual orientation.

KEY TERMS

Clitoral orgasm. A female orgasm that is the result of stimulation of the clitoris.

Ejaculate. The emission of seminal fluid during the male's orgasm. "Ejaculate" is sometimes used as a noun to refer to the seminal fluid and/or sperm emitted during orgasm.

Hymen. A lacy membrane that obstructs the entry to the vagina. Presence of the hymen was believed to be a sign of virginity. However, it often parts during the developmental years, long before sexual behavior usually occurs.

Psychosexual. Refers to sexual behavior that has both psychological and physiological aspects.

Vaginal orgasm. A female orgasm once presumed to be due to stimulation primarily of the vaginal walls. In fact, "vaginal" orgasms are due to stimulation of both the clitoris and the vaginal walls. Many experts think that stimulation of the clitoris is the most important factor in all female orgasms.

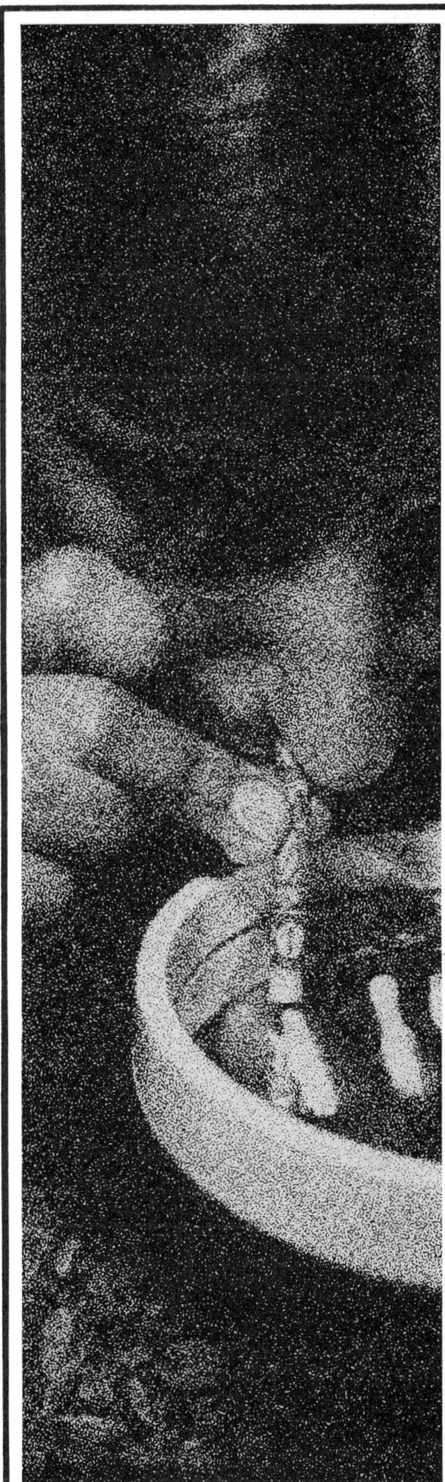

10

Substance abuse

- Alcohol: central nervous system depressant
- Other sedatives
- Narcotic analgesics (opioids or opiates)
- Major stimulants
- Hallucinogens
- Cannabis sativa (marihuana)
- General factors in substance abuse
- Key treatments
- Summary
- Key terms

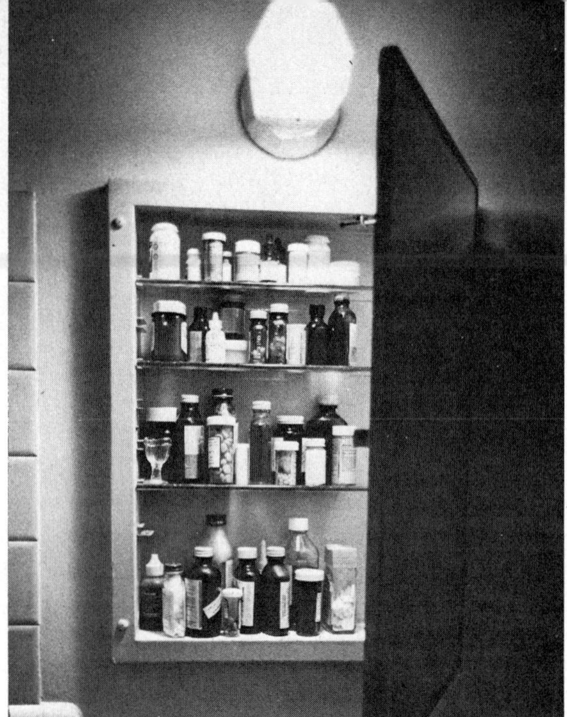

Do we live in a drug culture?

Throughout recorded history, and probably in prehistoric times, humans have sought substances which, if taken into the body, would alter their experiences. Such substances (drugs) usually have an initially pleasant effect, whatever their long-term consequences. This pleasurable effect has usually involved changes in perception of self and the environment, changes in physiological functioning of the body, changes in feelings, and changes in behavior. At various times in various cultures, the uses of drugs for such purposes have been condoned, condemned, promoted, or ignored. Their use has been seen as a gift of the gods or as a vice or criminal activity.

In the United States today, various subgroups manifest all these reactions to recreational drug use, depending on the drug used; but many observers have noted that, in many ways, we in the United States live in a drug culture. A glance in the typical family's medicine cabinet provides superficial proof of the statement, and observation of advertisements for **over-the-counter drugs** suggests that we are only too ready to believe that drugs can solve most problems. It is apparent that negative attitudes on recreational drug use have more to do with the myths surrounding the drug being used than with the real dangers of a particular drug. Alcohol, for example, is legal, widely used, and probably one of the more dangerous recreational drugs, but few people think of it in this manner. Marihuana is less widely used than alcohol, and its sale, possession, and use are against the law in most jurisdictions, although much less evidence exists that it is as dangerous as alcohol.

The use of drugs is widespread. Estimates of adult alcohol use range from 50 percent to 80 percent of all United States adult citizens, and drug use is significant in high school and even grade school. Table 10.1 shows the percentage of students who admitted drug use in a survey of 3402 students in grades 7–12 of eight midwestern schools (Seffrin & Seehafer, 1976). Such figures overlap to some extent, since most individuals who use drugs are polydrug users. They use more than one type of drug at the same time or during the same period (i.e., alcohol and marihuana or cocaine and heroin or other combinations).

Before considering the effects of the various drugs, two terms need definition: **tolerance** and **dependence.** "Tolerance" refers to the decreasing physiological and behavioral effect of a drug when it is administered (or used) repeatedly (see Figure 10.1). The drug user must continually increase dosage to obtain the same "high." Tolerance may peak and level off with some drugs, but with others, tolerance does not develop before lethal levels are reached. Some drugs apparently have no physiological tolerance effect, and increasing dosages are not required. We might think of tolerance as the body's way of compensating for some drugs in an attempt to maintain homeostasis.

Table 10.1
Percent of students reporting drug use in eight midwestern schools ($n = 3402$)

Substance used	*3 or more times per month*	*3 or more times per week*
Beer	19.2	6.1
Distilled spirits	11.8	3.1
Barbiturates	2.7	1.6
Amphetamines	2.0	1.6
Marihuana	4.7	4.0

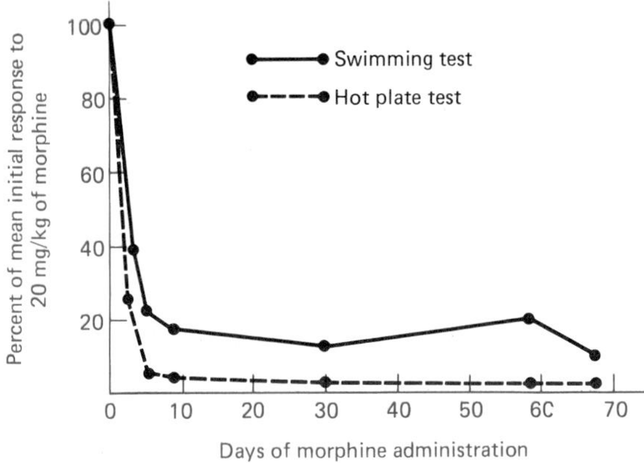

Figure 10.1. Example of the rapid development of tolerance to morphine in rats given daily doses. Test procedures consisted of measuring rats' escape behavior from a painfully hot surface, and measuring the speed with which they swam a straight alley maze. Within 10 days the constant dose of morphine lost over 80 percent of its effectiveness.
From: Kornetsky (1976, p. 130).

"Dependence" may be physical or psychological or both. Physical dependence is present when the withdrawal of the drug or abstinence from the drug results in a variety of unpleasant, sometimes dangerous physical reactions. Dependence apparently does not develop without prior development of tolerance, but tolerance may develop without a resulting physical dependence in some drugs (e.g., amphetamines). The withdrawal symptoms of physical dependence have often been described as being the opposite of the effects of the drugs. Psychological dependence may be present without physical dependence, but is always present when physical dependence exists. In psychological dependence, the individual needs the drug in order to cope, to function optimally from a subjective perspective. The terms "physical dependence" and "psychological dependence" are somewhat subsumed under the term "addiction," which most people erroneously use to mean physical dependence on a drug. One can be addicted because of psychological dependence alone.

In DSM-II (1968), alcoholism and drug addiction are listed under the broader category "Personality Disorder"; in DSM-III (1980), the category title is "Substance Use Disorders," and the central nervous system effects are included as "Substance Induced Organic Disorders." This important change is representative of the current flux in conceptualization of substance abuse. Most investigators no longer believe that the presence of a personality disorder is necessary for an addiction to develop. In the material which follows, the substance abuse disorders are organized by drug type and individual drugs. The major drugs abused are covered, but other substances can also be abused.

ALCOHOL: CENTRAL NERVOUS SYSTEM DEPRESSANT

While few people think of alcohol as a drug, it is a central nervous system depressant, and has profound effects on human functioning. Alcohol has been commonly used for thousands of years, ever since people learned that fermented fruit produces a beverage that has interesting effects on thinking, feeling, and behaving. At times alcohol's use was discouraged, sometimes informally and sometimes with the force of law. In the United States, the manufacture and sale of alcoholic beverages were prohibited by law (the Eighteenth Amendment) for 13 years, from 1920 to 1933. This law was no more successful in eliminating alcohol as a drug than today's laws are in controlling the use of illegal drugs such as heroin.

Since the repeal of Prohibition, alcohol has continued to play a major role in the lives of most Americans. It is a substance present at most family gatherings, parties, and holiday celebrations, and provides the focus around which many people's social lives revolve. Where does one go to meet friends after work or on a Saturday night or for entertainment? Why, to a bar or, as it is called by some, a cocktail lounge. By one estimate, over 80 percent of adults drink alcoholic beverages (Engs, 1977). The use of alcohol is common among teenagers. Margulies, Viessler, and Kanded (1977) found that 50 percent of first-year high school students drank, and the frequency increased to 75 percent during the senior year.

In spite of the widespread use of alcoholic beverages, the typical drinker is uninformed about alcohol's effects or about the etiology and consequences of alcohol use and abuse. Buckalew (1979) surveyed 190 high school, college, and graduate students and found that they averaged less than 60 percent correct answers on a test of these items of knowledge. The general populace is likely to have equally significant misconceptions and misinformation about alcohol use. Some common misconceptions are that coffee can sober a person who is drunk, and a person gets drunker on mixed drinks than on beer.

Most people report that they drink "for fun," because the use of alcohol facilitates social interaction (Trice & Beyer, 1977). Brown and her colleagues (1980) studied 440 male and female drinkers to determine their expectations for reinforcement from the use of alcohol (in effect, they asked Why do you drink?). They found that females expected generally positive social experiences, such as pleasure enhancement. Women believed that alcohol would act as a positive transforming agent: Their future would seem brighter; their conversation would be more stimulating; they would feel good; they would be better able to express their feelings, be more confident, less anxious, and, to some extent, sexier and more romantic. While males had the same expectations, they were more likely to also expect alcohol to be physically arousing (both sexually and otherwise) and to enhance their sense of powerfulness and aggression. Brown and her associates also found that less experienced drinkers had global expectations while experienced drinkers had more specific, refined expectations, usually of power enhancement and increased aggressiveness. As we shall see, numerous studies have demonstrated that one's expectations are important factors in how one behaves when intoxicated.

The almost universal use of alcohol by virtually all levels of society has contributed to an acceptance of the drug for recreational purposes by people who would be horrified if someone suggested that they use any other drug, such as marihuana, cocaine, or LSD, in a similar manner. In fact, the human misery that results from the use and abuse of alcohol *far* outweighs the adverse effects of all other abused drugs. It has been estimated that there are 10 million alcohol abusers in the United States, who may be physically dependent upon the drug, and 18 million problem drinkers, who have five to six drinks daily (Chambers & Griffey, 1975). However, physical dependence or **alcoholism** is not the only problem that may result from alcohol use. Of the 50,000 highway deaths each year, 50 percent are alcohol related. The primary drug implicated in criminal activity is *alcohol*, not heroin or the other drugs (NIAA, 1978). Even moderate use of alcohol under certain circumstances may lead to problems (see Table 10.2). Several studies have identified a **fetal alcohol syndrome** in infants born to mothers who drink heavily during pregnancy (K. L. Jones & Smith, 1973; Mulvihill & Yeager, 1976; D. W. Smith, Jones & Hanson, 1976); one-third of the newborn infants of female alcoholics have physical abnormalities and about one-half manifest mental deficiency. E. L. Abel (1980) reports estimates of from 4000 to 5000 such births per year. Some concern now exists about the effects of even moderate daily drinking on the unborn child, or fetus. In spite of the many possible adverse effects of alcohol ingestion, both on a short-term and chronic basis, drinking is such an ingrained pattern in our culture that significant changes in consumption are unlikely to occur in the near future.

Social Drinking vs. Alcoholism

How much drinking is too much? This question has been considered by many individuals, who usually answer "A lot more than I drink!" A consistent finding has been that people whom others would define as having a serious drinking problem or even a physical dependency deny the problem to themselves. Harford, Dorman, and Feinhandler (1976) have demonstrated that patrons in bars consistently made more and more errors in their estimates of how much they had drunk as the actual number of drinks increased. Apparently our self-perceptions of our drinking behavior become less reliable the more we drink! Typical male drinking behavior was studied by Vogel-Sprott (1974), who found that young males (age 18) drank about once per week, males

Table 10.2
Percent of students who drink at least once a year (n = 883) reporting alcohol-related problems at least once in past year and in lifetime

	Past year	*Lifetime*
Hangover	57.6	73.7
Nausea and vomiting	37.8	69.7
Driving after drinking	51.0	68.4
Driving after excessive drinking	30.8	50.8
Driving while drinking	25.7	45.7
Missing class because of hangover	16.8	24.2
Coming to class after drinking	10.9	21.9
Fighting with someone after drinking	9.1	19.4
Being criticized by date because of drinking	10.0	18.9
Missing class after drinking	10.6	18.6
Damaging university property, setting off false fire alarm, because of drinking	8.8	17.6
Knowing of problem with drinking	8.5	16.2
Having trouble with the law because of drinking	3.5	9.2
Receiving a lower grade because of drinking	4.1	8.7
Having trouble with school administration because of drinking	1.8	3.8
Being arrested for driving while intoxicated	1.8	2.5
Losing job because of drinking	.5	.9

From Engs (1977, p. 2150).

from 35 to 45 drank over three times per week, and men in their midsixties reduced their frequency to once per week. He suggests that further clarification of normative drinking behavior would be helpful in defining problem drinking.

Because of the lack of norms in this area, the definition of terms is somewhat subjective. One way of conceptualizing the range of drinking behaviors from social to abusive follows:

1. Social Drinking. Occasional drinking in social situations such as parties, dinners, and during joyous occasions when the intoxicating properties of alcohol are unimportant, but may secondarily enhance the occasion.
2. Intoxicant Drinking. Frequent drinking with the goal (overtly or covertly) of becoming intoxicated to enhance functioning, reduce tension, anxiety, boredom, or have "more" fun.
3. Problem Drinking. Drinking that causes problems (work, marital, social) or is used to escape from existing problems.
4. Serious Problem Drinking. Drinking that is hidden from others, becomes a preoccupation, and leads to guilt. Begins to seriously interfere with functioning (days missed from work, occasional intoxication on the job). Drinking approaches a daily basis.
5. Alcoholism. Usually involves daily drinking and periods of intoxication, benders, loss of control, loss of self-esteem, guilt; life becomes centered on the next drink. The drinker starts insuring a supply (carrying it around, hiding bottles), neglects nutritional needs. Increase in tolerance.
6. Chronic Alcoholism. Loss of control, craving, daytime drinking on a regular basis, almost constant high levels of alcohol in blood, major prolonged episodes of serious intoxication. Major disruptions of life: loss of jobs, dissolution of family life, divorce.

Many authorities have discussed similar stages of drinking, which imply a steady progression from one level to the next in the development of alcoholism. However, it appears more typical that behaviors overlap between stages (Mulford, 1977), and people may move between stages at different points in their lives (Fillmore, 1974). However, when an individual has the subjective experience that drinking cannot be controlled, experiences amnesia for the "night before," craves alcohol, and cannot abstain due to physiological after effects or **withdrawal** symptoms, the label of alcohol dependence or addiction clearly applies (Edwards, 1975), no matter what progressive stages the individual has gone through.

Short-Term Effects (Intoxication)

The short-term effects of alcohol depend upon various factors. Of major importance is the **blood alcohol content** (BAC), or percent of alcohol in the blood, which varies by body weight and number of ounces of alcohol ingested. For example, a 150-pound person would be more intoxicated by five bottles of beer than a 260-pound person who drank seven bottles of beer in the same period. (See Highlight 10.1 and 10.2 for additional data.)

When ingested, alcohol is rapidly absorbed into the bloodstream from the stomach, small intestine, and colon. Absorption rate can be influenced by the presence of food in the stomach (slowed), especially milk, but the variances are small. Once absorbed, the alcohol is quickly carried to the brain, where it has a depressant effect on the central nervous system. This

HIGHLIGHT 10.1

WHAT IT TAKES TO GET DRUNK: NUMBER OF DRINKS[1] NEEDED FOR THE PERSON'S BODY WEIGHT

Blood alcohol content (percent of alcohol in blood) and characteristic behavior	*Person's weight (pounds)*						
	100	125	150	175	200	225	250
.02 Slight changes in feeling, elation			1	1¼	1⅓	1½	1⅔
.05 Warmth, relaxation, impulsiveness	1¾	2⅓	2¾	3⅓	3¾	4⅓	4½
.10 Emotion and behavior are exaggerated (talkative, noisy, or saddened); judgment seriously affected, impaired coordination; legally intoxicated	2¾	3½	4⅓	4¾	5½	6½	7
.15 Legally intoxicated; gross intoxication seriously affects all faculties	4½	5¾	6	8	9⅓	10½	11½
.30 Stuporous	9½	11½	14	16½	18½	20½	22
.40 Unconscious, on verge of death	12½	15½	18½	21½	24½	27½	30½

[1]One "average drink" means one beer, one six-ounce glass of wine, or one highball (containing one ounce of 86 proof alcohol); doubles or mixed drinks, such as martinis, contain two to three or more times as much alcohol as the "average drink."

HIGHLIGHT 10.2
CAN ALCOHOL SNEAK UP ON YOU?

The average healthy liver metabolizes approximately only one ounce of 86 proof alcohol per hour. Steady drinking for a period of hours, even if at a moderate rate, can result in a surprisingly high level of intoxication or BAC level, which the individual may be unprepared for. Assume, for example, that a 150-pound individual arrives at a party at 7:00 P.M. and drinks three drinks per hour, a moderate rate of consumption in the setting:

7:00 P.M. to 8:00 P.M. Drinks three drinks, liver metabolizes one; by 8:00 P.M., person has two ounces of 86 proof alcohol in the blood. BAC is over .04 percent alcohol.

8:00 P.M. to 9:00 P.M. The two drinks in the body system are supplemented by three more; one is metabolized. By 9:00 P.M., person still has four drinks in the body system. BAC is almost .09.

9:00 P.M. to 10:00 P.M. The four drinks in body system at 9:00 P.M. are supplemented by three more; one is metabolized. At 10:00 P.M., six are still present in the body. BAC is .13; person cannot drive legally.

A rate of two drinks per hour would result in the following BAC:

Time	7 P.M.	8 P.M.	9 P.M.	10 P.M.	11 P.M.	12 A.M.
Drinks in body	1	2	3	4	5	6
BAC		.04	.065	.087	.11	.13

Even at a low rate of only two drinks per hour consumption, by midnight the individual is legally intoxicated. If drinking stops at midnight, the person will remain legally intoxicated for almost two more hours, and the body will not be free of alcohol until approximately six o'clock in the morning. The only way to reduce an intoxicated state is to allow time to pass without consuming more alcohol. Although it is a common belief that drinking large amounts of coffee or engaging in exercise will help a person to "sober up," all such things do is temporarily stimulate the individual, who may then *feel* less intoxicated. The physiological effects of intoxication are not diminished.

Many people underestimate the amount they drink. Next time, keep track, and you might be surprised to find out how intoxicated you *really* are!

depression of the activity of the cortical centers allows the unrestrained activity of other areas of the brain, and is experienced *subjectively* as stimulation. The intoxicated individual manifests impaired judgment, poor self-control, and impulsive behavior. Cognitive abilities are seriously impaired (E. Parker & Noble, 1977), time perception is speeded up (Tinklenberg, Roth, & Kopell, 1976), and aggressiveness is increased (Zeichner & Pihl, 1979). Although subjective sexual interest is increased, the ability to be physiologically aroused by sexual stimuli is decreased (Briddell & Wilson, 1976; G. T. Wilson & Lawson, 1978). Motor coordination is impaired; there is slurred speech, unsteady gait, double vision, and enlargement of surface blood vessels, which gives a sense of warmth and a flushing of the skin. The individual often *feels* relaxed, more adequate, and able to do things that are not possible when sober; for example, tell jokes, dance, or argue; manifest belligerence or aggression.

Questions remain in regard to whether all these manifestations are due to the biochemical effects of the alcohol (Briddell & Wilson, 1976; G. T. Wilson & Lawson, 1978; Zeichner & Pihl, 1979). At low to moderate alcohol levels many of the behaviors of the individual may be a result of personal expectations of what one ought to be like when drunk. Perhaps we learn to behave "like" a drunk when we drink, and can modify our behavior in line with individual circumstances at lower levels of intoxication, while at more intoxicated levels, the biochemical effects predominate.

Once intoxication has been achieved, continued drinking in amounts large enough to raise the blood alcohol level leads to extreme interference with cognition and motor coordination. The sensation of pain and cold continues to be blunted, and sedation and sleep will result. If ingestion is rapid and extreme, the central nervous system depressant effects may be so profound that coma and death result. Each year several such cases of alcohol deaths are reported. They often occur on college campuses because of excessive drinking in response to hazing or dares.

When clinical levels of intoxication are reached, abstinence often results in a hangover. The cause of a hangover is suspected to be a cellular reaction to the decrease in blood alcohol level. Symptoms include headache, dizziness, tremor, nausea, pallor, and sweating. No effective remedies for hangover exist.

Effects of Chronic Alcohol Abuse

Frequent use of large amounts of alcohol leads to physical tolerance. The tolerance is not comparable in degree, however, to the tolerance developed to the opioids. Rather large amounts of alcohol are required for tolerance to develop. On the average, probably *more* than three shots of whisky, half a bottle of wine, or four glasses of beer on a daily basis is necessary (U.S. Department of Health, Education and Welfare, 1974). Major abuse of alcohol leads to physical dependence. When physical dependence develops, people drink in a manner that appears to be out of control; they seem to "crave" alcohol.

Loss of Control and Craving. Loss of control and craving are considered important diagnostic signs of alcoholism. *Craving* is defined as an overwhelming sense of a need for alcohol, while *loss of control* is usually defined as an inability to stop drinking once the first drink has been taken. Both behaviors have been considered by some researchers to be related primarily to physiological factors. However, some research indicates otherwise. Ludwig, Wikler, and Stark (1974), for example, propose that craving may be a conditioned response to internal (subjective or physiological) stimuli and environmental stimuli (the setting of a bar or tavern). It may not simply be a response to physiological alcohol need. They have some evidence to support their view. D. W. Goodwin and his colleagues (1974) have suggested that loss of control is due to the intoxicated person "forgetting" the consequences of heavy drinking. If this is the case, the loss of control would not occur after the traditional first drink, but only after the individual has become intoxicated. Maisto, Lauerman, and Adesso (1977) have shown that alcoholics' loss of control may be due to their expectation that they *will* lose control. Maisto et al.'s study found that alcoholics drinking a placebo which they believed contained alcohol drank more (i.e., "lost control") than when they were drinking an alcoholic beverage they believed was alcohol free. Similar results were obtained by Asp (1977), who described it as a reward-expectation effect (i.e., the alcoholic expected a rewarding experiential change after ingesting the drug). Such studies suggest that even after physical dependence has developed, nonphysiological factors may be extremely important in precipitating or maintaining drinking behavior.

Withdrawal, Chronic Brain Syndrome, and Other Results of Alcohol Abuse. Once physical dependence has developed, and an individual has the subjective experience of loss of control and craving, alcohol consumption is likely to be extremely heavy. If abstinence is attempted, withdrawal symptoms occur within a few hours. In withdrawal, tremors, nausea, anxiety, weakness, and perspiration are present. Soon there may be muscle cramps and vomiting, and the tremors become so coarse that motor movements such as lifting a glass become difficult. As withdrawal progresses, **acute hallucinosis** may develop, in which hal-

Chronic alcoholism is extremely disabling.

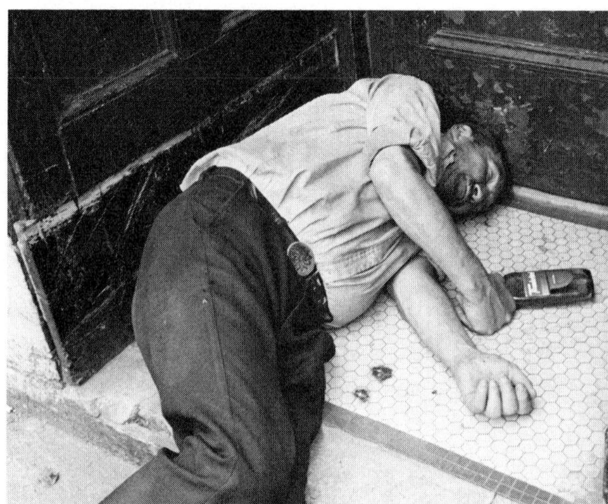

lucinations of critical voices are heard discussing the subject's weaknesses, innermost thoughts, and sexual problems. The voice may become extremely threatening and the subject often becomes terrified. Delirium (a confused, disoriented state) may also occur; exhaustion and seizures ("rum fits") are common. Cardiovascular collapse may follow, and death is then likely. If death does not occur, recovery is usual in five to seven days.

Delirium tremens ("DTs") may occur in withdrawal, or even following a long drinking bout in the chronic alcoholic. The tremens begin with anxiety, insomnia, illusions, hallucination; then tremor, rapid heart rate, and hypertension; followed by disorientation, motor excitement, and coma. During DTs hallucinations of bugs, snakes, and other terrifying sights are common. The delirium may last about one week and occurs in about 5 percent of alcoholics. The probable cause is a disturbance of brain cell metabolism from long-term abuse of alcohol.

A small portion (about 1 percent) of alcoholics manifest Korsakoff's syndrome, a chronic brain disorder resulting from brain cell destruction from a deficiency of vitamin B1 or the toxic effect of alcohol (opinion is divided on the etiology) (Freund, 1973). The following case illustrates the common features of the syndrome. Before the signs of Korsakoff's syndrome appeared, this 65-year-old man manifested delirium tremens for about a week after he stopped drinking.

> As he began to recover [from delirium tremens], he displayed the clinical signs of Korsakoff's syndrome. His memory for recent events was extremely poor and he [unknowingly filled the gaps with fabrication. A defect of nerve function called polyneuritis] was manifested in diminished sensation and muscular weakness. He was also disoriented for time and did not even know what year it was. Asked to subtract 7 from 100 successively—i.e., 93, 86, 79 and so on—his responses were "93, 89, 72. . ." [The 100-minus-7 test is a standard, quick method of appraising intellectual impairment.] He maintained that nothing was the matter with him except that he must have been hit on the head, and he contradicted reality by denying both his alcoholism and marital discord. He had amnesia for his wife's divorce suit.
>
> The patient was injected with large doses of vitamins, after which there was a marked and rapid improvement in intellectual functioning. . . . Vocabulary was relatively well preserved but there was considerable impairment in the nonverbal components of intelligence, a pattern typical of brain syndromes. Memory remained fairly poor and he showed evidence of concrete thinking and [repetition]. Emotionally, however, he began to approach normality as his excitement dissipated. His wife dropped the divorce proceedings and he returned home after two months but was unable to resume his law practice. (E. Rosen, Fox, & Gregory, p. 308, 1972)

Bolter and Hannon (1980) have reviewed studies of brain damage in alcoholics and concluded that while ample evidence demonstrates that alcohol consumption leads to significant brain damage, the specific areas damaged cannot yet be localized. Some investigators have proposed that the primary damage is in the right hemisphere. However, Ellenberg et al. (1980) found that for most alcoholics, the damage is diffuse in both hemispheres. In older alcoholics, they did find evidence of greater deficits in right hemisphere functions. Ellenberg et al. also found that verbal and visual concept deficits were recoverable in most younger alcoholics (under age 40) — regardless of the length and severity of their drinking—while irreversible deficits were seen primarily in older alcoholics.

Abuse of alcohol leads to several related difficulties. Since alcohol is metabolized by the liver, that organ may be damaged by the constant demands placed on it by alcohol abuse. The alcohol abuser may develop liver **cirrhosis,** a condition in which liver cells are damaged and replaced by scar tissue. Some investigators believe the alcohol directly causes cirrhosis; others think that nutritional deficits are at fault. Nutritional deficits in alcoholics are common, since alcohol's calories have no nutritional value. Excessive drinking also impairs the body's ability to fight disease because of impairment of white blood cell effectiveness. Some investigators have even found evidence for direct or indirect chromosomal damage from alcohol abuse (Obe & Herha, 1975).

Factors in Chronic Alcohol Abuse

Given that a majority of United States citizens drink, it is clear that the use of alcohol does not automatically lead to alcohol dependence. This simple observation suggests that there must be something different about individuals who do become alcoholics. For some reason, they are unable to drink in moderation, as most other people do. Factors that have been examined in terms of their relationship to alcohol abuse include physiological differences, psychological issues, and the impact of society and culture on the individual drinker.

Physiological Differences. Many investigators have suggested that there may be genetic differences between alcoholics and nonalcoholics, since alcoholism tends to run in families. D. W. Goodwin (1979) reviewed the available evidence and concluded that substantial evidence indicates that some (though not all) alcoholics have inherited a predisposition to alcohol abuse. He focused on Danish adoption studies which examined male and female children of parents hospitalized for alcoholism. The children had been adopted by other persons. The adoption limited the possible negative effects of the environment of an alcoholic parent on the children. The results of these studies can be summarized as follows:

1. Sons of alcoholics were about four times more likely to be alcoholic than were sons of nonalcoholics, whether raised by nonalcoholic foster parents or raised by their own biological parents.
2. Sons of alcoholics raised by their alcoholic parents differed from unadopted controls only with regard to alcoholism. They did not have a higher incidence of other disorders than did the controls.
3. Of the adopted daughters of alcoholics, 2 percent were alcoholic and another 2 percent had serious problems from drinking. In the adopted control group, 4 percent were alcoholic. Between .1 percent and 1 percent of Danish women are alcoholic. Thus, both in the proband (children of alcoholic parents) and the control groups, a higher than expected prevalence of alcoholism was found. The only fact known about the controls' biological parents was that they did not have a hospital diagnosis of alcoholism. Perhaps some of these biological parents were unidentified alcoholics, and thus more likely to have alcoholic offspring.

Recent evidence strongly supports D. W. Goodwin's data (Cadoret, Cain, & Groves, 1980). Other evidence indicates that genetic predispositions are not present in all alcoholics. Frances, Timm, and Bucky (1980) studied 7064 military men admitted to naval residential programs for the treatment of alcoholism. In this project, the incidence of a familial history of alcoholism was determined, and differences between alcoholic men with such a history and those who had no such history were examined. Frances et al. found that 48.8 percent of the men had a history of familial alcoholism. They also found that men who had such a history tended to report more severe alcohol-related physical and psychological symptoms. The *absence* of a family history of alcoholism in over 50 percent of the men suggests that genetic influences may be present in some alcoholics, but not in others.

D. W. Goodwin (1979) has proposed that what may be inherited is a "tolerance" for alcohol. One must be able to drink large quantities of alcohol to be an alcoholic, and evidence exists that many individuals are unable to imbibe without becoming extremely intoxicated, vomiting, or passing out. Others seem to have greater capacity and can "handle their liquor." Goodwin (1979) uses this evidence and proposes the following formulation of the development of alcohol abuse:

1. The potential alcoholic must be able to drink a lot (i.e., lack an intolerance for alcohol).
2. Some people experience more euphoria from alcohol than others do. This factor is also quite possibly under genetic control. Because euphoria is a positive reinforcer, presumably people who experience the most euphoria are the ones most likely to drink.
3. Like most drugs of abuse, alcohol is quickly absorbed and eliminated; the [positive] effects occur rapidly and disappear rapidly. Experimental studies indicate that alcoholics experience dysphoric [unpleasant] as well as euphoric effects from alcohol. Those individuals who experience the most euphoria (because of genetic factors) quite possibly also experience the most dysphoria. The *cure* for the dysphoria is more alco-

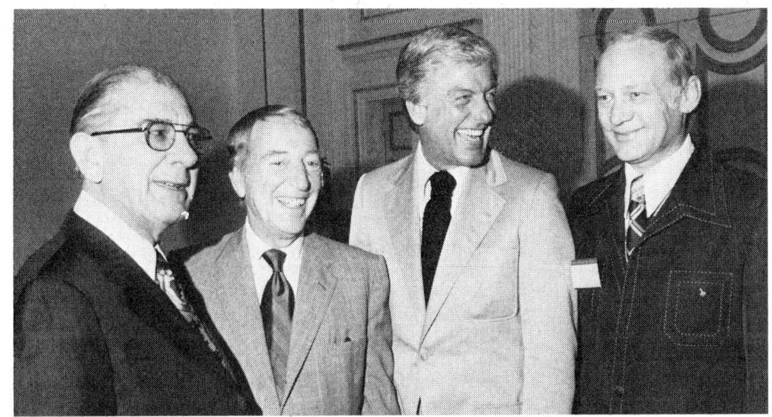

Alcoholism does not respect wealth, prominence, or class. At the 1976 Conference of the National Alcoholism Council, several prominent personalities openly discussed their battle with alcoholism. Left to right: Wilbur Mills, Congressman; Garry Moore and Dick Van Dyke, television celebrities; and Edwin "Buzz" Aldrin, ex-astronaut.

hol. After a few drinks, such people may drink more to relieve the dysphoria than to restore the euphoria. In any case, during a single drinking period there may be two reinforcers involved: production of euphoria and reduction of dysphoria. This peak-valley effect may explain loss of control. The height of the peak and the depth of the valley may be genetically controlled.

4. For reasons described above, alcohol in genetically susceptible individuals may be massively reinforcing. The reinforcements occur during the individual drinking periods and most strikingly "the morning after," when the "hair of the dog" swiftly relieves that formidable dysphoria known as a hangover. When loss of control leads to binge drinking, withdrawal symptoms occur (a super hangover). (p. 60)

While the data in these studies are impressive, Schaefer (1978) believes that apparently genetically related differences can be explained by other means, and disappear when more refined physiological measurement techniques are used. Of course, genetic differences may not account for the large proportion of persons who become alcoholics without a biologic history of familial alcoholism. Further research in the area can be expected.

Psychological Factors. The traditional psychoanalytic conception of alcoholism revolves around the concept of fixation at the oral stage of development. Frustration or indulgence at this stage leads to dependency needs in adulthood, which if frustrated lead to a regressive behavior: drinking to satisfy the repressed oral dependency needs. The liquor bottle becomes the mother's breast. The lack of success of psychoanalytic therapy with alcoholics has been advanced as evidence that these theories have little to do with reality (Schuckit & Hoglund, 1977).

Some investigators have proposed that people who become alcohol dependent may share significant personality traits, which differentiate them from nonalcoholics, and may lead to the problem drinking behavior. In other words, they have asked, Is there an **alcoholic personality?** Many studies have found consistent trait similarities. A 30-year prospective study by M. C. Jones (1968, 1971) found that males who became problem drinkers were impulsive, extroverted, and overemphasized their masculinity; women who became alcoholics were vulnerable, dependent, withdrawn, and sensitive to criticism. However, women who were total abstainers also had these traits. Other studies have also found higher levels of impulsiveness, lack of conformity, gregariousness, and interpersonal shallowness in alcoholics (M. F. Schwartz & Graham, 1979). Negrete (1973) concluded that common traits include withdrawn behavior, depression, hostility, passiveness, and dependence, but there is no "typical" alcoholic personality. Zimering and Calhoun (1976) agree and conclude that the "alcoholic personality" (or traits) may be triggered by specific environmental stresses. A major problem for the theory of an "alcoholic personality" is that most studies have been performed on alcoholics, and alcoholism may lead to the *traits,* not vice versa. In addition, as Krauthamer (1979) has pointed out, the generalizability of such studies is limited by the subject populations, which are usually drawn from institutionalized alcoholics.

Learning. Some studies have suggested that alcoholics have learned to use alcohol to reduce or avoid stress or anxiety, and that when people lack other coping mechanisms, drinking becomes a problem because it is such an effective (short-term) coping approach (e.g., Kean & Lisman, 1980). Maloof (1975) has demonstrated that alcohol decreases the effects of physiological stressors. He has concluded that drinking helps alcoholics cope with stress by affecting their cognitive appraisal of stimuli, and that alcohol's **analgesic** (pain-reducing) effect lessens the impact of emotional stressors, particularly those related to undesirable life events. These stressor-suppressor effects were not apparent in most normal controls. But when these effects were present, the normal control was found to be similar to the alcoholics in drinking behavior and attitudes about alcohol. Mules, Hague, and Dudley (1977) obtained high life change scores for alcoholics, *but* these alcoholics consistently rated life change events as requiring less adjustment than did controls. In effect, alcoholics may underestimate the stressfulness of events and find themselves more stressed than they expected. Levenson et al. (1980) found some significant physiological effects of alcohol on lowering the magnitude of response to stress. The data support the popular notion that alcohol is an effective tension reducer—at least in the short run.

The relationship of tolerance and dosage level to the tension-reducing effects of alcohol has been clarified by Lipscomb et al. (1980). They found that subjects become *more* anxious in stressful social situations with low doses of alcohol than with no alcohol or with high dosage. High tolerance subjects were more anxious at low doses than low tolerance subjects; but at high doses, no differences between high and low tolerance subjects were apparent. The data suggest that high tolerance subjects in stressful social situations would be more motivated to drink much more than low tolerance subjects, since the highs would be more anxious after one drink than the lows, and continued drinking would provide a greater (more rewarding) *relative* decrease in anxiety for the high tolerant subjects. These results suggest how people may acquire an abusive style of drinking.

Recent research has implicated the individual's perception of stimulus cues as an important factor in the etiology of alcoholism. If one has deficits in the perceptions of such cues, then behavior change may be difficult. Buck (1979) found that alcoholics are more responsive to external cues than normal controls. That is, alcoholics would be more likely to drink in response to external cues (such as being in a bar, having a bottle of alcohol present) than normals. Tucker, Vuchinich, and Sobell (1979) have obtained similar results. They found that alcoholics would drink more than nonalcoholics, even when both were at the same level of intoxication. The probability of a deficit in alcoholics' perception of internal cues has been demonstrated by Lipscomb and Nathan (1980). High tolerance subjects (such as alcoholics) were found to be substantially less accurate in judging their BAC level than low tolerant subjects (such as nondrinkers). The low tolerant subject's sensitivity to internal cues of intoxication may serve as brakes or moderators of drinking behavior. Without this ability, the high tolerant subject may continue in a cyclical fashion to drink heavily and to increase alcohol tolerance until alcohol dependence develops.

Sociocultural Factors. Significantly different rates of alcoholism between some cultures have led some theorists to consider cultural differences as factors in the development of alcoholism. In some cultures in which drinking occurs in moderation in the home, alcoholism is usually lower than in cultures in which light-to-moderate family drinking is infrequent, and primary drinking is done outside the home (Cahalan, 1978).

In the United States, alcohol is a common social facilitator and is an accepted aspect of our lives. A few evenings of observing television advertisements provide a glimpse of just how accepted and promoted alcohol is. If our culture were not so accepting of alcohol as a recreational drug, perhaps the problems of abuse might not be so widespread and severe.

The development of alcoholism in any culture is a complex phenomenon. The research reviewed in this section suggests the following tentative conclusions about why people become addicted to alcohol:

1. Some people appear to have a physiological predisposition to alcohol abuse which may involve a peak-valley effect. Drinking leads to greater **euphoria** and more **dysphoria** (intense unpleasant feelings) in these individuals than in the norm.
2. Individuals with a physiological predisposition find drinking massively reinforcing because it has positive effects and serves as a way to avoid unpleasant consequences. Others may have no physiological predisposition but may learn that drinking "solves" such emotional problems as anxiety, depression, and the experiences of stress. They may model a family member who uses alcohol this way, or may learn this behavior through experience.
3. Physiological predisposition and learning lead to heavier alcohol use and development of tolerance. Increased tolerance requires heavier drinking to obtain equivalent levels of reinforcement. Frequent drinking behavior may sensitize the person to external drinking cues, and tolerance may decrease sensitivity to internal warning signs of intoxication, leading to even more frequent heavier drinking. Finally, physical dependence occurs, and avoidance of withdrawal becomes a significant factor.

OTHER SEDATIVES

Sedatives, which have a central nervous system depressant effect similar to alcohol, are commonly used. In the 1850s, chemical substances known as bromides were discovered. They quickly became popular as sedatives, substances that induce relaxation, drowsiness, and finally sleep. Bromides, however, had quite negative side effects and were very toxic. By 1903 Fischer and Von Mering introduced barbital as an alternative, a derivative of barbituric acid (Kornetsky, 1976). In 1912 phenobarbital was introduced and remains a commonly used barbiturate. To date, more than 2500 **barbiturates** have been synthesized (Kornetsky, 1976).

Barbiturates

Medically, phenobarbital and other long-acting barbiturates are used for the control of epileptic seizure disorders, while short-acting barbiturates are used as sedatives when sleeplessness is a problem. These short-acting drugs, such as Seconal and Tuinal (see Highlight 10.3) are often abused. Bayh (1972) estimates that 1 million Americans are dependent upon barbiturates.

The effects of the barbiturates are somewhat state dependent. Taken immediately prior to bedtime, they promote sleep. However, tolerance develops with prolonged use for this purpose. When the usage is stopped, sleep is often restless with unpleasant dreams, which often leads to a return to the sedative.

When barbiturates are abused to obtain a "high," the effects are quite similar to alcohol —a release of inhibitions, a mild euphoria, clouded consciousness, labile emotions; and often slurred speech, unsteady movements, and impaired memory. These effects become apparent at dosage levels of approximately 100 mg

HIGHLIGHT 10.3
STREET NAMES OF BARBITURATES

General terms	Downers, Goofballs, Barbs, Candy, Peanuts, Sleepers, Stoppers	Tuinal Barbiturate-amphetamine mix—	Christmas Trees, Double Trouble, Jelly Beans, Rainbows
		Methaqualone	Ludes, Sopers
Specific Barbiturates		Secobarbital	Red Birds, Red Devils, Reds
Amobarbital sodium	Blue Angels, Blue Birds, Blue Devils, Blues	Pentobarbital sodium	Yellows, Yellow Birds, Yellow Jackets, Yellow Submarines
Seconal	Bullets, Pinks		

(milligrams). Tolerance requires increasing dosages for the same effect. When levels reach 400–600 mg per day, withdrawal effects from physiological dependence become apparent if drug use stops. Symptoms of withdrawal include severe anxiety, muscle weakness and tremor, nausea, seizures, insomnia, and psychosis. Abrupt withdrawal may be fatal for chronic abusers. The physical dependence is obviously very significant.

Long-term abuse of the barbiturates may also lead to chronic brain damage (Judd & Grant, 1975). E. Rosen et al. (1972) illustrate many of the withdrawal effects that appear following long-term abuse of barbiturates in the following case:

> . . . the patient developed signs of an acute brain syndrome. She had a marked tremor and was unsteady on her feet. She hallucinated, thought she heard the voice of her husband telling her that he was coming to get her in a taxi and she cried out to him. Soon she began seeing people climbing trees and looking through the windows at her. She became violent and abusive to the staff. Even after receiving sedative medication she remained restless, muttering to herself incoherently. Her tremor increased, her face became flushed and she began to perspire excessively. At times she twitched convulsively. A little later she began picking up imaginary objects and muttering "thank you" as if someone were handing them to her. Later she was observed reaching for an imaginary glass and drinking from it. She ate imaginary food and picked imaginary cigarettes out of the air; she heard nonexistent doorbells and an ambulance siren. Following several injections of a phenothiazine tranquilizer, her hallucinations ceased and she again became rational. . . . (pp. 317–318)

The combination of barbiturates and alcohol is particularly dangerous. These two substances together are "synergistic"; that is, they multiply each other's effects, rather than act additively. Many suicides are due to this combination, as are many accidental "ODs" (overdoses). Marilyn Monroe reportedly died of a combined dose of barbiturate and alcohol. The dangers of barbiturate abuse have led in recent years to the use of other sedatives such as methaqualone.

Methaqualone

A synthetic sedative, methaqualone is sold under the brand names Quaalude, Sopor, and Parest. It is commonly called "ludes" on the street and has been heavily abused. Therapeutic dosage is in the 150–300 mg range (Kornetsky, 1976). Abuse of ludes leads to a mildly euphoric high; a greater dosage results in the intoxicated state described for the barbiturates. Large dosages lead to delirium, coma, and death. Methaqualone also has a tolerance effect and physical dependence, and is frequently implicated in suicide and overdose deaths (Horvey, 1975).

NARCOTIC ANALGESICS (OPIOIDS OR OPIATES)

Many people associate the common term "drug addict" with abuse of heroin, a derivative of morphine. Morphine is an alkaloid isolated from opium in 1803 by a German pharmacist, and narcotic drugs are called **opioids** or **opiates** because of this relationship. Opium is obtained from the unripe seed capsule of the opium poppy plant. The capsule is cut and its milky juice collected, air dried, and powdered. From this powder morphine (and also codeine) can be extracted. For many centuries, opium was used as a medicinal analgesic. It was followed in the 1800s by the highly effective use of morphine for this purpose. However, recognition of the addictive properties of morphine stimulated the discovery of heroin, which was at first incorrectly believed to be an effective analgesic with no addictive (physical dependence) properties.

Opium was used in the Middle East for thousands of years for medicinal purposes, and probably also used (or abused) for recreational purposes. Chinese laborers introduced opium abuse to the West, especially America. Working as imported laborers, they established opium dens in the communities where they lived. The drug's use spread to Europeans and North Americans partly because of its easy availability. Opium was sold in drug stores without prescription, and was a common ingredient in patent medicine. Laws did not pro-

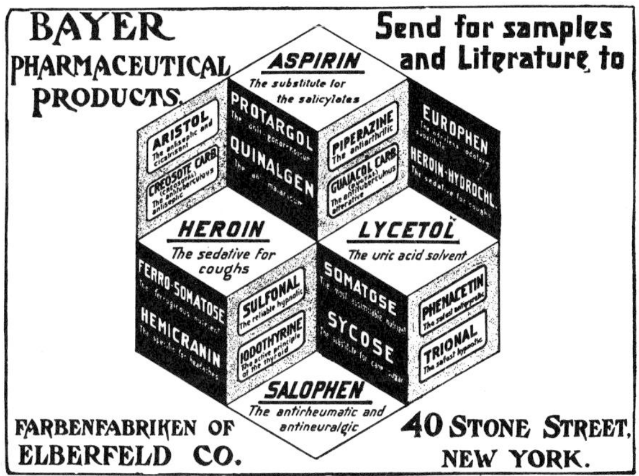

Early patent medicines often contained heroin.

hibit its use, and opium users remained in the mainstream. Opium use was considered to be a "vice" about equivalent to the use of alcohol.

The discovery of opium's derivative, morphine, was hailed as a medical breakthrough. In conjunction with the newly developed hypodermic syringe, morphine was widely used in the United States Civil War for pain relief in wounded soldiers. Many became physically dependent on morphine. As noted above, heroin was first believed to be a nonaddicting alternative to morphine. Several years' use, however, proved this belief to be in error. By 1914, the Harrison Act was passed to prohibit the unrestrained marketing of narcotic drugs.

Attitudes toward nonmedical drug use were changing, and increasingly stiff penalties were legislated against the now illicit use of drugs. Today, an estimated 50 percent of police personnel are involved in dealing with drug and drug-related illegal activities. This approach has been relatively unsuccessful (Schur, 1969). In the late 1960s and early 1970s, there were approximately 450,000–600,000 heroin addicts in the United States (M. H. Green & Dupont, 1974; E. Kaufman, 1976) and probably 2 million occasional users.

Immediate Effects of Opioids

Since heroin is the most abused opioid, it will be the focus of this discussion, although morphine and the synthetic opioids have similar properties.

Heroin may be taken orally, smoked, sniffed ("snorted"), injected intravenously ("mainlined"), or injected subcutaneously ("skin popped"). Snorting is the common route in the early stages of use, and for long-time occasional users, though many progress to *mainlining* (see Highlights 10.4 and 10.5). People who are physically dependent on heroin almost always inject it intravenously. The immediate effect is a euphoric "rush," which has been compared to a sexual orgasm, followed by a milder euphoric high. But some users do not experience the "rush" and, in fact, become nauseous. The milder euphoric high lasts four to six hours. During this time, the individual feels relaxed, free of anxiety and tension, and is lethargic, apathetic, and withdrawn. There may be drowsiness, slurred speech, inattention, and poor memory, and the pupils of the eyes are constricted. The milder high is followed by a letdown, mildly depressed feeling, which may encourage another dose of heroin. Physical dependence on heroin develops quickly, but not all heroin users become dependent.

D. H. Powell (1973) studied occasional users of heroin ("chippers") who had never been physically dependent on the drug. He found that their ability to avoid dependence seemed related to their purposeful avoidance of involvement in the drug culture (the large majority of their acquaintances were "straight") and their constant vigilance and control over the

HIGHLIGHT 10.4
STREET NAMES OF OPIOIDS

Opium	Wen Shee, Black Stuff	Heroin	"H," Horse, Noise, Scag, Smack, Shit, Dust, Speedball, or Dynamite (heroin and cocaine mix)
Morphine	Cube Juice, Emsel		

frequency of their drug use. This group of chippers was described as intelligent; usually anxious and tense; lacking a strong sense of well-being; and below nonuser peers in degree of socialization, maturity, acceptance of responsibility, and achievement. However, group members were higher in self-acceptance, independence, and flexibility. Their motives for occasional heroin use were to "feel better" (reduce anxiety, tension, and dysphoria), and enjoy the feeling of well-being the drug gave them.

Effects of Chronic Opioid Use

Tolerance to morphine and heroin develops rapidly. In a study with laboratory rats, Kornetsky (1976) found that daily doses of morphine led to approximately an 80 percent tolerance for the dose in less than 10 days (see Figure 10.1). Development of tolerance leads to the use of larger and larger doses to obtain an effect as strong as the initial doses; however, eventually the high disappears, no matter how much heroin is used. At this point addicts report that they use the drug to avoid the pain of withdrawal. Physical dependence also develops rapidly when heroin is injected intravenously, and becomes apparent upon withdrawal of the drug. When dependence is present, as little as 6 hours abstinence can result in the initial symptoms of heroin withdrawal—tearing eyes, a runny nose, yawning, and sweating. Within 24 hours the subject becomes restless, anxious, and experiences muscle twitches and tremors, pain in the back and legs, hot flashes, and chills. During the next 24 hours, there is nausea, vomiting, itching, diarrhea, and dehydration. Heroin withdrawal has been compared to a severe case of the flu and is not fatal. The symptoms disappear after 7–10 days. Withdrawal is so unpleasant, however, that addicts go to great lengths to obtain heroin to avoid it.

The major dangers of chronic heroin use are not due to the drug, but to the need to stay supplied with the drug. This need leads to social problems, including criminal acts to finance the exhorbitant cost of the habit. Most heroin "habits" cost from $150 to $250 per day, and few people can earn this amount, plus additional money to live on, in legal occupations. If heroin were legal, these problems would not exist; of course, others might. As Highlight 10.6 indicates, heroin addicts cannot afford to lie around, since they must find the money and source for their next hit.

The major physical danger from heroin addiction is the possibility of hepatitis or other infections from "shooting up" with unsterile needles, and lowered resistance to physical diseases between "hits" (doses) or during withdrawal. Although much has been made of deaths from heroin overdoses, such deaths probably occur very infrequently (Brecher, 1972). In fact, "heroin" deaths are most often due to toxic effects of the substances used to "cut" (dilute) the heroin before it is sold on the street.

Factors in Narcotic Dependence

The development of narcotic dependence (addiction) is not the result of one factor. Physiological issues, psychological issues, and sociological issues are important.

HIGHLIGHT 10.5
HEROIN-RELATED TERMS

Booting	Pulling blood into syringe after injecting heroin
Chipper	Occasional heroin user
Cop	Procure
Dope	Heroin
Hustling	Selling drugs
Get Off	Become euphoric
Junkie	Heroin addict
Rush	Paroxysmal (recurring) pleasurable sensation of brief duration
Shoot up	Inject (drugs) intravenously
Snorting	Inhaling
Straight	Nondrug using
Works	Apparatus for injecting drugs

HIGHLIGHT 10.6
DOING BUSINESS

The ghetto heroin addict is often an energetic businessperson. Most heroin addicts have to be fairly active in order to obtain the money to purchase the drug. The following "schedule" of a Puerto Rican heroin addict reveals this high activity level, along with some of the hazards and risk taking involved.

7:30 A.M. An "eye opener"—not a shot of liquor but heroin.

8:30 A.M. Meets with friends—all addicts—in side-street taverns. Discusses possible "hits" to get merchandise to pawn.

9:30 A.M. Gets burglar tools including small crowbar and screwdriver he hid the night before in tenement back hall garbage can.

10:00 A.M. Breaks into fourth floor apartment of downtown apartment house after knocking at door and getting no answer. . . . He makes off with some rings and a small TV set.

11:00 A.M. He pawns the TV and the rings at a downtown shop. Net proceeds: $50. Often he has to commit several additional robberies to net this amount.

11:15 A.M. Taxies to 125th Street, makes his connection with a pusher, buys nine bags of diluted heroin.

11:34 A.M. Goes to his apartment for a second shot. Goes out again.

12:30 P.M. Two burglaries. During one of these, an old man came into the room and Juan, suddenly terrified, struck. Later he was quoted as saying, "I hope that old man was okay. I didn't stop to look at him, man, I was scared. . . ."

1:00 P.M. After pawning more stolen goods, he goes for more heroin from the pusher.

2:00 P.M. Juan meets his wife and they go to a cheap downtown movie. Relax. Juan is high on heroin now and does not care about the movie. . . . He and his wife meet with other addict friends in "shooting gallery" uptown. . . .

5:30 P.M. Someone has lost his "hypo" needle. Juan lets the addict use his but will wash it carefully later. The danger of infection—and possibly death—from a contaminated needle is a high risk in the addict world.

7:00 P.M. to closing. This is dream time for Juan and his associates and friends. Now he loses himself and his pain in his world of dreams. (adapted from Jeffee, 1966, pp. 49–51)

Physiological Issues. Only recently have the physiological mechanisms of narcotic dependence been clarified. Pert and Snyder (1973) have found that the brain has specific receptor sites, into which the opioids fit, like keys into locks. Akil et al. (1978) suggest that the brain produces its own opiate-like substances, called **endorphins;** and they speculate that a deficit in endorphins could result in the opiates taking their place when used, leading to a craving for the drug. Snyder (1978) has identified the opiate peptides involved in this process as **enkephalins,** which are concentrated in portions of the brain that mediate pain perception, emotional behavior, and other functions altered by opiates; and "beta-endorphin," which is localized in the pituitary gland and the hypothalamus. He reports that animal studies have supported the notion that the opioid-like peptides produced by the brain are addicting, just as are the opioids of morphine and heroin, and that human studies remain to be done to further clarify the opioid addicting process. The use of opioids may lead to a reduction in the body's ability to produce its own opiate peptides, leading to an increased need for external opioids (tolerance). Subsequent abstinence would leave the opioid receptor sites vacant and cause the withdrawal symptoms. However, before definitive answers are available, much more research will be necessary (S. Watson & Akil, 1979).

Psychological Issues. For many years, some investigators have proposed that narcotic addiction (and addiction to other drugs) was related to an "addictive personality." Sutker and Archer (1979), for example, suggest that people with antisocial personality disorder are vulnerable to addiction because of the thrill-seeking character of their lives. Berzins and colleagues (1974), in a study of 1500 male and female addicts, concluded that only 7 percent of the subjects could be described as having antisocial personalities and used drugs to further pleasure seeking and to reduce feelings of hostility and resentment. Their study identified a second group, which used drugs to handle feelings of anxiety, tension, and depression. The third and largest group (60 percent) had no consistent personality patterns. Most addicts do not share a personality pattern that leads to addiction. Many different types of individuals use drugs to meet a variety of needs.

In addition to studies of personality traits, others have investigated whether psychopathology leads to heroin addiction. Steer and Schut (1979), for example, studied 157 male and 57 female heroin addicts and compared them with 6000 psychiatric patients on their results from the Brief Psychiatric Rating Scale. They found that while none of the addicts showed levels of thought disturbance comparable to the psychiatric patients, the following symptoms were present in the addicts: anxious depressive, 35.1 percent; hostile depressive, 16.6 percent; retarded depressive, 9.5 percent; hostile and suspicious, 6.6 percent; blunted affect/no depression, 26.5 percent

One might conclude from these data that people become addicted because they are trying to deal with a preexisting emotional disorder. A major confounding factor has been present in most of these studies, however. Gendreau and Gendreau (1973) have pointed out that such studies have focused on subjects who volunteered for treatment. When Gendreau and Gendreau examined a group of addicts who had not volunteered for treatment, and compared them to nonaddicts, they found no significant difference in levels of psychopathology. Kojak and Canby (1975) compared American servicemen in Thailand (where heroin is available and cheap) who used heroin to those who did not; they found no differences in levels of psychopathology or personality patterns in these subjects, who had not volunteered for treatment. The main differences they did find involved intelligence levels (the heroin dependent group was of average intelligence, the nonusers were 10 points higher); the users had less education and poorer work records and had used more drugs prior to military service. A similar study of black heroin users confirmed that addicts volunteering for treatment manifest significantly more pathology than those who do not seek treatment (Robinowitz, Woodward, & Penk, 1980). Apparently, most addicts (except for their drug addiction) are no more psychologically disturbed than nonaddicts. Such studies do not indicate that personality variables are not important in addiction, but that the subgroup of addicts not in treatment must be studied more extensively. One cannot generalize data on addicts in treatment to all addicts, when studies have demonstrated these significant differences.

"Shooting Up."

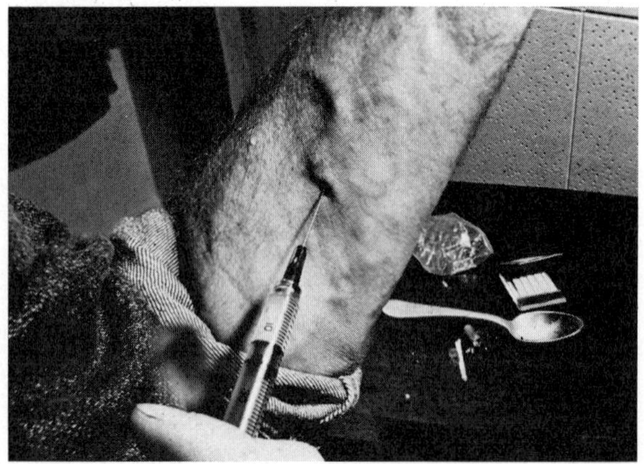

Learning. Richard Solomon (1980) proposes that heroin addiction (and other drug addictions) is learned. Solomon's *opponent process* theory proposes that the human brain functions to suppress intense affect, whether positive or negative, so that behavior will not be disrupted. The ingestion of a drug produces an intense affect which is ultimately suppressed by an opponent process, and followed by an unpleasant state. The unpleasant state motivates continued drug use to return to the pleasant drug intoxication, and a resequencing of the opponent process. Solomon (1980) describes the process as follows:

> The first few self-doses of an opiate (if the dosage is the right size) produce a potent pleasure called the "rush," followed by a less intense state of euphoria. . . . When the drug dose loses its effect because of metabolic destruc-

> tion, the user goes into a state of mild discomfort with both physiological and psychological aspects. . . . The psychological aspect is called craving and refers to an aversive state. Most organisms will perform an operant [behavior] if it will get rid of an aversive state. Thus, drug users tend to redose because this is the surest and quickest way to get rid of the physiological and psychological aspects of withdrawal aversiveness. A slower way is merely to let time go by because the withdrawal aversiveness will slowly die away; but this method is less preferred.
>
> . . . The onset and maintenance of the opiate first produce a peak of State A (the rush), followed by a decline in intensity (euphoria), the first sign of habituation. Drug-event onset functions as a positive reinforcer. Then, after the drug "wears off," State B, an aversive craving state, called the withdrawal syndrome, emerges. Finally, the aversiveness disappears with the passage of time. In such a case, there are two motivational events capable of reinforcing [behaviors]: the *onset* of State A and the *removal* of State B.
>
> If self-doses are frequently repeated, however, two correlated changes in affect then occur: (a) The rush is no longer experienced and euphoria is often absent (loss of euphoria); and (b) the withdrawal syndrome becomes much more intense, both physiologically and psychologically, and its duration lengthens dramatically. Thus, the positive reinforcer loses some of its power, but the negative reinforcer gains power and lasts longer. . . . Thus, the motivation in drug use changes gradually, with successive doses, from positive to aversive control. The user not only becomes drug tolerant but also becomes more intolerant of drug termination or absence. (p. 696)

Solomon's notions remain highly theoretical, although research is currently under way in this area, with quite supportive results.

Sociocultural Issues. Many authors have focused on sociocultural issues in heroin and other drug abuse. Chein et al. (1964) and Freudenberger (1975), among many others, have noted that drug abuse is epidemic among the poverty stricken and socioculturally alienated, even though their studies spanned a decade. Schur (1969) notes that even in poverty cultures, not all persons become addicts, and that those who do are to some extent "taught" to be addicts. However, once the individual has entered the drug subculture—whether for reasons of peer pressure, experimentation, or to seek relief from an unpleasant life situation—many forces interact to maintain the drug use behaviors. As we have already noted, ours is a drug-oriented culture.

MAJOR STIMULANTS

Of the commonly used major stimulants, **cocaine** and **amphetamines,** cocaine is by far the oldest. The Indians of the South American Andes have chewed the leaves of the coca shrub for their euphoriant effects since before the Spanish Conquest in the 1500s, perhaps as long as 3000 years ago (Guerra, 1971). Current estimates are that as many as 90 percent of the men and 20 percent of the women in the northern Andes continue the practice (S. Cohen, 1975). By the late 1800s, cocaine was a common ingredient in many patent medicines, and was an important part of the formula for the manufacture of Coca-Cola (Kornetsky, 1976).

The amphetamines are a more recent discovery, synthesized in 1927 by Gordon Alles. This drug, under the trade name Benzedrine, was used in a nasal inhaler to cause vasoconstriction (decrease in blood flow) of the nasal mucosa and the symptomatic relief of respiratory inflammation (Kornetsky, 1976). Its stimulant properties were discovered by users of the over-the-counter drug, some of whom chewed the wick of the inhaler to increase the dosage level and subsequent stimulant effect. By the mid 1930s, the stimulant properties of amphetamines had been formally identified by medical research, and they were no longer legally sold as nonprescription drugs. The central nervous system–stimulating effects have led to their use to stave off fatigue in soldiers (in World War II, both Allied and Axis powers routinely doled these substances to their troops) and by long-haul truck drivers, who called them "bennies" (see Highlight 10.7).

Cocaine

Cocaine is white powder that is either "snorted" (sniffed) or injected; in recent years, it has become an "in" drug among those who

HIGHLIGHT 10.7
STREET NAMES OF STIMULANTS

Cocaine	Coke, Flake, Snow, Nose Candy, Bernice	Amphetamines	Bennies, Black Beauties, Uppers, Speed, Bombida (injected amphetamines), Lid Poppers, Splash

can afford it. Cocaine is sometimes used simultaneously with other drugs, for example, "speedballed" with heroin when both are injected at the same time. Use of cocaine alone produces a four-to-six-hour euphoriant effect, labile emotions, increased intellectual functioning, hyperactivity, heightened alertness, suppressed appetite, lessened need for sleep; and some have reported heightened sexual pleasure (S. Cohen, 1975; Post, 1975).

An early advocate of the benefits of cocaine was Sigmund Freud, who declared:

> I take very small doses of it regularly against depression . . . with the most brilliant success. [The effects are] exhilarating and lasting euphoria, which in no way differs from the normal euphoria of a healthy person. . . . You perceive increase in self-control and possess more vitality and capacity for work. . . . This result is enjoyed without any of the unpleasant after effects that follow exhilaration brought about by alcohol. . . . Absolutely no craving for the further use of cocaine appears after the first, or even repeated, taking of the drug. (E. Jones, 1953, pp. 54–56)

Freud later became disenchanted with the drug and stopped using it. He was right when he described a lack of craving for the drug, at least in terms of physical need. One does not develop tolerance to cocaine, and no withdrawal symptoms appear upon termination of use. There is no physical dependence, but S. Cohen (1975) has pointed out that discontinuing cocaine after consistent use sometimes results in depression, which can be "cured" through readministration, possibly leading to psychological dependence.

Chronic cocaine use may lead to unpleasant and even dangerous, side effects. The sniffing of cocaine leads to marked nasal vasoconstriction which may ulcerate and perforate the nasal septum. Intravenous injection avoids this consequence and, in addition, leads to a rush of feeling often likened to an orgasm. While common dosage levels are 50–100 mg, dosages as low as 20 mg may lead to cocaine poisoning, in which the individual becomes excited, anxious, confused, and may have sensations of crawling insects on or under the skin. Some deaths have been reported in these cases. Chronic use may sometimes lead to **cocaine psychosis,** characterized by paranoid ideation (the "bull horrors") and auditory, visual, and olfactory hallucinations (Post, 1975). Some cases of extreme violence have also been reported.

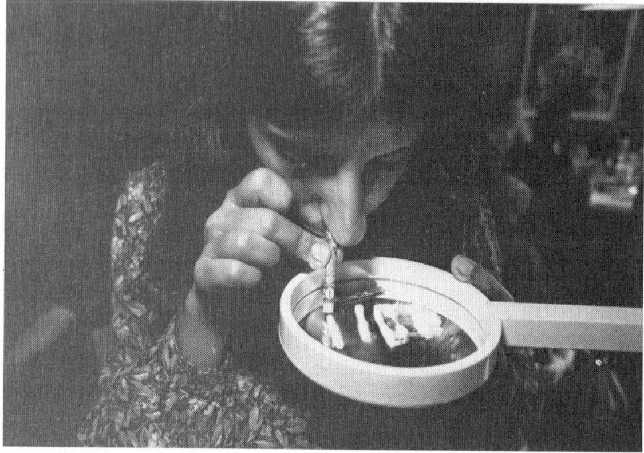

Snorting "coke."

Amphetamines

The amphetamines are central nervous system stimulants which may be taken either orally or intravenously; when not abused, the route of administration is almost always by mouth. A typical dose of 5–30 mg reduces fatigue, elevates mood, reduces appetite, leads to a sense of alertness and confidence, and improves the ability to concentrate. However, performance is not improved beyond a level the individual can achieve when rested and highly motivated without the drug. The stimulant effects have made amphetamines popular among people who want or need a little extra "zip" to complete a task when fatigued, such as truck drivers, college students studying for exams, or athletes. The appetite suppressant effect of these drugs led to their widespread use as diet pills in the 1960s and 1970s; and their popularity for this purpose may have contributed to their availability for abuse.

J. C. Kramer, Fishman, and Littlefield (1967) found that abusers began with oral doses, building up to 150–250 mg per day, and then usually switched to doses of 20–40 mg taken intravenously three or four times per day. Physical dependence or addiction does not occur. In most cases, no physiological withdrawal symptoms appear when the amphetamine is stopped. However, rapid withdrawal has been reported to lead to diarrhea, cramps, nausea, and at times convulsions (Kunnes, 1973). When abused, the amphetamines lead to increased blood pressure, rapid speech, tremors, an excited mental state, confusion, irritability, and sleeplessness. The "speed freak" may inject so much amphetamine that the excited state lasts for several sleepless days (a "run"), followed by total exhaustion ("crashing") and several days of prolonged sleep. The unpredictability of amphetamine abusers' has consigned them to the fringes of the drug culture. Even those who abuse other drugs consider speed freaks to be courting disaster.

Chronic abuse of amphetamines can lead to **amphetamine psychosis** (Snyder, 1973), which some investigators believe can be used as a model for paranoid schizophrenia. The former's symptoms include paranoid ideation; delusions; fear; stereotypic compulsive behavior; visual, tactile, olfactory, and auditory hallucinations; and, in some individuals, sexual excesses. The symptoms do not include formal thought disorder or the flattened affect characteristic of schizophrenia; and the presence of the visual, tactile, and olfactory hallucinations is not commonly seen in the schizophrenic. The presence of clear consciousness, good orientation, and hyperacute memory is also characteristic of amphetamine psychosis. Some investigators have suggested that amphetamine induced psychotic behavior is a function of sleep deprivation, overstimulation, or a "latent" schizophrenia. Griffith et al. (1972), however, have demonstrated that the primary factor is the presence of the amphetamine chemical in the brain. They administered 10 mg of amphetamine by mouth every hour to four volunteers who had been found free of previous schizophrenic tendencies. All subjects manifested psychosis between two and five days after the start of the experiment. Two became psychotic on the second day, having missed only one night's sleep. These results indicate that the primary factor was the action of the amphetamines. Since the use of amphetamines may lead to acute or chronic psychosis, violence, and postwithdrawal suicidal depression, the U.S. Federal Drug Administration has placed this drug on the list of drugs with a high potential for abuse.

HALLUCINOGENS

The **hallucinogens (psychedelic drugs)** are chemical substances that distort sensory processes. The effects include perceptual distortions in which the individual sees or hears things in unusual ways, including "hearing" colors and "seeing" sounds (synesthesia). The user often experiences rapidly changing emotions, feelings of detachment from reality, and depersonalization. Objects may seem brighter, more sharply defined, and may have special mystical meaning. There usually is a small decrease in level of task performance (Pittel & Hofer, 1973); increased blood pressure and body temperature, and nausea, weakness, and giddiness (Barber, 1970). Although intensively studied, the pharmacological and physiological mechanisms of these drugs are not fully understood. In fact, similar altered states of consciousness can occur without these drugs in conditions of sensory deprivation, sensory bombardment, and trance experiences (Ludwig, 1966). That fact does not imply, however, that the hallucinogenic drugs are not the primary causal factors in the states which accompany their use.

Many hallucinogenic substances exist. Commonly used substances include **mescaline, psilocybin,** and **LSD.** Some less well-known hallucinogens are bufotenine and DMT, found in cohoba snuff; harmine, from the South Amercian caapi vine; nutmeg; American Tropical Morning Glory seeds; and the synthetic STP (Kornetsky, 1976). In addition, marihuana in large dosages has a hallucinogenic effect.

Two of the most ancient hallucinogens are mescaline, in the peyote cactus button; and psilocybin, in the Psilocybe Mexicana mushroom. Both substances have been used for centuries in religious rites by Native Americans of the United States Southwest and Mexico and, in fact, can still legally be used in religious rites by members of these religious sects. As early as the 1920s, medical researchers began to explore the use of these drugs in an attempt to relate their action to schizophrenia (Kluver, 1966). Not until 1943 were the psychedelic properties of the synthetic LSD (lysergic acid diethylamide) discovered.

LSD

Albert Hofmann, a Swiss chemist discovered the hallucinatory powers of LSD by accident. His report summarizes the effects of the substance (Hofmann, 1959):

> In the afternoon of 16 April, 1943, when I was working on this problem, I was seized by a peculiar sensation of vertigo and restlessness. Objects, as well as the shapes of my associates in the laboratory, appeared to undergo optical changes. I was unable to concentrate on my work. . . . With my eyes closed, fantastic pictures of extraordinary plasticity and intensive colour seemed to surge towards me. After two hours this state gradually wore off.
>
> The nature and course of this extraordinary disturbance immediately raised my suspicions . . . that the lysergic acid diethylamide, with which I had been working that afternoon, was responsible . . . I decided to get to the root of the matter by taking a definite quantity of the compound in question.
>
> After 40 minutes, I noted the following symptoms in my laboratory journal: slight giddiness, restlessness, difficulty in concentration, visual disturbances, laughing.
>
> At this point the laboratory protocol ends. The last words are hardly legible and were written only with the greatest difficulty. It was now obvious that LSD was responsible for the earlier intoxication . . . I lost all count of time. I noticed with dismay that my environment was undergoing progressive changes. . . . Space and time became more and more disorganized and I was overcome by a fear that I was going out of my mind. . . . My power of observation was unimpaired. I was not, however, capable by any act of will, of preventing the breakdown of the world around me. . . .
>
> At the height of the experience, the following symptoms were most marked:
>
> Visual disturbances, everything appearing in impossible colours, objects out of proportion. At times the floor seemed to bend and the walls to undulate. The faces of the persons present changed into colourful grimaces.
>
> Marked motor restlessness alternating with paralysis. Limbs and head felt heavy as if filled with lead and were without sensation. My throat felt dry and constricted.
>
> Occasionally I felt as if I were out of my body. I thought I had died. My ego seemed suspended somewhere in space, from where I saw my dead body lying on the sofa. (pp. 240–258)

Hofmann had unknowingly taken a very large amount of the drug.

In the 1960s, the street use of hallucinogens appears to have been facilitated by the actions of two Harvard University psychologists, Timothy Leary and Richard Alpert (later to be known as "Baba Ram Dass"). Their personal use of the drug outside a research setting and their advocacy of its "mind-expanding" powers resulted in a scandal culminating in their dismissal from Harvard, and their subsequent notoriety in the media. In wake of these events, many "counterculture" people began "tripping" on LSD, mescaline, and psilocybin, in an apparent search for inner creativity and meaning. Whether meaning was found is not clear, but creativity is definitely not enhanced under the influence of the drug (Rinkel, 1966).

The effects of LSD upon any individual (whether one has a "good trip" or a "bummer") at any time appear to be state dependent. That is, these effects are dependent upon the individual's personality (Jarvik, 1968); his or her expectations, attitudes, and motives (Barber, 1970); and the amount of anxiety about results. When circumstances are positive, the trip is likely to be a positive experience, although even experienced "trippers" who have never had a bummer may find themselves having an experience filled with terror. Attempts to find personality correlates with psychedelic drug usage have been relatively unsuccessful, although Khavari, Mabry, and Humes (1977) have found that users of LSD are interested in new and unusual experiences, anxious, introverted, and have little need for social approval.

An interesting aspect of psychedelic drug use is the **flashback,** a sudden and unexpected recurrence of aspects of a drug trip that happened days, weeks, months, or even years before. Flashbacks cannot be (or are very unlikely to be) drug induced, since all measurable traces of LSD disappear from the body in eight hours, and no consistent evidence of cerebral damage from the psychedelics has been found (M. Wright & Hogan, 1972). Heaton and Victor (1976) have proposed that individuals who engage in "loose thinking," have defects in reality orientation, and expect to have a flashback, will do so. Naditch and Fenwick (1977) found that flashbackers were more likely to feel a lack of control over themselves, had less coping skills, more evidence of disorder thinking, were more maladjusted, had used LSD more often, and had had more adverse reactions than nonflashbackers. Other researchers have suggested that flashbacks are a result of attentional deficits caused directly or indirectly by LSD. However, Matefy, Hayes, and Hirsch (1979) found that both flashbackers and nonflashbackers had better attention skills than nondrug users. Matefy et al. suggest that heightened sensitivity to cues and role enactment may result in a reenactment of the drug experience.

No evidence exists for the development of tolerance or physical dependence on the major hallucinogens. Major negative effects while individuals have been "tripping" include self-mutilation, suicide, and violence (S. Cohen, 1970), and the development of psychotic states which are not easily reversible after the effects of the drug wear off. At one point, the threat of chromosomal damage was raised as a danger in the use of LSD (M. M. Cohen, Marinello, & Bork, 1967), but no substantial evidence for this claim has surfaced. However, future research may provide support for these findings.

Angel Dust

PCP is an extremely dangerous drug. This street drug is known as "angel dust" and "hog," among other phrases. Its actual name is phencyclidine hydrochloride. Available as a crystaline powder in tablets or capsules, it can be inhaled, smoked in marihuana, swallowed, or injected. It is useful as a tranquilizer in animals, but has very serious negative consequences when used by humans (S. Cohen, 1977). It is unclear whether tolerance and physical dependence develop, although Showalter and Thornton (1977) have indicated some preliminary evidence to this effect.

Doses of 1–5 mg result in a euphoria, which at times includes numbness, emotional lability, and general disinhibition of behavior. Larger doses of 5–15 mg lead to a confused, "drunken" state. At this point, there may be a perception of bodily distortion, reduction in the ability to speak, and feelings of terror and disorientation. High dosages may lead to major psychotic episodes, and dosages of 1000 mg to coma and death. Chronic use may result in chronic states of depression, anxiety, possible organic brain syndrome including memory gaps, and recurrent psychotic episodes. PCP is clearly a very hazardous drug.

CANNABIS SATIVA (MARIHUANA)

Commonly called **marihuana** (sometimes spelled *marijuana*), the cannabis sativa, or Indian hemp, plant produces several effects when used as a drug by humans. It has often been considered a mild hallucinogen, but usually has this effect only when consumed in large doses. Marihuana (see Highlight 10.8) is a preparation of the resin from the flowering tops, leaves, seeds, and stems of the hemp plant. The active chemical ingredient is delta-9-tetrahydrocannabinol (THC), and its concentration varies with the conditions under which the plant is grown, with plants from warmer climates supposedly being more potent (e.g., "Acapulco gold," "Maui wowie"). Marihuana is usually smoked or sometimes mixed in food, such as brownies, and eaten. The typical hand-rolled "joint" contains approximately 1 percent

HIGHLIGHT 10.8
MARIHUANA-RELATED TERMS

Joint or jay	Hand-rolled marihuana cigarette
Hash	Hashish or charas
Marihuana	Grass, Weed, Hay, Tea, Pot (from the Mexican *potaguaya*)
OJ	Joint dipped or smeared in opium
Bhang	Marihuana brewed as tea (East Indian term)
Ganja	Potent form of marihuana smoked in India or Jamaica

THC, or about 7.5 mg but dosage varies considerably.

The historical use of marihuana (Kornetsky, 1976) is fascinating. It was used medicinally 4000 years ago in China (Culliton, 1970), and later in the Middle East. Its more negative reputation may have begun in the Middle Ages, when it was associated with an Arabic sect of hired killers known as "Hashshashins," from which we get the Anglicized word "assassin." Introduced to Europe in the 1800s, it was used recreationally by Parisian writers who formed the Club of the Hashish Eaters (hashish, or "hash," is the solidified resin of the hemp plant). It also was used medicinally to treat migraine, insomnia, menstrual cramps, coughs, and asthma (Synder, 1971).

In the United States, Indian hemp had been grown since Colonial days to provide hemp fibers for the manufacture of rope. Marihuana was used from the 1800s to 1937 as a prescription medicine. The nonmedicinal use of marihuana as an intoxicant has been primarily dated to its use by Mexican workers in the early 1900s, and seems to have been stimulated by the Volstead Act, which prohibited alcohol's use as a legal intoxicant. After the formation of the Federal Bureau of Narcotics in 1930, marihuana was erroneously listed as a **narcotic** (a drug which induces relaxation and sleep); by 1937, almost all states had laws against its production, sale, possession, and use. In describing the marihuana "drug fiend," the FBI said, "He becomes a fiend with savage or 'caveman' tendencies. His sex drives are aroused and some of the most horrible crimes result. He hears light and sees sound. To get away from it, he suddenly becomes violent and may kill"

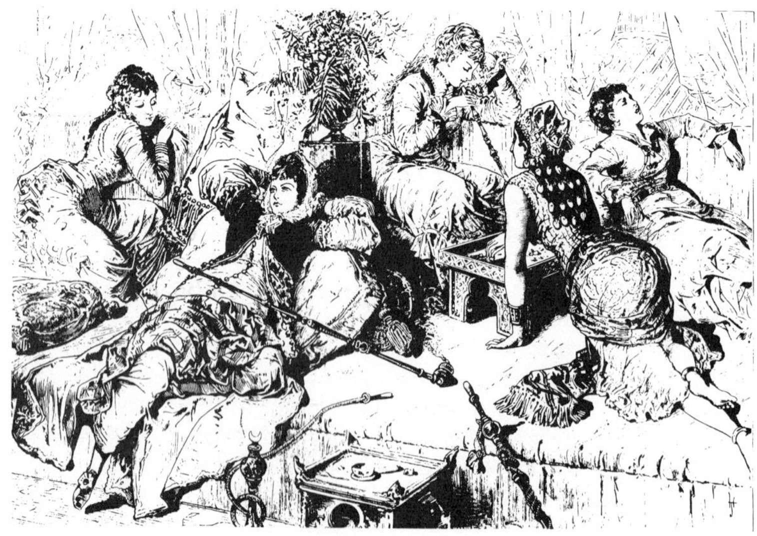

This 1876 drawing, "Hasheesh Hell on Fifth Avenue," indicates that drug usage was considered to be a problem in our society long before the 1960s.

(Grinspoon, 1971). A rather dramatic overstatement! In some states, possession was made a felony subject to life imprisonment, laws which are now being changed.

In the 1960s, marihuana use became popular among college students. The use of the drug by white middle-class educated youths led to its greater general acceptance as a social intoxicant. By the late 1970s, marihuana use had become even more common, with 48 million persons in the United States estimated to have used it at least once. There were 16 million current users in 1978 (NIDA, 1978). However, Trice and Beyer (1977) have pointed out that there is no "marihuana generation." Most of today's users of marihuana use alcohol more frequently than marihuana, although the use of marihuana will probably continue to become more common as time passes, and the drug becomes more widely acceptable.

Immediate Intoxicant Effects of Marihuana

When marihuana is smoked, the short-term effects occur rapidly, peaking in 30 minutes and lasting approximately two to three hours. If taken orally, the onset is slower, but the effects last longer. Physical effects are relatively small: heart rate increases; the capillaries in the eyes dilate, giving a bloodshot appearance; the mouth becomes dry; appetite increases; urination frequency increases; small increases in blood pressure occur; and the respiratory passages widen (Tashkin, Shapiro, & Frank, 1974). However, chronic heavy use seems to lead to significant respiratory obstruction (Tashkin et al., 1976), possibly from inhalation of the smoke residue.

The immediate intoxicant effects include euphoria; intensification of perceptions, such as increased intensity of color and sound; a preoccupation with visual and auditory stimuli; a sense of well-being, floating, sociability, and relaxation; somewhat slowed motor coordination; and feelings of indifference or apathy. In addition, in THC intoxication, time seems to pass more slowly, in contrast to alcohol intoxication, where time seems to pass more quickly (Tinklenberg et al., 1976). The intoxicant effects may also be negative. They may involve panic, paranoid-like thoughts, dysphoria, the feeling that one is dying or going crazy, and serious impairment of judgment. For most regular users of marihuana, the positive effects are predominant.

The effects of marihuana on an individual at a particular time depend upon a variety of factors. Extremely high dosage levels often lead to LSD-like experiences. Lesser, but still high, dosages are reported to produce dulled attention, fragmented thought processes, rapid emotional changes, and memory problems. At these higher dosage levels, the reactions are determined primarily by the drug; at more moderate dosage levels, the quality of the experience and the degree of the "high" is quite sensitive to other factors (Carlin et al., 1975). Low to moderate doses of marihuana may result in a high level of intoxication *if* the individual *expects* this, or if the social setting facilitates it. The reverse appears also true: If one is intoxicated on a moderate dose of marihuana, one can bring onself "down" if the need arises, a phenomenon which is not possible when the dosage is high. At the dosage levels typical for the social user, it has been demonstrated that the marihuana user's subjective assessment of the degree of intoxication and quality of the experience are very dependent upon expectation, and the facilitation of the environment (Galanter et al., 1974).

These factors may help to explain a number of issues in marihuana use. For example, first-time users of marihuana seem to have to "learn" how to get high, and the experiences tend to be more positive if the new users are in the company of others who have experienced the positive effects. Negative, intensely anxious reactions are more common among first-time users who are fearful and worried about possible negative effects, especially when they are alone during the first trial use (a more common situation when the first-time user is middle-aged and trying to "get on board the drug culture"). The subjective experience of enhanced creativity, perception of profound meanings, and enhancement of human relationships may also be due to expectation and set. Braden, Stillman, and Wyatt (1974) found no enhancement and a decrease in creativity in subjects intoxicated by marihuana; and Galanter et al. (1974) found marihuana-intoxicated subjects to be far more self-involved than other-involved (i.e., they were more detached from others while intoxicated than when in their normal state).

Social Marihuana Use vs. Chronic Abuse

With so many drugs available including the legal intoxicant, alcohol, why do some people use marihuana, and why do some use marihuana socially at low to moderate levels and others use it chronically at higher levels? Such a complex question cannot be answered adequately yet, but factors regarding marihuana use and abuse have been identified. Initial use of marihuana appears to be a function of availability, peer pressure, and subcultural sanction. In addition, people who are oriented towards seeking novel experiences appear more likely to try marihuana and other drugs (Feeney, 1976; D. L. Graham & Cross, 1975). Beyond the need to seek new experiences, Khavari et al. (1977) found that marihuana users have a high need for social approval and a tendency to be socially uninhibited. These two factors differentiated marihuana users from other drug users, as did the presence of lower levels of anxiety.

The social user of marihuana uses it occasionally to obtain pleasurable feelings, or becomes intoxicated occasionally in certain social settings. This user appears to be very like the social drinker. Social use lacks a compulsive, habitual quality. The chronic high frequency user (in our culture) who gets high daily, or frequently during a week, or who "binges" on marihuana (uses high dosages) may be like the problem drinker or alcoholic. Such an individual is altering his or her consciousness in order to change an unpleasant reality; and is likely to be using the drug as an escape, perhaps to avoid anxiety, isolation, alienation, or other problems.

Much concern has been expressed over the abuse of marihuana by adolescents. The following case illustrates some typical behaviors which are of concern.

> K., a white 17-year-old male began using "pot" at 14. In the medium-sized midwestern city in which he lived, marihuana was easily available. His use of "pot" increased gradually for several years, becoming his primary recreation with his friends. His preference became smoking and getting high, rather than doing schoolwork. His grades, below average to begin with, slipped drastically and his problems in school, including many "detentions" for "disruptive" behavior, led to his dropping out. He was not interested in working, and spent his days "zonked" at home with several buddies, also dropouts. His single parent (mother) worked and was out of the house. He entered treatment after he had tried to decrease his frequency of smoking for several months without success. He was frightened by the prospect of dependence on the drug, and the possibility of "what it might do to my head if I keep up at this rate." His goal was to return to "social" smoking.

Effects of Chronic Marihuana Use

Research and clinical studies have consistently demonstrated that people who use marihuana do not become physically dependent upon the drug, regardless of dosage levels and frequency of use. When use is discontinued, no physical withdrawal symptoms appear. For some time, controversy has existed over whether physical tolerance develops to THC, the active ingredient in marihuana. The latest research reported by the National Institute on Drug Abuse (NIDA, 1977) has confirmed that tolerance does develop with prolonged use. However, some few chronic users apparently develop a sensitivity to the drug, and need less THC to achieve an intoxicated state than was needed during their initial trials. The existence of this "reverse tolerance" remains a controversial issue.

Several investigators (e.g., Maugh, 1974a, 1974b; Nahas, 1975) have asserted that chronic use of marihuana leads to such disastrous consequences as: 1. impairment of cellular-mediated immunity to disease; 2. the development of chromosomal abnormalities that could lead to genetic damage; 3. decreases in hormones leading to impotence, sterility, and growth deficiencies; 4. increased incidence of lung cancer; and 5. the development of an amotivational syndrome. The evidence for these claims has been equivocal, with the weight of the data favoring the conclusion that these long-term effects are unlikely. The National Institute on Drug Abuse (NIDA, 1977) says that such long-term damage *may* occur. However, two major studies—one in Jamaica (V. Rubin & Comitas, 1975) and one in Costa

Rica (Doughty et al., 1976)—involving thousands of male and female heavy marihuana users (males used an average of nine joints per day in the Costa Rican study) found no support for these claims.

The issue of the amotivational syndrome has been clarified recently. In this syndrome, the chronic THC user supposedly loses all interest in doing anything except using drugs, becomes lethargic, morally deteriorates, manifests general personality deterioration, and moves on to stronger, more dangerous addictive drugs. The Jamaican and Costa Rican studies found no support for the deterioration of motivation or personality, or for the theory of progression to hard drug use; and their conclusions are generally supported by most recent studies. However, acute marihuana intoxication has a detrimental effect on motivation, as demonstrated convincingly by Pihl and Sigal (1978). They caution that to conclude that their data support the notion of a chronic marihuana-induced amotivational syndrome would be hasty. Their data suggest that a chronically intoxicated marihuana user would not be strongly motivated to engage in productive activity; but only the most extreme chronic marihuana users would be intoxicated continuously.

Future research may prove that prolonged use of marihuana has significant adverse effects on the human body. Mann (1980) reports recent findings that marihuana smoking may result in sinusitis, pharyngitis, bronchitis, asthma, and emphysema to a greater degree than found in heavy tobacco smoking. He also reports that consistently smoking 2 joints per day produces 25 percent more airway resistance than smoking 1.5 packs of cigarettes per day for the same period. Whether consistent long-term use of marihuana produces serious chronic health problems is still arguable, but more definitive answers may be available in the near future.

GENERAL FACTORS IN SUBSTANCE ABUSE

Whether an individual abuses a specific drug or becomes addicted to it is a function of many factors. The factors in the following list are significant in the abuse of some drugs, or important for some individuals:

1. Possible physiological predispositions. May be particularly important for some people in addiction to alcohol.
2. Physiological changes. Apparently important in alcoholism and heroin addiction. In the future mechanisms like the opioid receptors that are important in heroin addiction may be found for other substances.
3. Sociocultural sanctions. Sanctioned drugs are easily available, even promoted, like alcohol. If a predisposition exists, easy availability makes the individual more likely to use the drug.
4. Social pressure. When peers use drugs, the need to belong may be an important factor in initial drug experiences. This factor also makes it more likely that vulnerable people will be exposed to potentially addicting drugs.
5. Psychological vulnerability. Drugs can provide an escape from anxiety, depression, and stress. Individuals may discover too late that their solution to these problems has become an even more significant disorder. In the future, more subtle psychological vulnerabilities may be found for drug users; these would help us understand why most depressed, anxious, or stressed people do not become drug abusers in spite of easy availability, social pressure, or possible physiological predispositions.

KEY TREATMENTS

The treatment of substance abuse is a major focus of some private and public agencies. The long-term effects of drug abuse on addicted individuals, families, and society have made abuse an important public health problem. Millions of dollars are spent each year to try to solve the problem. The two drugs which have received the most attention in terms of development of treatment techniques are alcohol and heroin.

Alcohol dependence

With 18 million heavy drinkers and approximately 10 million alcoholics in the United States, the development of effective treatment programs is critical. Unfortunately, the most common form of treatment is medical **detoxification** (simple withdrawal under medical supervision), with no follow-up treatment; the individual often is withdrawn from alcohol (over 7–14 days), refuses further treatment, and hits the streets. This cycle may occur many times before some alcoholics decide to seek further treatment (others never do). An additional medical approach sometimes used is the administration of disulfiram (Antabuse). It is given orally or surgically implanted under the skin for long-term effect. On disulfiram, an individual who drinks even a swallow of alcohol becomes quite sick. It seems to be an effective deterrent as long as the individual takes it; however, most users soon stop, and the drinking cycle begins again.

Psychotherapy. Traditional individual psychotherapy has been relatively ineffective with alcoholics. Group approaches have reportedly better success rates, especially when used in residential programs. In recent years, family therapy has become quite common, and some have reported positive benefits for alcoholics (Janzen, 1977). Others are less positive (Dinaburg, Glick, & Feigenbaum, 1977) especially when therapy has been on an outpatient basis. The need for change in the family members of alcoholics is vividly illustrated by McDaniel (1976), who reports a woman who received much sympathy and attention because of her unhappy marriage to an alcoholic. When her husband stopped drinking, others' sympathy and attention to the wife disappeared. On his first anniversary of abstinence, she placed a bottle of whisky before him, ostensibly to celebrate his abstinence, but perhaps in reality to tempt him to reconstitute the drinking pattern.

Behavior therapy. Behavioral treatment approaches have become more prevalent in recent years for the treatment of alcoholism. Informally, behavior therapy has been around for centuries. In 1694, Ambrose Stegman, a German physician, reported an attempt to treat a female alcoholic by mixing in her beer and wine a substance that would cause her to vomit (the clever women switched to other alcoholic beverages). Peters (1976) has noted that Anton Chekhov's story "A Cure for Drinking" describes the use of aversion therapy in the 1800s to treat alcoholism.

Association of an aversive electric shock with drinking behavior has been quite successful in obtaining immediate reduction in drinking, but relapse is common. Michaelson (1976) has suggested that the long-term effects of this aversive therapy could be enhanced through follow-up treatment.

W. R. Miller (1978) compared three behavioral approaches: A. aversive shock (counterconditioning using self-administered electrical stimulation); B. behavioral self-control training including self-monitoring; and C. a controlled drinking composite including: 1. blood alcohol awareness training, 2. aversive counterconditioning, 3. self-monitoring, and 4. rate-control training. All produced significant reduction in weekly alcohol consumption and peak blood alcohol concentration. Gains were maintained at a one-year follow-up, but aversive counterconditioning used alone was least useful (see Figure 10.2). Sobell and Sobell (1978) also used a combined behavioral approach. It included aversive shock when subjects chose straight liquor rather than mixed drinks, and when they drank too fast. Sobell and Sobell also provided videotape feedback to subjects about their drinking behavior, and

Figure 10.2. Controlled Drinking Therapies. Mean self-report of weekly alcohol consumption.

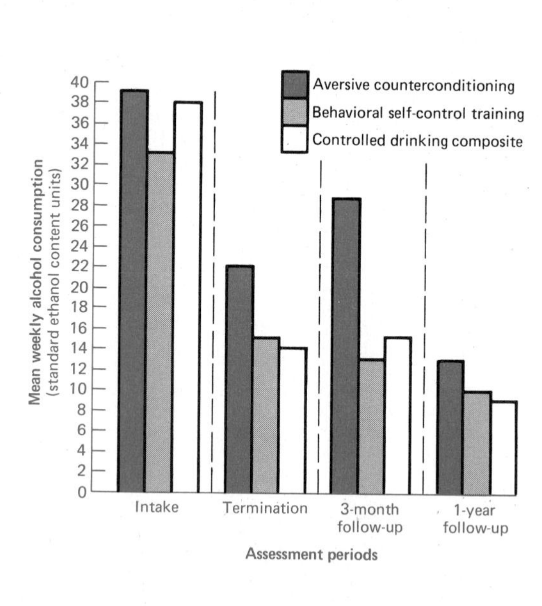

From: W. R. Miller (1978, pp. 78–79).

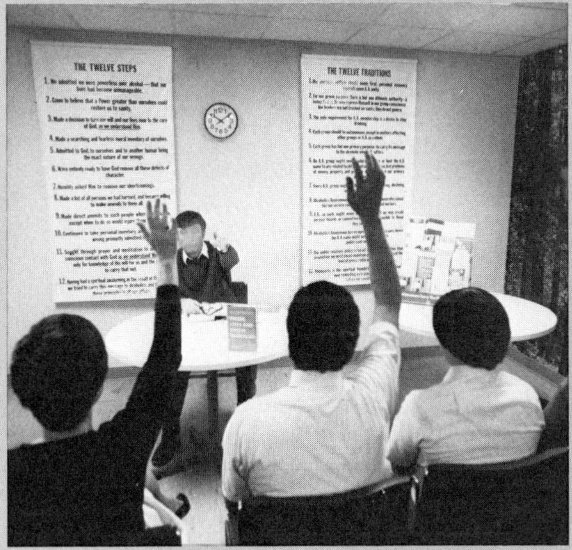
THE TWELVE STEPS
THE TWELVE TRADITIONS

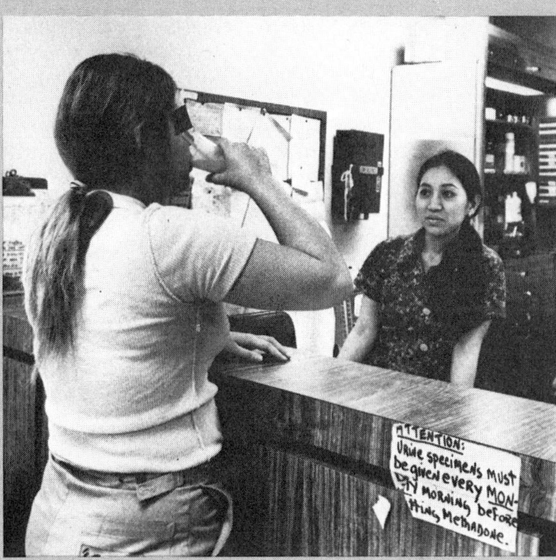
ATTENTION:
Urine specimens must
be given every MON-
morning before
methadone.

Alcoholics Anonymous is a well-established self-help organization for recovering alcoholics. **(left)**

A former heroin user taking a dosage of methadone at an inpatient treatment center. The use of methadone prevents withdrawal symptoms when heroin use is stopped. However, it is by no means a cure—the methadone must continue to be taken as a maintenance treatment, or withdrawal symptoms will occur. **(right)**

helped subjects identify stimuli that led to drinking. The subjects were also extensively trained in ways to solve problems and to assert themselves. The study demonstrated that alcoholics can dramatically reduce the frequency and amount of drinking. The major impact of this study was its comparison of controlled drinking and abstinence as treatment goals. Sobell and Sobell found that alcoholics who achieved controlled drinking with their approach, had a better prognosis than those who attempted to attain and maintain abstinence. Their publication of these findings resulted in an uproar, since most treatment approaches require total abstinence as a goal, and the results challenged the common assumption that a recovered alcoholic would lose control if social drinking was attempted. Controlled drinking may be possible for some alcoholics, but not others (W. R. Miller & Joyce, 1979).

Self-help groups. A well-known approach to alcoholism is **Alcoholics Anonymous** (AA), organized in 1935 by two alcoholics who were trying to stay "dry." Today, there are over 40,000 different AA groups in the world. Basically, AA is a self-help organization which focuses on helping members to: 1. admit they have a drinking problem, 2. make amends for the problems they have caused, and 3. commit themselves to a "higher power" (who some choose to call God). AA has abstinence as a goal, and members try "one day at a time" to accept that they can never drink again. Members stand ready to provide support to those in crisis, and to help each other avoid the bottle and learn to live by new rules. The approach is reported to be more successful than traditional professional approaches, and tens of thousands of people have been helped by this organization. However, Bebbington (1976) has pointed out that the structure of AA, with its lack of membership lists and case history files, prevents accurate evaluation of its effectiveness. AA's effectiveness must be taken on faith, an important ingredient in its overall approach.

Heroin dependence

Once the opioid-dependent individual has been detoxified (completed withdrawal), several approaches may be tried to help him or her readjust to an addiction-free life. Unfortunately, most approaches have been relatively unsuccessful. Currently, the two major approaches are the therapeutic community and methadone maintenance.

Methadone maintenance uses a synthetic narcotic (methadone) that prevents heroin craving (Dole, Nyswander, & Warner, 1968). This oral drug is also addicting but produces no "high" (unless used in extremely high doses). Addicts who are maintained on methadone receive daily doses while they undergo rehabilitative treatment to reorient their life-styles away from the drug culture, provide job skills, and deal with interpersonal problems. **Therapeutic communities** are oriented around drug-free treatment of addicts in residential programs. Participation is voluntary and includes confrontation of "addict behavior" in group settings. The confrontation is often brutal (perhaps necessarily so) and demanding of a change of life-style. Both approaches have been relatively successful with addicts who stay with the programs. However, dropout rates for these types of programs appear high. Appel and Kaestner (1979) studied dropouts and found that they had poorer interpersonal and emotional problem-solving skills than addicts who remained in good standing. Appel and Kaestner have suggested that treatment approaches focus on these problems.

A major evaluation of therapeutic communities and methadone maintence programs (Bale et al., 1980) found that participants who had been in therapeutic communities longer than seven weeks or who were continuing in methadone maintenance were more likely to be working or attending school, and less likely to be in jail, using heroin, or convicted of a serious crime than those who had only been detoxified. However, Bale et al. found that therapeutic communities had a dropout rate of 61 percent; methadone programs had a dropout rate of 69 percent. Only 18 percent of the patients assigned to the therapeutic communities actually entered treatment, and only 30 percent of those assigned to the methadone program actually entered treatment. Of the total addict population surveyed, only 10.3 percent entered and *stayed* in treatment for the recommended length of time. The data clearly suggest that although these two treatments are somewhat successful, the large majority of addicts either will not or cannot take advantage of them. Until some way is found to maintain addicts in treatment, the dropout rates of over 90 percent in some programs will prevent real impact on the heroin addiction problem through treatment modalities (Hollister, 1978).

It is unfortunate that so little can be said about the successful treatment of alcohol, heroin, and other drug abuses. These major psychosocial problems cause an incredible amount of misery. Although many individuals could benefit from the treatments described, most drug abusers do not seek treatment. Of those who do, most drop out. The lack of impact of treatment and the ineffectiveness of legislation against drug traffic leave drug usage as a major social problem.

Summary

1. The recreational use of drugs, including alcohol, is widespread in our culture. Frequent users of some drugs may develop tolerance and physical dependence. Tolerance refers to a decrease in effect over time when equivalent amounts of the drug are used, or the need to increase the dosage of a drug to continue to obtain equivalent effects. Physical dependence exists when drug abstinence results in unpleasant or dangerous physical reactions. Psychological dependence exists when the person has unpleasant psychological reactions when not using the drug.

2. Alcohol is a central nervous system depressant. As many as 10 million people may be addicted to alcohol. Abstinence from chronic alcohol abuse is likely to result in serious withdrawal symptoms. Chronic use has many negative psychosocial effects, and can result in organic brain disorders, such as Korsakoff's syndrome, or in physical deterioration.

3. A physiological predisposition to alcohol addiction may be genetically transmitted in some people. The predisposition may be a tolerance for alcohol, or a peak-valley effect in which the person experiences extremes of euphoria and dysphoria related to drinking.

4. There is no evidence for an alcoholic personality, but many alcoholics are impulsive, depressed, or passive; and drinking seems to help them "solve" or avoid problems. Some people may abuse alcohol because they learn it decreases the effects of stress and reduces tension. Alcoholics have a deficit in perception of internal cues of intoxication, and are more sensitive than nonalcoholics to external cues for drinking. Our culture makes alcohol readily available to individuals predisposed to have drinking problems.

5. Heroin is an abused drug of the opioid family. It causes a euphoric, drowsy, floating feeling. After frequent use, many people no longer have the euphoric effect, but continue to take the drug to avoid unpleasant feelings. Heroin addiction is a limited problem compared to alcoholism, but there are hundreds of thousands of heroin addicts.

6. The human body produces natural substances very much like heroin, called enkephalins, which fit into receptor sites in the brain. Heroin may take the place of these enkephalins and lead to addiction. Psychological factors are also important. The euphoric feeling of heroin use is a powerful reinforcer. Physical tolerance requires larger doses, and physical dependence results in unpleasant withdrawal symptoms. The addict avoids giving up the drug because it would be painful. Drug-taking behavior is further reinforced by peers in the drug culture.

7. Cocaine and amphetamines are major stimulants.

8. Hallucinogens are chemical substances which alter perceptions to the extent that hallucinations occur. The hallucinogens include LSD, PCP (angel dust), and several other natural and synthetic substances.

9. Marihuana is a hallucinogen when taken in large doses. At more common dosage levels, it usually produces euphoria, mild perceptual distortion, relaxation, and self-involvement. It can produce such negative effects as panic and paranoid feelings in some individuals.

10. At moderate dosage levels, the effects of marihuana are related to the user's expectations and set.

11. Social marihuana use occurs for the same reasons as social drinking: availability, peer pressure, and subcultural sanction. Marihuana users may, in addition, be seeking novel experiences. Chronic high frequency users may be trying to alter their reality. They seem to be trying to escape temporarily from anxiety, isolation, alienation, or other problems. Few long-term effects of chronic marihauna abuse have been demonstrated. Some research suggests that possible effects may be an increased likelihood of physical illness and chromosomal damage.

12. Alcoholism and heroin addiction are the two substance abuse problems which have received the most attention. Traditional psychotherapy has not been particularly successful with either disorder.

13. Detoxification is the first step in the treatment of all drug-abusing individuals. Often it is the only step, since the individual may refuse further treatment.

14. Behavior therapy with alcoholics has included aversive counterconditioning, self-control training, blood alcohol awareness training, self-monitoring, and rate-control training. Individual behavioral approaches have been very successful in immediate reduction of frequency and amount of drinking. Long-term gains have been maintained best by individuals treated by a combination of behavioral approaches. Treatment with these procedures may allow some alcoholics to become social drinkers.

15. Alcoholics Anonymous is a self-help group with an approach to alcoholism that has been reported to be very successful. The goal is total abstinence from drinking alcohol. Because of the nature of the organization, accurate evaluation of AA's effectiveness has been impossible.

16. Heroin addiction has been treated primarily by drug substitution (e.g., methadone maintenance programs) and therapeutic communities. Individuals who stay in treatment in these programs appear to be fairly successful in avoiding heroin addiction. However, 9 out of 10 people who enter these types of treatment programs drop out before the treatment is complete.

KEY TERMS

Amotivational syndrome. A group of behaviors consisting of a reduction in motivation towards socially valued goals and an increase in laziness, lethargy, and social withdrawal, which some people believe is a consequence of addiction to certain drugs.

Analgesic. Pertaining to a reduction in sensitivity to pain.

Dysphoria. A very unpleasant group of feelings that produce misery.

Euphoria. A sense of elated well-being.

Narcotic. A group of sedative drugs which reduce pain and induce sleep.

Over-the-counter drug. A drug that can be purchased freely, without a doctor's prescription.

Psychedelic drugs. Drugs which have an effect on mental processes. The term is commonly limited to hallucinogens such as LSD.

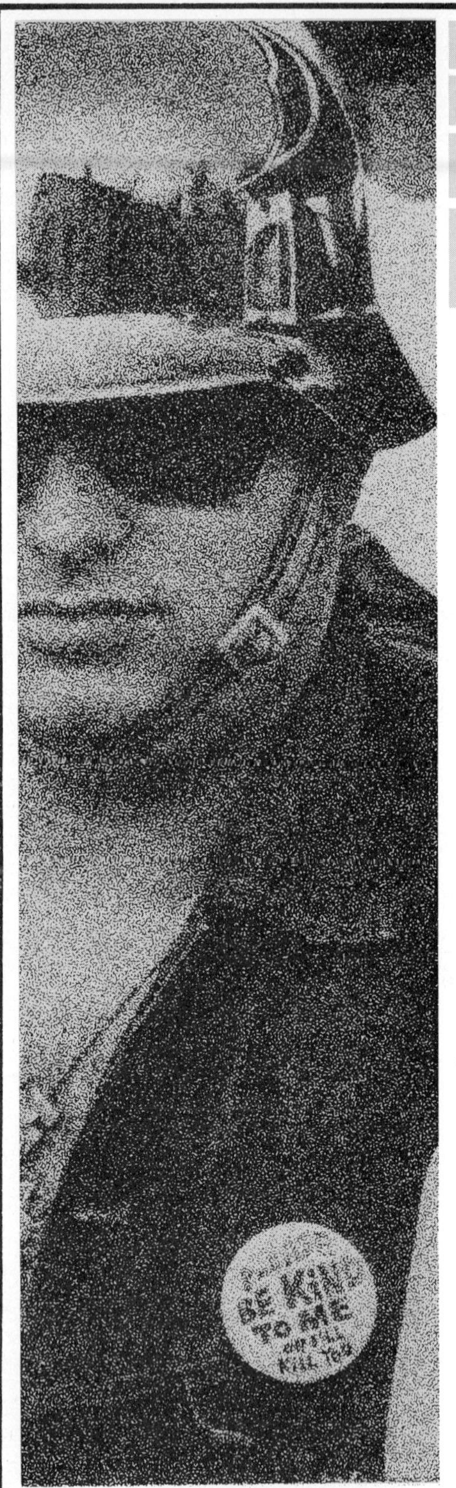

11

Personality disorders

- Personality disorders and DSM-I, DSM-II, and DSM-III
- Patterns of personality disorder
- Etiology of the personality disorders
- The antisocial personality disorder
- Etiology of the antisocial personality disorder
- Key treatments
- Summary
- Key terms

The relatively *enduring* patterns of thinking, perceiving, and behaving manifested by an individual have been described as **personality traits** by many psychologists. When such traits are problematic, that is, when they cause significant impairment in social functioning or result in subjective distress, they are diagnosed as a **personality disorder.** Central to the notion of personality disorder is that the traits which lead to problematic behavior are *not* a result of episodic emotional problems. The traits and behaviors are pervasive and long-lasting aspects of the individual's life.

Although the concept of personality disorder is relatively modern, the behaviors placed in these categories have long been recognized. Philippe Pinel, the early French psychiatrist, for example, described the behavior we now call the **antisocial personality disorder** as *manie sans délire* ("mania without insanity") and the English psychiatrist, Prichard, in 1835, called it "moral insanity." However, psychologically unsophisticated individuals have identified people with personality disorders throughout the ages with a variety of unscientific, but descriptive, categorizations: hermits, loners, clinging vines, eccentrics, liars, and swindlers.

Many of the disorders discussed in previous chapters are psychologically painful, acute in onset, and **ego alien** (unlike one's self, not acceptable). In contrast, personality disorder is long standing, and **ego syntonic** (accepted as a part of the self). The individual with a personality disorder rationalizes the problematic behavior as being "just the way I am," and is likely to resist change, since the behavior pattern is deeply ingrained.

PERSONALITY DISORDERS AND DSM-I, DSM-II, AND DSM-III

The identification of disorders of personality is relatively recent. In 1968, the first edition of the *Diagnostic and Statistical Manual* (DSM-I) of the American Psychiatric Association was revised (DSM-II), and gave more emphasis to personality disorders. In DSM-II (1968), the personality disorders are listed and described, along with the disorders of sexual deviation, alcoholism, and drug dependence, under the general category of "Personality Disorders and Certain Other Non-psychotic Mental Disorders." The most recent edition of this manual (DSM-III, 1980) groups the sexual disorders, alcoholism, and drug dependency in categories distinct from the personality disorders. It also deletes several previously used categories, and adds some newly identified ones (see Table 11.1). As in other sections of the manual, the criteria for diagnosis have been made much more specific.

In Chapter 4, the multiaxial diagnostic system of DSM-III (1980) was described. In this system personality disorder may be diagnosed in conjunction with another disorder. The primary rationale for this approach is to ensure that preexisting personality disorders are not overlooked when another clinical disorder is diagnosed (see Highlight 11.1). Frances (1980) suggests that this method will enhance the reliability of diagnoses of personality disorder, although some diagnostic problems remain. He notes (as have many others) that the personality disorders are probably no more than the severe *variants* of *normally* occurring personality traits that are distributed continuously and without clear boundaries to indicate pathology. The traits are not clearly distinct from normal functioning. For example, just how *dependent* must one be to have a **dependent personality disorder?** While DSM-III attempts to delineate clear criteria, terms that are used such as "inflexible" and "maladaptive" and phrases such as "inability to function effectively" are open to subjective interpretation.

In the following section each personality disorder that is identified in DSM-III is described. These descriptions are followed by a section which presents some of the etiological factors believed to be important in the development of the disorders. By necessity, this material is general. Little research has been conducted on most of the personality disorders. This section is followed by extensive presentations of the characteristics of antisocial personality disorder and the major research relevant to its etiology. The antisocial personality is the most extensively studied personality disorder, and illustrates that research on the other disorders may be equally revealing.

Table 11.1
Classification of personality disorders in DSM-II and DSM-III

DSM-II (1968)	*DSM-III (1980)*
Asthenic personality	No longer used
Inadequate personality	No longer used
Explosive personality	No longer used
Cyclothymic personality	Considered an affective disorder (cyclothymic disorder)
Obsessive-compulsive personality	Redefined as compulsive personality disorder
Hysterical personality	Redefined as histrionic personality disorder
Not in DSM-II	Schizotypal personality disorder
Not in DSM-II	Avoidant personality disorder
Not in DSM-II	Borderline personality disorder
Not in DSM-II	Narcissistic personality disorder
Not in DSM-II	Dependent personality disorder
Paranoid personality	Paranoid personality disorder
Schizoid personality	Schizoid personality disorder
Antisocial personality	Antisocial personality disorder
Passive-aggressive personality	Passive-aggressive personality disorder
Sexual deviation	Now in different category
Sexual orientation disturbance	Now in different category
Alcoholism	Now in different category
Drug dependence	Now in different category

PATTERNS OF PERSONALITY DISORDER

While all personality traits can be described as deeply ingrained habits or patterns of behavior apparent at an early age, the patterns manifested by those with a personality disorder have the additional characteristic of being "troublesome." These inflexible patterns prevent appropriate adjustment to the demands of life in a complex society, and most frequently disturb the individuals *around* the person labeled as having the personality disorder: coworkers, friends, and relatives. The person manifesting the problem behavior is often not bothered by the behavior, or is troubled primarily by other people's reactions. The person experiences the behavior patterns as consistent with the self, as "normal," and often sees the problems as due to others' behavior. Persons who manifest personality disorders tend to have problematic relationships with others, rarely see themselves at fault, blame others for their problems, and are self-centered. A striking characteristic is the repetitious nature of their relationship with others: Their life-long pattern of behavior suggests that experience does not cause them to modify their behavior to achieve more appropriate human relationships.

Paranoid Personality Disorder

Paranoid psychosis (see Chapter 14) involves an extreme break with reality, characterized by fixed, complex, false beliefs (delusions). The individual with a **paranoid personality disorder,** however, does not have delusions or other symptoms of psychosis. The major characteristics include pervasive suspiciousness and mistrust of others which is not warranted by the available evidence, hypersensitivity and vigi-

HIGHLIGHT 11.1
A MULTIAXIAL DSM-III DIAGNOSIS

A clinician who must diagnose an extremely disturbed psychotic individual will be interested in the individual's prepsychotic behavior for a variety of reasons. From examination of the individual in an interview, possible psychological testing, and the receipt of information from the client's relatives, the clinician may find long-standing patterns of **premorbid** behavior characteristic of a personality disorder. Since this information is important to postpsychotic adjustment, the clinician will most likely want to provide a diagnosis of both the current major disorder and the premorbid personality disorder. In such a case, the first two DSM-III (1980) axes might appear as follows: Axis I: Schizophrenic Disorder, Paranoid Type; Axis II: Schizotypal Personality Disorder.

lance, and restricted emotional responsiveness. While people sometimes should be suspicious (e.g., perhaps when buying a used car), individuals with a paranoid personality disorder are suspicious of others even when evidence indicates the unreasonableness of their attitude. In fact, they will respond with suspicion to those who challenge or argue about their distrusting approach.

Such individuals approach new situations with extreme caution and often expect some threat. Their **hypervigilant** attitude and sensitivity may allow them to "tune into" threats which most of us would ignore. This hypersensitivity often leads to their beliefs being confirmed. For example, an individual who is suspicious of others is likely to rebuff their overtures of friendship. The individual may then rationalize that co-workers are unfriendly because they are jealous or trying to make him or her look bad with the supervisor. The person's subsequent reaction to co-workers may be so negative that they may well complain to the supervisor, whose attempt to counsel the employee may confirm his or her original suspicions.

Persons with a paranoid personality often seem cold, aloof, humorless, and lacking in tender, warm feelings. When confronted, they are often argumentative and easily angered, extremely critical of others, and unable to accept criticism gracefully. While such individuals rarely desire or are required to obtain treatment because of this disorder; its characteristics can have profoundly negative effects on their adjustment and that of those around them. Zentner (1980) describes a situation in which a paranoid personality disorder complicates a work setting:

> A nurse, who had always been concerned that taking orders from her superiors might put her in a humiliating position, had a new supervisor whom she admired. The new supervisor was well thought of in hospital circles, and the nurse wished to impress her. She was very careful to make clear to the supervisor that she would follow her orders, simply because she liked her and she wanted to, rather than as an "underling."
>
> Although the supervisor seemed to have positive feelings for the nurse, she obviously did not single her out over anyone else; de-

The characteristics of personality disorder are often apparent in childhood or adolescence. The individual with a paranoid personality disorder often feels that others are talking about him or her.

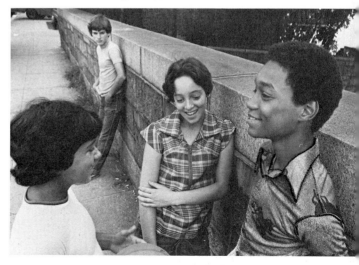

spite the nurse's wishes, it was clear that she was not a special favorite. At this point, the nurse began to get very concerned that perhaps the supervisor might be taking advantage of what she considered her "complacency" in following orders. She not only began to look for signs that the supervisor was taking advantage of her and did not care for her, but began to anticipate such symbols.

Within a relatively short time the client changed from simply longing for the supervisor's approval into being suspicious of her. The nurse became angrier and angrier. Instead of complying with routine assignments, she began to refuse them, feeling that she now had proof that the supervisor was trying to "reduce" her in some way. In a relatively short time the supervisor had gone from a person to be admired and a person from whom one would seek approval to a potential enemy. (p. 144)

Even more problematic are the difficulties of family life with someone who has a serious paranoid personality disorder. The more intense and intimate the relationships with such an individual, the more likely they are to be stormy and disruptive. Such individuals are easily slighted and quick to take offense; unless they have absolute trust in an individual (an unlikely event), they easily become jealous or suspicious of what other family members are doing "behind their backs."

Schizoid Personality Disorder

Individuals with a **schizoid personality disorder** can best be described as "loners." They are withdrawn and reserved, have few (if any) close friends, are seclusive, and usually involve themselves in solitary pursuits. They seem to have a defective capacity to form meaningful social relationships and, in fact, do not want to. Their isolation from others is ego syntonic in that it does not appear to concern them. Such people usually have no feelings of warmth or tenderness towards others, and are indifferent to other people's feelings and to praise and criticism. They are often unable to express feelings of hostility, seem self-absorbed and detached from what is going on about them. The stereotype of the absent-minded scientist reflects this pattern of personality disorder. Most such individuals do not achieve an adequate occupational adjustment, unless their occupation can be done in relative social isolation. Some individuals who manifest schizophrenia appear to have had a premorbid personality disorder of this type.

The following case illustrates the social isolation, aloofness, detachment, and lack of interpersonal relations of the individual with a schizoid personality disorder. Note also that the individual did not seek treatment, but became involved with the police and was hospitalized because of his mother's intervention.

Raymond A., a twenty-two-year-old unmarried man was admitted the first time to the psychiatric unit of a county hospital after having been arrested for disturbing the peace. Unemployed, he was living in the suburban middle-class home of his parents when he was arrested. . . .

Raymond's early years were uneventful, except that it was noted that he never displayed much emotion, even when it seemed evident to outsiders that he must be heartbroken. He made a good school adjustment, becoming an early favorite of teachers because of his quick mind. Socially, however, he chose to remain a lone wolf. . . . He never displayed any interest in the opposite sex and once confided in his mother that he feared that females might be sexually aggressive if he dated them.

After being graduated from high school . . . he attempted to find work with which he would be happy but seemed to drift aimlessly from one job to another. . . .

About three months before his hospital admission Raymond gave up any attempt to find work and began saying that anyone who had to work to earn his own living was a failure in life. He became personally untidy and unkempt. The same clothes were worn for days on end, and most of his time was spent alone in his room, where he practiced his trumpet-playing and wrote long essays to express his philosophy of life. He refused to alter these habits and resented any attempt by his mother to clean his room or to persuade him to change his clothes and be neater. He spoke of wanting to remain by himself forever in his own room and began refusing his mother admittance.

On Christmas Eve Raymond was repeatedly invited to participate in the family celebration that was taking place in his house, but he refused. Finally, harried by his mother's persistence, he slipped out his bedroom window

> and was later arrested by police on the complaint of neighbors that he was parading down the middle of the street playing his trumpet. Raymond's mother convinced the police that he should be placed in a hospital where he might be observed for a psychiatric disorder.
>
> During the thirty days that he was hospitalized Raymond was as indecisive about the course his life should take as ever. He offered various unrealistic plans which would take him out of his home town, the state, and even the country. Although he felt he should spend much of his time writing, he eschewed the idea of attempting to sell what he wrote and seemed to have no idea how he could support himself—nor was he greatly concerned. After a thirty-day period of observation he was released from the hospital on the grounds that he did not display a severe enough disorder to warrant his remaining. (Zax & Stricker, 1963, pp. 192–194)

The schizoid personality disorder displays the social isolation, withdrawal, and detachment of the schizophrenic. However, the major bizarre symptomatology of schizophrenia is absent. Schizoid individuals do not have hallucinations, delusions, or the other major signs of schizophrenia.

Schizotypal Personality Disorder

The similarity between the schizoid personality disorder and the **schizotypal personality disorder** illustrates the difficulty the diagnostician faces in making an accurate diagnosis. In both disorders, social isolation is common, there is constricted affect, and the individual appears cold and aloof. However, the schizotypal individual manifests oddities of thought, perception, speech, and behavior similar to those of a schizophrenic, but less severe. "Magical thinking" may be present, so that the individual may feel she or he has telepathy or a "sixth sense," or may be extremely superstitious. There may be **ideas of reference,** the belief that others are talking about one behind one's back or that the news reporters are making cryptic comments about one in their news reports. There may be **illusions,** the misinterpretation of real stimuli (such as interpreting a gust of wind as the touch of an angel or the devil).

The individual's speech may be strange, with poorly expressed concepts, odd word usage, or vagueness. Speech may be circumstantial or overelaborate or metaphorical. At times, emotion may be inappropriate rather than simply constricted; for no apparent reason, the individual may become angry or depressed or elated, making interpersonal interactions difficult. In addition, the individual may manifest suspiciousness and seclusiveness, and may be hypersensitive to criticism, real or imagined. As with the schizoid personality disorder, schizotypal characteristics may be apparent in the **premorbid** personality of people who later manifest schizophrenia, but the major signs of schizophrenia are not present.

Avoidant Personality Disorder

A disorder which may appear similar to the schizoid and schizotypal disorders is the **avoidant personality disorder.** Again, social withdrawal is a predominant feature. However, in avoidant personality disorder, the individual withdraws to avoid rejection, shame, or humiliation, to which he or she is extremely hypersensitive. In contrast to the schizoid individual, the avoidant personality strongly desires human relationships; subjective distress at the inability to face the demands of relating to another is common. Totally uncritical acceptance by another person is necessary for such an individual to become emotionally involved. The person with an avoidant personality disorder has extremely low self-esteem, undervalues actual personal achievements, and engages in a great deal of self-criticism. As Frances (1980) notes, some have argued that the major difference between the schizoid and avoidant personality disorders appears to be in motivation for human interaction: The schizoid does not want human relationships; and the avoidant personality wants them, is unable to manage them, and therefore avoids them. This motivational assessment may be unreliable in clinical practice, but may be quite important in terms of treatment: The distress experienced by the individual who manifests an avoidant personality disorder may be a motivator for treatment.

Borderline Personality Disorder

An individual with a **borderline personality disorder** manifests instability in behavior, mood, and self-image. Relations with others are intense but unstable, "burning out" rapidly. Impulsive and unpredictable behavior may be accompanied by rapid shifts in mood, from normal to dysphoric (dejected), or the manifestation of anger or lack of control (temper tantrum). The individual may have identity disturbances manifested as questions of self-image, sexual orientation, and values. Solitude cannot be tolerated and there may be frantic efforts to find companionship. At times, such individuals may engage in suicidal gestures and self-mutilation.

The rock musician-singer-composer, Jim Morrison, who died in 1971, has been described by Hopkins and Fine (1977) in a manner evocative of the borderline personality disorder:

> Morrison's sexual behavior and experience [is revealed] through the disclosure of a previous "lover" (Wolfe, 1971). She claims that he was "mostly impotent, often taking hours," sometimes giving up. And besides the sadomasochistic games he enjoyed (talking dirty to her, spanking her, telling her what a bad girl she was—"it excited him"), he would blame her for his sexual failures, occasionally getting violent enough to leave bruises after beating and choking her. She recognized in Morrison the brute and the baby, co-existing: ". . . . a lot of roughing up, then the sudden collapse, whimpering, 'I need someone to love me, please take care of me, please don't leave me. . . .' "
>
> . . . . Jim Morrison was quite obviously a desperate and despairing young man, and nowhere is this reflected more poignantly than in his poetry. He often adopted the poetic posture of being-on-the-outside looking in—not uncharacteristic of the [borderline] condition. These persons often refer to their experience of feeling withdrawn and cut off from outer reality. Morrison mused (meaning himself no doubt), "People have the feeling that what's going on outside isn't real, just a bunch of staged events." Morrison desperately wanted to "Break on Through." And other songs as well as the poetry communicate that he didn't like being where he was—he wanted to be someplace else. To escape "Way back deep into the brain, Back where there's never any pain." (pp. 425–426)

Some controversy remains in regard to this category. As Appelbaum (1979) has noted, a wide variety of syndromes have in the past been covered by the term "borderline syndrome." One can well ask, Borderline to what? normality? psychosis? In the development of the diagnostic criteria for the disorder described here, one term used by the architects of DSM-III was "unstable personality disorder" (Spitzer, Endicott, & Gibbon, 1979). This label was used to distinguish borderline personality disorder from the schizotypal personality disorder, which some have considered a borderline schizophrenic disorder. Unfortunately, the use of the term "unstable" was rejected, and the term "borderline" is commonly used, despite its confusing connotations.

Histrionic Personality Disorder

The central feature of **histrionic personality disorder** is overly dramatic behavior, emotional display, rapidly changing affect, shallowness of feeling, verbal exaggeration and impreciseness, and a tendency to be dependently demand-

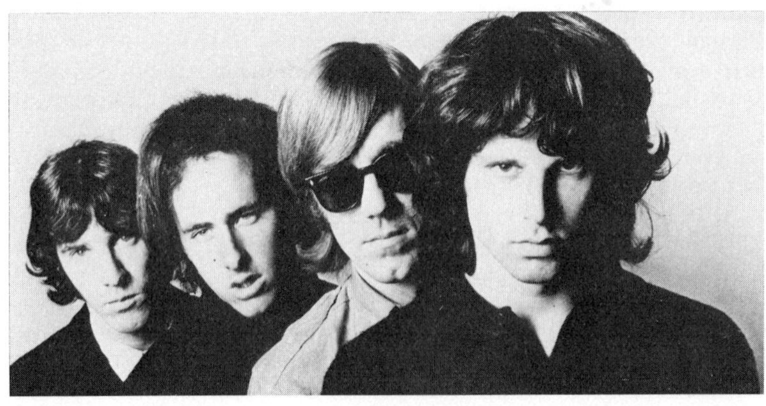

Jim Morrison, far right, with his rock group, the Doors.

ing. Minor events may provoke major displays of emotion and behavior in those who manifest this disorder. Their exaggerations may give the impression that their suffering is extreme, their joy Olympian, and their boredom cataclysmic. They crave stimulation and excitement and may create it when it is not present.

While charming and appealing on first acquaintance, and easy to befriend, persons with histrionic personality disorder often drive people away with their self-centeredness, constant demands for attention, and their manipulative behaviors. As a stereotype of this individual, one can think of the swooning, flirtatious Southern belle or the Shakespearian ham actor. The disorder is more frequently diagnosed among females than males. When diagnosed among males, it is sometimes associated with a homosexual arousal pattern.

In the past, an individual with these traits was labeled a **hysterical personality.** This term has been described by Chodoff (1974) as "one of the most loosely used phrases in the lexicon of a profession not famous for the scientific rigor of its concepts. . . . I have had the impression that susceptible young male [psychiatrists] classify as a hysterical personality any reasonably attractive woman with whom they come into therapeutic contact. . . . It has already been suggested that all we are doing with the term is giving a name to some of the ways in which women have to behave in order to get by in a male-oriented society." (p. 1076) Criticisms such as Chodoff's have led to an emphasis on behavior and faulty interpersonal relationships that lead to either significant impairment in social or occupational functioning or subjective distress as critical criteria before the diagnosis can be made.

Narcissistic Personality Disorder

The person with a **narcissistic personality disorder** has a grandiose sense of self-importance, is preoccupied with fantasies of unlimited success, and needs constant attention and admiration. The extreme self-absorption and self-centeredness of such individuals led to the disorder being named after the Greek figure Narcissus, who fell in love with his own image reflected in a pool of water, and subsequently starved to death when unable to pull himself away from the sight. Self-centered individuals appear to desire to be always on center-stage, and feel entitled to the admiration of others. When such admiration is not automatic, they often react with surprise and anger.

Criticism is difficult for narcissistic individuals to take, and even slight criticism may result in strong feelings of unworthiness. The narcissistic personality disordered individual may respond with either cool indifference to slights or with feelings of shame, humiliation, or rage. Such persons may exploit others for their own ends; they have little regard for the feelings of others. No one is as important to them as they are themselves. Their relationships with others often alternate between overinvolvement and abandonment, and they are unable to empathize or appreciate the feelings of others. Strean (1972) provides the following example of such an individual:

> Mrs. A. B., age 37, an attractive, well groomed woman, came to a family agency because her husband was "not stimulating me enough and my kids do not need me so how do I go about getting a divorce?" Her description revealed that her husband was essentially a considerate man who catered to his wife incessantly, often calling her "princess." Mrs. B.'s sons also sounded like fairly normal boys who indulged and adapted to their mother's whims—but Mrs. B. wanted more. "[An income of $50,000] a year is not enough these days and he is not enough of a swinger," she said of her husband. The client was constantly fantasizing having an affair and leaving her family. . . . "Nobody gives me what I want. My husband is not considerate, neither are my boys, nor my friends, and you do not seem to understand. Please try to understand!" The [caseworker] told Mrs. B. that she would like to understand and asked what she should understand first.
>
> Although Mrs. B. spent a number of intake interviews castigating the worker for not coming up immediately with answers to her plight, she did explore her dissatisfactions in her marriage with the worker. As she verbalized her powerful wishes for constant admiration, affection, and "power" which she felt all women received, she did ask the caseworker, on hearing herself verbalize her demands, "Do you think I am asking for too much?" When the worker asked, "Don't you?" Mrs. B. went

on to describe how she was the darling of her parents, teachers, neighborhood, etc., and felt so frustrated that this did not continue in her married life. (p. 274)

Dependent Personality Disorder

The major feature of the **dependent personality disorder** is giving up the responsibility for important aspects of one's life to others. This occurs because of a lack of self-confidence or an inability to function independently. The inability to be self-reliant leads persons with this disorder to subordinate their own needs to ensure the presence of others who will take care of them. The disordered individual fears to make demands on others, feeling that this might jeopardize the relationship and result in abandonment. Such individuals have poor self-esteem, and experience themselves as helpless, incompetent, or stupid. The dependence may be so extreme that even simple decisions are impossible (such as deciding the color of clothing to wear, where and what to eat), much less major decisions (such as where to live, what kind of job to have). The dependence may lead these persons to live under what most of us would consider to be intolerable circumstances. A wife may remain with an abusing husband, for example.

> Mrs. Ball, a woman in her midthirties, with three children, had spent many years in an unpleasant marriage with a mildly abusing and unfaithful husband, who finally divorced her to live with a girlfriend. During the marriage, she had been a subservient housewife, catering to his every need, as long as he would specifically tell her what to do. At the time of the divorce, she panicked at the prospect of having to care for herself and three children, in spite of generous child support and alimony arrangements. Her dependency needs were eventually handled, however, by using a female friend as a "surrogate husband." The friend was called upon three to four times a day to make significant life decisions for her during the course of lengthy phone conversations, which totaled two to three hours of conversation a day. The problem was resolved (perhaps more permanently) after approximately two years when the woman remarried, to a man who is apparently able to tolerate (and perhaps desires) her extreme dependence.

Compulsive Personality Disorder

Individuals who are excessively preoccupied with orderliness, rules, details, and trivia may be manifesting a **compulsive personality disorder.** Such individuals are also restricted in their affective range, appearing relatively cold and humorless, often expressing an excessive devotion to work or "getting things done." Their perfectionistic attention to detail often results in neglect of the overall purpose of the endeavor with which they are involved. Such individuals often insist that there is one right way to do things: *their* way. They often appear stiff and unbending in their social relationships.

The need to follow specific procedures and details takes its toll when the unexpected occurs. The compulsive person is unable to be flexible, may follow procedures that are no longer effective. Novel situations may result in major indecisiveness, since the usual routines no longer apply. In severe cases, even simple decisions may lead to rumination and worry about the "right" response, and the project or behavior may never be completed.

Mild compulsive traits are functional in our society in many endeavors, such as college studying, bookkeeping, and housekeeping. However, in the compulsive personality disorder, the compulsiveness is so extensive that it seriously interferes with the individual's ability to complete tasks or to relate warmly with others. Compulsive personality disorder differs from the obsessive-compulsive anxiety disorder in that it is an enduring personality style which has been present for most of the individual's life, rather than a new problem. The following case presents an individual with a compulsive personality disorder whose compulsive traits worked well in his occupation. Yet these traits led to a restricted life-style and an inadequate relationship with his spouse.

> Kenneth Reilly was a fifty-year-old executive with one of the largest newspapers in the country . . . he was universally admired for his editorial competence, his uncanny memory for facts and figures, and his ability to spot an error that everyone else had missed. The section of the paper for which he was responsible was rated as most reliable by leaders in the business and financial world. . . . For the

most part, however, he remained aloof, retaining a few old cronies whom he could dominate easily and who were sufficiently flattered by his occasional benefactions of free tickets to the theater or sporting events or tips on the stock market to put up with his oddities.

Ken did not ordinarily waste many words on his wife and when he did speak to her it was likely to be in an articulately insulting fashion. "Mary, you silly bitch," he would say at breakfast, "I've told you a thousand times I like four-minute eggs, and I'm damned if I know why I have to eat hard-boiled eggs half the time. At your age and with a college degree, it's a Christ-like miracle that you haven't learned to tell time." (This on the first occasion in months that his eggs had not been cooked for exactly four minutes.)

To his co-workers and subordinates he was crisp and efficient and reasonably patient as long as they did their work well, but fiercely sarcastic to any evidence of laziness, inefficiency, or ineptitude. There was no assignment to which he was not himself equal but he expected others to meet the recurring high demands of topflight newspaper work without complaint or special incentive. As one may imagine, he was admired and envied but little loved.

His compulsivity was manifested by his extreme rigidity, organization, and orderliness, his emotional coldness (except toward classical music) and his lack of involvement with others, the extraordinary regularity of his habits (symphony on Monday, opera on Wednesday, bridge on Friday . . . in addition, he spent his vacations in the summer always at the same resort, took a winter vacation to coincide with a banker's convention in Florida, Arizona, or California, never included his wife in his winter vacation, always bought his suits in the same men's store, and in a hundred other ways showed his penchant for unvarying routine), and his domineering insistence that every detail in the management of his home and work and recreation conform to his expectations. (R. J. McCall, 1975, pp. 247—248)

Passive-Aggressive Personality Disorder

The seemingly contradictory term **passive-aggressive personality disorder** describes an individual who is presumed to manifest covert aggression through a passive-resistant response to the demands placed upon him or her. This indirect resistance to typically accepted societal demands is manifested both occupationally and socially, though usually seen most clearly in the former environment. The passive resistance is usually manifested by procrastination, dawdling, stubbornness, intentional inefficiency, or "forgetfulness." To the individuals manifesting the behavior, the problem appears to be that promotions are not forthcoming, raises are not obtained, and social relationships are poor, since others become angered that they are always late for social engagements or rarely follow through on social commitments. These individuals are rarely aware that their own behavior is the source of the problem, and often think others "expect too much" of them.

The following individual manifests a number of these characteristics:

> B. is always 30–45 minutes late for work, always 10–15 minutes late for meetings. When given a deadline for a project, he is always delayed. Unless reminded frequently, the work is forgotten. His work has a high incidence of being "lost in the mail." When completed, it is superficial and simplistic, but just acceptable. At home, he forgets important dates, buys the wrong things when he goes shopping for his wife, and is often late for supper. His wife says, "I just can't count on him, so I do it myself." His passive resistance and stubbornness have led to a stormy series of arguments, during which he righteously feels that people are unreasonable to ask him to be more conscientious.

Antisocial Personality Disorder

The individual who manifests chronic and continuous antisocial behavior which violates the rights of others is often labeled an antisocial personality disorder. Due to the major social consequences of this form of behavior, this is one of the most studied of the personality disorders, and will be given special treatment later in this chapter.

ETIOLOGY OF THE PERSONALITY DISORDERS

With the significant exception of antisocial individuals (discussed in the next section), people who have personality disorders have not been studied to any substantial degree. Because the disorders are ego syntonic, only a small proportion of these individuals has been seen by clinicians or researchers. Much of our understanding of these disorders remains speculative.

Millon (1981) has compiled a major text which draws together much of what is known about disorders of personality. He emphasizes that a broad range of factors including biological predisposition, **temperament,** early childhood experiences, and the impact of self-perceptions in adulthood are important in the development of adult personality. After an extensive survey of these factors, he notes:

> That early experience plays a decisive part in determining personality is assumed by psychiatrists and psychologists of all theoretical persuasions. The "hard data," the unequivocal evidence derived from well-designed and well-executed research, are sorely lacking, however. There are findings that show no substantial difference in deleterious childhood experiences between normal persons and psychiatric patients. It is known also that adults who have been reared in devastating childhood environments not only survive but thrive, whereas others, raised under ideal conditions, often deteriorate into severe pathological patterns. Clearly, the events and sequences involved in producing pathology are awesomely complex and difficult to unravel. Only minimal reference to specific research has been made . . . lest the reader be led to believe that there are supportive data from well-designed studies. The author believes that the notions presented here are fundamentally sound and justified. Nevertheless, the reader should approach them as propositions to be sustained in future research. (Millon, 1981, pp. 103–104)

Many ideas exist about why some individuals develop exaggerations of the personality traits seen in normal people. Two factors that seem very important are temperament and learning. We do know that children are born with different temperaments. Some infants are quiet, some active; some are timid, others bold; some are unresponsive, some emotional. Millon (1981) suggests that temperamental states, which may be genetically transmitted, may interact with certain types of life learning experiences to result in specific personality trait exaggerations. For example, a gentle, fearful infant raised by overprotective parents might develop an image of self-doubt and a need for special care by others, which we would call a dependent personality. An emotionally reactive infant raised by parents who use minimal negative reinforcement and who positively but erratically reinforce the child for certain approved behaviors (being pretty, doing well) might grow up to be histrionic.

For most of the recognized personality disorders, temperament conditions are purely speculative. The only personality disorders in which any hard data support temperament as a factor are the schizoid, avoidant, schizotypal, and antisocial personality disorders. The first three are associated with predispositions similar to those found in schizophrenia. These types of predispositions will be covered extensively in Chapters 12 and 13.

Antisocial personality disorder also appears to have an important relationship to temperament variables. Because of the frequency with which antisocial individuals break the law, this personality disorder is of significant social concern, and has been studied extensively. In the remainder of this chapter, antisocial personality disorder will be covered intensively. When comparable clinical and research attention has been given to the other personality disorders, we may be able to say as much about their etiology as we can about the antisocial personality.

THE ANTISOCIAL PERSONALITY DISORDER

The antisocial personality disorder has over the years also been known as **sociopathy** or **psychopathy.** These patterns of behavior onset prior to the age of 15 and in childhood are characterized by theft, fighting, truancy, lying, and stubborn resistance to authority. However, not all children who manifest these behaviors develop into antisocial personalities. When the behaviors continue into adolescence, early sexual promiscuity may appear, along with the abuse of substances such as alcohol or other drugs. In early and mid-adulthood, the disor-

HIGHLIGHT 11.2

In this photo, 36 convicts are marching. According to traditional criteria of antisocial personality disorder, 11 convicts would be diagnosed as manifesting an antisocial personality disorder. DSM-III's more general criteria would lead to 29 convicts being diagnosed as having an antisocial personality disorder. Based on Guze et al. (1969) and Frances (1980).

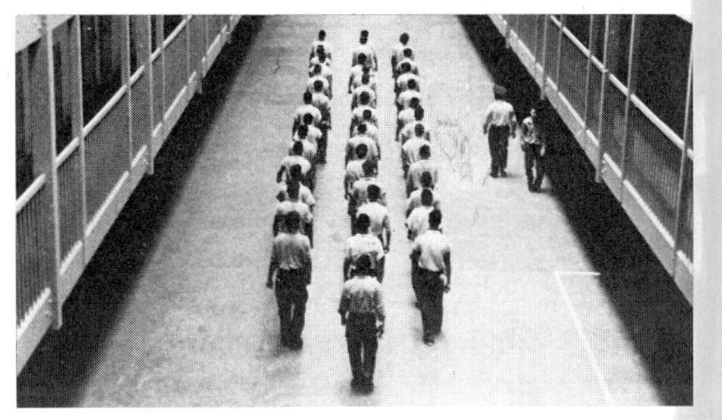

der is characterized by DSM-III (1980) as involving at least four of the following nine manifestations after age 18:

1. Inability to sustain consistent work behavior.
2. Lack of ability to function as a responsible parent.
3. Failure to accept social norms with respect to lawful behavior.
4. Inability to maintain enduring attachment to a sexual partner.
5. Irritability and aggressiveness.
6. Failure to honor financial obligations.
7. Failure to plan ahead, or impulsivity.
8. Disregard for the truth.
9. Recklessness.

While these characteristics are typical of the antisocial personality disorder, they have been criticized for omitting several factors that many researchers and clinicians traditionally consider central to the definition of the disorder (Frances, 1980). The factors excluded from DSM-III include the individual's lack of **anticipatory anxiety,** inability to learn from experience, lack of guilt and remorse over transgressions, and lack of loyalty to others. When these traditional criteria are not used, but criteria similar to those of DSM-III are used instead, approximately 80 percent of imprisoned criminals fall into the category (Guze, Goodwin, & Crane, 1969). When the criteria excluded from DSM-III are added, only 30 percent of imprisoned criminals are diagnosed as having antisocial personalities (see Highlight 11.2).

The DSM-III (1980) criteria neglect the difference between the primary and secondary types of antisocial behavior. The **secondary antisocial personality** is characterized by antisocial behavior which is symptomatic of anxiety associated with frustration and inner conflict, and which seeks to reduce the anxiety or conflict. This secondary type is less likely to engage in antisocial behavior of the same severity and frequency as the primary type (Fagan & Lira, 1980). In most recent studies on the antisocial personality, the primary type has been studied in regard to the etiology of such behavior.

The **primary antisocial personality,** who is the focus of this section, has been described most comprehensively by Hervey Cleckley (1976) in his book *The Mask of Sanity,* first published in 1941 (see Highlight 11.3).

Not all the characteristics identified by Cleckley are seen in each individual. Since Cleckley's formulation of the antisocial personality, certain characteristics have been identified as particularly important. The *lack of remorse and shame* after committing a reprehensible act is one. Another is the *apparent inability to learn from negative experiences.* Punishment of the antisocial personality has historically been an ineffective change strategy. Some researchers, as we shall see, have tied the antisocial personality's *absence of anxiety* to this failure to learn to avoid punishment.

Two Cases

Before we examine the theories and research on the etiology of the antisocial personality dis-

HIGHLIGHT 11.3
CHARACTERISTICS OF THE ANTISOCIAL PERSONALITY DISORDER

One of the most extensive descriptions of the antisocial personality was developed by Hervey Cleckley, over forty years ago. He noted 16 characteristics. In the following list (based on Cleckley, 1976, pp. 337–364) the most salient characteristics are asterisked:

1. Superficial charm and good intelligence. Such individuals are friendly, alert, likable, and make good first impressions.
2. Absence of delusions and other signs of irrational thinking. They are logical thinkers, and their mood seems normal.
3. Absence of "nervousness" or psychoneurotic manifestations.* Such individuals do not show extremes of anxiety; they also appear to lack the common anxieties and worries that most of us feel. They are unusually poised in circumstances where most would be anxious. Under some conditions they may manifest tension and restlessness.
4. Unreliability. These individuals show no responsibility, even to those dependent upon them, such as children; their socially acceptable conduct may rapidly be replaced by irresponsible acts.
5. Untruthfulness and insincerity. They have a glib disregard for the truth, and may promise anything with no intention of following through.
6. Lack of remorse or shame.* Though blame may be accepted verbally, these individuals have no sense of wrongdoing or regret for behaviors that harm others.
7. Inadequately motivated antisocial behavior. Major risks may be taken for minimal reward or for no reward.
8. Poor judgment and failure to learn from experience.* Though intelligent and able to reason, these individuals may impulsively take risks, and seem unable to learn from past negative experiences.
9. Pathologic egocentricity and incapacity for love. Though capable of "liking" others, these individuals seem incapable of the deeper emotions of love and tenderness; rather, they are extraordinarily self-centered: "The world revolves around Number One." They can pretend to be in love to gain their own ends.
10. Poverty in major affective reactions.* They seem not to feel the major emotions of anger, joy, and sorrow, but are adept at acting "as if" the emotions are felt.
11. Specific loss of insight. These individuals cannot see themselves in an experiential sense as others see them. Intellectually, they can explain their behavior, and often use sophisticated psychiatric or psychological terminology.
12. Unresponsiveness in general interpersonal relations. Although courtly and considerate when something is to be gained, these persons rarely show genuine kindness, or honor others' trusts.
13. Fantastic and uninviting behavior with drink and sometimes without. Social conventions are often ignored, particularly when these individuals are drinking, usually with the intent to embarrass or humiliate others.
14. Suicide rarely carried out. Though some such individuals make a suicidal threat or gesture when it will serve their own ends (especially when incarcerated), they *very* rarely carry out the act.
15. Sex life impersonal, trivial, and poorly integrated. Sexual behavior begins early, tends to be promiscuous, and is oriented totally towards physical satisfaction with an absence of emotional meaning.
16. Failure to follow any life plan. The process of working towards long-range goals is usually absent. Success in a field of work is accidental, since these individuals live totally in the present.

order, two cases are worth reviewing. The first example is an individual with an antisocial personality who has managed to avoid criminal conviction and psychiatric hospitalization. In this sense, the case is unusual: Most people studied with this disorder have been available only because they were imprisoned. The second case is a more typical one: The individual is treated subsequent to criminal charges. However, we should be aware that *most* antisocial personality disorders probably never do come to our attention.

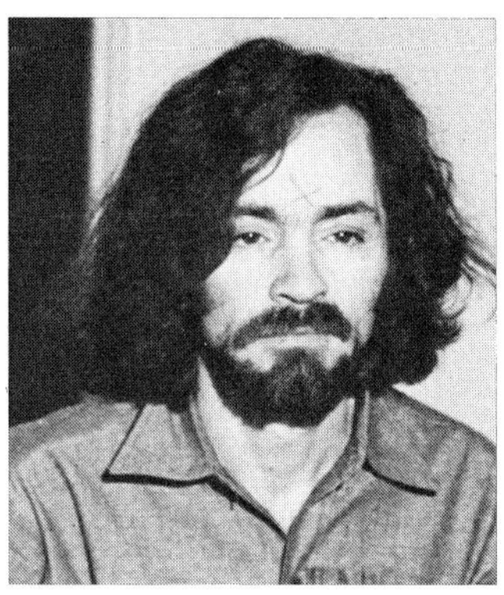

Charles Manson, the charismatic mastermind of the Tate-LoBianco murders, manifests many of the features of the antisocial personality disorder. To this day, he feels no guilt or remorse for his actions.

Dan F. Psychologist Elton McNeil (1967) became acquainted with Dan F. socially and developed an unusual relationship, in which Dan volunteered an extraordinary fund of information about his life in the "straight" world:

> Dan F. was not a patient of mine but he probably told me more about himself and was less defensive than most of the patients I had treated. He was a well-known actor, a "personality" who had appeared on national television a number of times but had never really made it big on what he called the "boob tube." He made a lot of money, had a handsome wife, a big house in an exclusive suburb, drove a beautifully appointed Mercedes, and couldn't care less that there were other people in the world. . . .
>
> One night a colleague of Dan's committed suicide. . . . Later, when I brought it to his attention, all he could say was that it was "the way the ball bounces." At the station, however, he was the one who collected money for the deceased and presented it personally to the new widow. As Dan observed, she was really built and had possibilities.
>
> He was adept at office politics and told me casually of an unbelievable set of deceptive ways to deal with the opposition: character assassination, rumor-mongering, modest blackmail, seduction, and barefaced lying were the least of his talents. His most spectacular device was to enlist the help of A to "get" B and, as the plot progressed, to implicate A to the station manager in a subtle fashion as the culprit: "I don't like to mention this, Mr. Manager, but lately A has been complaining about B behind his back, and I wouldn't put it past him to try to make trouble for B. If they can't get along with each other there may be trouble for you." It always worked since station managers seemed to spend their lives uncovering plots and counterplots on the part of the talent. . . .
>
> In a strange way, Dan has been brutally honest with me. He has openly confessed shortcomings that others would hide in shame but the appropriate emotions simply never appear. It is impossible to distinguish between emotionally important and unimportant events with him. I sometimes think he has substituted practiced social skill for all emotional experiences. He is as much at home in the social swim of an executive's twenty-room mansion as he is in a bar where as many women as men are tattooed. He speaks the several languages of class, caste, and occupation with ease and great fluency. He is a chameleon with a sixth sense that few other human beings possess.
>
> What is the most likely fate of Dan F? It would be pleasing and comforting to most of us if we could believe that one day he will be punished for his behavior. There is very little likelihood that this will happen. Dan is successful in a material sense and doing very well for himself professionally. Canny and junglewise, he is firmly ensconced in a business in which being cool produces a profit. . . .
>
> Dan was also victimized by his impulsiveness and inability to tolerate frustration for long. He moved too fast and with too little wisdom when the impulse struck him and the outcome was sometimes painful even to him. He resentfully reported several incidents in which he paid dearly for some momentary transgression that escalated to unpredicted heights and cost him more than he was interested in paying. He never quite knew how he got into these jams and, most often, blamed the stupidity of others for his predicament. (pp. 83–90)

This remarkable case depicts an individual who in spite of (or perhaps because of!) antisocial personality disorder characteristics exists quite successfully, leaving a trail of psychological pain and anger behind him. Obviously high intelligence may contribute to his ability to stay out of serious trouble. However, his callous disregard for others is quite characteristic of the antisocial personality disorder.

Donald S. The case of Donald S. is more typical of the type of antisocial personality disorder seen by clinicians. This individual's behavior is characterized by law breaking, and legal consequences:

> Donald's misbehavior as a child took many forms including lying, cheating, petty theft, and the bullying of smaller children. As he grew older, he became more and more interested in sex, gambling, and alcohol. When he was 14 he made crude sexual advances toward a younger girl, and when she threatened to tell her parents he locked her in a shed. It was about 16 hours before she was found. Donald at first denied knowledge of the incident, later stating that she had seduced him and that the door must have locked itself. He expressed no concern for the anguish experienced by the girl and her parents, nor did he give any indication that he felt morally culpable for what he had done. His parents were able to prevent charges being brought against him. Nevertheless, incidents of this sort were becoming more frequent and, in an attempt to prevent further embarrassment to the family, he was sent away to a private boarding school. His academic work there was of uneven quality, being dependent on his momentary interests. Nevertheless, he did well at individual competitive sports and public debating. He was a source of excitement for many of the other boys, and was able to think up interesting and unusual things to do. Rules and regulations were considered a meaningless hindrance to his self-expression, but he violated them so skillfully that it was often difficult to prove that he had actually done so. The teachers described him as an "operator" whose behavior was determined entirely by the possibility of attaining what he wanted—in most cases something that was concrete, immediate, and personally relevant.
>
> When he was 17, Donald left the boarding school, forged his father's name to a large check, and spent about a year traveling around the world. He apparently lived well, using a combination of charm, physical attractiveness, and false pretenses to finance his way. During subsequent years, he held a succession of jobs, never staying at any one for more than a few months. Throughout this period he was charged with a variety of crimes, including theft, drunkenness in a public place, assault, and many traffic violations. In most cases, he was either fined or given a light sentence. . . .
>
> After being charged with fraud Donald was sent to a psychiatric institution for a period of observation. While there he came to the attention of a female member of the professional staff. His charm, physical attractiveness, and convincing promises to reform led her to intervene on his behalf. He was given a suspended sentence and they were married a week later. At first things went reasonably well, but when she refused to pay some of his gambling debts, he forged her name to a check and left. He was soon caught and given an 18-month prison term. . . .
>
> It is interesting to note that [at age 30] Donald sees nothing particularly wrong with his behavior, nor does he express remorse or guilt for using others and causing them grief. Although his behavior is self-defeating in the long run, he considers it to be practical and possessed of good sense. Periodic punishments do nothing to decrease his egotism and confidence in his own abilities, nor do they offset the often considerable short-term gains of which he is capable. However, these short-term gains are invariably obtained at the expense of someone else. In this respect, his behavior is entirely egocentric, and his needs are satisfied without any concern for the feelings and welfare of others. (Hare, 1970, pp. 1–4)

How many Dans and Donalds are there? One recent estimate (DSM-III, 1980) suggests that 3 percent of males and 1 percent of females manifest behavior which would place them in this category—an astonishing figure of over 8 million U.S. citizens!

The Humanness of the Antisocial Personality Disorder

To many, the terms used to describe antisocial behavior suggest that such individuals are less than human: "a monster empty of human compassion," in the words of Elton McNeil (1967, p. 91). They are condemned, rather than understood as individuals (Vaillant, 1975). Certainly, it is difficult to see the humanness of individuals such as Charles Manson, the charismatic figure who directed the brutal murders of actress Sharon Tate and four others; or of the Reverend Jim Jones, who was ultimately responsible for the murder and suicide of hundreds of his followers—men, women, and children. It would be difficult even to appreciate the humanness of Dan F., if one bore the brunt of his manipulation.

Yet one authority, William Reid (1978), believes that the person with an antisocial personality does feel emotional pain. He or she may feel the "objective" anxiety of acute loss, the anxiety of waiting for trial, the concerns of the moment; at least this seems so when these issues are measured in terms of how strongly the individual tries to escape from the situation. Particularly when success is elusive or fades away, often as years go by and the individual ages, Reid suggests that the antisocial person deteriorates into inadequacy and depression. To suggest that the individual with an antisocial personality disorder may suffer in the long run does not minimize the misery this individual's antisocial behavior inflicts on society and the persons around him or her. Rather, it seeks to present a more balanced picture of the disorder.

ETIOLOGY OF THE ANTISOCIAL PERSONALITY DISORDER

Why individuals manifest an antisocial personality disorder has been considered from a variety of approaches. Five factors that may be involved in the etiology of antisocial behavior include heredity, cortical correlates, avoidance learning, autonomic nervous system underarousal, and the role of the family and environment.

The large majority of the studies done on psychopaths or sociopaths have used institutionalized subjects as the experimental group (such as Donald S., not Dan F.) because of their ready availability. This raises the issue of the degree to which such sociopaths are representative of the total population of sociopaths at large in the society. Some clinicians believe that institutionalized sociopaths are by definition not very successful at their behavior, since they have been caught! Recently, Widom (1977) developed a method of recruiting noninstitutional sociopaths. She ran an ad in an "underground" newspaper, which read:

> **Are you adventurous?**
> Psychologist studying adventurous carefree people who've led exciting impulsive lives. If you're the kind of person who'd do almost anything for a dare and want to participate in a paid experiment, send name, address, phone, and short biography proving how interesting you are to. . . .
>
> [A later version read:] Wanted charming, aggressive, carefree people who are impulsively irresponsible but are good at handling people and at looking after number one. Send name, address. . . . (p. 675)

During an eight-month period, 73 responses were received; 23 males and 5 females were selected for study based on the degree to which they appeared to typify the characteristics of antisocial personality identified by Cleckley (see Highlight 11.3). These subjects were assessed on a variety of measures; and almost 80 percent manifested the characteristics of antisocial personality usually cited in the literature. The success of Widom's selection process provides a way to select noninstitutionalized antisocial personalities for study and contrast to institutional populations.

Heredity or Genetic Abnormality?

Genetic studies of the antisocial personality have focused on criminal populations. Early research frequently found a greater concordance for criminal behavior in identical twins rather than in fraternal twins. (Identical twins have an identical genetic makeup, while fraternal twins have a genetic makeup no more similar than ordinary siblings.) However, the twins in these studies were raised by their biological parents, who may have treated the identical twins more alike than the fraternal twins. In addition, criminal behavior may not necessarily be a result of antisocial personality disorder.

Recent adoptee studies have continued to support the notion that heredity may play a part in this disorder. A major study in Denmark by Fini Schulsinger (1972) examined biological and adoptive relatives of 57 antisocial adoptees and 57 matched controls. He found the frequency of all mental disorders to be higher among the biological relatives of the antisocial probands (subjects) than among their adoptive relatives or than among either group of relatives of the controls. The differences are even greater when only antisocial disorders were considered. Antisocial personality disorder was five times more prevalent among the biological fathers of antisocial adoptees than among their adoptive fathers or among biological fathers of the control subjects (Rainer, 1979). Similar evidence in regard to criminality has been found by Hutchings and Mednick (1974), who found a significantly higher rate of criminality in the biological relatives of criminals adopted as infants, than in the adoptive relatives or the general population. Recent evidence from United States adoptee studies also supports the possibility of an inherited predisposition in antisocial behavior (Cadoret, 1978; Cadoret & Cain, 1980).

A genetic abnormality that has been linked with antisocial behavior, criminality, and violence is the XYY "super" male. Normal female cells have two X (female) chromosomes (XX); normal male cells have one X and one Y (male) chromosome (XY). The extra Y chromosome of the XYY male has been considered by some to be more prevalent in people with antisocial personality disorder and in criminals than in the normal male population. In the normal male population, most studies indicate that the incidence of XYY males is 1.3 per 1000; however, some researchers (Gardner & Neu, 1972; Jarvik, Klodin, & Matsuyama, 1973) have reported incidences of up to 19 per 1000 in antisocial and criminal populations in institutions. The typical XYY male described in these studies is more violent than average, tall, and below average in intelligence.

A more recent study by Witkin et al. (1976) examined all males born between 1944 and 1947 in Copenhagen, Denmark. From 31,436 men, 4,591 were selected who were over six feet tall to ensure an adequate sample of XYY men. Twelve were found (2.9 per 1000). Of the 12, over 40 percent (5 subjects) had been convicted of at least one crime, while less than 10 percent of XY males had been convicted of a crime. The data show that XYY males are more likely to be convicted of a crime than XY males, but of the 12 XYY men, only 1 had been violent. A major finding of the study was that low intelligence was related to higher rates of criminality; in fact, less intelligent individuals such as XYY males may simply have been caught more frequently than criminal XY males, accounting for a higher prevalence of XYY men in prison. The variable of lower intelligence confounds the available data, leaving the XYY theory of antisocial behavior in doubt. However, the evidence for a predisposition to antisocial personality disorder based on general genetic factors remains substantial (Cloninger, Reich, & Guze, 1978).

Cortical Correlates

The EEG (electroencephalogram) has been used to study the electrical cortical activity of people with antisocial personality disorders. Many studies have found several abnormalities in the brain waves of many antisocial individuals: for example, slow wave activity, which is often found in children but is rare in adults, and positive spike phenomena from the **temporal lobe** (a section of the brain located in the area of the temple), which may be associated

Figure 11.1. EEG waveforms.
Notice the similarity between a child's EEG and adult abnormal slow waves.

Four-Year-Old Child

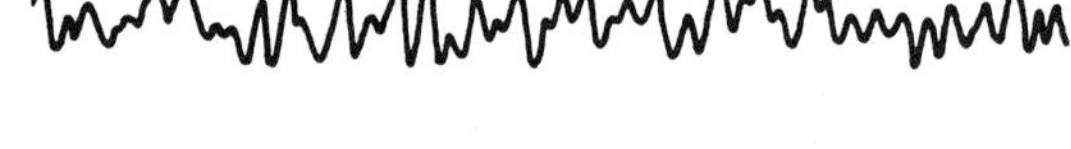

Adult, Abnormal Slow Wave

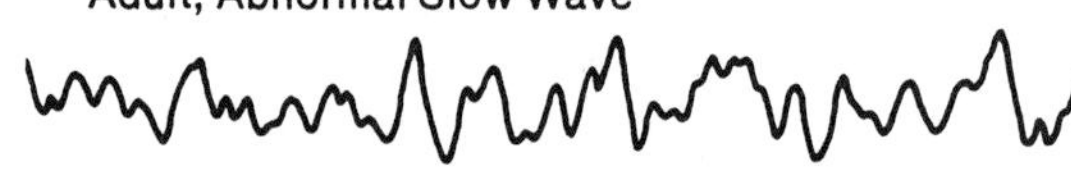

Adult, Abnormal 6/sec. Positive Spikes

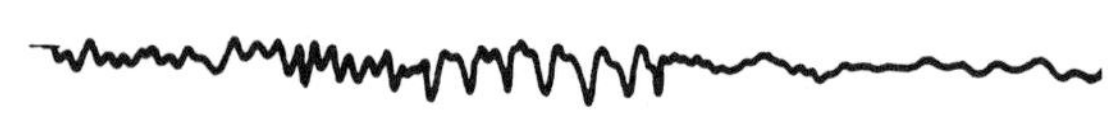

Adult, Abnormal 14/sec. Positive Spikes

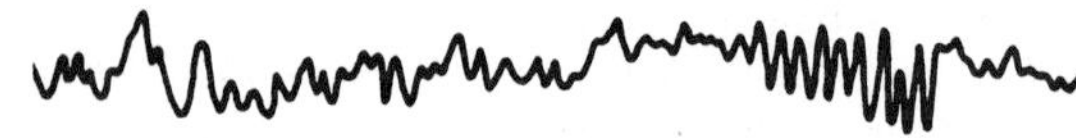

Based on Hare (1970, p. 29).

with impulsive aggressive behavior (see Figure 11.1) (Hare, 1970; Schwade & Geiger, 1965). In a review of studies, Ellington (1954) found that 31–58 percent of antisocial individuals manifested some form of EEG abnormality.

In evaluating the data, Hare (1970) suggests that the slow wave activity may represent a maturational retardation, or lack of development of the brain, in adult antisocials, and some of their behaviors may reflect the lack of control seen in some children who have maturationally less developed brains than adults. In addition, Hare suggests that the added factor of positive spike activity reflects a dysfunction in the temporal and **limbic systems** (which appear to have an inhibitory function on behavior) making it difficult for antisocials to learn to inhibit behavior that is likely to lead to punishment. These factors may lead to impulsive behavior even when punishment is threatened.

In considering these theories, one must keep in mind that many people with antisocial personality disorders do not show EEG abnormalities. In addition, some 15–20 percent of the normal population do show abnormal EEGs with no apparent impact on their behavior. The data do not support a clear relationship between abnormal EEG activity and antisocial personality disorder (I. Greenberg, 1970).

Autonomic Nervous System Underarousal

The individual with an antisocial personality disorder has consistently been described as not reacting emotionally to the environment to the same degree as normals. Quay (1965) has suggested that a lowered state of autonomic nervous system arousal is responsible for many of these individuals' characteristics:

> It may be possible, then, to view much of the impulsivity of the [antisocial personality, the] need to create excitement and adventure, [the] thrill-seeking behavior, and the inability to tolerate routine and boredom as a manifestation of an inordinate need for increases or changes in the pattern of stimulation. We are suggesting that the level and variability of sensory inputs, which are necessary for the maintenance of pleasant affect are much greater for the [antisocial personality] than for the ordinary individual. . . .
>
> What may account for this apparent pathological need for sensory input? Two possibilities suggest themselves. The first is that basal reactivity to stimulation is lowered so that more sensory input is needed to produce efficient and subjectively pleasurable cortical functioning. A second possibility is that there is a more rapid adaptation to stimulation which causes the need for stimulation variation to occur more rapidly and with greater intensity. (p. 181)

Under normal circumstances, the antisocial personality may not be autonomically aroused to an optimum level for adaptive functioning. Hare (1970) reviews much of the research on the autonomic functioning of these individuals, and concludes:

> During periods of relative quiescence [antisocial] subjects tend to be [less active than normal] on several indices of autonomic activity, including resting level of skin conductance and autonomic variability ("spontaneous" fluctuations in electrodermal and cardiac activity).
>
> Although these findings must be interpreted with caution, they are at least consistent with most clinical statements about the [antisocial personality's] general lack of anxiety, guilt, and emotional "tension."
>
> The situation with respect to autonomic responsivity is more complex. Nevertheless, it appears that [these individuals] may give relatively small electrodermal responses to "lie detection" situations and to situations that would ordinarily be considered stressful. They may also exhibit rapid electrodermal recovery at the termination of stressful situations.
>
> Finally, there is some evidence (although scant) that [they] give a blood pressure response to injection of [a drug that increases parasympathetic activity and causes a drop in blood pressure] that is indicative of rapid homeostatic recovery. . . . (p. 57)

Hare (1978) has suggested that people with antisocial personality disorder are underaroused because their sensory input is inhibited ("tuned out"). Thus, normally unpleasant stimuli do not have the same impact on them as on normally aroused individuals. The warning signals must be much more intense before they are perceived by the antisocial individual; driving 90 miles per hour on a motorcycle on a winding road, compared to driving 57 miles per hour on a highway. The underarousal can lead to impulsive, reckless, risk-taking behavior before sensory input is experienced as a warning signal. Thus, the individual engages in "sensation-seeking" behavior to reach a level of arousal that most normals usually experience.

Numerous studies have suggested that the differences seen in antisocial personalities' autonomic arousal and reactivity may be due to a relatively unalterable physiological deficit (genetic factors, cortical damage, or cortical immaturity). A study by E. P. Steinberg and Schwartz (1976) suggests that this may not be the case. They used biofeedback training to determine if antisocial people could learn to modify their autonomic nervous system functioning. The study demonstrated that resting levels of spontaneous electrodermal skin resistance responses and heart rate for antisocial personality disorders and normal controls were comparable. Before biofeedback training, both groups could produce increases in heart rate when told to do so, and these increases were identical in magnitude. However, before training, simple instruction to increase electrodermal activity was effective only with the control group. The antisocial individuals were unable to do it. After training, the ability to modify electrodermal activity improved in both groups; and at this point, the antisocial individuals could not be differentiated from normals on this response. Steinberg and Schwartz tentatively conclude that "these data further support the hypothesis that differences in reactivity between [antisocials] and [nonantisocials] depend on their interaction with particular stimulus conditions in the environment, rather than on an all-inclusive physiological deficit that prohibits the attainment of high levels of responsivity in the [antisocials]" (p. 414). Perhaps learning is as important as biological predisposition in the development of psychopathy.

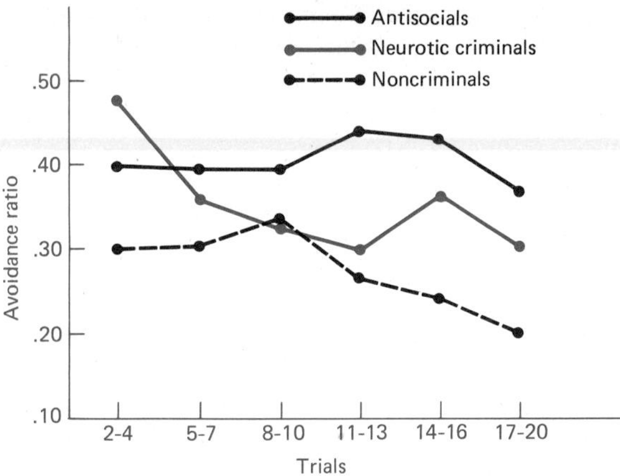

Figure 11.2. Avoidance learning and antisocial personality disorders.
Avoidance ratio (electrically shocked errors divided by nonshocked errors) as a function of a number of trials. A decrease in the ratio indicates learning to avoid shocked errors.
From Hare (1970, p. 80) based on Lykken's data.

Avoidance Learning

Antisocial individuals do learn, but their learning seems to be most effective when it is due to positive reinforcement. When negative consequences are involved, antisocial individuals do not appear to be able to profit from experience. A major theory about antisocial behavior is that individuals who have low levels of anxiety while in a resting state or when faced with stress are less likely to learn to avoid behaviors that have negative consequences.

Mowrer's (1947) two-factor theory of avoidance learning has figured prominently in the development of this concept. The first factor (or stage) consists of *cues* becoming associated with the punishment of a response, and thereby obtaining the capacity to elicit conditioned fear responses (anxiety). The second factor (or stage) consists of the reinforcement of *avoidance* of punishment by fear (or anxiety) *reduction.* If the antisocial personality does not become anxious when threatened by punishment (or in the presence of cues), the cues cannot become conditioned to anxiety, and avoidance does not produce fear or anxiety reduction. Avoidance behavior is not reinforced.

In a classic study, Lykken (1957) tested this assumption under well-controlled conditions and found that primary antisocial individuals performed poorly on avoidance learning tasks, compared to normal controls and other criminals (see Figure 11.2). In addition, the former showed less overall anxiety on a number of measures, and less electrodermal skin response reactivity to a stimulus associated with an uncomfortable electric shock than the controls did. Lykken's results were subsequently confirmed by other investigators (Chesno & Kilmann, 1975; Schmauk, 1968).

Schachter and Latané (1964) added an interesting dimension to Lykken's work. Using a similar format, they reasoned that if antisocials are not affected by avoidance learning because they have little anxiety, the creation of anxiety ought to enhance their ability for such learning. In their study, they injected either a placebo (inert substance) or adrenalin into antisocials, non-antisocial criminals and normal controls, and tested them on a task consisting of the avoidance of an unpleasant electric shock. **Adrenalin** is a hormone which has effects similar to sympathetic nervous system activity, and results in physiological changes like those experienced when a person is anxious. The results indicated that the placebo had no effect; but when injected with adrenalin, the antisocials (who could now be considered anxious) improved their performance on the avoidance learning task. The non-antisocial criminals' avoidance learning was disrupted by the adrenalin (see Figure 11.3). These results strongly support the notion of an avoidance learning deficit in antisocials because of low anxiety levels.

Schmauk (1970) has further clarified the factor of avoidance learning in a study using different kinds of punishment: monetary fines, social disapproval, and electric shock. He found non-antisocial controls to be superior to antisocials in avoidance learning when the punishment was physical or social. However, antisocials were superior in avoidance learning when the punishment was tangible, such as loss of money. Thus, antisocials apparently can learn to avoid punishment when they perceive its negative consequences as important. An additional factor in antisocials' avoidance learning has recently been identified by R. A. Siegel (1978): the *probability* of punishment or negative consequences. In this study, the negative consequence was the loss of tokens (poker chips) which were redeemable for money. The three groups studied included antisocial offenders, non-antisocial offenders, and nonoffenders. The task was a simple card game in which the probability of negative consequences could be manipulated by the experimenter. Ten 40-card decks of playing cards were used, with each deck "stacked" so that they varied in probability of negative consequences by 10-percent increments from zero probability to 100-percent probability. The subject would turn each card over, receive a token for number cards, and lose one token for face cards. The more face cards in a deck, the greater the probability that the individual would experience a net loss of tokens. Each subject could stop playing a deck at any time (the avoidance of negative consequences or "inhibition" of behavior).

Siegel found significant differences between the groups (see Figure 11.4). When the likelihood of punishment (for a punishable response) was low, (10–30 percent), neither antisocials or non-antisocials were likely to inhibit their punishable responses. When the punishment was virtually certain, all would inhibit their responses. However, in the middle ranges (40–80 percent), when the likelihood of

Figure 11.3. Avoidance learning in antisocial individuals given adrenalin.

Effects of placebo and adrenalin administration on avoidance learning, in antisocial and non-antisocial men.

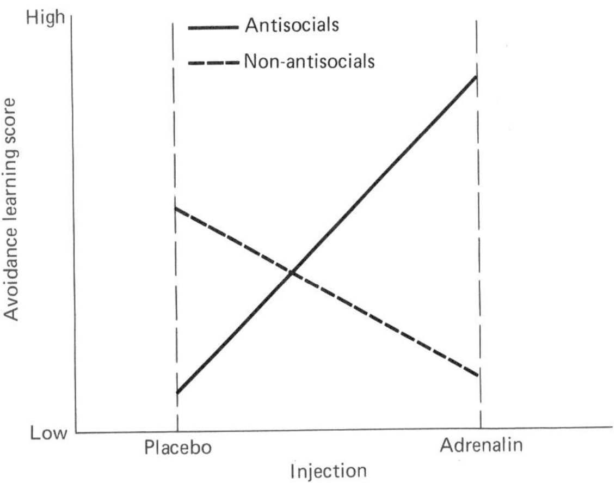

Based on Schachter and Latané (1964).

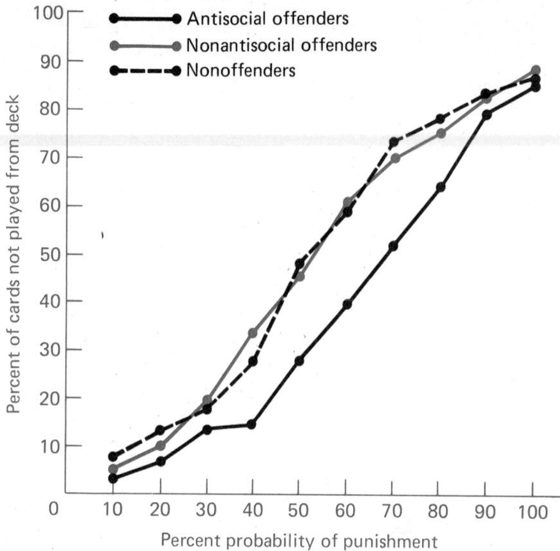

Figure 11.4. Suppression (or inhibition) of behavior as a function of probability of punishment (negative consequences) for antisocial offenders, non-antisocial offenders, and nonoffenders.

From R. A. Siegel (1978, p. 518).

punishment was uncertain, antisocials were much less likely to inhibit their punishable responses than non-antisocials (both normals and those convicted of criminal offenses). In this study, Siegel found that the presence or absence of anxiety, guilt, or depression did not distinguish between the antisocial and non-antisocial groups, and suggests that antisocials' cognitive estimates of the likelihood of being punished are an important variable in whether behavior is inhibited. Apparently, the psychopath who believes that punishment is a certainty can inhibit the behavior. The importance of cognitive factors has also been examined by Heilbrun (1979), who found that in a population of white male antisocials, the brighter antisocials were less impulsive and more conforming to general societal expectations than the less intelligent subjects. Subjects with higher intelligence may be able to judge the likelihood of punishment better than those of low intelligence, and may be able to learn to avoid at least some socially unacceptable behaviors. Heilbrun suggests that intelligence is a variable which must be controlled in future studies of antisocial behavior.

Family and Environment

The individual with an antisocial personality disorder has been described as suffering from a defect of the socialization process. Since parents are the individuals primarily responsible for the socialization of children, parent-child relationships are often seen as important in the development of antisocial behavior. Among the earliest theories which emphasized the interactions between parents and antisocial offspring was the psychoanalytic approach. Many psychoanalysts have described antisocial personalities as people with inadequate ego and superego processes. The faulty superego (conscience) allows the id impulses to dominate the personality, so that the demand for immediate gratification is not mediated by the ego and dominates the individual's behavior. Because of faulty superego processes, the antisocial behavior does not result in guilt. In this theoretical formulation, the necessary socialization does not occur during childhood because of faulty parent-child interactions, and the child does not internalize the parents' socioculturally acceptable values. Little direct support for this theory exists.

The presence of disruptive relationships in the families of many antisocial people is well established, however. S. Green (1964) reports that more than twice as many antisocials as "neurotics" or controls lost one or both parents early in childhood. Robins (1966) found, in addition, that most antisocials' fathers were either antisocials, alcoholics, or both, and presumably did not provide a very good role model. In her prospective study, detailed records of family interactions had been previously obtained for children found to have antisocial features 30 years later. In addition to the fathers' antisocial behavior or alcoholism, disciplinary processes in these families were either inconsistent or absent. The finding of inconsistent or absent discipline is interesting in the light of R. A. Siegel's findings (reported earlier) that adult antisocials are less likely to inhibit their behavior than normals when the likelihood of pun-

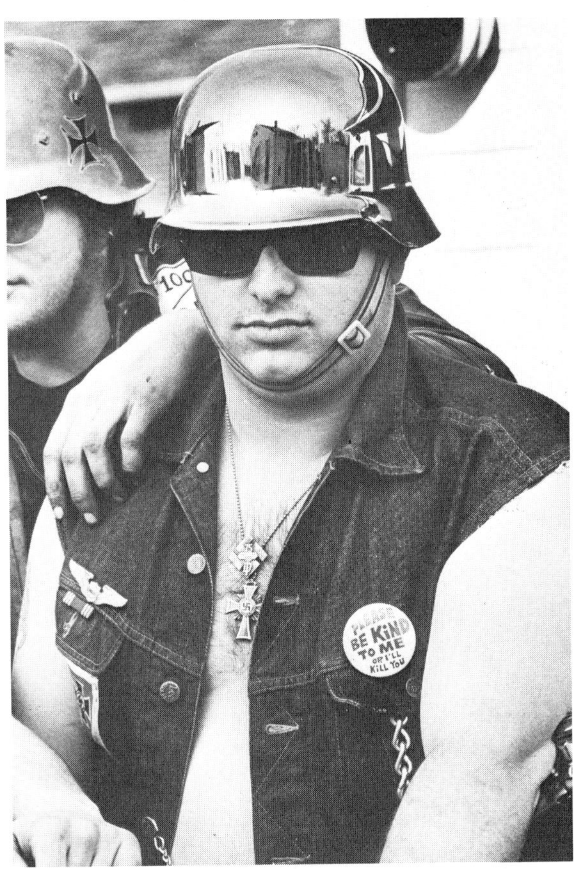

Is this man exhibiting an antisocial personality disorder? Or does he just fit our stereotypes?

ishment is unpredictable (inconsistent). Of course, discipline is inconsistent in many families in which the children do not become antisocial. These studies highlight three factors: 1. faulty parental models (one or both parents antisocial); 2. parental inconsistency in discipline; and 3. parental loss through death, divorce, or abandonment.

Variables of the broader environment have also been implicated by some theorists (R. J. Smith, 1978). The antisocial personality disorder appears to be more frequent in the lower socioeconomic classes. Perhaps the chaos and disorganization of poverty, with the breakdown of social norms and alienation from the mainstream of society is a factor. The general materialistic and self-centered nature of American culture has also been described as a factor. Some investigators (Zuckerman, Eysenck, & Eysenck, 1978) have reported tentative cross-cultural differences in sensation-seeking behavior between Westerners (American and British subjects scored higher) and Easterners (Japanese and Thais scored lower). An interesting discovery was that scores on a sensation-seeking scale appear to vary more with subjects' age within samples than scores varied between samples. The data on aging is supportive of clinical experience: Antisocial personality disorder is rare in the elderly. The tentative data from this study are minimally supportive of cross-cultural factors in psychopathy. The evidence tends to be confounded by other variables.

Conclusions

Most individuals who develop an antisocial personality appear to have an inherited predisposition to a lower level of autonomic nervous system arousal. This lowered arousal level makes avoidance learning unlikely. Some types of punishments or threats of punishment have less impact on the individual's behavior. If such an individual is raised by parents who engage in antisocial behavior, he or she has role models to copy. The subsequent childhood antisocial behavior is likely to be inconsistently disciplined by the parents. At times, the antisocial behavior will be positively rewarding for the individual, and this will make it more likely to recur. As the person is reinforced for unacceptable behavior, it is not surprising that he or she might see socially conforming individuals as "squares." Unlike most people, the threat of punishment does not outweigh the immediate gains of impulsive self-centered behavior. The brighter antisocial person can modify such behavior to avoid outright criminal activity or, more likely, to avoid being caught. The less bright individual is likely to be more impulsive and have poorer judgment, and thus is more likely to come to the attention of the criminal justice system.

KEY TREATMENTS

The treatment of personality disorder has traditionally been difficult. Such individuals usually do not perceive themselves as needing to change, and, therefore, lack motivation to do so. Even when they seek treatment, the long-standing nature of the behaviors makes modification difficult. Little can be said about the treatment of most personality disorders, since we have such limited experience with them. The contexts in which most such individuals are seen for therapy are in couple's therapy, at the spouse's insistence; as a parent in family therapy, when a child's behavior results in a request for services; or at the instigation of a court of law. Among people convicted of crimes, the individual with the antisocial personality disorder is most frequently required to obtain treatment. Many such individuals end up in treatment settings in an attempt to avoid prosecution, as a consequence of a probation requirement, or subsequent to conviction for a crime; thus, there is substantial experience with the treatment of antisocial personality disorder unlike the other personality disorders.

The traditional psychotherapeutic approach usually focuses on the development of "conscience" in the antisocial person through the development of a meaningful relationship between the therapist and client, an exceedingly difficult task. It has had little apparent success (Craft, 1965), especially when attempted on an outpatient basis. Vaillant (1975) has noted that better, though not outstanding, success has been achieved in institutional settings when certain criteria are met:

1. The antisocial behavior must be controllable within the therapeutic environment.
2. The control must not be punitive, and the patient must have some hope of release if the behavior changes.
3. Once anxiety is manifested, it should not be controlled; rather, the therapist should assist the "antisocial person in living through it."
4. The therapist cannot take the subject's stories at face value (they are mostly fabrications, at least initially).
5. Substitute behaviors must be taught to replace the behaviors presented (such as lying, stealing, violence).
6. Confrontation of behavior works better than interpretation of motivations.
7. Peer group feedback is essential.
8. Gralnick (1979) has pointed out that interstaff communication is essential if the staff members are not to be manipulated.
9. Finally, Templeman and Wollersheim (1979) have emphasized that any approach to treating antisocial personality disorder must appeal to the person's self-interest.

Even when these criteria exists, the manipulative behavior of the individual with an antisocial personality disorder is difficult to deal with (Reicher, 1979), and success is difficult to achieve.

Certain behavioral treatment approaches have been applied to antisocial offenders with some success (Braukmann et al., 1975). However, a major problem with these approaches is that the behavior change often does not generalize to the noninstitutional environment (Beit-Hallahni, 1976). Once back on the street, the antisocial individual reverts to the old reinforcement contingencies. While one might expect the use of behavioral approaches that focus on the intensification of anxiety or on punishment systems that impact on the autonomic nervous system, such approaches are unlikely to be used because of their ethical implications. The application of punishment techniques to nonconsenting individuals is a violation of their rights, and is not permitted in most settings.

An approach that focuses on how antisocial persons think and what they believe about themselves and the world has been reported by Templeman and Wollersheim (1979). This cognitive-behavioral approach focuses on motivating these individuals to change by appealing to their self-interest. Templeman and Wollersheim (1979) provide a case example which illustrates this process:

> After working for six months with a young, bright, and psychopathic [antisocial] inmate and getting nowhere on his "personal problems," the therapist and client finally concurred that the client's number one goal was to get out of prison and to stay out. Together, therapist and client considered alternatives for achieving this. Both agreed that the client could break out and attain some short term freedom but that the odds of remaining free for very long were stacked against him. Working within the prison to earn a school furlough was another alternative but was problematic because of the client's overwhelming tendency to alienate prison officers by impulsively teasing them, talking back, testing limits, and occasional outright defiance of rules, which resulted in frequent disciplinary action, which in turn placed his application for furlough in jeopardy. After discussing the situation in just these

terms, the therapist asked the client to list the costs and benefits of every single decision he made throughout the week and write these lists down. Practice in doing this was offered in the therapy sessions. The client perceived the potential benefits of his acting out toward the guards as feeling superior to them, standing up for inmate rights, and increasing his status in the eyes of fellow inmates. The potential costs included lessening his chances for furlough, a closer monitoring of his behavior in the future, possible disciplinary action with resultant restrictions of his freedom, and increasing the likelihood of further confrontations with the guards. Poor decisions were challenged by the therapist with, "Is this getting you nearer your goal of freedom?" and the client was instructed to ask himself the same question. After several weeks of this, the client spontaneously remarked, "You know, I've decided it's more important for me to get out of here than to get even with the guards." He is now attending the University of Montana on a school furlough. Bearing in mind the anecdotal nature of the evidence, it nevertheless suggests that attitude change and subsequent behavior change in [an antisocial personality] may derive to some extent from practice in thinking in [different] ways. (p. 136)

The success of such an approach remains to be seen, but one might question whether this approach simply helps antisocial people to be more effective in their antisocial behavior! Is this individual becoming more like Dan F. than Donald S.?

Summary

1. In this chapter several relatively enduring patterns of thinking, behaving, and perceiving have been categorized as personality disorders because of the impairment of social functioning or the subjective distress which result from their manifestation.

2. In DSM-III, some disorders previously described have been eliminated, several new categories have been listed, and all have been defined with more concrete criteria. The disorders examined in this chapter include:

1. Paranoid personality disorder
2. Schizoid personality disorder
3. Schizotypal personality disorder
4. Avoidant personality disorder
5. Borderline personality disorder
6. Histrionic personality disorder
7. Narcissistic personality disorder
8. Dependent personality disorder
9. Compulsive personality disorder
10. Passive-aggressive personality disorder
11. Antisocial personality disorder

3. The etiology of many of the personality disorders remains obscure. With the exception of the antisocial personality, these disorders are seldom seen by clinicians and researchers.

4. The etiology of personality disorders as a group probably relates to temperament of the child, which interacts with a particular lifetime of experience. The factors result in the exaggeration of traits commonly seen in people who would not be described as disordered.

5. Special attention has been given to the antisocial personality disorder or, as it has often been known, the sociopathic or psychopathic disorder. This is one of the few well-studied (but still baffling) personality disorders.

6. The text has focused on the characteristics of primary antisocial behavior. These behaviors were defined by Cleckley over 40 years ago. In addition to overall antisocial behavior, Cleckley's criteria of lack of remorse and shame, the inability to learn from negative experience, and the absence of manifest anxiety are seen as important features of the disorder.

7. Studies on the etiology of the antisocial personality disorder suggest that: 1. there is an inherited predisposition to antisocial personality; 2. there may be cortical dysfunction in many people with antisocial personality, as evidenced by abnormal EEGs; 3. antisocial persons' autonomic nervous systems are hypoactive (i.e., they are usually underaroused); 4. they have difficulty in some types of avoidance learning, but seem able to inhibit their behavior when the stakes are apparently important to them; and 5. the presence of one or both parents who are antisocial and who provide inconsistent discipline or no discipline is associated with antisocial behavior in offspring.

8. Treatment of the personality disorders is difficult, since the individuals are often satisfied with their behavior. Most individuals with personality disorders do not seek treatment and those most frequently treated have an antisocial personality disorder and have been forced (usually by a court of law) to seek treatment.

9. Antisocial personality disorder is often treated in a prison setting. Treatment must set limits, but not be punitive. Therapists must be cautious not to be taken in by the manipulation of the patient, and therapy must appeal to the self-interest of the antisocial person. Even in controlled settings, treatment success is difficult to achieve.

10. Behavioral approaches that are used to treat antisocial personality disorders often meet with initial success, but the behavior change often does not generalize to the noninstitutional environment.

11. A successful cognitive approach has been reported which attempts to appeal to the antisocial individual's self-interest. However, it may simply be a process for making antisocial people into more successful manipulators, able to obtain their selfish ends without being detected.

KEY TERMS

Anticipatory anxiety. Anxiety that is felt in anticipation of some future unpleasant event, such as punishment.

Hypervigilant. The state of being extremely attentive to surrounding events.

Personality trait. A consistent, enduring, personality characteristic such as dependence, suspiciousness, orderliness, flexibility, openness, etc.

Premorbid. The period preceding the development of a disorder.

Psychopathy. A term commonly used in the past (and still on occasion) to refer to the pattern of behavior now called antisocial personality disorder.

Sociopathy. See Psychopathy.

Temperament. Biologically based dispositions which underlie the energy level and color the moods of the individual. For example, some infants have a quiet temperament, others are fearful, others are active, etc.

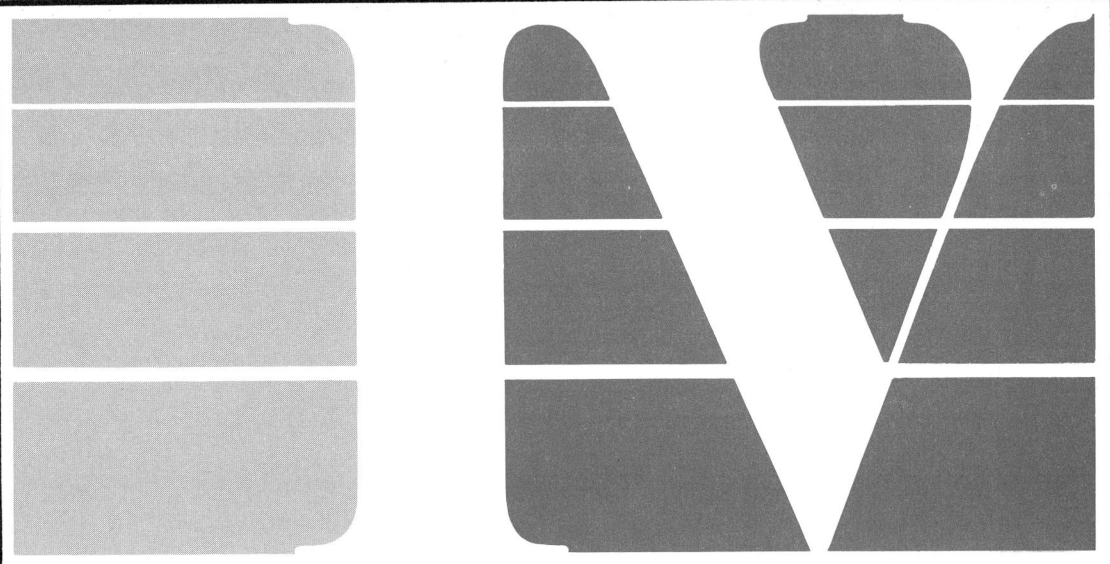

SCHIZOPHRENIA AND PARANOID PSYCHOSES

In this section we begin to examine psychological disorders in which individuals lose contact with reality, and so are unable to function effectively. Individuals who lose contact with reality and have severe problems such as hallucinations and delusions are often called psychotic. The unusual subjective experiences of such individuals, and their strange behavior, often require that they be temporarily or permanently hospitalized for their own protection, for the protection of others, and in order to receive treatment. Fully one-half of all individuals in public and private mental hospitals are given one of the diagnoses discussed in this section.

Schizophrenia is one of the major social and psychological problems of modern society. Its toll in human suffering is extreme. Chapter 12 presents the clinical features of the subtypes of this disorder. "Schizophrenia" literally means "split mind," and people often think the term refers to people with split or multiple personalities. Actually, the term refers to a split between thoughts and emotion in one personality, rather than to multiple personalities like those discussed in Chapter 8. Chapter 13 presents the major theories of schizophrenia, the research relevant to the etiology of the disorder, and various treatment approaches that are being applied to the disorder. Chapter 14 covers the severe paranoid disorders. The paranoid disorders are grouped with the schizophrenic disorders because a disturbance in cognition occurs in both these types of disorder. Yet the paranoid disorders differ substantially from schizophrenia, and thus require separate consideration.

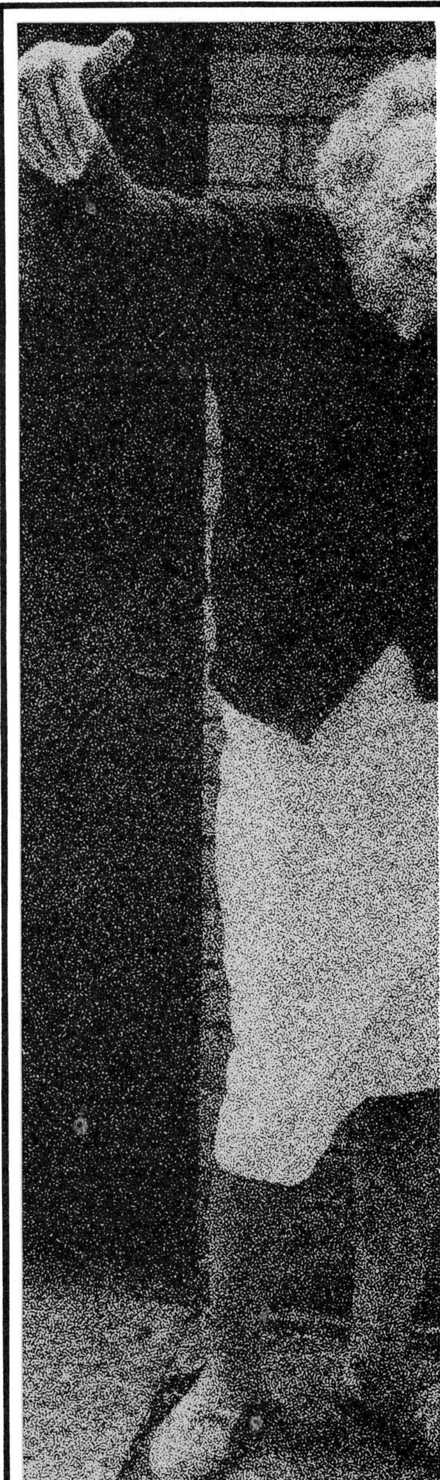

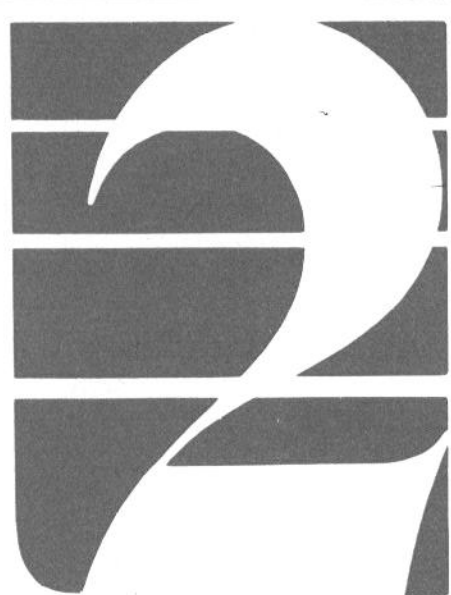

Schizophrenic disorders I: phenomenology

Of behaviors that we label abnormal, the behaviors characteristic of **schizophrenia** most closely approximate what most of us think of as "craziness." Schizophrenic behavior ranges, however, from mild to intense. Its most severe form involves a major personality disorganization and estrangement from what most of us consider "reality." Personality disorganization or decompensation means that the person who exhibits schizophrenic behavior shows a deterioration from a previous level of functioning. He or she can no longer perform life tasks as well as before the onset of the disorder. Work suffers, social relationships become stormy, all the individual's social roles become difficult and disorganized.

The disorganization and deterioration of behavior is particularly problematic for such persons' relatives—spouse, children, and parents—but also often impacts on others—friends and acquaintances, employers and supervisors, teachers, strangers, and frequently the police. Most of us may never have close contact with an individual who has a **schizophrenic disorder,** unless we go into one of the helping professions. However, since schizophrenic behavior appears in about 1 in 100 persons, there are estimated to be approximately 2–3 million such individuals in the United States (Dohrenwend & Dohrenwend, 1974).

The specific behaviors seen in the schizophrenic disorders are quite varied. You may be aware that people with such disorders engage in odd reasoning, and often steadfastly maintain strange beliefs. Sometimes they see or hear things that are not there. You may have some idea that their emotions seem difficult for them to control, or that they seem to have no emotions at all. Perhaps you have seen some people who have behaved very strangely, engaging in bizarre acts such as odd grimaces, repetitive movements, or who have been very oddly dressed, perhaps wearing several layers of winter coats in the summertime. Do such behaviors signify that the individual is manifesting a schizophrenic disorder? Not necessarily. There may be other explanations for such behaviors. However, all these behaviors are often seen in the schizophrenic disorders, along with other characteristics.

CHARACTERISTIC DISORDERS IN SCHIZOPHRENIC BEHAVIOR

Disorders of Thought and Communication

People who exhibit schizophrenic behavior usually have disorders in the form and content of their thinking, which are manifested in their language and communication with others.

Form of Thought. The schizophrenic seems to have trouble maintaining a coherent train of thought. Eugen Bleuler (1950) called this **derailment,** and Paul Meehl (1962) used the term "cognitive slippage" to describe the process. The term most commonly used is **looseness of association.** In this process, ideas shift from one subject to another which may be only slightly related, or which appear totally unrelated. Frames of reference may change and, in extreme cases, totally unrelated ideas may be jumbled together. It appears that the associations to thoughts which most of us can suppress burst through and distract the individual from the goal of the train of thought. One subject stated (B. Freedman & Chapman, 1973): "My mind was so confused I couldn't focus on one thing. I had an idea and I was wondering whether I should press charges and then all of a sudden my mind went to something pleasant, and then it went back to my work, and I couldn't keep it orderly" (p. 50).

R. W. White (1964) gives the following example, which illustrates the bizarre quality in speech that may result from derailment:

Interviewer (I). How old are you?
Patient (P). Why, I am centuries old, sir.
I. How long have you been here?
P. I have been now on this property on and off for a long time. I cannot say the exact time because we are absorbed by the air at night, and they bring back people. They kill up everything; they can make you lie; they can talk through your throat.
I. Who is this?
P. Why, the air.
I. What is the name of this place?
P. This place is called a star.
I. Who is the doctor in charge of your ward?

P. A body just like yours, sir. They can make you black and white. I say good morning, but he just comes through there. At first it was a colony. They said it was heaven. These buildings were not solid at the time, and I am positive this is the same place. . . . (p. 514)

In addition to the loose manner in which thoughts or concepts are associated, schizophrenic thinking may also be characterized by extreme concreteness and literalness. The concreteness of some schizophrenics and their difficulty in avoiding runaway associations in their thinking have led to their thought processes being described as "autistic." **Autism** means that they live primarily within themselves; that their thinking is dominated by their wishes, fears, fantasies, and inner life to a greater extent than the norm. Table 12.1 illustrates concrete and autistic responses to several proverbs.

A final problem in the schizophrenic thought process is the apparent lack of normal logic in reasoning. Schizophrenic behavior is often characterized by logic such as "The Virgin Mary was a virgin; I'm a virgin; therefore, I'm the Virgin Mary." This type of reasoning process leads to disorders in the content of thinking.

Content of Thought. Schizophrenics usually think that their problems are outside themselves. They have poor insight. Most schizophrenics have little or no awareness that their difficulties are of their own making. They deny that their problems are internal, but see them

Table 12.1

Types of responses to proverbs given by persons manifesting schizophrenic behavior

INSTRUCTIONS TO PATIENT: "I'm going to give you some sayings or proverbs and I want you to interpret them for me; that is, to explain them to me as if I were a child, and put the meaning in the most general way possible that applies to people or a lesson."

Proverb	Literal	Concrete	Abstract	Bizarre (austistic)
1. People who live in glass houses should not throw stones.	"People shouldn't throw rocks—they might get hurt, hurt people with the rocks, or break the glass."	"You're not always going to be the one looking out, other people will be looking at you occasionally."	"People who are easily hurt should not try to hurt others."	"You shouldn't do something like work for the FBI which will disrupt your life."
2. All that glitters isn't gold.	"It might be brass."	"Glitter doesn't mean it's worthwhile—it could be cheap."	"Everything may not be as it appears to be."	"There is so much to life and wonder and things beyond you can't put it into one ball and call it gold or precious."
3. A stitch in time saves nine.	"If you take one stitch for a small tear now, it will save nine later."	"If you do one thing right, you don't have to do the other eight."	"If prevention is exercised, a larger problem may be obviated."	"A collect phone call saves a dime."
4. Even monkeys fall from trees.	"They can miss a step when they're climbing trees."	"If you don't keep your feet flat on the ground, something can happen."	"Even people with expertise and talent make mistakes."	"We fall from grace as we believe not in Christ who was on the tree of the cross-ash."

Adapted from Kreuger (1978, pp. 196–197).

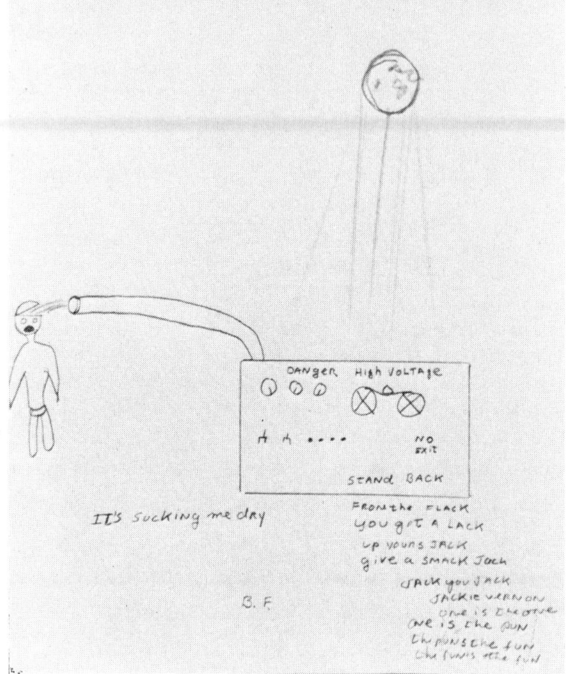
DANGER High VOLTAGE
NO EXIT
STAND BACK
IT'S sucking me dry
FROM the FLACK
you got A LACK
up yours JACK
give a SMACK Jack
JACK you JACK
JACKIE VERNON
B. F
The drawing and comment illustrate thought withdrawal and the incoherence of loose associations.

as imposed by outside agencies or other people. An individual interviewed by the author, when asked if she knew where she was (a midwestern state hospital) replied, "The jail for human meat." She explained angrily that she was locked up by the "Goldsteins" (her neighbors) who were after her money and that she could not be mentally ill because it is against her religion. She attributed a previous suicide attempt (in which she attempted to hack off her hand with a hatchet) to the effects of "electricity" used by the Goldsteins and her daughter. She was totally unable to accept that any of her problems were due to her own behavior, not the behavior of others.

A second type of problem in the content of thought is the maintenance of false beliefs, or **delusions.** In the example just given, the woman's neighbors were not after her money, and they had nothing to do with her being hospitalized—in spite of her convictions otherwise. To be a delusion, a false belief must be one that the person's culture does not accept; and it must be maintained in spite of evidence to the contrary. For example, some people might consider a belief in God to be false, but this belief is so widely held that it is not considered a delusion. However, if a person believes he or she *is* God, and this belief is not shared by others, we would consider the belief to be delusional. Delusional beliefs are "fixed," so that the individual maintains them even when others "prove" they are not true.

Delusions often begin as vague, unformed ideas that something is "not quite right," and may be preceded by ideas of reference. An **idea of reference** is a belief or feeling that events in the environment have a special reference to the individual. For example, a man at a party sees several people across the room having a conversation; without any evidence, he concludes that they are talking about him. As the ideas become more firmly entrenched, they attain delusional proportions. The delusions reported by schizophrenics have usually been described as "unsystematized and chaotic" compared to the "logical," complex, and systematic delusions described by the paranoid psychotic. In **paranoid psychosis,** the individual's delusions usually make sense if the basic premise is accepted (see Chapter 14). For example, a pure paranoid might have an elaborate belief, complete with a rationale, that the police are spying on her. She may know the names of the police, how they spy, when and where, and for what reason. In contrast, the schizophrenic—even with paranoid features—is more likely to report a strange belief with little clear rationale; for example, "somebody" is draining his brains with a cosmic vacuum cleaner.

Delusions of varying types have been identified as important aspects of problems in the content of thought. Highlight 12.1 presents some categories of delusional beliefs. In the section on the diagnosis of the schizophrenic disorders, the delusions considered primary in schizophrenia will be identified.

Many other types of delusional content, besides those described in Highlight 12.1, occur in persons who manifest schizophrenic behavior. These delusions are less common; they include **somatic delusions** (false beliefs about the body, such as the belief that one's brain is rotting) or **nihilistic delusions** (the belief that one is dead or has ceased to exist, or that one's en-

HIGHLIGHT 12.1
CATEGORIES OF DELUSIONAL BELIEFS

1. Persecutory delusions. These false beliefs involve the notion that some person or agency is plotting against the subject, manipulating events, spreading lies, trying to kill the individual, and so on.
2. Delusions of reference. Common events are given special symbolic meaning in regard to the subject. For example, one subject who saw flags being flown at half-mast on a state holiday at a mental hospital (coinciding with his twentieth birthday) concluded that this was a signal that his life was half over and he would die when he reached 40.
3. Grandiose delusions. The belief that one is a very special person, for example, God, or a new Messiah, or that one has done or knows something particularly significant such as how to cure cancer. Such a delusion may be combined with persecutory ideation, as in the patient who knew the "secret to world peace," but was being kept locked up by "warmonger capitalists, pinkos, and Fidel Castro."
4. Delusions of influence and control. These delusions are considered very common and characteristic of schizophrenia. They are among the symptoms emphasized by the German psychiatrist Kurt Schneider (1959), who called them first-rank symptoms, and contrasted them with second-rank symptoms, which are less unique to schizophrenia and are often seen in other diagnostic groups.

A. Thought broadcasting. The belief or experience that one's thoughts are broadcast into the external world where others can hear them as they occur. One subject experienced this visually as a shimmering in the air as her thoughts left her head.

B. Thought insertion. The belief that thoughts are being inserted into one's mind by an external agency. The thoughts are often "bad." One subject asked his therapist to call the subject's uncle to ask that the uncle stop putting thoughts about homosexual behavior in the subject's head.

C. Thought withdrawal. The experience that thoughts are being taken away or stolen. A patient reported that her thoughts were disappearing like "popping soap bubbles," and that this was being done by "invisible acupuncture."

D. External control. The belief or experience that feelings, impulses, actions, or thoughts are not under one's control, but are imposed by an external source. In one or more of these areas, the patient experiences no self-volitions, and feels unable to prevent the occurrence or to take responsibility for it. In an extreme example, a woman reported that the devil filled her with hate and made her kill her children, while she was helpless to stop herself.

vironment and the people in it no longer exist). Also less frequent, though by no means rare, are **delusions of jealousy** (an unwarranted, extreme belief that one's spouse or lover is having an affair), and religious delusions.

Disorders of Perception and Sensation

One of the more dramatic disorders seen in schizophrenic behavior are changes in perceptions. These changes include distortions of real stimuli **(illusions),** and perceptions in the absence of external stimuli **(hallucinations).** Such distortions may occur in all sensory areas. B. Freedman and Chapman (1973) provide two examples of mild sensory distortions reported by people diagnosed as schizophrenic; the first is a visual disturbance, the second an auditory one:

> Maybe I'm not very sensitive to sight. . . . I have been [sort] of a little blurry. . . . I keep thinking maybe I'm tired. . . . the other night in front of the television, I felt a sort of blurring like that. (p. 51)

> I have trouble understanding things people say anyway, particularly like records. It's like things come in loud and clear but the words don't come in straight. . . . like songs. . . . it comes in loud enough in my ears, but I can't understand the words. . . . I have the same trouble if people don't speak very distinctly to me, and really look at me and really get my attention, I've really had it. . . . (p. 52)

Other perceptual experiences may include distortions such as changes in odors or the taste of food (e.g., food does not taste or smell "right"). Some experience distortions of touch (feeling numbness or tingling sensations).

More intense distortions of perceptions, called *illusions,* may occur. In an illusion, the individual misinterprets real stimuli. Many of us have had this experience. For example, we may walk into a darkened room and "see" a menacing figure moving in the corner. The percept may seem quite real for a moment, until we recognize that the figure is a curtain blowing in a breeże from an open window.

Hallucinations consist of perceptions in the absence of any external stimuli. They have often been compared to "dreaming while awake," since they seem to be exaggerations or altered forms of the normal dream process. The unusual nature of hallucinations has led to a major interest in the study of hallucinatory mechanisms (see R. K. Siegel & West, 1975). Hallucinations may occur in any of the sensory realms, although auditory hallucinations seem to be the most frequent, and visual hallucinations the second most common. Auditory hallucinations usually consist of hearing voices, which speak to or comment about the person. Often the voice or voices are recognizable as a relative or neighbor; or they may be interpreted as being the voice of God or the devil. Sometimes the voices are unrecognizable or cannot even be understood: They are an indistinguishable mumble. Voices may say something uncomplimentary about the person ("You're a bastard"), tell the person to do something ("Don't leave your room"), or say something that the person may come to believe ("You're the Virgin Mary"). The voices may discuss very private aspects of the person's life, such as sexual or hygiene habits. Other auditory hallucinations are simple sounds: roaring, banging, or rumblings.

Visual hallucinations may be frightening or pleasant. An individual may see a vision of a religious figure or a demon. The following case is from the author's files:

> A young woman in her 20s was continually confronted by the visual perception that snakes and worms were emerging from the walls, attempting to bite or grasp her as she walked down halls. As she walked, then ran wildly, the "slimy creatures" would withdraw behind her, but new ones would emerge in front of her. As she moved, the floor before her would crack and chasms would open. Her ears were assailed by moans and shrieks issuing from the chasms, along with a foul odor that she described as a "combination of warm shit and rotten garbage."

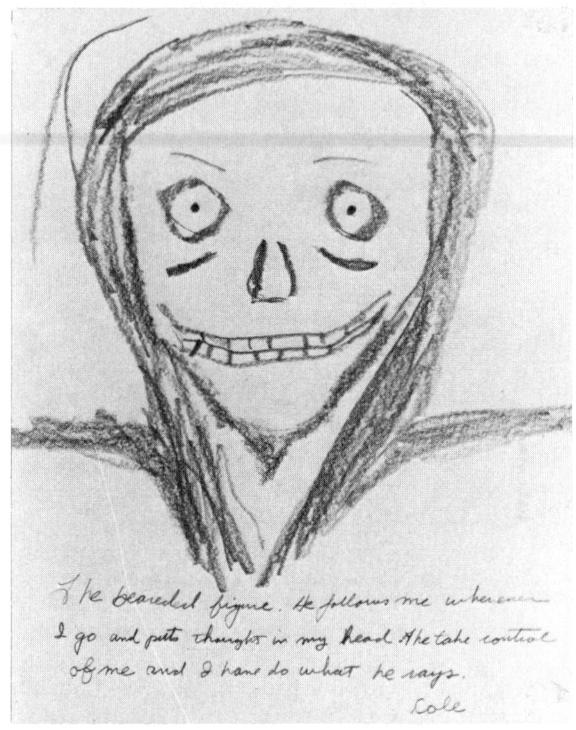
The bearded figure. He follows me
I go and puts thoughts in my head. He take
of me and I have do what he says.
Cole
The drawing and comment by a person with a schizophrenic disorder illustrates the experience of thought insertion and delusions of being controlled by an outside force.

In this case, as in many others, visual hallucinations were accompanied by hallucinations in other sensory areas. When hallucinating, people may become frightened or angry and respond behaviorally. They may talk back, argue, stare as if seeing something, run in fear, or physically attack a nonexistent threat. Many studies (e.g., Larkin, 1979) have indicated that the more vivid and complex hallucinations are usually seen in acute schizophrenic disorders (where the onset of symptoms has been sudden) rather than in persons who have had many episodes of such behavior or who have manifested the disorder for a long period (i.e., chronic disorders). Hallucinations may cause problems when their content (especially in auditory hallucinations) directs the person to engage in unacceptable behavior (such as violence).

Do hallucinations have to be present for an individual to be diagnosed as a schizophrenic? No, other criteria may be sufficient. Nor does the presence of hallucinations mean that a person has a schizophrenic disorder. Hallucinations may be due to known brain injury or to brain deterioration or other organic factors (see Highlight 12.2). A. G. Goldstein (1976), an experimental psychologist, has recounted his personal experience of hallucinations while hospitalized for a back injury. His hallucinations were visual and auditory, and he experienced odd physical sensations. As his experiences progressed, he was able to realize that they were not real, yet the perceptions were as vivid and "solid" as if the events were actually happening. He has attributed his experience to a combination of lack of sleep due to intense pain, the use of sedative and pain-killing drugs, and the stress of anxiety over his injury.

Disorders of Affect or Emotion

Disorders of **affect** were identified in people with schizophrenic disorders by both Emil Kraepelin and Eugen Bleuler around the turn of the nineteenth century, and less formally even before then. Many contemporary observers have noted that schizophrenic individuals seem to have a defect in their capacity to experience pleasure. This pervasive lack of enjoyment of most or all aspects of life has been called **anhedonia.** Some investigators consider anhedonia to be one of the primary deficits in schizophrenia (e.g., Meehl, 1962). Harrow et al. (1977) have found that anhedonia is most characteristic of people with long-term schizophrenic behavior, rather than acute first-episode disorders. Although it may also appear in nonschizophrenic disorders, they confirm that anhedonia is a significant issue in schizophrenic behavior.

In addition to anhedonia, or lack of pleasure, individuals with a schizophrenic disorder appear to have quantitative differences in affect. They often have "shallow" or **blunted affect.** This term refers to a reduced emotional responsiveness. Such individuals may be described as "stony" or "cold." When this affective disorder becomes severe, these persons are often said to have "flat affect"; they appear to be apathetic or indifferent, and show virtually no emotional response. Individuals with shallow or blunted affect seem very similar to an animated store-window mannequin or robot.

At the other extreme, many schizophrenics manifest **inappropriate affect.** These individuals may laugh, grin, or giggle when discussing events that normally arouse emotions of sorrow or sadness, such as the death of a loved one; or they may break into tears when talking about neutral events. Rage and anger may also be inappropriately expressed. These responses which may be quite disconcerting to an observer may also be **labile;** that is, they may change rapidly. The individual may giggle one moment, cry the next, and then suddenly fly into a rage. The unpredictability of such behavior makes social interactions very difficult.

A fourth disturbance of affect seen in many schizophrenics is an exaggerated "ambivalence." Ambivalence is a term used to describe a state in which two conflicting emotions are experienced towards an object, event, or person at about the same time. While most of us may feel slight ambivalence, such as liking and disliking a particular person, or the different behaviors of that person, ambivalent feelings in schizophrenics are pronounced. They may have strong feelings of love and hate towards a parent, for example. These conficting emotions may lead to inconsistencies in behavior. The schizophrenic may be strongly attracted to mother and behave very dependently, like a young child, and in the next moment, may verbally or physically attack or withdraw from mother.

The degree of affective disorder, particularly anhedonia and blunted or flat affect, has been considered by some to be a significant indicator of the severity of the schizophrenic disorder. The greater the degree of anhedonia and affective blunting, the more severe the disorder is often considered. The more the individual retains reasonable emotional responsiveness, the

HIGHLIGHT 12.2
VISUAL HALLUCINATIONS

Many investigators have studied the hallucinatory experience by studying the effects of the hallucinogenic drugs, such as LSD and THC. Most workers report that the majority of visual hallucinations in these drug-induced states consist of perceptual distortions or visions of geometric forms. The visual hallucinations of persons manifesting schizophrenia are usually more personalized. The perceptions involve people, voices, or experiences that are threatening, frightening, or have special meaning for the person. The illustration of objects and geometric shapes is an artist's interpretation (adapted from R. K. Siegel & Jarvik, 1975) of a subject's visual experience while taking the drug THC. The subject gave the following report: "And then my eyes again, a hexagon, a little hexagon—whoa—here comes a big hexagon! He is pushing those little hexagons aside because he doesn't fit. My God! He split up the whole, all the little hexagons are going out to the right, all out the funnel, they all disappeared, nothing left but a plastic sink." (R. K. Siegel & Jarvik, 1975, p. 118).

The illustration of a person (adapted from Wadeson & Carpenter, 1976, p. 322) is a schizophrenic man's drawing of a hallucination he saw while in the hospital. He described his vision of God surrounded by light in a seclusion room dormitory as follows: "I saw a vision of God in the hallway [seen through the window of the seclusion room door]. He was transparent, and there was light all around Him. He told me I should pray. I thought it was real. It lasted about half an hour." (Wadeson & Carpenter, 1976, p. 320). In another instance, Mao Tse Tung appeared and instructed the patient how to bring peace to the world. The patient was reassured by this comforting message and enjoyed his special status in this regard. He said Mao Tse Tung's face appeared on the wall: "He told me in Chinese to keep peace in the world. It was a surprising psychic communication. . . . I felt important" (Wadeson & Carpenter, 1976, p. 320).

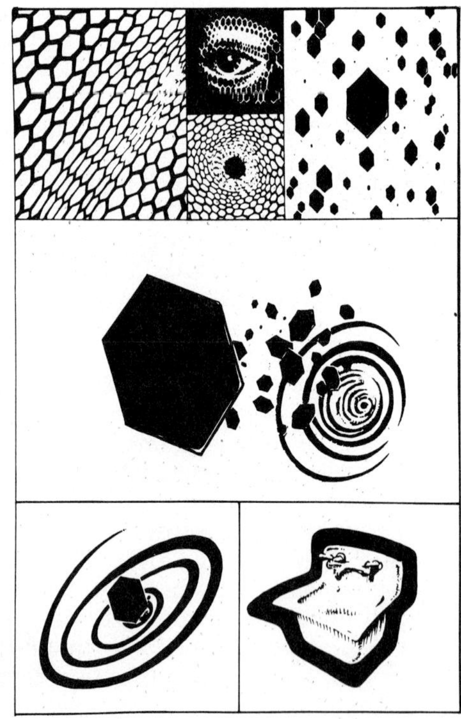

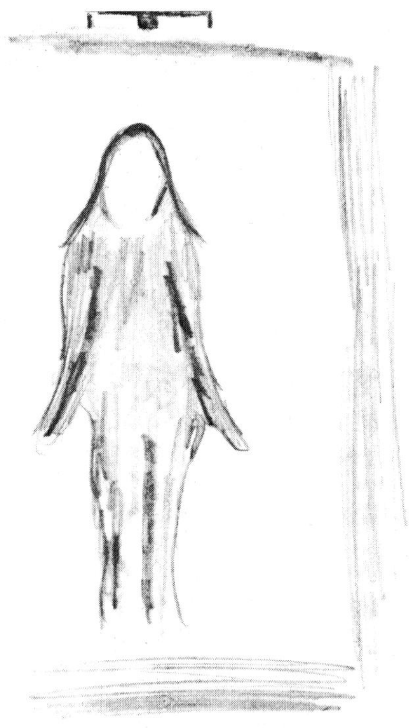

less severe the disorder and the greater the likelihood of a successful treatment (M. McCabe et al., 1972).

Disorders of Motor Behavior

The disorders described so far require fairly close contact for observation. One must be able to interact with the subject and engage in communication to determine the presence, absence, and severity of many of these behaviors. Disturbances in motor behavior, however, are obvious physical manifestations that can be observed visually. Most disorders of motor behavior are not dramatic. Individuals may appear somewhat agitated or excited. They may pace, grimace, or fidget; and those in **catatonic excitement** may become extremely agitated and manifest strange mannerisms. At the other (and more common) extreme, physical movement may be slowed (motor retardation) and, in rare instances, a person may become immobile. In **catatonic immobility,** the person may adopt an unusual posture or position and hold it for long periods without moving. In this condition, an individual may be moved into a different position—much as one would mold a wax figure—and will hold the new position for long periods.

The catatonic patient may assume an unusual posture and then hold it for hours.

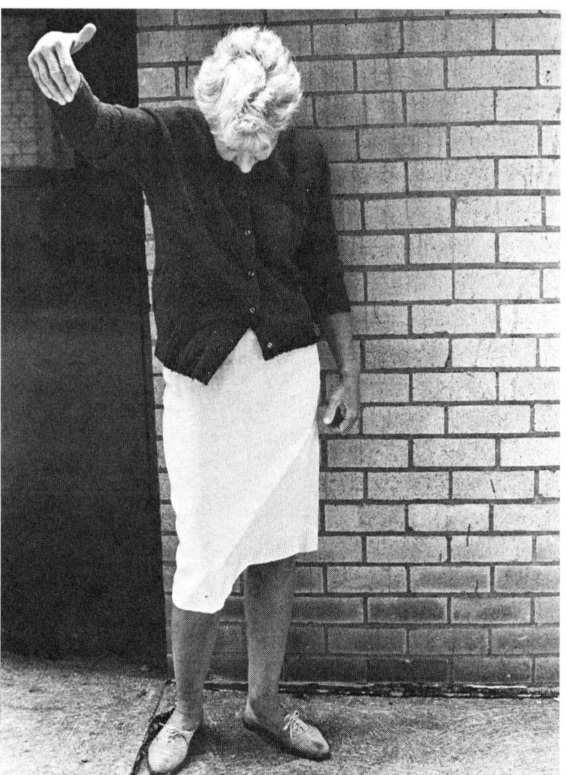

One unusual pattern of behavior is **echopraxia,** in which the individual "echoes" the behavior of another. If someone scratches, so does the patient. When manifested verbally, this mimicking is called **echolalia,** (the person may parrot another's speech). A more common behavioral manifestation in long-term schizophrenic disorders is **stereotypic behavior,** in which the individual engages in an unusual repetitive behavior. These stereotypic behaviors often seem to have symbolic significance for the individual. For example, a patient walking across a hospital's grounds would stride a dozen paces, stop, take two steps back, one forward, turn to face the sun, make complicated hand gestures, continue for another dozen paces, and repeat the sequence over and over. Upon inquiry, he confided that if he did not behave this way, some catastrophe would occur to the world. The nature of this catastrophe had not yet been "revealed" to him.

Disorders of Socialization

The manifestations of schizophrenic behavior described so far certainly contribute to the withdrawal from social contact that usually characterizes the disorder. The oddities of schizophrenic thinking, speech, emotion, and behavior usually make others uncomfortable in interactions with someone manifesting these behaviors. The individual may have a continually decreasing social network, but is unlikely to reach out for human contact to reverse the process. Many such individuals begin to pull away from or avoid social contacts long before their disorder becomes obvious. This decreasing contact allows even more autistic thinking, that is, more unusual personalized thinking unique to the individual. Consider the following individual:

> P. had "always" been a "loner," according to his parents. He had few friends in school and only dated occasionally, but was not particularly unusual. He was "simply shy." After

> graduation from high school, he held a few short-term jobs while supposedly deciding whether to go on to college. During this period he became more and more quiet, spending long hours each day in his room listening to music. Yet his behavior was not bizarre, and he could still communicate well with his parents when they forced the issue. After being out of work for several months, he abruptly announced to his mother that he was going to his room. He did not leave his room again for approximately eight months. His mother brought food for him and left it at his door. After her departure, he would open the door, take the food, and leave the dirty dishes from the previous meal in return. His parents presumed he toileted in the nighttime, for they never saw him. Their main concern was that he played his stereo at full volume continuously. It was later found that during the three-quarters of a year in self-imposed isolation in his room, his thinking had become more and more schizophrenic. He developed a delusion that the verses of his favorite hard rock group's songs were guiding his life and future behavior. He finally realized that the words of one song were ordering him to kill his mother. One night he left his room and attacked his sleeping mother with a kitchen knife, wounding her. He was subsequently hospitalized with a diagnosis of schizophrenia and found not guilty of the assault by reason of insanity.

While the great majority of people with a schizophrenic disorder do not act out this violently, the progressive social withdrawal illustrated is common.

The most common behavioral manifestation of a disorder in socialization is the occurrence of a wide range of socially inappropriate behaviors or the absence of socially conventional behaviors. Self-care and hygiene behaviors are often neglected. Such individuals do not dress appropriately, care for their hair, bathe regularly, or respond with common polite conventions. They may have crude manners, not respond to greetings, not feed themselves, or not bother to use table utensils. They may masturbate in public, or "lose" control of bowel and bladder functions. The erosion of the social amenities and the presence of such inappropriate behavior have been attributed to the negative effects of hospitalization by some psychiatrists and psychologists (such as Szasz and Sarbin), but these behaviors are also seen in people with a schizophrenic disorder who have never been hospitalized.

ARE SOME CHARACTERISTICS OF SCHIZOPHRENIC BEHAVIOR MORE IMPORTANT THAN OTHERS?

Are the behaviors often seen in individuals with a schizophrenic disorder seen *only* in schizophrenia? Many formal studies and clinical observations indicate that some, if not most, of the behaviors described are also seen in some other psychotic and nonpsychotic disorders. As we discovered in Chapter 4, it is important to be able to identify the behaviors that are primary signs of a particular disorder, so that we can validly and reliably distinguish the disorder from other types. Since the time of Emil Kraepelin clinicians and researchers have attempted to do this with what we call schizophrenia.

By 1898, Kraepelin had distinguished schizophrenia, which he called "dementia praecox," from manic-depressive psychosis and several other disorders. His term sums up the primary characteristics which he felt separated this disorder from others: "Dementia" meant an irreversible, progressive deterioration of thought processes and behavior; the term "praecox" meant that the dementia had an early onset. Kraepelin also identified many of the behaviors discussed above—hallucinations, delusions, stereotypic behavior, disordered affect—but he did not feel that these were critical to the diagnosis of the disorder. A problem with his definition, which Kraepelin recognized, was that about 13 percent of the persons diagnosed by his criteria recovered without any deterioration or lasting major defect. This finding conflicted with his concept of the disorder as irreversible and progressive.

By 1908, Eugen Bleuler suggested a new way of defining this disorder (M. Bleuler, 1979), and coined the term we still use, "schizophrenia." Bleuler rejected the idea that the disorder was irreversible (probably because of his observations of the 13 percent who recovered). Rather than focusing on outcome, he focused on a split ("schizo") of thinking ("phrenia") from other functions of the personality in this disorder. We should note that the term does not mean "split personality," as is commonly assumed. Bleuler identified behaviors which he considered to be primary signs of the disorder vs. those he considered to be a result of these primary defects.

The signs which Bleuler considered to be primary in schizophrenia, and not in other disorders, can be remembered easily as the four As: 1. affect (flat, blunted, or inappropriate); 2. associations (loose, derailed, or fragmented); 3. ambivalence (usually to an extreme degree); 4. autism (unusual self-centered thinking).

Bleuler saw other schizophrenic manifestations—such as hallucinations, delusions, withdrawal, and strange behavior—as being due to the disturbances in the four As. The secondary signs could also be present in other disorders, for other reasons, and thus were not considered to be primary signs of schizophrenia. Their presence in an individual was supportive of a diagnosis of schizophrenia; but even if the secondary signs were absent, schizophrenia could be diagnosed if disturbances of affect and associations were present with ambivalence and autism. Bleuler's conception of primary and secondary signs became commonly accepted and formed the basis for the diagnosis of schizophrenia by psychiatrists, psychologists, and other mental health workers. More recently, other criteria have been identified as primary signs of schizophrenia in a number of important cross-cultural studies.

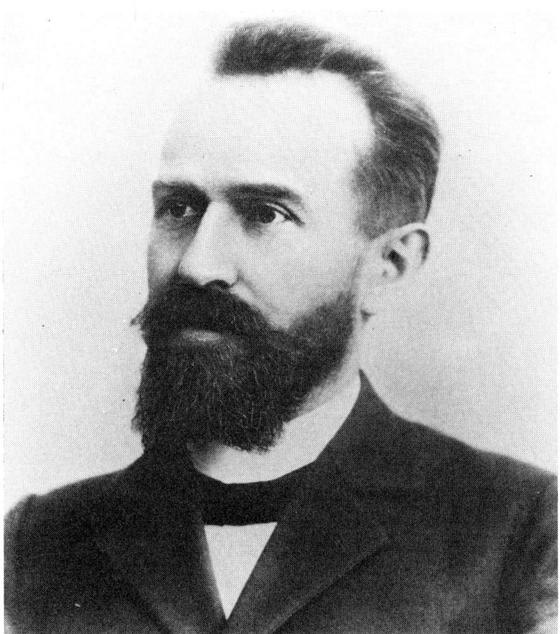

Eugen Bleuler, inventor of the term "schizophrenia."

Cross-cultural Differences in the Diagnosis of Schizophrenia

From Bleuler's time into the 1970s, there has been some disagreement on the significance of various symptoms in the diagnosis of schizophrenia. Highlight 12.3 contrasts the North American definition of schizophrenia, which was common in the past, with the British/European definition. These differing definitions appear to have had significant impact on the identification and study of schizophrenia. The British/European definition was based on the identification of specific critical signs. In the United States, the definition was broader, and resulted over the years in a consistent increase in the number of people included in the category. For example, in the 1930s, about 20 percent of the patients at the New York State Psychiatric Institute were diagnosed as schizophrenic. In the 1950s, this percentage leveled off at about 80 percent. During the same period, the percentage of patients diagnosed as schizophrenic at Maudsley Hospital in London fluctuated very little (Kuriansky, Deming, & Gurland, 1974). This discrepancy was studied by J. E. Cooper and colleagues (1972), who studied the diagnoses given to consecutive admissions to psychiatric hospitals in New York and London. Their own team of psychiatrists interviewed the admissions and compared the diagnoses they assigned with the diagnoses given by the hospitals' psychiatrists. The project staff, which consisted of both American and British psychiatrists who had been trained together, made diagnoses that were more in accord with the British hospital psychiatrists. A large proportion of the cases identified by the New York hospital staff as having schizophrenia (42 percent) were diagnosed by the project staff as manifesting an affective illness. The considerable differences of opinion between

HIGHLIGHT 12.3
NORTH AMERICAN VS. BRITISH/EUROPEAN DEFINITION OF SCHIZOPHRENIA

The DSM-II (1968) definition of schizophrenia presents the American viewpoint:

> This large category includes a group of disorders manifested by characteristic disturbances of thinking, mood, and behavior. Disturbances in thinking are marked by alterations of concept formation which may lead to misinterpretation of reality and sometimes to delusions and hallucinations, which frequently appear psychologically self-protective. Corollary mood changes include ambivalent, constricted and inappropriate emotional responsiveness and loss of empathy with others. Behavior may be withdrawn, regressive, and bizarre. (p. 33)

The *British Glossary* (1968) provides the British/European definition of the disorder.

> [An illness] characterized from the outset by a fundamental disturbance of the personality involving its most basic functions, [which] give the normal person his feeling of individuality, uniqueness, and self-direction. . . . [The patient has] explanatory delusions that [his] thoughts etc. are influenced by outside forces which may be natural or supernatural. . . . Hallucinations are common, predominately auditory, in the form of "voices" which may comment on the patient's thoughts and actions, and somatic or tactile. [There are] unpleasant sensations which the patient may be unable to describe in ordinary language and which again usually [have] delusional interpretation. An important symptom of schizophrenia, not however evident in all cases, is a curious disturbance of thinking. . . . Peripheral, marginal, and irrelevant features of a total concept, [normally] inhibited . . . are brought to the forefront and utilized in place of the elements relevant and appropriate to a given situation. Thus thinking becomes vague, elliptical, and obscure and its expression in speech [is] often incomprehensible. Sudden breaks in the flow of thought ("blocking") are frequent, and there is difficulty in retaining thoughts, which is often interpreted delusionally as "thought withdrawal" by outside agencies. Hearing one's thoughts spoken aloud is common and is believed to be diagnostically significant. . . . The patient [may] believe that every-day objects and situations, e.g. statements in the press, possess a special, usually sinister, meaning especially intended for him. The affective state becomes capricious and often inappropriate to a given situation. (pp. 97, 98)

the New York and London hospital psychiatrists on the use of diagnostic criteria of schizophrenia led to the question of which approach might be better. A clear point in favor of the British/European system is that this approach seems to generate a more reliable diagnosis. Wing et al. (1967) found reliabilities of 92 percent for the British approach, while A. T. Beck et al. (1962) found reliabilities of 53 percent for the American approach.

J. E. Cooper et al.'s work suggests that the populations diagnosed as schizophrenic around the world differ to a significant degree because of the broadness or narrowness of the diagnostic criteria. Many researchers' and clinicians' concern over this cross-cultural variability in diagnosis stimulated a major study by the World Health Organization; this study was called the International Pilot Study of Schizophrenia (Sartorius, Shapiro, & Jablensky, 1974).

The International Pilot Study of Schizophrenia began in 1966 in selected centers in nine countries. These countries differed widely in sociocultural and economic characteristics: Colombia, Czechoslovakia, Denmark, India, Nigeria, China, the Soviet Union, Britain, and the United States. Psychiatrists from these centers were jointly trained to reliably use the same assessment instruments. Among the questions the study tried to answer were whether there were identifiable schizophrenics in each country, and whether certain behaviors were characteristic of schizophrenia, regardless of the cultural environment in which the schizophrenic lived. During the course of the study, 1202 patients were examined throughout the nine centers, and 811 were diagnosed as schizophrenic. Of these 811, about half had clear-cut diagnoses. These patients with a definite diagnosis of schizophrenia shared the characteristics indicated in Table 12.2. Carpenter, Strauss, and Bartko (1974) used a computer analysis with the study's data to generate 12 symptoms which could be used to differentiate between schizophrenia and other disorders. These symptoms are listed in Table 12.3.

Studies such as those described above demonstrate that when exact criteria are used as the signs of the presence of schizophrenia, the disorder can be diagnosed with some accuracy. In addition, they demonstrate that schizophrenia, when identified in this manner, occurs with approximately equal frequency in various parts of the world and shows many of the same manifestations. The data generated in these studies were a significant factor in the development of diagnostic criteria for schizophrenia in the latest revision of the *Diagnostic and Statistical Manual* of the American Psychiatric Association (DSM-III, 1980; see Highlight 12.4).

SUBTYPES OF SCHIZOPHRENIA

So far, the major focus of this chapter has been on the general disorder of schizophrenia. Beginning with Kraepelin, however, the disorder

Table 12.2
Percent of individuals with specific characteristics when a diagnosis of schizophrenia is certain

Characteristic	*Percent*
Lack of insight	97
Auditory hallucinations (minimum of sounds)	74
Verbal hallucinations (minimum of words)	70
Ideas of reference	70
Delusions of reference	67
Suspiciousness	66
Flatness of affect	66
Voices speaking to the patient	65
Delusional mood	64
Delusions of persecution	64
Inadequate description	64
Thought alienation	52
Thought spoken out loud	50
Delusions of control	48
Hearing voices speak full sentences	44
Poor rapport	43

Based on Carpenter, et al. (1974, p. 47).

Table 12.3
Differential symptoms of schizophrenia

Restricted affect	Elation (−)[1]
Poor insight	Widespread delusions
Thought broadcasting	Incoherent speech
Waking early (−)[1]	Unreliable information
Poor rapport	Bizarre delusions
Depressed appearance (−)[1]	Nihilistic delusions

Based on Carpenter, et al. (1974, p. 47).
[1]A minus sign (−) indicates that an absence of this symptom is necessary for diagnosis to be made.

of schizophrenia has been split into subtypes. The differentiation of these subtypes has usually been based on behavioral characteristics considered to be more prominent in one subtype or another. Kraepelin identified three types: the hebephrenic, the catatonic, and the paranoid. Eugen Bleuler added the simple type. In DSM-III (1980), the simple type has been redefined as a personality disorder (the schizotypal personality disorder) and the behaviors identified as hebephrenic are now called the disorganized type. These changes from DSM-II (1968) are in addition to the increase in specificity of diagnostic signs and the general narrowing of the definition of schizophrenia. Although some have considered the subtypes as individually discrete disorders with differing etiologies, many workers consider the subtypes simply as descriptive clusters of behavior (Carpenter, Strauss, & Mulch, 1973; J. S. Strauss & Docherty, 1979). After the subtypes currently listed in DSM-III have been described, several other important dimensions of the schizophrenic disorders will be presented.

Disorganized Type

Previously called **hebephrenia,** the disorganized type of schizophrenic behavior is marked by incoherence and flat, blunted, inappropriate, or silly affect. Such individuals appear to have regressed to infantile levels of behaving. They are among the most impaired individuals who develop a schizophrenic disorder. Onset is usually early (e.g., in adolescence) and the disorder progresses slowly with behaviors becoming more and more disorganized as time passes. These individuals' affect is often

HIGHLIGHT 12.4
SCHIZOPHRENIA AND DSM-III

DSM-III has incorporated many of the findings of the International Pilot Study of Schizophrenia. The primary features of schizophrenia as defined in DSM-III are much more specific than in DSM-II (1968) and include a number of Kurt Schneider's first-rank symptoms. The DSM-III (1980) diagnostic criteria for a schizophrenic disorder follow:

A. At least one of the following during a phase of the illness:
(1) bizarre delusions (content is patently absurd and has no possible basis in fact), such as delusions of being controlled, thought broadcasting, thought insertion, or thought withdrawal
(2) somatic, grandiose, religious, nihilistic, or other delusions without persecutory or jealous content
(3) delusions with persecutory or jealous content if accompanied by hallucinations of any type
(4) auditory hallucinations in which either a voice keeps up a running commentary on the individual's behavior or thoughts, or two or more voices converse with each other
(5) auditory hallucinations on several occasions with content of more than one or two words, having no apparent relation to depression or elation
(6) incoherence, marked loosening of associations, markedly illogical thinking, or marked poverty of content of speech if associated with at least one of the following:
(a) blunted, flat, or inappropriate affect
(b) delusions or hallucinations
(c) catatonic or other grossly disorganized behavior

B. Deterioration from a previous level of functioning in such areas as work, social relations, and self-care.

C. Duration: Continuous signs of the illness for at least six months at some time during the person's life, with some signs of the illness at present. The six-month period must include an active phase during which there were symptoms from A, with or without a prodromal or residual phase, as defined below.
Prodromal phase: A clear deterioration in functioning before the active phase of the illness not due to a disturbance in mood or to a Substance Use Disorder and involving at least two of the symptoms noted below. ["Prodromal" refers to the period prior to the development of major symptoms.]
Residual phase: Persistence, following the active phase of the illness, of at least two of the symptoms noted below, not due to a disturbance in mood or to a Substance Use Disorder. ["Residual" refers to symptoms that remain after major symptomalotogy has diminished.]

Prodromal or Residual Symptoms
(1) social isolation or withdrawal
(2) marked impairment in role functioning as wage-earner, students, or homemaker
(3) markedly peculiar behavior (e.g., collecting garbage, talking to self in public, or hoarding food)
(4) marked impairment in personal hygiene and grooming
(5) blunted, flat, or inappropriate affect
(6) digressive, vague, overelaborate, circumstantial, or metaphorical speech
(7) odd or bizarre ideation, or magical thinking, (e.g., superstitiousness, clairvoyance, telepathy, "sixth sense," "others can feel my feelings," overvalued ideas, ideas of reference)
(8) unusual perceptual experiences, (e.g., recurrent illusions, sensing the presence of a force or person not actually present). (pp. 188–189)

strange, with periods when for no apparent reason they burst out laughing. Delusions and hallucinations when present are fragmented and simple (for example, a female believing that she is pregnant because she has been hugged). The disorder is severe, and the likelihood of recovery is poor. The case of Pam is typical:

> Pam is a 24-year-old white female who has been hospitalized nine times, the current time continuously for five years. Pam is now very regressed and has been so for the entire five-year stay at her current hospital. Although her behavior still fluctuates somewhat, she is often awake at night, drinks many cups of coffee, and vomits it as she walks. She babbles, hugs and kisses staff and other patients, and sometimes becomes aggressive. She is usually bizarre and overactive; her speech is disconnected and confused. Giggling, she speaks in fragments about delusions and hallucinations which involve mythology, demonology, and

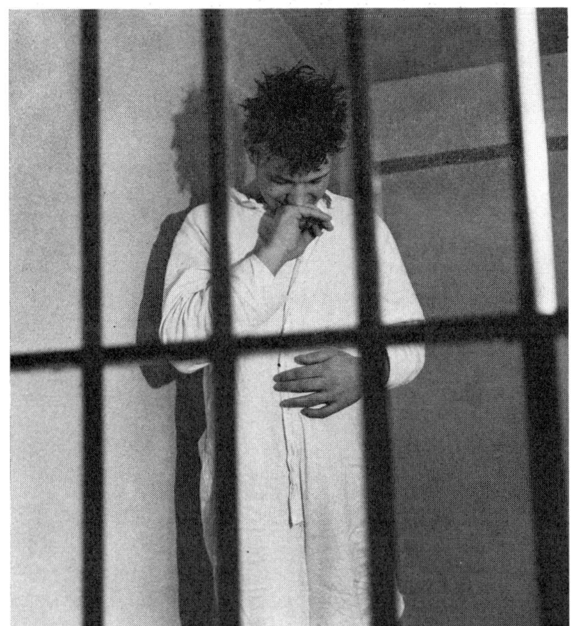

Posturing, grimacing, and smirking are symptomatic of the disorganized type of schizophrenic disorder, formerly known as hebephrenic schizophrenia.

sexual behavior. She ingests objects such as pens, pencils, and screws, and has placed many foreign objects in her vagina and rectum, including broken glass and paper clips. She often sleeps on the floor, and plays like an infant in the toilet. Her extremely disorganized behavior continues in spite of treatment with psychotherapy, various major tranquilizing medications, and an intensive behavior modification program.

Catatonic Type

Catatonic schizophrenia is characterized primarily by psychomotor disturbance. There may be a stupor, physical rigidity, excitement, posturing, or oppositional behavior (in which the person does the opposite of what is desired). The individual may rapidly swing between motor retardation and excitement. In the withdrawn phase, mutism (the absence of speech) is common. The onset of these symptoms may be quite sudden. One may see **waxy flexibility:** The limb of a subject who is immobile may be raised by someone else and will stay in that position for extended periods. In excitement, the patient may become very agitated, shouting, pacing, talking nonstop. Angela, the patient in the following case, was diagnosed as paranoid schizophrenic on her first admission to a hospital. On her second admission, described below, the catatonic symptoms became obvious. This overlap of symptoms is not unusual in actual cases.

After being discharged from her first hospital admission, Angela obtained a good job at a large accounting firm. She worked for about a year, but again became withdrawn. One day her supervisor found her standing immobile in the hall with her hands stretched over her head. She remained in this position for 10–15 minutes, unresponsive to the intervention of the supervisor. She finally responded and was sent home to "regain her composure." Several hours later, she was found walking nude down a highway by a passerby. She would not talk, but continually flapped her arms above her head and crowed like a rooster. After admission to the hospital, she continued to display catatonic symptoms. She refused to eat and was alternately immobile and agitated. She was mute and would walk only with assistance. If left standing, she would remain in that position for hours until staff placed her in a chair.

Angela was unresponsive to staff and had to be dressed, bathed, fed, and taken to the bathroom by staff. In an excited episode, she attacked staff. Several months of psychotherapy resulted in major improvements, and Angela was discharged.

Paranoid Type

In **paranoid schizophrenia,** the major signs are persecutory or grandiose delusions, or hallucinations with persecutory or grandiose content. In some cases, delusions of jealousy may be prominent features. The case of Carl ("Spirit Boy") Johnson follows:

This 43-year-old male called himself "Spirit Boy" since before his admission 17 years ago. At that time he was confused, manifested irrelevant speech, lacked insight, was unkempt, and showed an absence of affect. He had a nihilistic delusion that most people were dead, and grandiosely believed that he "owned" Chicago. He believed that he could communicate with ghosts or "spirits." During the interview, he brought in the ghost of his father, conversed with him, and then invited God to join the interview. (Carl graciously interpreted

God's side of the interview, since the psychologist could not see or hear Him.) During the interview, Carl stated that he was married to the movie star Kim Novak and was a friend of the late President John F. Kennedy. Carl was also planning to run for "governor of the world." Carl would provide no history of his life before his hospitalization, and none was available from other sources.

Seventeen years after this admission, Spirit Boy is essentially unchanged. His associations remain loose, his affect is flat, and his speech is still somewhat incoherent. He hallucinates "spirit" voices, which tell him what to do. His eyes become glazed when this happens and he now attacks other patients and staff, throwing them in the air. (He is 6 feet, 4 inches tall and weighs 350 pounds.) When he hallucinates and attacks people, he is acting upon a delusion that "gangsters" are invading the ward. These "gangsters" look exactly like the staff and patients, and they even have the same faces. But they are impostors, and Carl's voices tell him to protect himself against them. In the 17 years that Carl has been hospitalized, he has received virtually every available treatment with little success.

The paranoid subtype is one of the most commonly diagnosed schizophrenic disorders. The individuals often have had a fairly well-organized personality before the onset of the disorder, and usually do not become as disorganized as the catatonic or disorganized type. They are, however, often suspicious, angry, and hostile. People with this disorder may occasionally act on their delusions or respond to their hallucinations in a violent manner. Although most do not engage in extreme acting out, some (such as David Berkowitz, New York's "Son of Sam" killer, or the murderer of rock star John Lennon) may engage in senseless violence. Paranoid schizophrenic behavior is distinguished from paranoid psychosis by the presence of schizophrenic symptoms such as alterations in affect, looseness of associations, and thought withdrawal or insertion. The individual with a pure paranoid disorder does not manifest these symptoms. However, these symptoms are often of less magnitude in the paranoid schizophrenic than in the other types of schizophrenia. This fact has led some workers to conclude that paranoid psychosis and paranoid schizophrenia are points on a continuum of behavior, although many clinicians and researchers feel the data are too uncertain to derive such a conclusion (Swanson, Bohnert, & Smith, 1970; Tanna, 1974).

Undifferentiated Type

As noted in Angela's case, the individual may manifest different subtypes of schizophrenic behavior at different times. As you read Arty's case, note the broad range of symptoms.

Arty is a 61-year-old white male who was admitted to the hospital at the age of 28. The onset of his illness followed a broken relationship with a girlfriend. He became careless, neglected his appearance, and began mumbling and giggling in a bizarre manner. Most of his time was spent kneeling in prayer or reading religious material. At admission he was incoherent; his affect was flat with the exception of occasional giggling. In 33 years of hospitalization he has manifested a variety of symptoms and behaviors. He believes that people talk about him on television, and spy on him by listening to radio broadcasts. He usually does not discuss these ideas, and his speech is often not understandable. He wanders about, touching and handling objects such as light switches and telephones, and must be watched lest he eat from garbage cans. He wears multiple layers of clothing such as a long-sleeved shirt, an undershirt on top of it, and then a tie. He frequently wanders into residential neighborhoods and takes small objects from people's yards, but returns later with an item to replace them—usually a park bench, piece of wood, or human feces. The owners of the residences are predictably annoyed when this occurs.

Arty engages in stereotypic posturing and mannerisms, and on some days sits immobile for hours staring off into space. He occasionally becomes agitated and excited. When he can be encouraged to talk, his language can only be understood with great effort by the interviewer. At these times, Arty reveals that he is God's number one missionary and that we are keeping him from "his appointed rounds," since neither "rain, nor sleet, nor feet" should keep him from "spreading the gospel through his sharing with others." Arty knows that we are in the employ of the "Red consumers" (Communists) and keep him locked up because he is a threat to our Godless world domination. Arty rarely talks about these issues, since he is a "fatulist" (fatalist) like "Billy

Gram" (Billy Graham), whose name often elicits an associative train: "Billy Gram, billy club, belly button, who has it, where is it, I don't have it."

Arty's behavior is not more characteristic of the paranoid subtype than of the catatonic or the disorganized. He shows features of all three categories; this type of behavior is categorized as **undifferentiated schizophrenia.**

In addition to these four major subtypes of schizophrenic behavior, DSM-III also has a category called the "residual type." This term is used to categorize an individual who has had a schizophrenic episode in the past but who now has no prominent psychotic symptoms. However, these cases manifest some continuing deficits such as blunted affect, withdrawal, or illogical thinking.

OTHER DIMENSIONS OF SCHIZOPHRENIA

When Kraepelin asserted that true schizophrenia always has a deteriorating course, and Bleuler disagreed, they identified a significant dimension of schizophrenia which has been the subject of much study. Since their time it has been extensively documented that some individuals who manifest schizophrenic behavior do recover completely or almost completely, while others seem to deteriorate in spite of most efforts at treatment. Are these two groups of persons different in some significant way? Many researchers and clinicians think so.

The Process-Reactive Dimension and Premorbid Competence

Schizophrenic behavior has an insidious onset in some people. The behaviors develop over long periods, becoming more and more obvious as time passes. Ultimately, the individual develops a clear-cut schizophrenic disorder. Other individuals have a sudden onset of the behaviors, which appears at times to follow a significant increase in stress in the individual's life. In the first case, we often describe the development of the disorder as being representative of a growing "process" of schizophrenia.

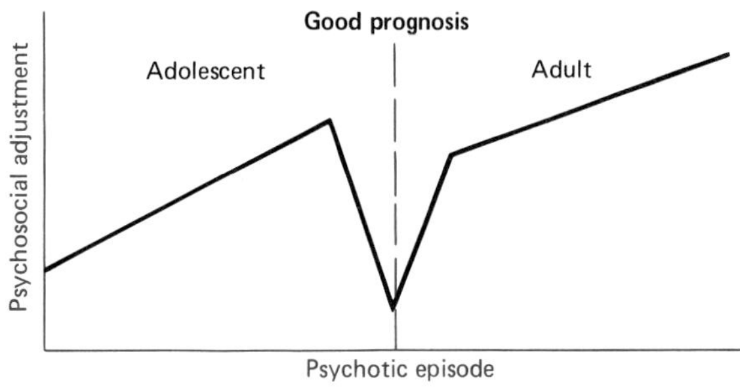

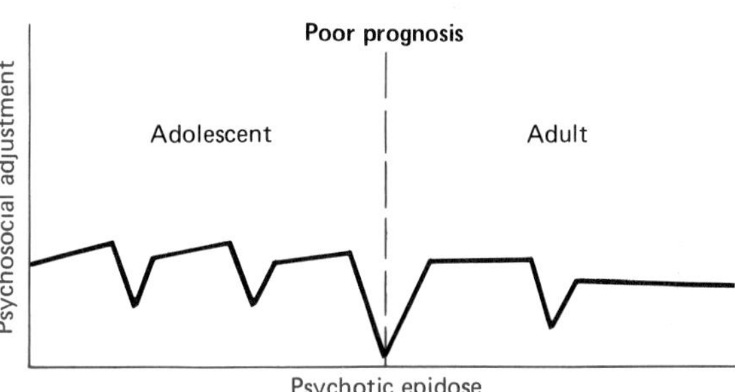

Figure 12.1. Process-reactive and premorbid dimensions and prognosis.
The individual who has a good premorbid development and a sudden, reactive onset of schizophrenia is more likely to have a good prognosis than an individual who has a poor premorbid development with a slow, insidious onset of the psychosis. Adapted from the *Schizophrenia Bulletin*, (1977, pp. 180–181).

In the second case, the schizophrenic disorder is described as "reactive" (see Figure 12.1). A major finding has been that process schizophrenics tend to have a poor prognosis: They are not likely to recover from the disorder. Persons who manifest a reactive disorder are more likely to recover (Houlihan, 1977). Table 12.4 lists the typical differences found between people whose disorder is of the process or reactive types.

Research, such as that by A. B. Heilbrun and Heilbrun (1977), has found differences in the delusions of process and reactive types. A reactive onset was found to be associated with delusions that were more extensive, had greater variety, were more oriented toward the environment, better integrated, more logical, and less autistic than the delusions of the process group. This finding is quite interesting be-

Table 12.4
Case history criteria for differentiating process and reactive schizophrenia

Process schizophrenia	Reactive schizophrenia
BIRTH TO THE FIFTH YEAR	
a. Early psychological trauma.	a. Good psychological history.
b. Physical illness, severe or long.	b. Good physical health.
c. Odd member of family.	c. Normal member of family.
FIFTH YEAR TO ADOLESCENCE	
a. Difficulties at school.	a. Well adjusted at school.
b. Family troubles paralleled with sudden changes in patient's behavior.	b. Domestic troubles unaccompanied by behavior disruptions. Patient had "what it took."
c. Introverted behavior trends and interests.	c. Extroverted behavior trends and interests.
d. History of breakdown of social, physical, mental functioning.	d. History of adequate social, physical, mental functioning.
e. Pathological siblings.	e. Normal siblings.
f. Overprotective or rejecting mother. "Momism."	f. Normal protective, accepting mother.
g. Rejecting father.	g. Accepting father.
ADOLESCENCE TO ADULTHOOD	
a. Lack of heterosexuality.	a. Heterosexual behavior.
b. Insidious, gradual onset of psychosis without pertinent stress.	b. Sudden onset of psychosis; stress present and pertinent; later onset.
c. Physical aggression.	c. Verbal aggression.
d. Poor response to treatment.	d. Good response to treatment.
e. Lengthy stay in hospital.	e. Short course in hospital.
ADULTHOOD	
a. Massive paranoia.	a. Minor paranoid trends.
b. Little capacity for alcohol.	b. Much capacity for alcohol.
c. No manic-depressive component.	c. Presence of manic-depressive component.
d. Failure under adversity.	d. Success despite adversity.
e. Discrepancy between ability and achievement.	e. Harmony between ability and achievement.
f. Awareness of change in self.	f. No sensation of change.
g. Somatic delusions.	g. Absence of somatic delusions.
h. Clash between culture and environment.	h. Harmony between culture and environment.
i. Loss of decency (nudity, public masturbation, etc.).	i. Retention of decency.

From Kantor, Wallner, and Winder (1953, pp. 157–162).

cause people who manifest paranoid schizophrenia, which is characterized by these types of delusions, are also more frequently reactive types and generally have a better prognosis than persons manifesting the other subtypes. The overlap is not total, however. Some reactive schizophrenics are not of the paranoid type, and some process schizophrenics are.

Both clinical observation and research have demonstrated that people who develop schizophrenia are not necessarily clearly process or reactive in the onset of their disorder. This dimension seems to be a continuum on which people fall, rather than two discrete types of onset.

The process-reactive dimension has also been discussed in terms of **premorbid competence,** the individual's level of adjustment before the onset of symptoms. The person at the reactive end of the continuum has a good premorbid adjustment, and fits the description of **reactive schizophrenia** in Table 12.4. This person was relatively competent at dealing with life before the onset of the disorder; and did acceptably well in school, in social relations, in work, and marriage. The individual with a poor premorbid personality has a long history of behavioral problems, poor social relationships, family troubles, and a poor work history. Such a life-style indicates a lack of coping skills. Almost by definition, the **process schizophrenic** has a poor premorbid personality, since the gradual onset of the disorder is likely to begin in early adolescence.

What is the significance of these data? Over the years, the research has been quite convincing that the process-reactive, poor premorbid–good premorbid dimensions are related to prognosis or likelihood of recovery (Garmezy, 1970; J. S. Strauss et al., 1977; J. S. Strauss & Docherty, 1979). Many clinicians and researchers have become convinced that the process type is one disorder, and reactive schizophrenia with a good premorbid personality is another disorder. If this is true, these disorders may have differing causal factors. One significant factor, which will be examined in depth in the next chapter, involves the degree of biological predisposition present. The process schizophrenic may have a greater biological vulnerability to schizophrenia than the reactive schizophrenic.

The evidence for these dimensions is so convincing that DSM-III (1980) now categorizes the person who has a first episode of schizophrenic behavior as having a **schizophreniform disorder.** Only after the behavior has lasted at least six months is the person diagnosed as having a schizophrenic disorder. This is one approach (perhaps not the best) for differentiating beteen the poor long-term prognosis of narrowly defined schizophrenia and the likelihood of a better long-term outcome for the reactive, good premorbid schizophrenia.

Primary vs. Secondary Underlying Deficits

A major issue in the study of schizophrenic behavior is which of the characteristics are basic deficits, and which of the behaviors are secondary to the basic deficits. Some researchers have studied very basic behaviors in schizophrenia in an attempt to clarify the process by which more global behaviors such as hallucinations and loose associations might develop. It will be helpful to an understanding of schizophrenic behavior to briefly examine some of the research done on basic deficits.

Attention: Reaction Time and Distraction. One of the defining characteristics of schizophrenia is an impairment in perceptual functioning. Could this impairment be due to some deficit in the individual's ability to attend to environmental stimuli? Some research seems to suggest that this is the case. For example, since the 1930s, David Shakow, a psychologist, has been studying the phenomenon of alertness and readiness to respond in an attempt to measure the degree to which people with schizophrenic disorders are able to focus attention on various stimuli.

Reaction time is the interval between the onset of a stimulus and the subject's response. Schizophrenics usually have slower reaction times than normals, and chronic schizophrenics are slower than acute schizophrenics (Shakow, 1963). In some studies, the subjects were provided with a preparatory period before the onset of the signal to respond. For example, a green light would be flashed signaling that a red light was about to be flashed. The green light is the preparatory signal. The red light in this case would be the signal to respond. Studies such as these found that chronic or process schizophrenics' performance decreased as the preparatory interval lengthened. They did not appear to be able to maintain their attention on the task. Several investigators have suggested that this is a result of the schizophrenic being unable to avoid attending to distracting stimuli (Neale, 1971).

Recently studies of attention have been extended to **high risk populations** (Asarnow, Steffy, & MacCrimmon, 1977). Asarnow and colleagues, for example, studied the biological children of mothers who had had schizophrenia. Children of schizophrenic mothers have an increased risk of developing the disorder, and thus compose a "high risk" population. The children, who had been raised away from the mothers in foster homes, were compared with foster children whose biological parents had not been diagnosed as schizophrenic, and with a control group of children living with their biological parents. Using several measures of attention deficit, Asarnow et al. found that many high risk children showed attention deficits similar to those found in schizophrenic adults. In a later study, Asarnow and MacCrimmon (1978) used the same tests on hospitalized schizophrenics, remitted schizophrenics (free of major symptoms), and a control group. Once again the hospitalized schizophrenics' performance deteriorated, when distractions increased, to a greater degree than the controls. The remitted schizophrenics who showed no current major symptomatology did as poorly as the hospitalized schizophrenics (see Figure 12.2). This study not only supports the previous work but also suggests that the deficit in attention is not due to the presence of symptoms such as hallucinations and affect disorder. The deficit is present even when these symptoms are not. Some investigators consider this deficit to be a primary factor in schizophrenic vulnerability, rather than a result of the schizophrenic disorder (Cromwell et al., 1979).

A major problem in attention deficit studies is that many of the tasks used to measure attention do not correlate with each other (as we would expect them to, if they were measuring the same thing). The lack of correlation between measures weakens the conclusions of the studies (L. J. Chapman, 1979); but as the measures continue to be refined, support for the existence of an attention deficit continues to mount (Kornetsky & Orzack, 1978).

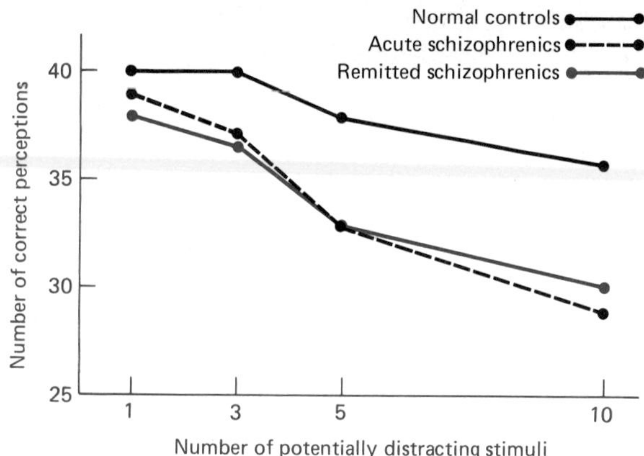

Figure 12.2. Response to potentially distracting stimuli by normal controls, acute, and remitted schizophrenics.

For each group, $n = 20$.
From Asarnow and MacCrimmon (1978, pp. 597–608).

Cognitive Factors. Schizophrenics appear unable to screen out irrelevant stimuli. We may ask, then, what they do with stimuli once they are perceived. When we are experiencing a number of inputs, we usually organize the stimuli into a coherent whole. In a sense, we filter out what is not relevant to the organization. Schwartz-Place and Gilmore (1980) have suggested, based on their research, that the perceptual deficit seen in schizophrenics is due to an inability to organize incoming data at an early stage of the perceptual process, resulting in disorganized thinking.

The disorganization of the cognitions of schizophrenics has been studied by many researchers. L. J. Chapman and J. P. Chapman (1973), for example, have proposed that a major problem for schizophrenics is that they *yield* to normal internal associations. This suggests that all of us could have loose associations, but most of us do not allow (or are able to prevent) these associations from intruding into our thinking. Our thinking and speech are strongly influenced by our perception of the context in which we are operating. In the context of writing a poem, we can think and write in obscure symbolism, rhyme, and use odd grammar. When writing a term paper, we strive for clarity and communication of data. The schizophrenic seems to be unable to stay within the context required.

Chapman and Chapman have demonstrated that the schizophrenic is less able to ignore noncontextual meanings of words (Rattan & Chapman, 1973). For example, if you asked someone to hand you a screwdriver while you were fastening a board in place, they would hear your communication in that context. A person with a schizophrenic disorder might hear your request in this context, but associate the term "screwdriver" with "screw" and respond as if you had made a sexual comment or request. Chapman and Chapman see these types of errors by schizophrenics as being a difference in the frequency with which normal associations are made, rather than a qualitative difference in thinking. If schizophrenics make many more associations than do normals, their thinking and language may appear extremely different from normal.

Some investigators have attempted to find out if "schizophrenic" associations can be induced in normal subjects. Levitz and Ullmann (1969) demonstrated that normal subjects could learn to give more uncommon responses on a word association test and on a projective test when given appropriate instructions and social reinforcement. They suggested that this finding was consistent with the notion that schizophrenics learn to associate loosely. A later study by Meiselman (1978) found that when normal subjects were induced to let themselves associate freely by acting like the common stereotype of a mentally ill person, their associations became more uncommon, and their response latency or reaction time slowed (see Figure 12.3). Remember, this deficit in reaction time is a common finding in schizophrenia. However, previous work (R. H. Price, 1972) has shown that while schizophrenics who manifest little pathology (healthy presenters) could modify their associations in either direction (toward either more common or more uncommon responses), schizophrenics who have more symptomatology could not change the level of their associations in either direction. Meiselman has interpreted this finding and her own research to suggest that reaction time deficits are a function of making uncommon associations, and uncommon associations are not the primary deficit in schizophrenia. The difficulty with which schizophrenics modify their associations, and the ease with which normals do so, suggests that individuals who develop schizophrenic disorders have a more basic deficit, which limits their associative flexibility and results in more autistic associations.

In this brief section on "primary" deficits in schizophrenia, we have begun to touch on the area of causal factors in schizophrenia. Are reaction time deficits, distractibility, or intrusive normal associations the causal factors in schizophrenia, or must we look further? While these deficits are important characteristics of schizophrenic disorder they also are likely to be the result of more primary problems in schizophrenia. In the next chapter, we will explore some of the current etiological factors in schizophrenia. However, before moving on, we must consider the typical outcome for individuals who manifest schizophrenic behavior.

LONG-TERM OUTCOMES OF SCHIZOPHRENIA

The British/European definition of schizophrenia, which has been adopted in DSM-III (1980) is narrower than the previous definition used in the United States. As we have seen, this definition results in the identification of a group of

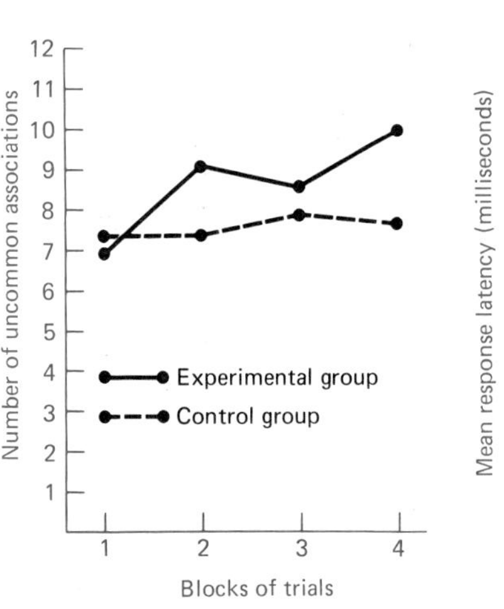

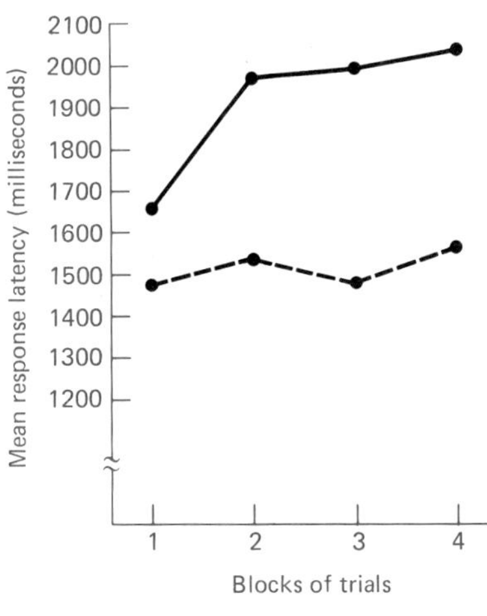

Figure 12.3. The effects of inducing "schizophrenic" associations in normal subjects. Uncommon associations for experimental and control groups across blocks of trials show that subjects in the experimental group (told to associate "like a mental patient") produced significantly more uncommon associations as they became more experienced at the task. The mean response latencies for experimental and control groups across blocks of trials show that as associations became more uncommon in normals (in the experimental group), the response latency, or reaction time, increased.
From Meiselman (1978, p. 292).

individuals with a relatively poor prognosis. This is not to say that individuals do not recover some level of functioning after or between major episodes of schizophrenia. We have already noted that most people with schizophrenic disorders are not continuously hospitalized. Many of these individuals live marginal lives, residing in boarding homes or transient hotels. Others live independently and, while they may not be fully contributing members of society, they manage to get along. Some schizophrenics recover completely, although they are not in the majority.

Achté et al. (1979) followed up first admission of schizophrenics to a Finnish psychiatric hospital from 1950 to 1970. They followed the admissions for five years to determine outcome and found that 20 percent could be considered to be completely recovered at the five-year point. During the study period, they found that the percentage of people still requiring hospitalization had decreased from 22 percent in 1950 to only 6 percent in 1970. From 1950 to 1970, many more community support arrangements had been developed which provided nonhospital settings in which schizophrenics with moderate symptoms could reside. As noted, about 2–3 million people have a schizophrenic disorder in the United States; and at any one time, about 200,000 persons are in mental hospitals. Obviously, most people who have a schizophrenic disorder are not hospitalized continuously.

Many variables seem to interact to determine which patients admitted to a mental hospital will recover enough to be released. Many workers feel that the presence of flat affect is a very negative sign. Some research has demonstrated that if emotions are present, the individual is more likely to respond and recover (Knight et al., 1979). Other work has demonstrated that the presence or absence of emotion is not the most significant factor in the outcome of the disorder, but implicates psychotic disorganization as a major factor (Gift et al., 1980). A large survey of 1500 patients in 1966 was followed up seven years later to examine chronicity (Pokorny et al., 1976). It found a number of variables to be significant in the likelihood that, once discharged from a psychiatric hospital, a person would remain out. These factors included the length of hospitalization, the patent's relatives' attitudes about release, the patient's social adequacy, and the patient's degree of conceptual disorganization. The study by Gift et al. (1980) found that the degree of affective deficit was unrelated to prognosis, and supported the idea that the degree of disorganized thinking may be a major factor. Knight et al. (1979), who had found that affective deficit was important, also found that the degree of interpersonal competence of the individual was significant in whether he or she would have a poor or good prognosis. Although affective deficit and its relationship to long-term outcome remains questionable, such studies allow us to describe the individual who is likely to have a better outcome. This person probably shows only minimal flatness of affect, and is still able to relate somewhat adequately to others—at least when the cognitive disorganization is not too severe. This person's relatives (a social-emotional support group) have a positive attitude towards his or her release. Finally, the individual has not had a lengthy hospitalization.

The most frequent outcome for an individual who manifests a schizophrenic disorder is a life of struggle with being different, lonely, alienated, and often disturbed. They have difficulty in maintaining adequate relationships with friends, and often exhaust their families' resources. Schizophrenia can take a dreadful toll. The 2–3 million people with schizophrenic disorders in the United States lead lives of quiet desperation, struggle, and little drama. This bleak outlook must be balanced by the fact that some individuals make dramatic recoveries. A case reported by Betz (1980) illustrates the remarkable adjustment of a man 25 years after a severe catatonic disorder. This is an appropriate case to close this chapter, since it demonstrates that not all schizophrenic disorders result in chronic life problems.

> On admission in 1955, the patient . . . expressed feelings of loneliness and tension, stating: "A dream world is about the only place I could live. Things outside are too tough." In an initial, strategy-planning clinical conference, the Chief Psychiatrist said: "One

kind of treatment was tried, namely helping him float and hold a job—that did not work. Best now to get into active treatment." During his 28 months as an inpatient, three changes of doctors . . . occurred—after 7 months, 19 months, and 25 months.

During the first year his course was stormy, with negativistic, resistive, combative, self-destructive, and catatonic behavior. He attempted to chew off a finger, [chewed] his lips and tongue, continually bruised his head against the wall, rubbed his eyes until they were seriously inflamed, ground his teeth forcibly to the point of [physical damage], spit, attacked attendants and his therapist. . . . This state persisted month after month. Patient is quoted as saying: "I am disgusted and shuddering at every ray of sunshine that comes into this room." During the seventh month he became acutely catatonic, speaking in a low harsh voice with an eerie effect. He was described by a staff member as "one of the sickest patients I have seen." Over several weeks he was given a course of insulin treatment, combined with ECT.

As several months passed the more distressful psychotic manifestations abated and some communication began. He became interested in a student nurse and in his doctor. He liked the head nurse, and he wrote to his sister. He said that he had "never enjoyed pleasure," that he seemed "to thrive on hating people."

Nineteen months after admission, his first therapist wrote: "Making significant contacts with other patients. Enjoys being taken care of and babied. Asserts his independence by resenting boundaries." Twenty-five months after admission, his second therapist wrote: "A severe schizophrenic. Petulant that his therapist hasn't pampered him."

At this point a new therapist took over. The patient talked freely with him about difficulties he had had with his preceding therapist, and was bothered by the intensity of his feelings. He became more at ease, and more active. He began job hunting, with success. Three months later he was discharged "much improved," and transferred to outpatient status, but without change of therapist. His improvement was seen as "a reorganization of his character structure with widening of horizon of interest and activities, and testing out different patterns in interpersonal relationships."

[The patient was transferred after 23 sessions to a new therapist, Dr. S.] Subsequent notes in this patient's record are sparse but informative. He did call Dr. S. and maintained regular contacts . . . over a period of four years, at intervals of about every three months. [Dr. S.] reports that he showed no evidence of psychotic difficulties during this period, although his temperament remained quite inward and uncertain, particularly in situations requiring, or arousing, some aggressiveness.

During the first year he changed jobs to one with better pay and additional benefits, and remained in this job. Toward the end of the first year he married the landlady's daughter. Although there were tensions in the marriage, they seemed realistic and he managed them well. His wife was employed and he assumed a number of domestic tasks, as helping with the cooking.

He became the father of two sons, and formed a warm attachment to his children. He and his wife had continued to live in her mother's house, but with the birth of the second child they bought a house of their own.

During the fourth year, Dr. S. felt that the patient was really functioning in an autonomous way, and that therapy, indeed, was no longer needed. This was discussed with the patient, and by mutual agreement, goodbye was said without making a "next" appointment.

More than 20 years later (in 1978), in the interest of follow-up information, Dr. S. called the patient by telephone. His response was open and warm. He expressed surprise that he was "remembered," and seemed pleased. He said that he was doing well, and had had no health problems. He was still employed in the same firm, and still living in the same house. His wife had died suddenly a few years ago, presumably of a cerebral hemorrhage, while their sons were in their teens. He has continued to maintain the household and look after the sons who are still living with him. He was asked about his parents, and said that his father had died many years ago, but that his mother and his sister were still living, and he and the children made trips to see them each year. It seemed evident to Dr. S. that his image of himself was not that of an ex-patient. A few months later, Dr. S. met him by chance. He was well groomed and confident. The encounter confirmed and strengthened the impression gained during the earlier follow-up telephone conversation. (pp. 253–259)

Summary

1. Schizophrenic behavior can be extremely incapacitating, and affects about 1 in 100 persons. The characteristic disorders seen in schizophrenia include the following.

1. Disorders of thought and communication, such as problems in associative thinking, concreteness and literal thinking, and incoherence. In addition, problems in content of thought, such as delusions, are often present.
2. Disorders of perception and sensation, such as illusions and hallucinations.
3. Disorders of affect or emotion, including possible flatness of affect, blunting, inappropriate affect, and ambivalence.
4. Disorders of motor behavior, including unusual mannerisms, stereotyped behavior, agitation, or immobility.
5. Disorders of socialization are primarily manifested in withdrawal from social contact.

2. The critical characteristics of the schizophrenic disorders have been the subject of much disagreement in the past. Bleuler identified the four As as being primary: affect, associations, ambivalence, and autism.

3. The differences in definition between the British/European and North American concepts of schizophrenia contributed to the implementation of the International Pilot Study of Schizophrenia by the World Health Organization. This cross-cultural study derived critical characteristics which were present in most individuals with schizophrenia, regardless of the cultural context in which they lived. These data contributed to the adoption of a narrower definition of schizophrenia, which is reflected in the third edition of the *Diagnostic and Statistical Manual* (DSM-III, 1980).

4. Particular patterns of symptoms have been linked together by clinical and research data into particular subtypes of the schizophrenic disorder. The current diagnostic types consist of the: 1. disorganized type, 2. catatonic type, 3. paranoid type, 4. undifferentiated type, and 5. residual type.

5. Other dimensions of schizophrenia which have been studied include premorbid personality and the process-reactive dimension. These two factors are related to some extent.

6. The individual with a well-functioning personality prior to the development of schizophrenia is more likely to have a sudden (reactive) onset of the disorder, and to regain a higher level of function after the disorder is treated.

7. The person with a process schizophrenic disorder is usually described as someone who has a poorer premorbid personality and whose schizophrenic behavior is slow in onset and follows a deteriorating course.

8. The factors of premorbid personality and process or reactive onset are not totally correlated. The relationship of these factors to prognosis has led many investigators to conclude that two types of disorders exist which share similar symptomatology: schizophrenia and the schizophreniform psychosis. These disorders may, in fact, be opposite poles of a continuum.

9. Many investigators have tried to determine whether basic underlying psychological deficits in schizophrenia result in the behaviors which are more obvious to the clinician. Researchers have focused on possible deficits in attention and cognition.

10. Research demonstrates attention deficits in schizophrenia which are manifested in problems in reaction time and in the ability to avoid distraction. Other research indicates that people with schizophrenic disorders have difficulty in organizing or processing stimuli once the stimuli have been perceived.

11. The cognitive associative process has been studied by some investigators who believe that schizophrenic associations consist of an increased frequency of normal associations: Schizophrenics, unlike normals, may be unable to suppress excess associations.

12. Recent research suggests that while symptomatic schizophrenics associate more freely than normals, the major problem may be that they are unable to decrease the frequency of associations. These researchers suggest that we can all increase our associative frequency when the context is appropriate, such as writing a symbolic poem.

13. The long-term outcome of the narrowly defined schizophrenic disorder is bleak. Approximately 50 percent of people in mental hospitals are diagnosed as schizophrenic; but 2–3 million people in the United States are estimated to have this disorder. Most manage to live marginally in the community. In spite of the disorder's poor prognosis, some individuals recover completely. Those who do not recover lead lives of quiet desperation.

KEY TERMS

Affect. An emotion or subjective feeling which influences behavior.
Anhedonia. The inability to experience pleasurable feelings.
Delusion. A fixed false belief.
Derailment. Also known as "looseness of association." The inability to maintain a logical train of thinking without intrusion by irrelevant thoughts.
Hallucination. A perception or sensation in the absence of an actual stimulus.
Premorbid. Existing before the onset of a disorder.
Prognosis. A prediction of the likely course and outcome of a disorder.
Psychosis. A severe disorder involving loss of contact with reality.
Schizophrenia. A type of psychosis, consisting of several subtypes, which involves withdrawal from reality, emotional blunting or inappropriateness, and disturbances in thinking and behavior.

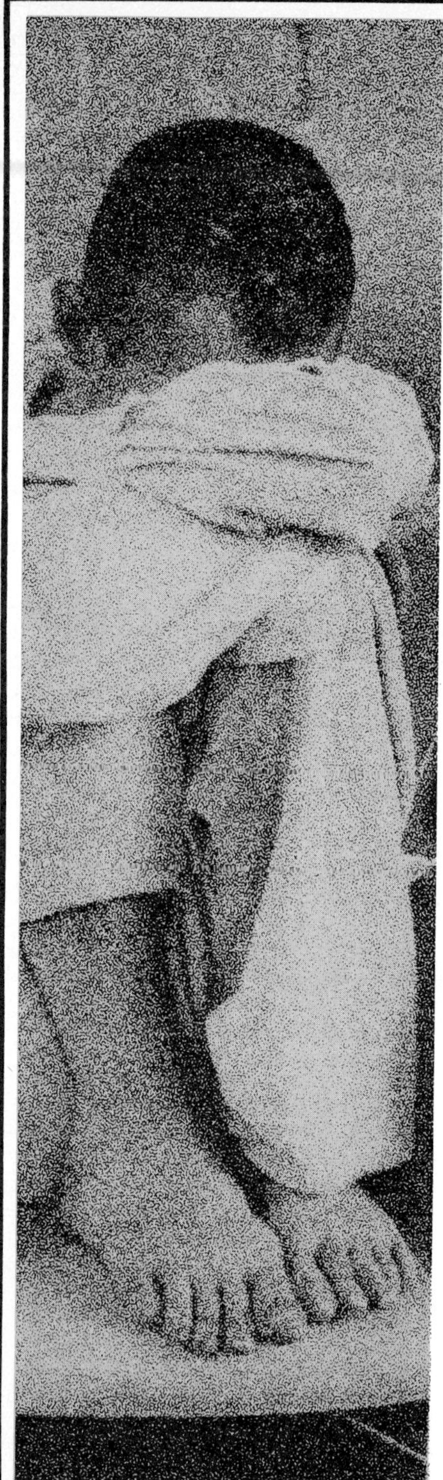

13

Schizophrenic disorders II: theories, research, and treatment

- General theories of schizophrenia
- Research on the heredity, biochemistry, and high risk factors of schizophrenia
- Where does schizophrenia come from? The vulnerability hypothesis
- Key treatments
- Summary
- Key terms

While schizophrenia can be described with some precision, less agreement exists in regard to its causes and treatments. Some theorists believe that such behavior is a function of biological abnormalities, that a deranged mind is due to deranged molecules. Others believe that the behavior is due to major problems in childhood experiences in the family. Some propose that schizophrenic behavior is learned, like many other behaviors. Others believe that the disorder is a way of coping with an insane society. Different theories of the cause or etiology of the schizophrenic disorders exist with varying degrees of supportive evidence. No single theory has received consistent or convincing support. In this chapter, the major theoretical formulations of schizophrenia will be described. In addition, the contributions of research to the understanding of the etiology of schizophrenia will be examined by focusing on three areas: heredity, biochemistry, and **high risk studies.**

Society has never had the luxury of sitting back and waiting for definite answers about the etiology of the schizophrenic disorders before attempting to do something about them. Schizophrenics' bizarre behaviors are disturbing to those around them, and we have seen that society has responded to these behaviors throughout history. Although we are not yet certain about the basic causes of schizophrenic behaviors, treatment approaches based on various theories and clinical experiences have been developed. Many of these approaches are helpful in reducing the problem behaviors of persons who manifest a schizophrenic disorder. The treatment of schizophrenic disorders will thus be considered in this chapter.

GENERAL THEORIES OF SCHIZOPHRENIA

Psychoanalytic Theory

Sigmund Freud was not particularly concerned with schizophrenia. His focus was on individuals who manifested less severe disorders, but he did speculate on the application of psychoanalytic theory to schizophrenia or, as it was then called, "dementia praecox." Based on his study of several individuals who manifested these behaviors, Freud proposed that schizophrenia was due to a massive regression to a period early in the oral stage.

At this early stage of development, the ego is very primitive. It has not yet developed adequate reality-oriented or **"secondary process" thinking.** The individual who has regressed to this primitive stage of development engages in **primary process thinking,** which is characterized by "wish fulfillment" and "primary narcissism." The individual withdraws from the external world and creates an inner world of fantasy and bizarre ideas and hallucinations. The strange ideas and hallucinations are symbolic of the id impulses, which overwhelm reality. According to Freud, in the psychotic individual, the ego is the servant of the id, rather than being a mediator between id impulses and reality.

The regression to this primitive state of functioning (which is normally characteristic of an infant during the first year of life) is due to an extremely severe state of anxiety. If the individual had developed a more adequate ego, the regression would not be so severe; the individual would have developed a neurosis rather than a psychosis. However, in schizophrenia, the individual's ego does not develop enough to mediate successfully between id, superego, and environment. Subsequently, when sexual or aggressive id impulses threaten to overwhelm the individual, the fragile ego crumbles and the massive regression occurs, since the ego withdraws from reality. Since attachments are withdrawn from the external world, including from a prospective therapist, Freud felt that psychoanalysis had little to offer in the treatment of schizophrenia. Later analysts were not so pessimistic.

In Chapter 12, it was noted that many researchers have found basic differences in attention and reaction time in people with schizophrenic disorders. Later in this chapter, we will examine other differences, including some psychological ones. Many of these differences were noted during Freud's time. A student of Freud's, Carl Jung, speculated on how these differences might occur. Contrary to Emil Kraepelin's suggestions, Jung proposed that an organic disorder did not result in schizophrenia. Jung said the mechanism was actually the re-

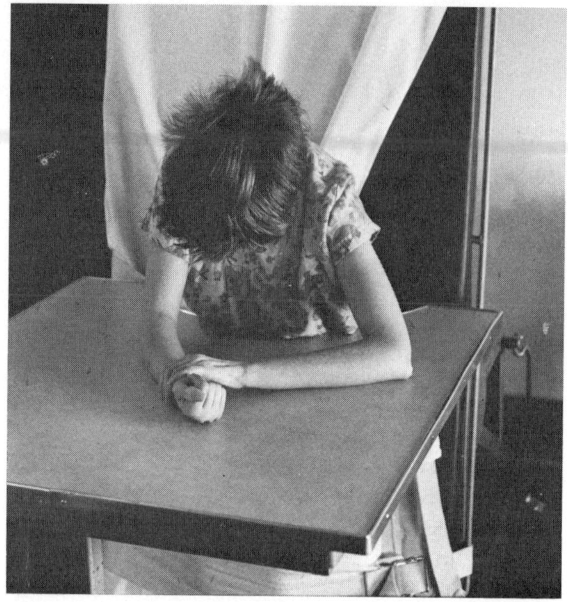

What causes schizophrenia? How can we explain a massive behavioral disorder which results in a lonely, disturbed life, usually led in the austere surroundings of a mental hospital?

verse. He proposed that the emotional disorder of schizophrenia produces an abnormal metabolism which causes physical damage to the brain (a psychophysiological disorder) (Arieti, 1966). This is a point worth keeping in mind when we study what others have said about biological factors in schizophrenia.

Although Freud and his students did not focus on the schizophrenic disorders, the later neo-Freudian Harry Stack Sullivan did. Sullivan (1953) was trained as an analyst, but later focused on the interpersonal relationships of people who became schizophrenic. Although he basically accepted the analytic conceptions of instinctual id impulses, unconscious processes, and regression, Sullivan believed that distorted interpersonal relationships lead to anxiety and regression. The most important interpersonal relationships are those between child and parent. Sullivan introduced the term **parataxic distortion** to describe what results when these critical early relationships are poor.

When parents treat children inconsistently or overpunitively or overindulgently, the child may experience "a disaster to self-esteem." To defend against this disaster, the person uses parataxic distortion; that is, the individual distorts subsequent interpersonal interactions. This distortion consists of an identification of one person (such as a girlfriend) with another real person (such as a mother), or fantasy person. When parataxic distortion is not corrected, the individual loses **consensual validation,** the recognition by others of the appropriateness of the person's thinking and behavior. Lack of consensual validation makes interpersonal relationships even more difficult, leading to more parataxic distortion. The individual spirals down into the distorted human relationships we call schizophrenia. Sullivan's emphasis on interpersonal relationships led to a great deal of later interest in the importance of family interaction and communication in the development of schizophrenia.

Interpersonal Theories

What factors present in familial relationships could lead to schizophrenia? Since disordered communication is commonly seen in schizophrenic individuals, some clinicians and researchers have studied communication patterns in schizophrenics' families to find out if they are different from families in which there are no schizophrenics. Anthropologist Gregory Bateson identified a communication pattern, which he called the **double bind,** that seemed to be frequent in the families of schizophrenics.

Double-bind Communication. Bateson and colleagues (1956) described double-bind communication between parents and their schizophrenic children. In this communication, the child (or adult child) is emotionally dependent on the parent, and the relationship is so intense that it is extremely important that parental messages be understood, since if they are not, psychological or physical punishment will follow. The parent, however, expresses two conflicting messages at the same time. Because of the importance of the relationship, the child (or adult child) cannot confront the parent's conflicting message, comment upon the conflict, ignore it, or escape from it. The individual is caught in a situation from which escape is impossible and in which punishment is likely. The contradictory messages may be verbal, or one message may be verbal with the other gestural. To illustrate double-bind communication, Bateson et al. (1956) give the following example of a young man in a hospital who was visited by his mother:

> He was glad to see her and impulsively put his arm around her shoulders whereupon she stiffened. He withdrew his arm and she asked, "Don't you love me anymore?" He then blushed and she said, "Dear, you must not be so easily embarrassed and afraid of your feelings." The patient was able to stay with her only a few minutes more. . . .
>
> Obviously, this result could have been avoided if the young man had been able to say, "Mother, it is obvious that you become uncomfortable when I put my arm around you, and you have difficulty accepting a gesture of affection from me." (pp. 258–259)

Bateson et al. point out that the schizophrenic has difficulty confronting and pointing out the double message to the parent. A lot of psychological strength is needed to deal with such situations—strength that a schizophrenic presumably has not developed.

The concept of double-bind communication in schizophrenic families has been especially appealing to clinicians who work with such families. Very often the communication patterns among these family members are disturbed and distorted. But does double-bind communication cause schizophrenia, or does schizophrenia cause distorted family communication?

Some workers have pointed out that all of us experience double-bind communications, yet only a few become schizophrenic. At least one study (E. V. Smith, 1976) has demonstrated that such messages can be upsetting. In this study, normal subjects were exposed to double-bind communications in punitive situations, and were found to experience significant increases in anxiety (see Figure 13.1). In addition, some subjects felt that the contradictory messages were meant to "trick" them, and continued to press the experimenter for fuller explanations of what was going on in the experiment, even after an explanation was given. This mystification effect of double-bind communication has been proposed as a factor in the development of schizophrenic thinking. A later study by S. S. Reilly and Muzekari (1979) is less supportive. They found that normal adults responded to both the words and the more subtle communications in mixed messages, but gave most weight to clues such as gestures and tone of voice. An unexpected finding was that both normal and disturbed children and disturbed adults attended only to the *words* of the mixed messages; they filtered out the contradictory message that was communicated with the verbal message. If people who develop schizophrenic disorders do not experience double binds, then using this concept to explain schizophrenic behavior is without merit.

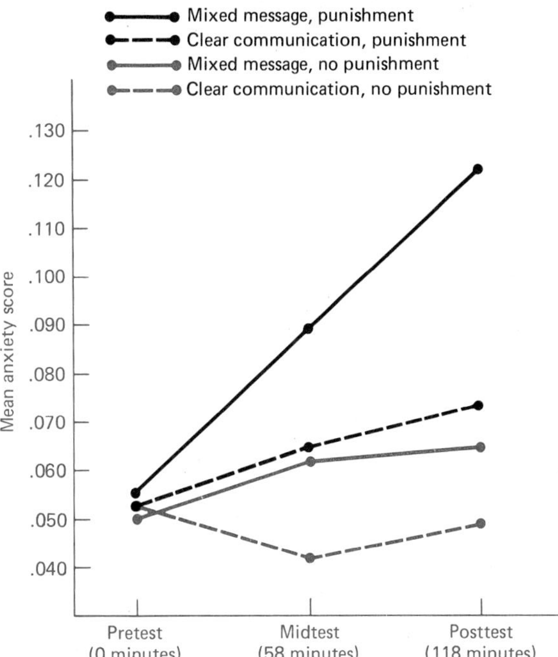

Figure 13.1. Effects of mixed messages and punishment on anxiety levels in normal individuals.

From E. V. Smith (1976, p. 361).

Family Relationships. In addition to double-bind communication, other factors in family relationships have been identified as important in the development of schizophrenic behavior. The noted psychoanalyst Frieda Fromm-Reichmann (1952), introduced the term **schizophrenogenic** to denote a particular type of mother which schizophrenics were sometimes observed to have. These mothers were described as extremely overprotective and intrusive. They were continually intruding into the life of their child, even when the child was an adult. The mother had to know exactly what her child was doing, thinking, and feeling at each moment. Such maternal behavior has been thought to prevent the child from developing a separate identity; and the offspring's lack of identity and lack of separateness are believed to lead to schizophrenia.

Little supportive research exists for the concept of a schizophrenogenic mother. In fact, some evidence shows that the overprotective and intrusive behavior of schizophrenics' mothers may be partly due to the fact that these women have a disturbed child. Klebanoff (1959) compared mothers of schizophrenics with mothers who had brain-injured and retarded children and found them all to be similar in levels of "overprotectiveness."

Although the idea of a particular type of mother (schizophrenogenic) has little support, investigators such as Theodore Lidz, Flech, and Cornelison (1965) have found that mothers of individuals who have developed schizophrenia are often unstable, intrusive women (see Highlight 13.1). They found that the fathers were also disturbed—either paranoid and aggressive, or passive, ineffectual, and distant. The parents' marriages were often marked by marital schisms. That is, there was overt conflict, with each parent trying to form an alliance with the children against the spouse. In some cases, there was marital skew, so that one parent passively accepted the bizarre behavior of the other parent. Lidz suggests that such families transmit irrationality to the children. These data were found in families that already had a schizophrenic child. What about families in which an adult child later becomes schizophrenic?

Several studies have examined interactions in families with problem children, only some of whom later were to become schizophrenic. W. McCord, Porta, and McCord (1962) found that a higher percentage of mothers of children who later became schizophrenic were overcontrolling, dominant, and affectionate than were mothers in control groups. Waring and Ricks (1965) compared the families of 50 problem children who later became schizophrenic with a matched control of 50 problem children who did not become schizophrenic. Their findings did not support the idea of a dominant, overcontrolling mother. In fact, the mothers in their study group were characterized as vague, withdrawn and inadequate. Waring and Ricks identified an interaction they called "symbiotic union" in about 35 percent of the families of those who later became schizophrenic. This symbiotic union involved an intrusive, overcontrolling style on the part of the parents. About 35 percent of the families who later had a seriously disturbed schizophrenic member also had a relationship characterized by minimal interactions, emotional distance, and distrust and hostility. Waring and Ricks called this "emotional divorce." The families were also characterized by a chaotic environment, which consisted of emotionally disturbed parents who neglected the child's basic safety and security needs, and "family sacrifice," which means that the child was effectively driven out of the home in adolescence. When family sacrifice occurred, the child usually manifested a less severe schizophrenic disorder.

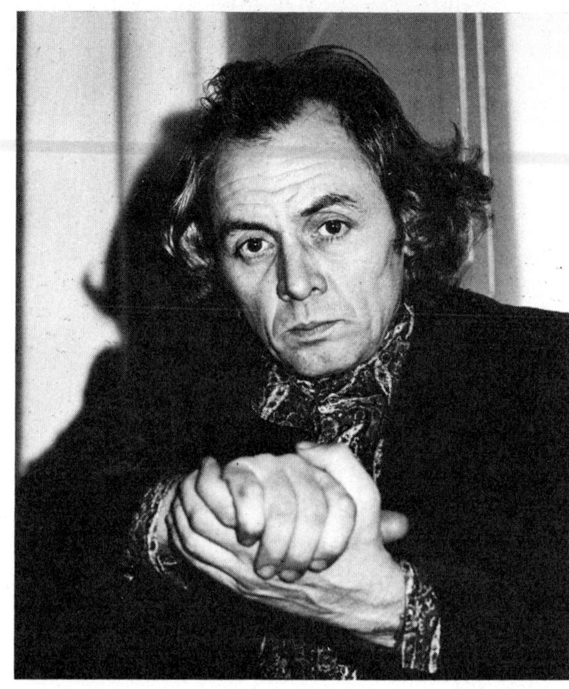
R. D. Laing, a British psychiatrist, believes that schizophrenia is an escape from life in an insane world.

HIGHLIGHT 13.1
RONALD LAING: THE MYSTIFICATION OF MAYA

R. D. Laing is a psychiatrist who believes that schizophrenia is an individual's adjustment to an insane environment, that of the "crazy" family. The families described by Laing (Laing & Esterson, 1971) sound very much like those seen by Bateson, Lidz, and others. Family characteristics include double-bind messages, irrational behavior, and chaos. In these families, says Laing, schizophrenic behavior is the only rational way to act.

In one example, the parents of Laing's patient Maya believed that she could read their thoughts. The parents conspired to test this possibility through a secret experiment which involved subtle attempts to control Maya's behavior. Maya manifested ideas of reference, which Laing concluded were due to the parents' "experiment." In fact, Maya's "ideas of reference" were accurate perceptions of the environment, says Laing. In family interviews, the parents engaged in a series of "knowing" winks, smiles, and nods when Maya would talk. In addition, they rarely accepted what she would say, even when her statements were about things only she could know accurately. They would "mystify" and "disqualify" her statements. For example:

1. Maya would say: she masturbated when she was fifteen. Parents would say: she did not.
2. Maya would say: she had sexual thoughts about parents. Parents would say: she did not.
3. Maya would say: she could remember attacking her mother. Parents would say: she could not remember.

Laing views schizophrenia as a psychological "trip." He sees the experience as valid, meaningful, and potentially beneficial—a possible growth experience through which the individual can become a better, more coping human being. While Laing's anecdotal evidence supports the existence of disturbed relationships in families of schizophrenics, there is little evidence that schizophrenia is a growth experience for most persons who manifest it.

These studies suggest that problems in family interactions are correlated with the development of schizophrenia. However, they do not demonstrate that problematic family interactions cause schizophrenia. D. Riess (1976) has pointed out that most studies of family interactions fail to meet the criteria for such proof: 1. the variables are not clearly defined, and are not measured by reliable and objective methods; 2. the causal role of the variables are not demonstrated by a. specifically linking them to schizophrenia as opposed to other disorders, b. showing that they have an impact on the individual *before* the onset of schizophrenia, and c. not confusing the effects of family interaction with the effects of another variable which is the "true" etiological agent.

Since 1976 better controlled studies have come closer to Riess's requirements (Liem, 1980). These studies have confirmed that schizophrenics usually grow up in families characterized by disordered communication and intrusive, overcontrolling, critical parents (e.g., Doane, 1978). Whether the disorders seen in these families lead to schizophrenia in one member, or are the *result* of schizophrenia in the affected member, has not been concretely demonstrated (see Highlight 13.2). Liem (1980) suggests that the distorted family interactions may be both a contributing factor to and a result of schizophrenic behavior in a family member. She suggests that disturbed family relationships are not the sole cause of schizophrenia, some other predisposing factor is also important; and she notes that a number of currently ongoing longitudinal studies may help to clarify the importance of disturbed family relationships in the development of schizophrenic behavior.

Schizophrenia as Learned Behavior

Can schizophrenia be learned? In a broad sense, some interpersonal theorists imply that schizophrenic behavior is learned from parents. In a more restricted sense, we can ask whether the principles of learning can be used as the primary etiological factor in the development of schizophrenic behavior. Some theorists strongly advocated an explanation of

HIGHLIGHT 13.2
IS THE COMMUNICATION DISTURBANCE IN THE FAMILY OR IN THE SCHIZOPHRENIC?

Joan Huser Liem (1974) wanted to find out the locus of the communication problem so often seen in families with a schizophrenic child. She selected families with a schizophrenic son and families with a normal son to participate in an identification task. Each "communicator" was to describe common objects such as a lamp and concepts such as "teacher," so that they could be identified by a listener. Five communications about three objects or concepts were tape-recorded in each session. Each normal son and each schizophrenic son took a turn in the role of "communicator," as did each set of parents.

Later, the parents and sons responded to these taped descriptions and tried to identify the object or concept being described. The parents responded to tapes made by their own son, by an unknown schizophrenic son, and by an unknown normal son. The sons responded to tapes made by their own parents, by unknown parents of a schizophrenic son, and by unknown parents of a normal son.

The parents of both normal and schizophrenic sons communicated quite adequately, as did the normal sons. However, "the communication disorder of schizophrenic sons had an immediate, observable negative effect not only on the parents of schizophrenic sons, but on all parents who heard and attempted to respond to them" (Liem, 1974, p. 445). Liem's study suggests that the disorder of communication seen in families of schizophrenic sons resides in the sons, rather than being a problem of the parents which *results* in a son becoming schizophrenic.

schizophrenic behavior based on learning theory. Consider the following example:

> In the early 1960s in a state mental hospital, a psychiatrist observes a female chronic schizophrenic patient who constantly and compulsively paces while holding a broom, but never is seen to sweep with it. The psychiatrist's opinion of the behavior is that "Her constant and compulsive pacing, holding a broom in the manner she does, could be seen as a ritualistic procedure, a magical action. . . . her broom would be then: (1) a child that gives her love and she gives him in return her devotion, (2) a phallic symbol, (3) a sceptre of an impotent queen. . ." (Ayllon, Haughton, & Hughes, 1965, p. 3).
>
> This psychiatrist's interpretation of the symbolic meaning of the patient's behavior arises from a psychoanalytic model of the development of schizophrenia. However, the psychiatrist did not know that psychologist Teodoro Ayllon and several colleagues had taught the woman to hold the broom, without sweeping, by reinforcing her with cigarettes when she did as they asked her to. Ayllon and colleagues believed that they had demonstrated how "schizophrenic" behavior arises in the world at large.

While this example demonstrates that schizophrenics can learn behaviors which appear odd when viewed out of context of the learning situation, it does not clarify how the primary forms of schizophrenic disorders might be learned.

Since Ayllon's experiment (or trick played on the psychiatrist), theorists have suggested how schizophrenic behavior might be learned. The social learning theorists Albert Bandura, Leonard Ullmann, and Leonard Krasner are among those who have suggested possible mechanisms.

Albert Bandura (1968) has proposed that hallucinations, delusions, ideas of reference, and other disorders seen in schizophrenia develop through a process of modeling and reinforcement. The data generated by studies of families described in the preceding section illustrates, according to Bandura's formulation, the disturbed parental models which are present in the families of those who become schizophrenic. Bandura also suggests that cognitive processes are quite important in learning to be schizophrenic. An individual might behave in an apparently disturbed manner because of fantasized contingencies and consequences. The consequences which are in one's fantasy may become so important and powerful that the consequences for "inappropriate" behavior in the environment are weakened and no longer affect behavior.

The theorists who have most strongly advocated a learning model of schizophrenic behavior are Ullmann and Krasner (1975). They take the position that schizophrenic behavior is primarily due to "the extinction of attention to social stimuli to which normal people respond." If one is not reinforced for attending to normal, usual social stimuli and, instead, attends to unusual external stimuli or internal stimuli such as one's own autistic thoughts, then one will manifest "loose associations" and strange speech patterns. The lack of attention to the social stimuli presented by other people will result in behaviors of aloofness and social isolation.

The disorders of affect present in schizophrenia are seen by Ullmann and Krasner (1975) as being due to a life-long absence of reinforcement for emotional expression. That is, they believe that some schizophrenics have not been reinforced for laughing, smiling, or crying. Inappropriate affect in others occurs because the individual was not taught to discriminate between stimuli. According to Ullmann and Krasner, hallucinations are learned by watching these types of behaviors being modeled in popular movies, reading about them, and seeing others manifest them. The experience occurs when the individual withdraws attention from the surroundings, focuses on internal stimuli, and no longer differentiates between what is real and what is imagined. Strange beliefs become delusional, according to their model, when the person discovers that: 1. talking about such ideas obtains attention, 2. the attention of others is found to be reinforcing, and 3. other more normal behaviors are not as effective in gaining reinforcing social attention.

Ullmann and Krasner (1975) have been extraordinarily successful at conceptualizing a theoretical framework for explaining schizophrenia from a sociopsychological framework. However, their concepts are not well documented with experimental evidence. Certainly, many behaviors (perhaps most) which schizophrenics manifest could be learned. However, Ullmann and Krasner's emphasis on a learning approach and their neglect of other variables are serious weaknesses in their conception of the development of schizophrenic behavior. We can return to our original example from Ayllon et al. and ask, Why did this woman so easily and willingly learn to engage in a purposeless, ritualistic, absurd act for the simple reinforcement of cigarettes? Why was she unable to find a more appropriate way to gain reinforcers? Was it because reinforcers were unavailable in any other way? Or was she amenable to learning this strange behavior because of some more primary deficit?

In Ullmann and Krasner's favor, they have focused attention on the social role behavior of schizophrenics. They have raised the question of the degree to which the bizarre behavior we see in schizophrenics is due to societal expectations of what a "crazy" person is "supposed" to be like. The idea that schizophrenia is a social role that people enact, rather than an illness, is shared by some other theorists (e.g., Perrucci, 1974; Scheff, 1975). In the following section, we will examine contributions to the theories of schizophrenia which have been the result of studies of the relationship of society and culture to schizophrenic behavior.

Sociocultural Theories of Schizophrenic Behavior

To what extent is schizophrenic behavior a function of the impact of society and culture? Thomas Scheff (1975) takes an extreme view similar to Ullmann and Krasner's and believes that schizophrenia is simply a label applied to deviant behavior. The individuals behave "as if sick." Sarbin (1969) suggests that schizophrenia consists of an individual behaving in a manner which meets the expectations of observers. If, for example, we expect schizophrenics to behave bizarrely, to hallucinate, and to have strange affect, then people who are labeled thus will behave in this manner. The integration of Ullmann and Krasner's sociopsychological learning theory with these concepts results in a model which purports to explain schizophrenic behavior as a learned response to society's reactions to deviance.

There is little question that some behaviors that individuals with schizophrenic disorders exhibit are learned. In addition, the incidence rates of schizophrenia have been reported to vary from culture to culture (H. B. M. Murphy, 1968). For example, one study found the incidence of schizophrenia per thousand adults to be 3.5 for Chinese adults and 13.1 for a traditional French-Canadian community. This substantial variation suggests that differences in these cultures may have influenced the amount of schizophrenia present. Or does it? Perhaps in the French-Canadian community, intermarriage led to a limited genetic pool, which resulted in a greater likelihood of a genetic predisposition to schizophrenia. Unfortunately, the data are not sufficient for us to make such a judgment.

A compounding problem in studies of cross-cultural incidence involves the diagnosis of schizophrenia. We do not know if schizophrenia in the Chinese sample and schizophrenia in the French-Canadian sample were diagnosed according to the same criteria. Perhaps the French-Canadian diagnosis included a broader spectrum of behavior in the criteria for schizophrenia and, therefore, found more schizophrenics in the population. You will recall that in the World Health Organization International Pilot Study of Schizophrenia (Sartorius, Shapiro, & Jablensky, 1974), when a well-defined narrow description of schizophrenia was used, the primary symptoms were present in subjects in all nine countries. Schizophrenia apparently exists in all cultures—from the extremely primitive to the most industrially advanced. While the major symptoms of schizophrenia seem common to all cultures, there is some evidence that the content of some symptoms, such as hallucinations or delusions, may be culturally determined. For example, religious delusions seem more frequent in Roman Catholic cultures, and are low in frequency in Buddhist cultures, (H. B. M. Murphy et al., 1963). A common delusion in individuals in Latin American countries is that of possession by the devil (León, 1975), a delusion not as frequently seen in the United States and Europe.

The importance of social factors in the development of schizophrenia has received support from studies of the incidence of schizophrenia in various socioeconomic classes. In one classic study, Faris and Dunham (1939), two sociologists, found higher rates for severe mental disorder in lower-class inner-city areas. The rates of schizophrenia decreased in higher-status areas at the fringe of the city. These findings have been frequently replicated. Does this imply that socioeconomic class membership is a factor in schizophrenia? Possibly, but another explanation has been advanced, called the **drift phenomenon.** Several studies (e.g., Gerard & Houston, 1953; L. Levy & Rowitz, 1973; R. J. Turner & Wagonfeld, 1967) have generated data that the higher proportion of people with schizophrenia in the lower socioeconomic classes may be due to the drifting of middle- and upper-class schizophrenics to lower socioeconomic neighborhoods after their schizophrenia develops. Many such individuals may find that their inability to work and support themselves, and their bizarre behavior, are more acceptable in the inner-city areas. The studies cited above found that the parents of schizophrenics were often from a higher socioeconomic class than the adult child who manifested the disorder. In other cases, the drift may have occurred across many generations. Schizophrenia may result in downward social drift.

Not all schizophrenics in the lower socioeconomic classes have drifted there. An alternative explanation of this higher incidence is that the stress of a lower-class life of poverty leads to more mental disorder. The concept that the stresses of poverty lead to schizophrenia is attractive to those who feel that no human being should be subjected to a poverty life-style, but the evidence for such a concept remains weak. The stresses of lower socioeconomic class membership may be a contributing factor, but they do not appear to be sufficient as a sole etiological explanation of schizophrenic behavior. The same can be said of the theory that schizophrenia is a result of society's reaction to social deviance—that the individual is behaving in the manner expected of someone who is labeled "schizophrenic." A satisfactory explanation of the major deficits in schizophrenia will require more than is offered by the theories presented so far.

Biological Theories of Schizophrenia

For at least a century many theoreticians have suspected that schizophrenic behavior is due at least in part to an underlying physiological disturbance of the human organism. Even in the absence of sufficient evidence, some theorists and clinicians took an extremely dogmatic view that this disorder was primarily caused by an organic malfunction. As we have seen, some proponents of psychosocial approaches have taken an equally dogmatic but opposite viewpoint. The biological perspective has conceptualized schizophrenia as caused by among other things, a genetic abnormality, toxins (poisons) in the blood, an infectious virus, a major vitamin deficiency, deterioration of brain tissue, and biochemical malfunction of neural transmission.

The early research which supported these ideas was often poor in its methodology, and subject to much criticism. The questionable nature of much of this research left great room for doubt about the findings. As a result, workers in the field continued for many years to conceptualize schizophrenia as an entirely psychosocial disorder. However, during the last 30 years, and especially during the last 15 years, some very adequate research has shown clearly that biological factors play an important role in the etiology of schizophrenia. We must be careful to remember that these biological factors are probably not the exclusive causes of schizophrenia. In the following section, the findings about biological factors in schizophrenia will be examined. The focus will be on heredity, biochemistry, and high risk studies in schizophrenia.

RESEARCH ON THE HEREDITY, BIOCHEMISTRY, AND HIGH RISK FACTORS OF SCHIZOPHRENIA

Heredity

For many years, responsible professionals have attempted to convince the public that mental illness is not inherited, since there is no evidence that a specific mental illness (e.g., schizophrenia) is *directly* transmitted genetically. However, substantial evidence exists that a predisposition to schizophrenia is due in some degree to genetic endowment. Before considering the implications of this evidence, we will examine how the data were determined.

Family Studies. In 1916, Rudin published the first of the family studies of schizophrenia. In a family study, the relatives of a person with schizophrenia (the index case, or **proband**) are studied to determine if they have a greater incidence of the disorder than the general population. If they do, the data are taken to indicate that the disorder has a genetic component. The risk of schizophrenia for different classes of relatives, as determined in two well-regarded studies, is shown in Table 13.1 (S. Kessler, 1980). For all the close relatives of a schizophrenic, the risk for schizophrenia is much higher than the general population's risk of about 1 percent. The risk for relatives is graded: Closer relatives show a higher risk than more distant relatives. We would expect this finding if genetic transmission were a factor. Close relatives share more genes than distant relatives.

Many family studies have found that even though most relatives of schizophrenics do not manifest schizophrenia, even these relatives manifest disorders called **schizophrenic spectrum disorders,** which include schizoid and inadequate personality disorders and "borderline" schizophrenia. These findings have been supported by a long-term study of 208 schizophrenic subjects, their 184 children, and 205 grandchildren. The study was conducted by Manfred Bleuler (1974), the son of Eugen Bleuler and a well-known psychiatrist in his own right. He found that the children of schizophrenics were 10 times as likely to become schizophrenic as children in the general population. However, he emphasized that of the 184 children of the schizophrenics, only 10 became schizophrenic, and 174 led reasonably adaptive lives. Of the 174, 18 percent had "unfavorable personality development," while in a control group drawn from the general population, 5 percent had unfavorable personality development. Bleuler feels that this is a much less pessimistic outcome than many other studies have found, and his study is quite significant in this respect.

Although the data from family studies suggest genetic transmission of a possible predisposition to schizophrenia, another interpretation is possible. Since the schizophrenic's children (and other relatives) are exposed to the family, their disordered behavior might be

Table 13.1
Estimates of the risk for schizophrenia among relatives of schizophrenics (percent)[1]

	D. Rosenthal (1970)	*Slater and Cowie (1971)*
Parents	4.2	4.4
Sibs (neither parent affected)	6.7	8.2
Sibs (one parent affected)	12.5	13.8
All sibs	7.5	8.5
Children	9.7	12.3
Children (both parents affected)	35.0	36.6–46.3
Half-sibs	—	3.2
Aunts and uncles	1.7	2.0
Nephews and nieces	2.3	2.3
Grandchildren	2.6	2.8
First cousins	1.7	2.9

From S. Kessler, (1980, p. 405).
[1]Risk in general population is usually estimated at 1 percent (Cancro, 1979).

due to disordered child-rearing practices and other influences of being raised by or having long-term relationships with a schizophrenic. Family studies cannot really separate genetic effects from psychosocial effects. Another approach must be utilized.

Twin Studies. Studies of twin pairs in which one twin is known to manifest schizophrenia have been implemented, since they control for the environmental factors which exist in family studies. Twin studies assume that each twin of the pair has such a similar environmental experience with the other that the environmental effects are cancelled out. Two types of twins are studied: monozygotic, or identical, twins, and dizygotic, or fraternal, twins. Identical twins have an identical genetic inheritance, and fraternal twins are genetically no more similar than ordinary siblings. If schizophrenia has a genetic component, then identical twins, but not fraternal twins, should be concordant. That is, if one twin has a diagnosis of schizophrenia, the other twin would be concordant if he or she had the same diagnosis. The concordance rates from a number of major twin studies are shown in Table 13.2.

The impressive differences in concordance rates for schizophrenia between identical and fraternal twins suggests a genetic factor in this disorder. However, the fact that the concordance rates for identical twins are less than 100 percent is strong evidence that genetic factors are not the only important factors. The data indicate that environmental factors play a major role in the etiology of schizophrenia.

Adoption Studies. Many investigators have criticized twin studies because sibling pairs are raised together, usually by the biological parents; thus, psychosocial environmental differences may *still* be a factor, even though we may assume that the co-twins have similar environments. In order to totally eliminate environmental factors, adoption studies have been utilized. The study of adopted biological children of schizophrenics should provide us with data free of the confounding issue of the psychosocial influences of life with a schizophrenic or disturbed parent. In adoption studies, the early removal of a child from a biological parent who is schizophrenic prevents the psychological transmission of the disorder.

An alternative method of study is to identify schizophrenic adults who were raised by adoptive parents and then determine the incidence of schizophrenia in the person's adoptive family and biological family. If a schizophrenic predisposition is inherited, more of these disorders should occur among the biological relatives of the adoptive schizophrenic than among the biological relatives of matched non-

Table 13.2
Concordance rates of schizophrenia in twin studies

Study	*Number of pairs of twins*		*Concordance (percent of twin pairs diagnosed as schizophrenic)*	
	IDENTICAL	FRATERNAL	IDENTICAL	FRATERNAL
Inouye (1961), Japan	55	11	60	18
Kringlen (1967), Norway	55	90	25	4
Tienari (1971), Finland	19	20	16	5
M. Fischer (1973), Denmark	21	41	24	10
Gottesman and Shields (1972), England	24	33	42	9

schizophrenic subjects. However, if schizophrenic disorders are psychosocially transmitted, more schizophrenic adults should have adoptive relatives (those who raised them) with schizophrenia than should matched nonschizophrenic subjects (D. Rosenthal, 1971).

One of the first studies to focus on adopted children of schizophrenic mothers was reported by Heston (1966), who studied a group of 47 individuals born to schizophrenic women in mental hospitals. The subjects had been separated from their mothers at birth and placed in foster homes. A matched group of 50 controls was selected from children whose mothers had no psychiatric disorder, but had placed them in the same foundling home (thus, the two groups of children had similar environments). Three independent psychiatric examinations were done on all subjects, including psychological testing on the Minnesota Multiphasic Personality Inventory (MMPI) and an IQ test. Five of the experimental group (10 percent) were diagnosed as schizophrenic, but none of the control group was found to have the disorder. In addition, the biological children of schizophrenic mothers were more likely to be diagnosed as mentally retarded, sociopathic, or neurotic. The study provided early support for the importance of genetic factors in schizophrenia.

More recent adoption studies have consistently supported Heston's findings. Beginning with David Rosenthal (1971), investigators have used an Adoptive Register and a Psychiatric Register in Denmark to study genetic contributions to schizophrenia. Denmark, a country with a great emphasis on social services, maintains accurate and comprehensive records of names, residence, and health statistics on its citizens. D. Rosenthal et al. (1975) identified almost 5,500 adoptees and their roughly 10,000 biological parents. The records of these parents and offspring were then extracted from a psychiatric registry, a listing of all persons in Denmark treated for psychiatric disorders. Such a project would be impossible in the United States, since the country lacks these types of central registries.

After searching the records, the researchers were able to identify 76 index cases: adopted offspring who had a biological parent known to be schizophrenic. The index cases were matched with 67 control cases: adopted offspring whose biological parents were known to be free of a psychiatric history. Of the adopted offspring of schizophrenic parents, 30 percent were found to have a diagnosis of schizophrenia or schizophrenic spectrum disorder, as compared to 17.8 percent of the controls. A later refinement of the criteria of schizophrenia or schizophrenic spectrum disorder led to percentages of 21.9 percent of index cases and 6.3 percent of controls manifesting the disorders (Haier, Rosenthal, & Wender, 1978).

In a variant of this type of study, Kety et al. (1976) used the same population to identify a group of adoptees who had become schizophrenic, and then tracked down their biological parents to see what percentage of these parents were schizophrenic. Kety et al. then compared

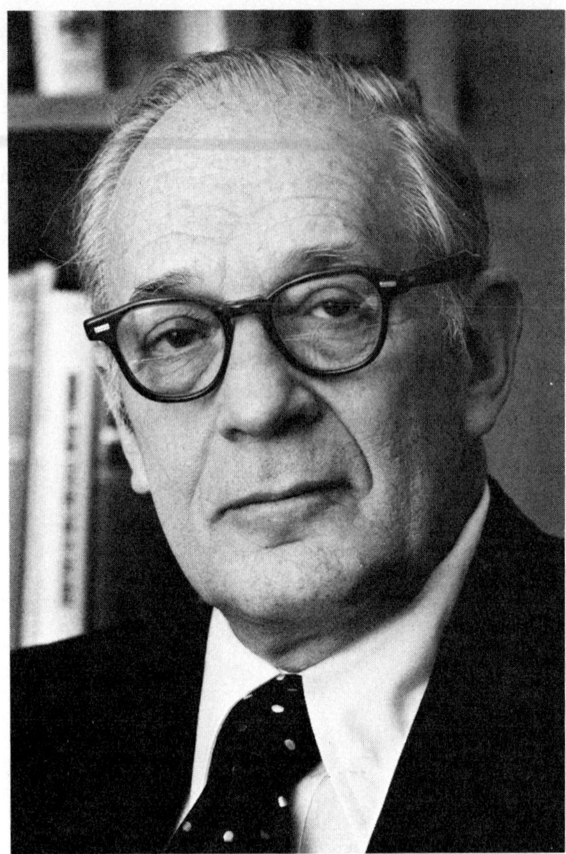

Seymour Kety, a researcher, who has studied genetic and other biological factors in schizophrenia.

these findings with a study of control adoptees' parents (the control adoptees had no psychiatric history). They found that the biological parents of schizophrenic adoptees were more likely to be schizophrenic than were the biological or adoptive parents of controls or the adoptive parents of the schizophrenics (see Table 13.3). In addition, the other biological relatives of the schizophrenic adoptees (such as sibs or half-sibs) were also more likely to manifest schizophrenic spectrum disorders than the adoptive relatives of the schizophrenics, or the biological relatives of the control adoptees. This finding has been given strong support by replication studies (e.g., Kendler, Gruenberg, & Straus, 1981a). If disordered child rearing were the primary issue, one would expect more disorder in the adoptive relatives than in the biological relatives, since the adoptees had been raised by and were in contact with the adoptive relatives, not the biological relatives.

Table 13.3
Parents diagnosed as definite or possible schizophrenics

	Number	*Percent schizophrenic*
Biological parents of schizophrenic adoptees	173	13.9
Biological parents of control (normal) adoptees	174	3.4
Adoptive parents of schizophrenic adoptees	74	2.7
Adoptive parents of control (normal) adoptees	91	5.5

From Kety et al. (1976).

While these studies demonstrate that psychopathology in biological parents is an important factor even when offspring are raised by "nonpathological" adoptive parents, what about the reverse? Is child rearing by a pathological parent likely to lead to schizophrenia in a child who is not likely to have an inherited genetic component? Wender et al (1974) studied this issue, once again using the Danish population. In this study, a group of 69 adoptees born to schizophrenic parents and a matched group of 69 control adoptees born to parents with no record of psychiatric problems were compared to 28 adoptees whose biological parents were not schizophrenic but who were *adopted* into families with a schizophrenic adoptive parent. This last group is called a cross-fostered group. The results of this study indicated that being reared by a schizophrenic adoptive parent does not increase the risk of schizophrenia in the offspring unless a genetic predisposition is already present.

Such studies cannot *prove* that there is an inherited predisposition in schizophrenia. However, these studies are very strong from a methodological standpoint, and many find them compelling. S. Kessler (1980) summarizes the prevailing opinion about genetic factors in schizophrenia:

> Individual studies—family, twin, adoption—all contain methodological problems and flaws, and can be subjected to greater or lesser

> criticism. Nevertheless, the overwhelming direction of the findings of all these studies, carried out in different countries and at different times, is remarkably consistent in confirming that genetic factors are involved in the etiology of schizophrenia. Also, these studies confirm that although in many cases a genetic predisposition to schizophrenia may be a necessary precondition, it is by no means a sufficient condition to produce the disorder. Both genes and environment play a substantial role in the etiology of schizophrenia. (p. 411)

Perhaps without *some* genetic predisposition a person will not become schizophrenic under any circumstances, no matter how great the stresses he or she may experience. With a moderate genetic predisposition, an individual may become schizophrenic or may not, depending upon the environmental contribution to the disorder. And if there is a strong genetic predisposition, a person may become schizophrenic under environmental conditions which might seem average to most of us.

Biochemistry of Schizophrenia

The possibility that individuals who manifest schizophrenic behavior are suffering from some biochemical malfunction has received a great deal of study. Many different factors have been identified as possible etiological agents, and in the excitement of the moment have been trumpeted by the popular press and media as the "cause" of schizophrenia. Unfortunately, most of these "discoveries" were not supported by further research.

For example, Heath and colleagues (1958) implicated abnormal plasma proteins (gamma globulins) in the blood as a causative agent. They isolated such a substance, called taraxein, in the blood of schizophrenics. In a startling experiment, they injected this substance (obtained from the blood of schizophrenic patients) into normal subjects (volunteers), who then displayed schizophrenic behavior. Although it created a major stir, this study has never been successfully replicated. Subsequent critics have suggested that Heath's original volunteer subjects somehow were aware of the experimenter's expectations of what the injections would do (produce schizophrenic behavior) and therefore behaved "schizophrenically" to meet those expectations.

Another example of a substance once implicated in the development of schizophrenics is nicotinic acid (part of the B vitamin complex). Hoffer et al. (1957) concluded that schizophrenia may be due to a vitamin deficiency. This line of investigation was partly stimulated by an awareness that such vitamin deficiency disorders as scurvy or pellagra, when severe, are associated with psychotic behavior. Hoffer (1966) administered large dosages of vitamins to schizophrenics and found that a large percentage improved in their behavior. His work resulted in an approach to the treatment of schizophrenia called **orthomolecular psychiatry,** which uses megavitamin (large dosages of vitamins) therapy. The approach and the underlying concept have not been adequately supported by research evidence, and several experts in biochemical psychiatry consider it essentially worthless (Ban & Lehmann, 1970; Ban, 1973). A small group of orthomolecular psychiatrists still maintain the approach, in spite of the surrounding controversy.

More current research on the biochemistry of schizophrenia has focused on the biochemical activity involved in the transmission of nerve impulses. Since no disorders of neural tissue (nerve cells and nerve fibers) have been reliably found in schizophrenics, many researchers have focused on substances called **neurotransmitters.** At the point where a nerve fiber ends, a small gap exists between it and the beginning of the next nerve fiber. This space is called the **synaptic cleft** (see Figure 13.2). When a neural impulse reaches a nerve ending, a chemical neurotransmitter is released across the synaptic cleft. This neurotransmitter activates the next nerve ending, sending an impulse on its way. Over 20 different chemical neurotransmitters have been identified, and they have different concentrations in various parts of the brain. One of the most important neurotransmitters in the research on schizophrenia is **dopamine,** a member of the chemical catecholamine family (Carlson, 1978).

Dopamine Theory. In the mid 1950s, the family of drugs called **phenothiazines** were found to have a significant effect on schizophrenic behavior. These drugs reduce the symptoms of flattened affect, withdrawal, and thought dis-

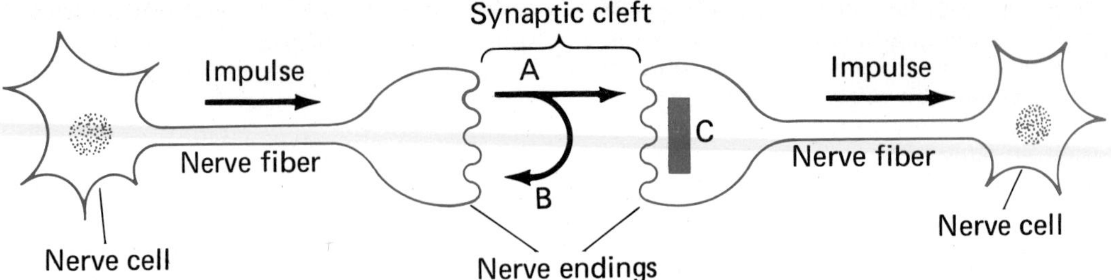

Figure 13.2. Neural transmission.
Neurotransmitter is released (A); some neurotransmitter is "saved" and stored by the re-uptake mechanism (B); neurotransmitter molecules travel across the synaptic cleft and attach themselves to a receptor site on the next nerve ending, activating a nerve impulse which travels along that nerve fiber (C).

order; they are less effective with delusions, hallucinations, and disorientation, and seem to have little effect on depression and anxiety. Although large dosages seem to have a sedative effect, (e.g., causing sleep), this does not seem to be the primary reason for their effectiveness with the schizophrenic behaviors. A great deal of research has demonstrated that phenothiazines primarily affect the transmission of neural impulses by dopamine (e.g., Horn & Snyder, 1971).

The research on the effects of the phenothiazines indicates that they block the receptor sites in the nerve endings which are sensitive to dopamine. Therefore, it has been suggested that at least some symptoms of schizophrenia are due to the presence of an excess of the neurotransmitter dopamine. This excess, when blocked by the phenothiazines, cannot overactivate the neural receptors, and symptoms are reduced.

Additional indirect support for this theory comes from the study of amphetamine psychosis. Behavior which is similar to paranoid schizophrenia occurs from the prolonged use of amphetamines (see Chapter 10). In addition, amphetamine use by individuals with a schizophrenic disorder can cause a dramatic increase in their symptoms (Angrist, Lee, & Gershon, 1974). These effects have been found to be due to something other than the general stimulating effects of the drug (Angrist & Gershon, 1970). The weight of evidence indicates that amphetamines block the re-uptake mechanism of both dopamine and another neurotransmitter, norepinephrine (Snyder, 1974). The stimulating effects of amphetamines seem to be due to the increase of norepinephrine, while the schizophrenic-like symptoms have been related to the increase in dopamine in the synaptic cleft (see Figure 13.2).

The research into the relation of dopamine to schizophrenia has suggested that an excessive production of dopamine is less likely to be the issue than is an excessive sensitivity to dopamine at the receptor site. That is, schizophrenics do not have too much dopamine, but are too sensitive to it (Post et al., 1975; Snyder, 1976).

What might cause the oversensitivity of neural receptor sites to dopamine? Some startling findings in brain chemistry have suggested some answers. In 1973 Solomon Snyder and Candace Pert of Johns Hopkins University announced that they had discovered opiate receptor sites in the brain. These sites were like molecular "locks," into which opiate molecules fit like "keys." This discovery was highly significant for theories of morphine and heroin addiction, as we have seen in Chapter 10. It has since been discovered that the human brain produces its own morphine-like substances, called **endorphins,** which fit into these opiate receptor sites (Hughes, 1975). Studies of the endorphins' effects on brain tissue have indicated that some endorphins affect the activity of dopamine (Loh et al., 1976). These discoveries have led to a great deal of research and speculation on the importance of endorphins to dopamine activity. Either a deficit or excess of endorphins can lead to heightened sensitivity of the dopaminergic receptors, and this sensitivity may be a contributing factor to the apparent overactivity of dopamine-sensitive neurons which appear to be present in schizophrenics (Volavka, Davis, & Ehrlich, 1979; S. J. Watson et al., 1979). These data remain highly speculative, and the specific findings vary from study to study. Many researchers who are investigating the relationship between endorphins and dopamine receptor sites urge that conclusions be postponed until more data are collected (Usdin, 1979; S. J. Watson & Akil, 1979).

The evidence supporting a theory of oversensitive dopamine receptor sites is not the only evidence available. The theory of an overabundance of dopamine in the synaptic cleft is still being studied by many researchers. For example, one group is focusing on the possibility that a deficiency of the enzyme monoamine oxidase may lead to an excess of dopamine in the cleft, and some research does support this theory (Wyatt et al., 1980).

Solomon Snyder investigates the effects of brain chemicals, like the model of the one he is holding, on schizophrenia.

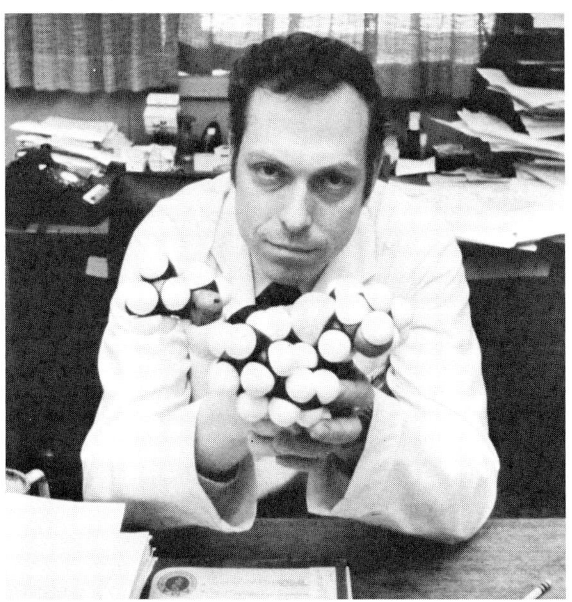

The biochemical theories of schizophrenia are quite complicated and difficult to understand unless one is well versed in biochemistry. Their very complexity may lead to an uncritical acceptance of a simplistic notion of causality—for example, that schizophrenia is a result of: 1. an excess of dopamine in the synaptic cleft or 2. a supersensitivity to normal levels of dopamine in the receptor site. While support is strong for these possibilities, we do not know yet that they are the primary cause of schizophrenia or whether they are secondary effects of some other factor. We do not know the answers to many questions. What is inherited? How does dopamine activity result in the symptoms of schizophrenia? This, too, cannot be answered as yet. Does dopaminergic activity precede the overt schizophrenia, develop as the symptoms develop, or follow their development? There is presently no answer to this question either. Many questions remain, and the biochemical research which is under way and which will proceed in the future may answer them soon; or these questions may be too complicated for answers in the near future.

Contributions from High Risk Research: The Danish High Risk Studies

The vast majority of research on the schizophrenic disorders has a common problem. Although it can often demonstrate significant differences between schizophrenics and nonschizophrenics, it cannot unequivocally reveal whether these differences are the cause or the result of the disorder. Why is this so? A primary factor is that the studies have been done on subjects who already have developed the disorder. We cannot tell, for example, if a problem in attention span displayed by schizophrenics existed in those same individuals before the onset of the disorder. Retrospective studies, in which one checks *back* into a person's history, are liable to be inaccurate, since the relevant data are not likely to have been kept with any accuracy.

Studies done on the adoptive children of schizophrenic mothers have already been mentioned. These studies were implemented in Denmark and other sites to deal with the problem of retrospective data (Mednick &

Schulsinger, 1968; Sobel, 1961). Studies of the children of schizophrenic parents are known as high risk studies, since the children are more likely to be at risk for the development of schizophrenia than children of nonschizophrenic parents; most genetic studies have found that 1 in 10 children of schizophrenic parents is likely to become schizophrenic. Based on this proportion, if we wanted to study 100 children who would later become schizophrenic, we would have to select 1,000 children from families with a schizophrenic parent. Our study would then have to be applied to *all* 1,000 children in order to obtain complete developmental data on the 100 who would later become schizophrenic. While this may seem like a great deal of work, if we decided to obtain our 100 children who would later become schizophrenic from the general population, we would have to implement our research with *10,000* children to obtain results on 100 who as adults would be schizophrenic.

The high risk studies have the advantage of saving time and energy when we want to study individuals who are not yet schizophrenic but who later will be. The primary procedure currently being used to select high risk children is, as we have noted, to identify schizophrenic mothers and select their children for study. The focus is on schizophrenia in mothers rather than fathers, since we can be sure that the mother contributed her genes to the child, while paternity is not always certain (a child could be the result of a union with someone other than woman's schizophrenic husband). Other procedures for identifying children at risk for schizophrenia could be used, such as identifying children of families in which there is double-bind communication. However, the genetic selection approach is most commonly used, partly because it has been so successful. It does have a distinct disadvantage: Only about 10 percent of people with schizophrenia have a parent (or parents) who has been diagnosed as schizophrenic. Thus, the results of these studies may not be generalizable to 90 percent of the persons who develop schizophrenia (Keith et al., 1976). This must be kept in mind while we consider the results of such studies, but most authorities believe that the results are generalizable to most people who develop a schizophrenic disorder.

The Initial Studies. The first major high risk study was initiated by Sarnoff Mednick, an American, and Fini Schulsinger, a Dane, in Denmark in 1962 (Mednick & Schulsinger, 1968, 1973; Mednick, Schulsinger, & Schulsinger, 1975). Important findings in this study have been reported by various groups of authors over the years. In this series of studies, 207 children (the high risk group) of schizophrenic mothers were compared to 104 children of nonschizophrenic mothers. Each high risk child was matched to a low risk child on a number of variables (e.g., age, social class, sex). The early studies found a number of differences in these two groups of children. For example, the high risk children had more often had difficult births (prematurity, oxygen deprivation, prolonged labor). At the time, a finding which created a great deal of excitement was that the high risk children manifested a mild disorder of association. They gave more rhyming associations, and associations to their own words, than low risk children. This seemed to support the idea that associative disturbance was not due to schizophrenia, but preceded it.

Within five years, some children were identified as showing very abnormal behavior (not necessarily schizophrenia). These 20 high risk subjects became known as the "HR sick group" and were matched with 20 high risk subjects who did not show problems in adjustment, called the "HR well group." In order to find out why these groups were different, the investigators turned to the data from five years before and compared the groups. They came up with a number of interesting findings.

Findings about Mothers. The schizophrenic mothers of the HR sick group were hospitalized when their children were younger than those in the HR well group, and they had had more severe symptoms. These mothers' hospitalizations had also occurred when the mother was younger, compared to the hospitalizations of the mothers in the HR well group. In addition, the HR sick group mothers had more difficulty with the birth of their child. A later study based on the same data (Talovic, 1980) found that HR sick group mothers were likely to have had a schizophrenic episode in childbirth, suggesting that their adjustment was even more tenuous than the mothers of the HR well group. The HR sick group mothers were more likely to have poorer relationships with males than the HR well group mothers. Taken together, these findings suggest that the HR sick group mothers were more adversely affected by their disorder than the HR well group, even though many of the immediate symptoms of psychosis in both groups of mothers were equally severe.

Associative Disturbances. Early assessment of the data indicated that the HR sick group children tended to drift away from stimulus words on an association test to a greater extent than the HR well group children. A reanalysis of these data (Griffith et al., 1980) has indicated, however, that these conclusions were in error. The associative deficits in the total high risk group were greater than in the low risk group; but when the HR sick group was compared with the HR well group, there was no difference in the amount of associative disturbance between the groups. This finding strongly suggests that associative disturbances do not differentiate the premorbid functioning of those who eventually become schizophrenic from the high risk persons who do not.

Physiological Differences. The HR sick group was found to have experienced more complications of birth or pregnancy (70 percent) than the HR well group (15 percent) or the low risk group (33 percent). In addition, the HR sick group tended to show signs of physiological overreactivity. They showed greater reactivity to stimuli, greater generalization of conditioning, and less adaptation to stimuli. These findings supported the theory of schizophrenia proposed by Mednick (1958). He had suggested that schizophrenia was due to heightened arousal or anxiety acting as a drive which would lead the individual to overattend to stimuli and be overwhelmed. Mednick suggested that the overarousal was due to brain damage from birth and pregnancy complications. The theory has found only limited support in other studies (P. Kessler & Neale, 1974; Salzman & Klein, 1978).

These Danish studies (and other high risk studies; e.g., Asarnow, Steffy, & MacCrimmon, 1977; Hanson, Gottesman, & Hester, 1976) are making major contributions to our understanding of the premorbid characteristics of schizophrenics. Perhaps this methodology will enable us to identify with more certainty the primary deficits of schizophrenia. The longitudinal approach to the study of schizophrenia can offer something that cross-sectional studies cannot. By following high risk individuals from early childhood, we may gain an idea of which deficits are present before the onset of a schizophrenic disorder, and which contribute to the development of the disorder. The potential for this type of research is so important that many research agencies are giving priority to new high risk studies.

WHERE DOES SCHIZOPHRENIA COME FROM? THE VULNERABILITY HYPOTHESIS

So far, we have reviewed a broad, possibly bewildering array of theories and research on the etiology of schizophrenia. We will soon look at some current treatment approaches for this disorder, but first we need to place the data and theories into a unified framework. For this purpose, the **vulnerability hypothesis** will be used. The lack of unquestionable evidence for any one theory of schizophrenia, and the presence of significant evidence for many major theories of schizophrenia, have led Joseph Zubin (Zubin & Spring, 1977; Zubin & Steinhauer, 1981) to propose that the important issue is not the presence of the disorder of schizophrenia, but persons' vulnerability to this disorder. Zubin and Spring (1977) state:

> The vulnerability model proposes that each of us is endowed with a degree of vulnerability that under suitable circumstances will express itself in an episode of schizophrenic illness. Each etiological model offers suggestions about the possible origins of such vulnerability.
>
> . . . there are two major components of vulnerability, the inborn and the acquired. . . . we have described inborn vulnerability as that which is laid down in the genes and reflected in the internal environment and neurophysiology of the organism. The acquired compo-

> nent of vulnerability is due to the influence of traumas, specific diseases, [birth] complications, family experiences, adolescent peer interactions, and other life events that either enhance or inhibit the development of subsequent disorder. (p. 109)
>
> [Figure 13.3] shows the hypothesized relation between life event stressors and vulnerability. As long as the stress induced by the challenging life event stays below the threshold of vulnerability, the individual responds to the stressor in an elastic homeostatic way and remains well within the limits of normality. When the stress exceeds threshold, the person is likely to develop a psychopathological episode of some sort. Further, we postulate that the episode is time limited. When the stress abates and sinks below the vulnerability threshold, the episode ends and the patient returns to a state similar to his pre-episode level of adaptation. (p. 110)
>
> . . . the challenge is to find ways of reducing vulnerability or improving the coping abilities and competence of the vulnerable poor premorbids so that the likelihood of future episodes can be reduced. Even if an episode does occur, the rehabilitated patient will have a better level of coping to return to when the episode passes. (p. 122)

The concept of vulnerability provides a framework from which we can attempt to understand the development of schizophrenic behavior, and from which we can attempt to help individuals who are vulnerable to the disorder. As Zubin has pointed out, not everyone who is vulnerable manifests the disorder. Those who do cannot postpone their need for assistance until research efforts reveal a primary deficit. Nor can society afford to simply lock such persons away until a cure is found.

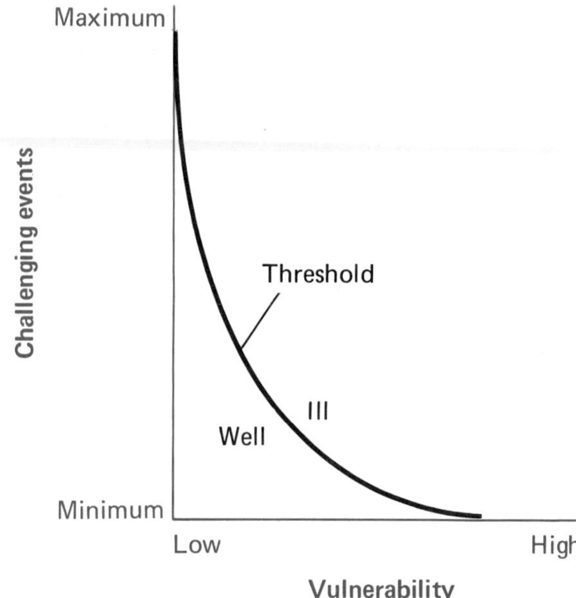

Figure 13.3. Relation between vulnerability and stress in the development of schizophrenic disorders.

When stress exceeds the vulnerability threshold, the individual will manifest the disorder. Individuals with low vulnerability must encounter maximum levels of stress before the disorder appears. Minimal levels of stress may lead to the disorder in persons with high vulnerability.

Adapted from Zubin and Steinhauer (1981, p. 481).

KEY TREATMENTS

A review of historical aspects of abnormal behavior (Chapter 2) over the ages has shown that a wide variety of strategies have been used in response to what we call schizophrenia. This remains true today. Many different treatment approaches are applied to schizophrenic behavior. When the behavior disorder is severe (as it often is), the individual is usually treated in a residential setting: a public or private mental hospital. However, most persons who manifest a schizophrenic disorder are not treated in these types of hospitals. Of the 2–3 million schizophrenics in the United States, at any one time only about 100,000 are hospitalized. The current total population of private and public mental hospitals in the United States is slightly less than 200,000, so we can see that schizophrenics make up about one-half of all those in these hospitals. Many criticisms have been raised regarding the appropriateness and effectiveness of treatment in mental hospitals. These issues are addressed in Chapter 21, since they are not specific to schizophrenia, but are relevant for persons who manifest any behavior that results in admission to a mental hospital. Here we concern ourselves with specific treatment approaches for schizophrenics either within residential settings or the larger, public community. These treatments can be separated into two broad categories: biologically focused treatments and psychosocially focused treatments.

Biologically focused treatments

Several theories propose that schizophrenia is due primarily to some dysfunction of human biology. However, the current biologically based therapies were not developed from research based on specific biological theories. The reverse occurred: Many theories were initially developed because these biological treatments worked. Later research was based on the theories, and new treatments have been developed specifically as a result of this theory-based research.

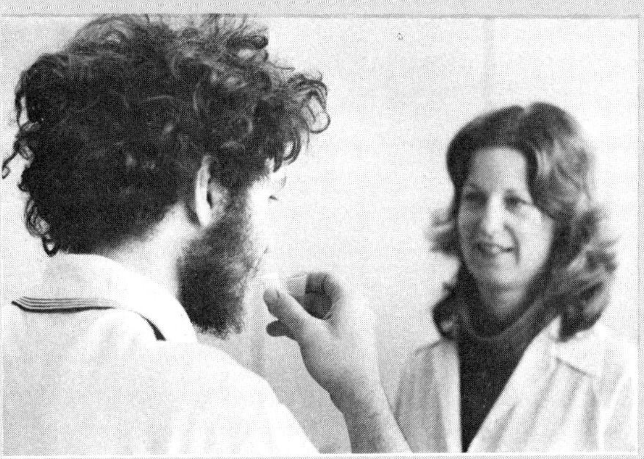

The use of major tranquilizers is a common treatment for reducing the symptoms of schizophrenia.

Chemotherapy. During 1950–1955, a family of drugs was discovered which led to major changes in dealing with persons who manifest schizophrenic behavior. These drugs are commonly (but mistakenly) called the major tranquilizers. Their tranquilizing effects are not their most important characteristic. They are more appropriately called the **antipsychotic drugs.** The most commonly used antipsychotic drug is a phenothiazine called chlorpromazine, which is sold under the brand name Thorazine. These drugs have been so important that the National Institute of Mental Health (1975) considers them one of the two most significant discoveries in the 25 years from 1950 to 1975.

The phenothiazines were among the earliest antipsychotic drugs used, and continue to be the most commonly prescribed. Since they are the most common, this discussion will focus on them. The phenothiazines can reduce psychomotor excitement, agitation, delusions and hallucinations, tension, combativeness, hostility, negativism, poor sleep patterns, and social withdrawal. However, they do not seem to lead to much improvement in insight, judgment, memory, or orientation.

In a controlled **double-blind study,** Spohn and associates (1977) studied the specific effects of the phenothiazines. A double-blind study is structured so that neither the experimenter nor the subject knows whether the treatment (in this case, the drug) is active or a **placebo** (a neutral substance which has no relevant biochemical effect). This type of study guarantees that neither the subjects' nor the experimenter's expectations will influence the results in a systematic way. In this study, 20 chronic schizophrenics were given a phenothiazine (chlorpromazine) and compared to 20 matched schizophrenic controls who received a placebo.

At the end of the study, the experimenters were informed which groups had received the actual medication. This treatment group was found to have significantly improved behavior, while the control group (who had not received the phenothiazine) had become worse. An eight-week period of medication had also led to the following specific changes: 1. the treated group was better able to attend to visual tasks requiring continuous concentration, 2. the treated group's ability to correctly perceive visual stimuli under varying lengths of presentation improved, 3. the treated group's physiological response to stressors decreased. Many studies have found similar results, which suggest that the antipsychotic drugs help the patient to filter out distracting stimuli. Most theorists (and much research) suggest that these drugs act by decreasing the activity of the dopaminergic system of neurotransmitters.

Much of the credit (or criticism) for the tremendous decrease in mental hospital populations since the mid-1950s must go to the antipsychotic drugs. The moderation of severely disturbed behaviors assisted many helping professionals to accept the notion that many of the patients residing in hospitals could live in the community. However, in order to maintain the positive drug-induced behavioral changes, the drugs must be taken on a long-term, maintenance basis.

Many people who are released from hospitals do not continue to take the medication, and their bizarre behavior usually returns shortly after its discontinuation. Even when the maintenance of medication is assured, the symptoms may return. Schooler et al. (1980) studied 143 patients who were discharged from a mental hospital, as recovered, and who received an injection of a phenothiazine maintenance dose every three weeks at a clinic to assure that they would receive the medication. She and her colleagues compared this group to a group of 147 patients who were also discharged but who were simply given oral medication refills to take home with them to be taken on their own (see Figure 13.4). After one year, only 38 percent of the patients given oral medication had maintained themselves outside of the hospital, and only 46 percent of those who were assured of taking injectable medication stayed out. While other factors may have influenced whether an individual was readmitted, it is clear that the taking of medication did not assure that the symptoms of schizophrenia would not return. Those who were not rehospitalized manifested significantly less psychotic symptomatology than those who were rehospitalized, but 54 percent of those who had taken the injectable medication did have a recurrence of symptoms *even* while taking the medication.

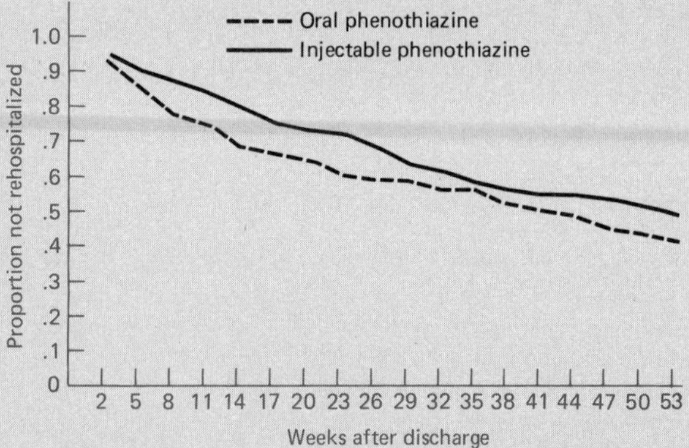

Figure 13.4. Proportion of patients maintaining themselves outside a mental hospital 53 weeks after discharge.

From Schooler et al. (1980, p. 19).

The antipsychotic drugs do not cure schizophrenia; nor can they turn a poorly adjusted, severely disturbed person into a well-adjusted, functioning community member. In this sense, the drugs are a temporary measure, although a valuable one.

A final comment on the antipsychotic drugs relates to side effects. Use of the drugs can result in many problems. There may be drowsiness, dry mouth, blurred vision, impotence, allergic reactions, weight gain, and uncontrollable trembling of the extremities. The disorder **tardive dyskinesia** sometimes occurs in people who take the drugs over long periods. This disorder is apparently irreversible and consists of repetitive involuntary facial movements such as smacking and licking of the lips, sucking movements, chewing movements, rolling and protrusion of the tongue, blinking, grotesque grimaces, spasms of facial muscles; and body movements such as jerking of the fingers, ankles, and toes, and contractions of neck and back muscles. Other major side effects of long-term use of the antipsychotic drugs may be discovered in the near future, since some people have been taking these drugs for more than 25 years.

Electroconvulsive therapy. In Chapter 2, we saw that **electroconvulsive therapy** (ECT or EST) was introduced in 1938 and was widely used in the treatment of schizophrenia. With the introduction of the antipsychotic drugs, there was a significant decline in the popularity of ECT (Fink, 1979). However, ECT is still used (though less so than in the past), particularly in private hospitals and by psychiatrists in private practice. Currently, about 25 percent of psychiatrists consider ECT an appropriate treatment for schizophrenia, and about 60 percent do not (ECT Task Force, 1978).

In the ECT treatment, the subject lies prone, electrodes are placed on one or both temples, and a "dose" of 70–130 volts is given from .1 to .5 seconds. The subject immediately becomes unconscious. With the use of a muscle relaxant drug, the seizure is only minimally noticeable as tremors in the hands and feet. After the treatment, the subject experiences a period of confusion and may have a memory loss of events preceding the treatment. Treatments are usually given several times per week until the problem behaviors or feelings dissipate, and maximum benefit is usually obtained in 5–10 treatments during a period of two to three weeks (Mehr, 1980).

Salzman (1980) has reviewed the use of ECT with schizophrenics; he attributes the renewed interest in ECT to concern over the possible long-term side effects of the antipsychotic drugs. He found that most studies on the effectiveness of ECT were poorly designed, and that it was difficult based on these studies to assess the effectiveness of ECT in comparison to the antipsychotic drugs. The well-controlled studies consistently found that the symptomatic response to ECT was inversely related to the duration of schizophrenic symptoms. That is, ECT worked better with acute-onset schizophrenics than with persons who had been manifesting the symptoms for a prolonged period. Furthermore, ECT worked best with persons who manifested affective and catatonic symptoms. With these types of persons, most studies (including the well-designed ones) demonstrated that ECT effectively reduced schizophrenic symptoms in 40–80 percent of the cases treated. Salzman notes that most studies suggest that ECT is effective for only about 5–10 percent of persons who have manifested schizophrenia for more than two years, and the relapse rates are high.

In a recent well-controlled double-blind study of ECT, P. Taylor and Fleminger (1980) found that patients treated with ECT were more greatly improved after 6 treatments and at the end of therapy (8–12 treatments) than the control patients, who had not received ECT. Both these groups of patients were concurrently treated with antipsychotic drugs. An interesting aspect of the study was the finding that 16 weeks after the beginning of the ECT treatments, the experimental and control groups no longer manifested significantly different degrees of pathology. In other words, the control group's improvement caught up with the group treated by ECT. This study suggests that ECT is of greater benefit only in the short run, and that patients who do not receive ECT improve as much in the long run. This likelihood is significant when one considers the apparently serious potential side effects of this treatment.

One controversial side effect of ECT is memory loss. Many mental health professionals and the public have been extremely critical of this technique, taking the position that the post-ECT loss of memory is sometimes permanent. Some have said the memory loss is cumulative, so that frequent ECT treatments could wipe clean the patient's memories. These claims appear to be exaggerated. The application of ECT disrupts the recall of some events which occurred a few days before treatment, and this memory loss is persistent. In addition, memories of events occurring many years before may also be disrupted, but these memories usually return within a few months after treatment (Squire, Slater, & Miller, 1981). Not all memories are affected, however. The fact that there usually is a loss of some memories, and that not all these memories will return, is an important consideration which must be weighed by therapists and clients before agreeing to this treatment.

Psychosocial treatment

Can the extremely disordered behavior of schizophrenia be treated psychologically? There is much controversy over this issue. Many clinicians (including the author) are convinced that psychosocial treatments have much to contribute to the treatment of schizophrenia. However, the application of these treatments to schizophrenia (and other major psychotic disorders) is an extremely difficult task.

Individual psychotherapy. The traditional psychoanalytic approach is difficult to implement with schizophrenic individuals. Schizophrenics' difficulty in making contact with other human beings necessitates a more active approach on the part of the therapist. In a sense, the therapist must impose himself or herself on the patient. The therapist cannot sit back and wait for the patient to make the first move. Two noted therapists who applied psychoanalytic concepts to the treatment of schizophrenia with some success were Freida Fromm-Reichmann (1952) and Harry Stack Sullivan (1953). Both were very directive, strong human beings with a deep concern for their patients. Both were adept at establishing a warm and giving relationship with the client, were able to tolerate extraordinarily bizarre behavior, and yet were able to see past the behavior to the essential humanity of the disordered individual.

Psychodynamic psychotherapy with individuals who have a schizophrenic disorder is a challenge. One noted therapist who specialized in this technique was Elvin Semrad. Semrad's approach has been reviewed by G. Adler (1979) and can be condensed into three basic points:

1. The therapist's empathic understanding allows the individual with schizophrenia to make human contact, and this contact interferes with the schizophrenic process.
2. Therapy must assist the patient in dealing with a previously unbearable reality, and in recognizing his or her own responsibility for the dilemma.
3. The therapist must both support and frustrate the patient. This creates a setting in which the therapist can help the patient focus on recognizing feelings. Once recognized, the patient's feelings can begin to be integrated into the rest of the personality. As the various aspects of the personality become reintegrated, the therapist can begin to withdraw from the relationship.

The primary issue for the therapist is to create an atmosphere of devoted acceptance and trust in an effort to "reach" the patient. The patient in this atmosphere retrains himself or herself to establish communication with others and to relinquish bizarre individualistic ways of living. With an increased ability to communicate, the patient, through the therapist, gains insight into the genetic and dynamic nature of his or her disorder, and gains self-esteem (Arieti, 1966, 1980). Other individually oriented psychotherapeutic approaches differ somewhat (e.g., the approach of Carl Rog-

HIGHLIGHT 13.3
TREATING SCHIZOPHRENIA BY CLEANSING THE BLOOD?

In 1977, a startling announcement was made. Wagemaker and Cade (1977) had treated a number of chronic schizophrenics with **hemodialysis.** In their uncontrolled study, the six patients treated showed excellent remission of symptoms. This was soon noted in the public media; and once again, many thought that the "cure" for schizophrenia had been found.

Hemodialysis is a medical procedure in which blood is removed from a patient, the toxins are cleaned from the blood by a series of filters, and the blood is returned to the body. The procedure is medically necessary to sustain life in people who have experienced failure of the kidneys, the organs which usually provide this function. The speculation about Wagemaker and Cade's work was that hemodialysis filtered some substance from the blood that caused the symptoms of schizophrenia.

In 11 studies, including Wagemaker and Cade's, 92 schizophrenics have been reported treated by hemodialysis. Of these, 22 improved, 21 partially improved, 47 showed no change, and 2 became worse (Fogelson, Marder, & Van Putten, 1980). While this may sound promising, in the first double-blind study of hemodialysis with schizophrenics, Diaz-Buxo and colleagues (1980) found no difference between patients who were actually dialyzed and those who were given sham dialysis (their blood was removed, but not filtered before being replaced). Diaz-Buxo et al. suggest that alternative explanations for the positive results from previous uncontrolled clinical studies could include: 1. the patients' expected that they would get better when treated with the very complex and sophisticated equipment necessary for hemodialysis; 2. the withdrawal of other medications may have led to improvement (some patients get better when antipsychotic drugs are stopped after having been taken for long periods); or 3. improvement may have been due to the positive effects of the intensive additional attention the patients received while they were being treated and studied.

This double-blind study does not prove that hemodialysis cannot help some schizophrenics, but it raises serious questions about the approach.

ers), but all share the goal of creating a trusting relationship between therapist and patient. When applied to schizophrenics, this goal requires active intervention by the therapist.

A question we must always ask is, Does it work? Mosher and Keith (1979) have reviewed the major outcome studies on psychosocial approaches to schizophrenia, and have found conflicting results. Unfortunately, many studies on the effectiveness of psychotherapy with schizophrenia are seriously flawed. Some provided insufficient exposure to the treatment; others did not adequately define the characteristics of the therapy, the patients, and the therapists; and still others measured success using criteria that were too broad. Many of the studies which demonstrated the utility of psychotherapy with schizophrenics treated patients who were suffering from acute rather than chronic disorders. Most studies have not demonstrated that significant change in chronic schizophrenics occurs through psychotherapy. Mosher and Keith conclude that traditional individual psychotherapy alone appears to be relatively ineffective with serious schizophrenic disorders. However, they found the data for intensive general psychosocial interventions more promising. When the psychotherapeutic approach utilizes extensive attention to the patient's social environment, as in family therapy, the studies tended to find that subjects changed in positive directions. These findings are reflected in the development of alternative treatment programs around the country for schizophrenics which focus

The effectiveness of psychotherapy in treating schizophrenia continues to be debated. However, many patients and therapists believe it is useful.

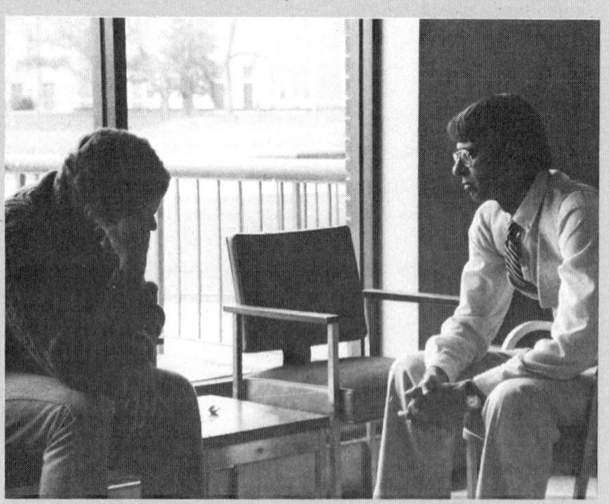

less on traditional individual psychotherapy and more on creating therapeutic environments. These systems-based approaches to the treatment of major disorders will be examined in some depth in Chapter 21.

After reviewing the same studies as Mosher and Keith, Donald Klein (1980) concludes that there is little evidence to support the idea that psychosocial treatments of schizophrenia "are of any clinical significance in reversing or ameliorating the course of the disorder." At the same time, he suggests that such treatments may be significant in helping people with a schizophrenic disorder to maintain themselves outside hospitals, or to avoid psychiatric hospitalization in the first place. A study by J. C. Beck, Golden, and Arnold (1981) found just such an effect in 27 individuals who were receiving long-term (over one year) psychotherapy. When compared to a matched group of individuals with schizophrenic disorders who were not receiving psychotherapy, 44 percent of the treatment group showed slightly greater improvement in overall behavior during the year. However, the improved subjects were still manifesting significant signs of schizophrenic disorders. They were not "cured," but the psychotherapy appears to have increased the likelihood that they could maintain themselves outside an inpatient setting.

If we again consider the vulnerability hypothesis of Zubin, it is perhaps clear why neither drugs alone nor psychotherapy alone is very successful in treating schizophrenia. When a disorder seems to result from many factors, one single approach to treatment seems unlikely to be successful.

Behavioral approaches. Can the application of therapy based on learning principles cure schizophrenia? It seems very unlikely, but time after time learning approaches have been very powerful tools for changing many behaviors seen in schizophrenics. The application of behavioral treatment to schizophrenics was identified by the National Institute of Mental Health in 1975 as one of the two most significant advances in the previous 25 years in the mental health field.

One of the first demonstrations of the utility of these approaches with schizophrenics was done by Teodoro Ayllon (Ayllon & Micheal, 1959; Ayllon & Azrin 1965). Ayllon's work resulted in the development of a **token economy** for the broad-scale treatment of schizophrenic patients in hospital settings. In a token economy, desirable behavior is reinforced both by social reinforcement (e.g., praise from staff members) and by tokens, which can be redeemed for special privileges or for commodities such as candy, cigarettes, and pop. Undesirable behavior is treated by the withdrawal of positive reinforcement (withdrawal of attention) or by punishment such as fines.

Many token economy programs are in effect now, and have led to significant behavior changes in many people. Typically, such programs result in less apathy, widened patterns of interest, more

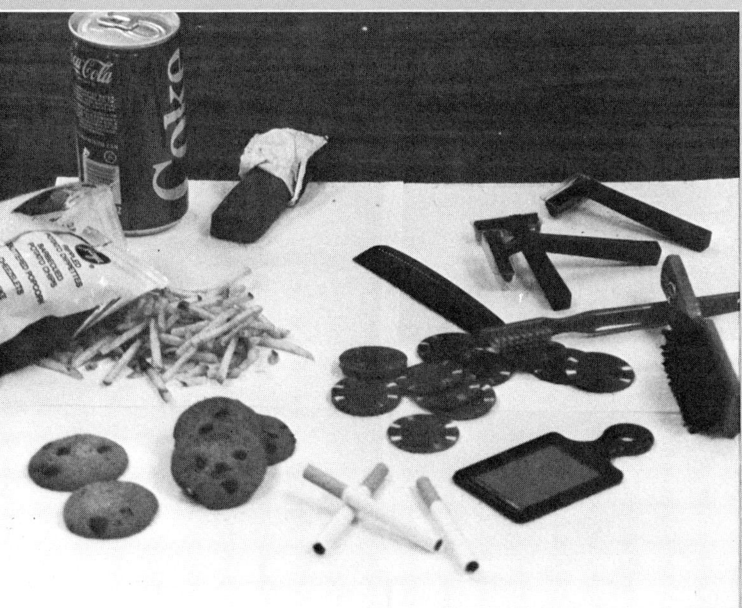

In treatment programs using token economies, tokens (for example, poker chips) are used as reinforcers for appropriate behavior. They can be redeemed for commodities, such as the items pictured, or for "intangibles," such as being allowed to attend special activities.

communication, less bizarre behavior, and increased levels of self-care skills (Atthowe & Krasner, 1968). The application of behavioral principles to residential groups will be examined in more detail in Chapter 21.

Specific problem behaviors can also be modified through the application of behavior principles. The basic principles of reinforcement are applied, just as in a token economy, but with the focus on one specific behavior in one specific individual. Matefy (1972) used these procedures with the following case:

> The patient was a 26-year-old woman who had been a patient at a state psychiatric hospital since 17 years of age and who had been diagnosed by the psychiatric staff as schizophrenic reaction–chronic undifferentiated. She was released once after a year's commitment only to be returned within a few months to the hospital where she has resided ever since. Her commitment was precipitated by increased general social withdrawal during her senior year in high school. She was described by the family physician as possessing paranoid and suicidal tendencies and being in a constant state of depression. At the hospital she was reported confused, incoherent and hallucinatory with impaired judgment and minimal powers of concentration. She seldom took part in hospital activities and was relegated to the back wards of the hospital. Perhaps most disturbing to the staff was the patient's apparent attempts to commit suicide by choking herself with her hands, nylon stocking, or other objects she could obtain. (p. 226)

The choking behavior was selected for modification as an initial approach. The patient was first baselined (a frequency count was taken of the behavior before intervention) and then was reinforced with a cigarette when she would go for two hours without choking herself. For this patient, cigarettes were a very desired item. After 13 weeks, the behavior dropped to zero, was absent for 8 weeks, reappeared for 2 weeks, then declined to zero at 24 weeks, and remained absent (see Figure 13.5). Concurrent with the reinforcement of the absence of the inappropriate behavior, the staff used withdrawal of attention to modify "psychotic episodes." When the patient behaved bizarrely, the staff would walk away from her. Other behaviors which then also disappeared included crying, fake heart attacks, claims that she was losing her mind, and urinating on the floor. Strong social reinforcement was given for positive behaviors such as sitting in chairs rather than on the floor, rátional speech, taking walks, and going to occupational therapy. The improvement in the patient's behavior allowed a significant decrease to be made in her antipsychotic medication. The patient was not cured, nor was her personality "reconstructed," but she was no longer as disturbed as she had been.

What about changing things that go on inside schizophrenics, for example, a delusion? From the behavioral perspective, it is not really important to change the delusion, but it is important to change the behaviors that represent the delusion. Does it matter whether a person has a delusion, when he or she never acts on it or talks about it? Liberman

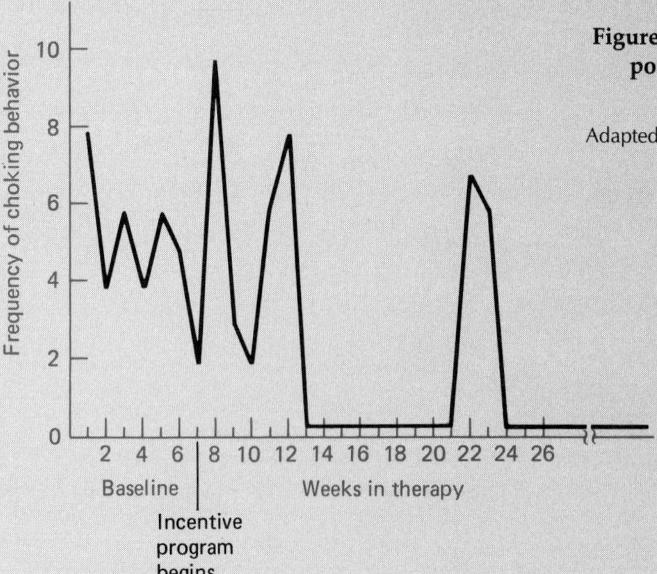

Figure 13.5. Reducing schizophrenic behavior by positive reinforcement in periods when the behavior (self-choking) was absent.

Adapted from Matefy (1972, p. 228).

(1976) has demonstrated that delusional speech can be eliminated from the behavior of schizophrenics by contingent attention. The patient is attended to when speaking rationally, and not given attention when speaking delusionally. Under these structured conditions, rational speech increases dramatically. When the contingencies are reversed—that is, irrational speech is attended to—the rational speech decreases, and the irrational speech increases. This seems to suggest that schizophrenics may talk about delusions to gain attention of mental health workers!

While these behavioral techniques may sound simple, they are quite difficult. Their successful use requires a great deal of planning, specification of techniques, and consistency in application. The successful rehabilitation of a schizophrenic individual using this approach requires complex staff efforts. Liberman (1976) considers major environmental manipulation to be a necessary part of the application of behavioral principles if the goal is more than changing an isolated behavior (see Table 13.4).

Since the behavioral approaches require exact specification of treatment goals and accurate data keeping, it is usually clear whether they are effective. Large numbers of studies have demonstrated the effectiveness of these techniques in changing much of the behavior manifested by schizophrenics. Studies have also demonstrated that 9–22 percent of schizophrenics are not responsive to this approach (Kazdin, 1973). This is to some extent due to the limitations of available reinforcers in most treatment settings.

Though approaches based on learning principles do not appear able to modify the primary deficit of schizophrenia, they hold promise for changing many of the behaviors that cause schizophrenics so much difficulty. A major problem for behavior modification approaches continues to be the lack of structured reinforcement systems in the community. Once discharged from a residential setting, patients may not find reinforcers in the community to help maintain the appropriate behavior; community structures may even reinforce the old maladaptive behavior. Such situations can lead to an increase in the frequency of problem behavior and the patient's readmission to a mental hospital.

The behavioral approaches described so far have focused on reinforcement contingencies for specific behaviors. They have tried to either train behaviors which are not present (behavioral deficits) or have tried to eliminate behaviors which are present (behavioral excesses). They have not tried to modify the schizophrenic's behaviors by modifying thinking processes. An approach that has tried to change behavior through this process has been devised by Meichenbaum (1977).

Table 13.4
Steps in the behavioral rehabilitation of chronic schizophrenics

Behavioral task	*Required activity*
Therapeutic goals	Define precisely the behavioral goals for each patient.
Therapeutic progress	Measure the frequency of the desired behaviors.
Reinforcement	Attach clear positive and negative consequences to adaptive and maladaptive behavior, respectively.
Shaping behavior	Use instructions and prompts to elicit the desired behaviors. Reinforce patients for making small, discrete steps in the desired direction.
Stimulus generalization	Structure the hospital setting to approximate the real world outside.
Training skills	Provide opportunities for patients to learn and practice vocational and housekeeping skills which have marketable value in the community or instrumental role value within the family.
Interpersonal goals	Prepare patients and significant others to live in mutually supportive ways in the community (prerelease training, aftercare). Teach significant others to use behavioral principles to maintain gains.
Community adjustment	Coordinate community resources to reinforce and back up the discharged patient's coping efforts.

From Liberman (1976, p. 193).

Many behaviors of schizophrenics are seen by Meichenbaum as being task irrelevant, and he has tried to teach schizophrenics to be more task relevant. Often our behavior is task irrelevant because our *thoughts* are task irrelevant. One cognitive behavior modification approach applied to this problem is **self-instructional training.** People with schizophrenic disorders are taught to monitor their behavior and thinking for task irrelevancies (e.g., bizarre thoughts or behavior). These behaviors are used as cues to begin saying a set of instructions to themselves (for example, "to be relevant and coherent," "to make myself understood"). These instructions are first modeled orally by an instructor. The clients then practice them out loud, and later practice saying them to themselves. These internal verbalizations are used as guides for behavior. For example, A. Meyers, Mercatoris, and Sciota (1976) taught individuals to repeat to themselves statements such as:

1. Don't repeat an answer.
2. I must pay attention to what others say. I must not talk sick talk.
3. The only sickness is talking sick. I mustn't talk sick.
4. I must stay on the topic.
5. Relax, take a few deep breaths.

Meichenbaum and Cameron (1973) also devised similar self-instruction statements and used this method to treat schizophrenics who engaged in "sick talk." The sick talk of schizophrenics who used self-instruction was reduced more than in a control group who simply practiced talking rationally and who were reinforced operantly for success. A major advantage of this approach is that clients carry the technique around with them. Since they are taught to reinforce their own behavior by self-praise, there is no need for an external complicated reinforcement system, and the behaviors may generalize to other settings (such as the community) when the individual is discharged from the treatment program.

Is schizophrenia treatable?

A variety of treatment approaches have been used with schizophrenics. All of these approaches seem to offer some benefits to those manifesting the disorder. One of the most beneficial approaches seems to be chemotherapy; but even this is not always successful, and antipsychotic drugs do not "cure" schizophrenia. Rather, they seem to primarily mask the symptomatology. The behavioral approaches have a major contribution to make in the modification of global and specific behaviors. They are useful both for decreasing inappropriate behaviors and teaching appropriate ways of behaving. The traditional individual psychotherapies seem least effective in treating chronic schizophrenia, but may have a place in working with acute schizophrenics. The critical evaluation studies of psychotherapy for use with schizophrenics have yet to be done.

Is schizophrenia treatable? Yes, certainly it is. Can this disorder be cured? At our current state of knowledge, the goal of "cure" still eludes us. Schizophrenia, particularly when it is the process type, is a disabling life-long disorder. The available treatments can reduce its impact, but do not seem to be able to return most schizophrenic individuals to an optimal level of functioning. This rather pessimistic assessment must be balanced by our awareness that some individuals with a schizophrenic disorder get better, even though the process may take many years. Unfortunately, the large majority of people with schizophrenic disorders, even when they are living in a community setting, lead lives of quiet desperation (Serban, 1980).

Summary

1. Contrasting theories have been proposed to account for the development of the schizophrenic disorders. Psychoanalysts have theorized that schizophrenia is due to major developmental problems early in life which result in the development of a weakened ego. The weakened ego allows the id processes to break through into behavior. Later neo-Freudian analysts have focused on the impact of distorted parent-child relationships.

2. Parent-child relationships have also been the center of attention of other interpersonal theories. Some parents seem to engage in double-bind communications with their children. The double-bind, conflicting messages may be communicated by a "schizophrenogenic mother." This type of overprotective, intrusive, mother, may have children who cannot separate their identity from her. This theory has little support in hard data; in fact, most evidence indicates that it is a relatively useless concept.

3. Other studies have demonstrated that the parental families of individuals with schizophrenia are usually chaotic and disturbed. Perhaps having schizophrenic offspring leads to chaos and poor communication in families.

4. Some theorists have proposed that schizophrenia is learned like any other behavior. Although many of the behaviors of schizophrenics have been learned, the basic deficit seems to require another explanation.

5. Like learning, sociocultural factors and expectations for the social role behavior also seem to have some impact on the type of behavior manifested in schizophrenic disorders. However, the basic symptoms of schizophrenia appear to cut across socioeconomic classes, subcultures, and national/cultural boundaries.

6. Many studies of twins and adoptive children of schizophrenic parents have consistently and convincingly demonstrated that there are hereditary factors in schizophrenia. At the least, there seems to be an inherited predisposition to schizophrenia, which may vary on a continuum from a strong predisposition in some persons to no predisposition in others.

7. Perhaps this predisposition is manifested as a biochemical disturbance. One major theory of schizophrenia is the dopamine hypothesis. This theory suggests that either an excess of the neurotransmitter dopamine or an oversensitivity of the dopaminergic receptors in the neurons is a primary factor in the manifestation of schizophrenic behavior.

8. The recent discovery of innate morphine-like substances in the brain called endorphins may result in new information about problems in neural transmission which are important in schizophrenia.

9. A major focus of recent research in schizophrenia has been on high risk studies. In these studies, children of schizophrenic mothers are examined longitudinally (over long periods) in an attempt to determine if basic deficits precede the development of overt schizophrenic behavior. Many of these studies have been conducted in Denmark, where these children are more easily identified and followed because of a national health register. Findings from these studies have indicated that these children differ from matched groups of children who do not have schizophrenic mothers.

10. In the high risk studies, children who became schizophrenic had mothers whose disorders were more severe, and often had birth complications. Some evidence exists that these children had early associative deficits. In addition, these children were likely to be physiologically more reactive to stimuli. As these children age and the studies continue, more data should become available.

11. The evidence for each theory of schizophrenia has led some to propose a vulnerability hypothesis, which states that people have varying vulnerabilities to schizophrenia. This vulnerability is most likely due to a combination of biological and psychosocial factors. As fas as we can tell, schizophrenia is not due to just one etiological factor.

12. Various treatment approaches have been applied to schizophrenia with varying degrees of success. Biological therapies, such as the use of antipsychotic medication and ECT, are common and often successful in attaining remission of most symptoms. However, a high percentage of those treated in these ways relapse.

13. The evidence is equivocal for verbal psychotherapies that focus on developing relationships and insight. They probably help, but we cannot say for sure. When used in conjunction with medication, the psychosocial approaches can help with the problems related to having a chronic disorder. Advocates of these approaches feel the methods are more powerful than most think; some psychotherapists are quite successful with the population they work with. We need more data to be able to draw a firm conclusion.

14. A very significant development since the 1950s has been the application of behavioral learning theory to the treatment of schizophrenia. Operant approaches for groups and individuals have dramatically changed many behaviors thought to be primary to schizophrenia. These approaches can clearly modify many of the disruptive disturbing behaviors we see in this population. The techniques do not, however, seem to be effective with about 10 percent of the people who manifest the disorders. Why this is so is not clear.

15. An approach that focuses on the cognitions of schizophrenics is cognitive-behavioral modification. This technique attempts to modify the thinking processes of schizophrenics so that they can change their own behavior. Some studies have demonstrated that the approach can succeed in modifying the behaviors of some individuals.

16. An advantage of the cognitive approach is that when it is successful, the individual may be able to maintain the behavior by self-reinforcement. If this is so there may be fewer problems postdischarge for schizophrenics who leave hospitals to live in communities without structured therapeutic reinforcement.

17. While behavioral approaches have made major contributions to the treatment of schizophrenic disorders, they still are not a panacea. Even when they have led to major behavioral changes in chronic schizophrenia, there are often residual symptoms (perhaps the basic deficits) which leave these individuals vulnerable to a recurrence of problem behaviors that often lead to rehospitalization. We still do not have a cure for this disorder.

KEY TERMS

Antipsychotic drugs. Chemical compounds which reduce or mask many of the overt symptoms of psychosis.
Dopamine. One of many neurotransmitters. A biochemical substance which is produced at one nerve ending and activates the next nerve ending.
Double bind. A type of communication in which two conflicting messages are given at the same time by the same person.
Electroconvulsive therapy. Treatment that administers electrical current to the brain in order to induce a disruption of nerve impulses.
High risk study. A study which selects its sample from an identified population known to be at risk for a particular disorder.
Primary process thinking. Thinking which is considered by psychoanalysts to be representative of primitive impulses. It is illogical and highly symbolic.
Proband. The individual in a genetic study with the characteristic that the researcher is interested in.
Token economy. A group-oriented treatment approach in which individuals receive tokens or other objects for performance of positive behaviors. The tokens can be withheld or taken away when the desired behaviors do not occur.
Vulnerability hypothesis. A hypothesis that people may have a combination of predispositions which result in varying degrees of vulnerability to the development of schizophrenia in the face of environmental stress.

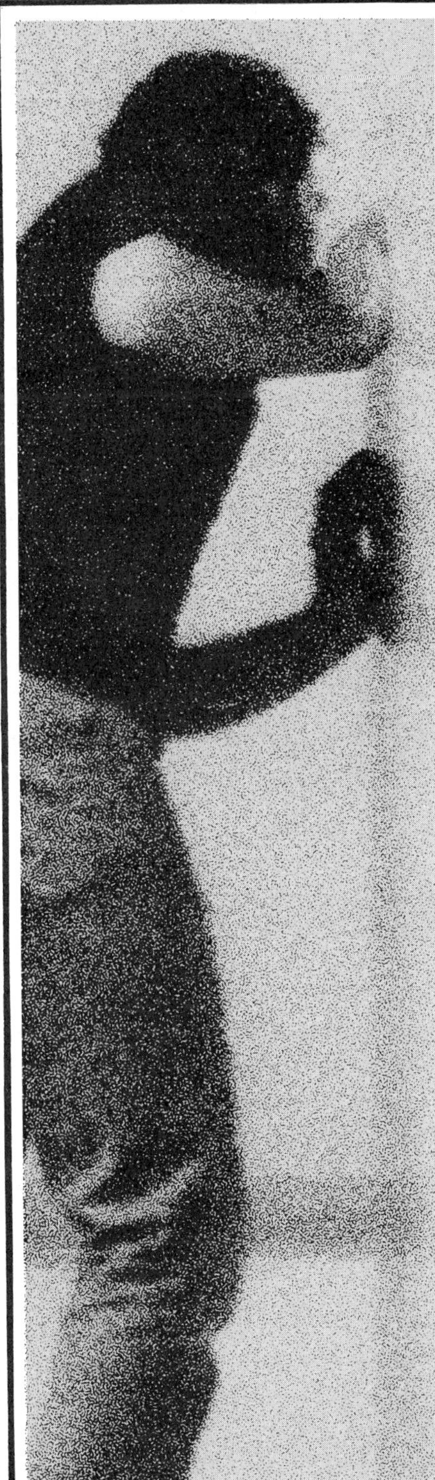

14

Paranoid disorders

- Paranoid behavior: a continuum?
- Types of paranoid disorders
- Etiology of paranoid disorders
- Key treatments
- Summary
- Key terms

All of us have probably experienced moments when we had suspicions that we could not confirm, when we had a sense that others were doing something "behind our backs," or that we were perceiving the "real truth" of a given situation which others did not perceive. Yet without proof to confirm our suspicions, we would eventually shrug them off. Or when the reality of the situation was made known to us, we would accept its validity. In any case, our "paranoid" suspicions would not characterize our typical behaviors.

Individuals with **paranoid disorders** have strong beliefs that seem impervious to reality. They have delusions or fixed false beliefs about being conspired against, followed, drugged, poisoned, harassed, cheated, or spied upon. They may have delusions of grandeur, which revolve around an exaggerated belief in their self-importance, such as having found a solution to war. These beliefs are maintained in spite of convincing evidence to the contrary. The false beliefs are so rigidly held that the paranoid disorders are often called paranoid psychosis because the individual is not in full contact with reality.

The reported incidence of paranoid disorders is low. Individuals with these disorders may come to the attention of a social agency when they begin to act on their beliefs. But such individuals almost never seek treatment on their own volition because they do not believe anything is wrong with them. Those with a paranoid disorder can often function reasonably well in society, since their personality is not significantly affected in areas outside the delusional content. Their affect is usually appropriate and realistic, their judgment remains good, and they are usually appropriately oriented (they know where they are, the time of year and day, etc.). Hallucinations may occur, but they are relatively rare. Capable of maintaining basic economic and minimal social skills, individuals with paranoid disorders are often able to avoid involuntary hospitalization.

PARANOID BEHAVIOR: A CONTINUUM?

The paranoid personality disorder (described in Chapter 11) and paranoid schizophrenia (discussed in Chapter 12) have similarities to the paranoid disorders. In all three cases there is suspiciousness, hypersensitivity, eccentricities of behavior, and seclusiveness. However, there are important differences. In the paranoid personality disorder, the symptoms consist of unrealistic suspiciousness, hypersensitivity, and restricted affect. These are enduring personality traits usually recognizable in adolescence and lasting through adult life. In contrast to the paranoid disorders, delusional beliefs are not characteristic of the individual with paranoid personality disorder. While some individuals with the paranoid personality disorder may develop a true paranoid disorder in later life, many do not; and some people who do develop a paranoid disorder do not have the signs of the paranoid personality prior to the development of their paranoia. In schizophrenia, paranoid type, the individual's thinking and behavior are much more disorganized, the delusions are much more bizarre and fragmented, and the thinking processes are not as logical or coherent as in the paranoid disorders. The onset of the paranoid schizophrenic disorder is usually in adolescence or early adulthood, while the paranoid disorders often begin in midlife. In contrast to the irrationality of schizophrenia, the thought processes of the individual with a paranoid disorder tend to make sense if the primary faulty assumptions are accepted; the deluded beliefs are usually elaborate and well organized. Table 14.1 summarizes the similarities and differences among the three groups of disorders. The similarities between paranoid personality disorder, the paranoid psychoses, and paranoid schizophrenia have led some clinicians (e.g., Meissner, 1978) to take the position that they are really the same disorder with a varying range of schizophrenic disorganization. Others (e.g., Tanna, 1974) maintain that the true paranoid disorders are distinct entities. The second perspective often views the paranoid personality as a premorbid basis for the final disorder. Figure 14.1 illustrates these differing conceptions of the paranoid disorders.

The position that the psychotic paranoid disorders are distinct from paranoid personality disorder and paranoid schizophrenia is supported by some interesting recent research. Chapter 13 reported on research which demonstrated a risk of schizophrenia in the biolog-

Table 14.1
Some similarities and differences between paranoid personality disorder, paranoid disorders, and schizophrenia, paranoid type

Similarities and differences	*Paranoid personality (see chapter 11)*	*Paranoid disorder*	*Schizophrenia, paranoid type (see chapter 12)*
Similarities			
Unwarranted suspiciousness	x	x	x
Hypersensitive	x	x	x
Eccentricities	x	x	x
Seclusiveness	x	x	x
Differences			
Onset	Adolescent to early adult, slow development.	Usually middle or late adulthood, slow but can be sudden.	Usually early adult; major symptoms can be sudden; disorganization can be over long period.
Delusions	No	Yes, concrete and well organized.	Yes, fragmented and bizarre.
Hallucinations	No	Occasionally, but usually not prominent when present.	Usually a prominent feature of the behavior.
Thinking process	Logical	Logical when basic premise is accepted.	Illogical, usually includes loosening of associations or incoherence.
Affect	Appropriate, may be restricted.	Appropriate within context of delusion. May be restricted.	Usually blunted, flat, or inappropriate.
Behavior	Organized	Organized, consonant with thinking.	Often disorganized.

ical relatives of individuals with schizophrenia greater than that in the general population. These biological relatives are at an even greater risk for what are called **schizophrenic spectrum disorders.** These disorders have some similarity to schizophrenia, such as schizotypal personality. If paranoid personality disorder and the paranoid disorders are milder variants of paranoid schizophrenia, then we would expect the frequency of these disorders in the biological relatives of people with schizophrenia to be greater than the frequency in the general pop-

Figure 14.1. Paranoid Disorders: Distinct entity or a point on a continuum?
Some clinicians view the paranoid disorders of paranoia, shared paranoid disorder, and paranoid state as a group of disorders distinct from schizophrenia, paranoid type, and paranoid personality disorder, although some behaviors overlap. Other clinicians view these three forms of behavior as points on a continuum of schizophrenic disorganization.

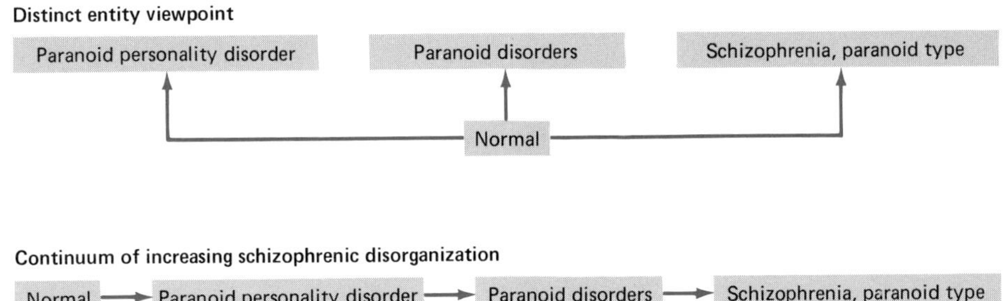

ulation. However, recent studies have not found the paranoid psychoses or paranoid personality disorder to have an increased frequency in the relatives of people diagnosed as having schizophrenia (Debray, 1975; Watt, Hall, & Olley, 1980). In addition, relatives of individuals with paranoid psychoses do not have an increased risk of schizophrenia (K. Kendler & Hays, 1981). A reanalysis of the subjects of a major study of genetic transmission of schizophrenia (the Danish adoption study discussed in Chapter 13) found the same result: Paranoid disorders were not more common in biological relatives of schizophrenics than in the general population (K. Kendler, Gruenberg, & Strauss, 1981b). K. Kendler et al. found that the incidence of paranoid psychoses in the general population was 2.2 percent. While definite conclusions are limited by a small sample size, this study and the others cited suggest that the paranoid psychoses are distinct from schizophrenia and more common than has been believed in the past.

TYPES OF PARANOID DISORDERS

Two primary subtypes of paranoid psychoses have been identified: **paranoia** and the **paranoid state.** These two types of paranoid disorders share a number of major characteristics (see Table 14.2). A third subtype, **shared paranoid disorder** (also called "folie à deux"), shares these major characteristics, but is very rare. Shared paranoid disorder is discussed in Highlight 14.1.

Individuals who develop a paranoid state or paranoia tend to share certain characteristics in their premorbid personality styles. Often these people are extremely sensitive to the reactions of others, are rigid, suspicious, and seem to be unable or unwilling to develop open, warm, and affectionate relationships with others.

Table 14.2

Major characteristics of the paranoid disorders

1. Organized delusions of persecution or jealousy, at times associated with grandeur.
2. Orientation and affect are appropriate.
3. Judgment is good except in areas of delusions.
4. Absence of the bizzare fragmentation of thinking processes manifested by schizophrenics (i.e., no extremes of affect, or bizarre mannerisms).
5. Hallucinations may be present, but are not a prominent feature.

Some exhibit what has been described as **magical thinking.** Wilder (1975) characterizes magical thinking as "thinking in terms of absolutes, in terms of omnipotence (all powerfulness) and omniscience (all knowingness), in terms of magic certainties, pleasant or unpleasant." For example, a magical certainty for some individuals might be the conviction "Everyone's out to get me." Magical thinking is not uncommon, it is demonstrated in beliefs in "lady luck," "knocking on wood," and in the common youthful "delusions" of immortality, free will, and unlimited personal potential (Bellak, 1970). Before the onset of the disorder, people who become paranoid also tend to be arrogant and dominating, infused with their own self-importance, and unable to accept blame for things that go wrong. Grunebaum and Perlman (1973) describe premorbid paranoids as individuals who have difficulty in realistically trusting others. They either trust too much or not enough; thus, they are likely to perceive others as "letting them down." After the letdown and disappointment, they overreact to the hurt.

Individuals who develop the disorder that we call paranoia gradually become more and more disturbed over time. The person who develops a paranoid state moves from the premorbid personality described above into a full paranoid experience in a short time, and this change is usually associated with an increase in environmental stressors.

Paranoia

In paranoia, the primary feature is the subtle, progressively damaging, **insidious** development of a lasting, relatively unmodifiable system of false belief which is accompanied by clear and orderly thinking in areas not related to the delusion. People with this disorder frequently consider themselves to have special powers or abilities, and their affect is appropriate to their belief system.

Such individuals are often socially isolated,

HIGHLIGHT 14.1
SHARED PARANOID DISORDER (FOLIE À DEUX)

"Folie à deux," loosely translated from French, means "insanity or folly of two." In this disorder, two people share (at least partly) a delusional system. Ordinarily one person develops an established paranoia. A second individual, as a result of a close, dependent emotional relationship, comes to share portions of the other's delusional system. The individual with the original paranoia is usually the dominant member of the relationship, and is generally the more disturbed of the two. The second person tends to be submissive and less caught up in the delusional system. If separated from the dominant member, this person's delusional beliefs will often rapidly disappear or diminish. Most reported cases are comprised of blood or marital relatives (i.e., siblings, spouses, parent and child).

Potash and Brunell (1974) have focused on the problem of the inability to express anger, and the mutually reinforcing communications in shared paranoid disorder. From their perspective, the shared paranoid behavior is an outward **projection** of intolerable anger and hostility toward each other. The partners have a dominance-dependence relationship that is desperately needed, and hostility must therefore be externalized outside of the relationship. This issue is then complicated by the reinforcing nature of the shared false beliefs, which leads to a self-perpetuating system of constant distortion. The shared beliefs provide a bond that further conceals the underlying deep hostility that each person feels towards the other.

appear eccentric, and seem seclusive. Their false beliefs usually lead them to engage in behaviors such as trying to bring legal action against those whom they see as being "against" them; complaining about injustice; and writing letters to various authorities. They can often maintain their day-to-day functioning for long periods before being labeled as "problems." They are difficult to live with, however, and create turmoil and disruption among family members and others with whom they have contact long before they are identified as having paranoia.

It is difficult to be sympathetic to paranoid individuals because of the anger, suspiciousness, and frequent rejection that they direct towards their companions. Others often lose sight of the subjective anxiety and terror with which a paranoid person must live. Lemberg (1978) provides a glimpse into the terrifying subjective experiences of a woman with paranoia, through excerpts from the diary which the woman kept for three years prior to hospitalization. This 37-year-old woman had a reasonably good adjustment until she was 32, when she began to have experiences of a paranoid nature, including persecutory hallucinations. She did not manifest the major personality disintegrations and formal thought disorder of schizophrenia. The following limited diary excerpts illustrate in her own words her view of what was happening to her. Her physical symptoms are described first, her auditory hallucinations second:

> Back burned in vicinity of kidneys, rectum and genitals burned whenever I urinate or have bowel movement. If taking a bath, body burned in entirety especially breasts. . . .
>
> Since first week of November being awakened two or three times a night. Caused to vomit.
>
> Head burned (extreme headaches at times over eyes) extremely painful.
>
> Chills, sweating spells extreme thirst at times. Heart palpitations accelerated—right arm unable to stand weight.
>
> Sudden pain in eyes—pupils hurt in light. Have to be close to read or look at television impossible only allowed to walk the floor or sit down or become quiet. vagina and rectum burned.
>
> Some or all of these things were repeated daily. Compiled from notes I have taken from what was being said.
>
> (male voice) I'm not gonna bother a man, get a husband you . . . bitch get a dog's ass.
>
> I hated everything you had, that car, I couldn't stand to see it.
>
> I got to get away. I won't enjoy this shit if I am caught.

(higher male voice) If you had had a . . . man in there, I wouldn't have bothered you. I am trying to make you lose your mind.

I hate you.

We have hurt your daughter's mind too. We started on the little bitch first.

I hate you.

Your mind's been opened with electricity. I wouldn't do a dog like this.

I'll sneak up behind you and cut your face up, you Goddam bitch. I got something to do it with. (Lemberg, 1978, pp. 461–464, spelling errors corrected.)

One can imagine how upsetting this woman found these comments. The hallucinations she experienced were consistent with her persecutory delusions that her male neighbor was intentionally tormenting her for sadistic sexual pleasure. She had complained of this to the Federal Communications Commission and the police, and had hired a detective to investigate him. Finally, she was "forced" to take matters in her own hands. At the urging of the "voices," she approached the neighbor and fired a revolver at his feet in what she stated was "self-defense." This act led to her hospitalization after court charges of "assault with intent to kill."

The somatic experiences and hallucinations she experienced provide some insight into the underlying self-degradation and self-hate of this woman. Projection of the horrid ideas onto others in the environment seemed to allow her to continue to value herself. She could perceive these horrid thoughts and fears as coming from outside herself, rather than as being reflective of her own concerns, fears, and suspicions about the kind of person she might "actually" be.

The following case illustrates a severe paranoia. The psychotic level of the disorder developed after the threat of rejection from an academic program in which the subject had invested many years of hard work. This threat appeared to be the "straw that broke the camel's back." The description of the subject's premorbid life-style, however, reveals a long-established paranoid personality disorder. This case provides an excellent example of **grandiose thinking** frequently seen in the paranoid disorders. The case also illustrates how a person with paranoid thinking incorporates unrelated events into an organized delusional system as proof of the false beliefs. In addition the person's ability to cover up the problem for a long period demonstrates that most functioning outside the delusional system remains intact.

The patient was a 23 year old graduate student in psychology. . . . Upon entry to graduate work, he showed a disposition toward avoiding assignments in favor of "creative" thinking mostly aimed at refuting accepted scientific principles. His arguments were based on possible but not probable lines of analysis. Facts were often twisted until they fit his preconceptions. He was always quite willing to argue but never willing to listen. *At mid-year, he was advised to reconsider his goal in education and encouraged to postpone completion of his degree until*

Early feelings of mistrust toward others may escalate into paranoid suspicions, as the individual matures. The negative response of others to these paranoid suspicions may only serve to reinforce the disordered individual's perceptions, such as the belief that he or she is being followed.

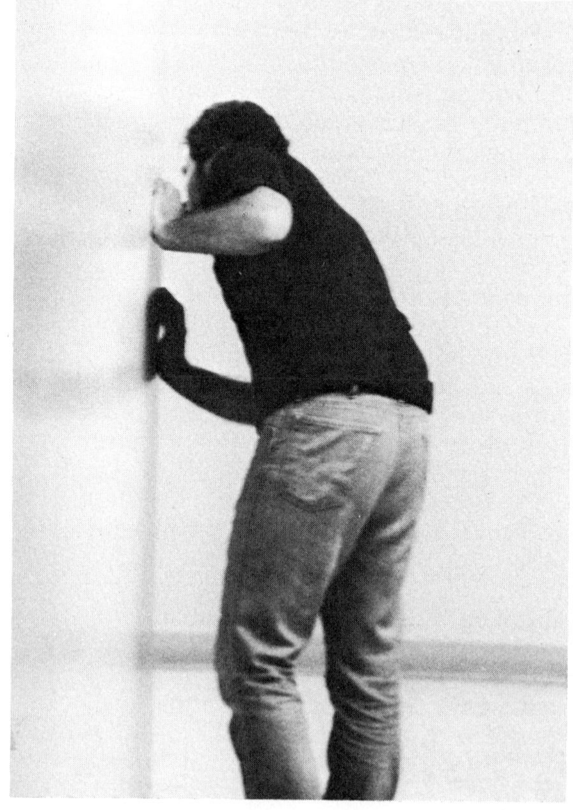

he was more certain of his choice of career. He refused to delay his education and continued in the department. Within weeks, a highly intricate delusional system evolved of a persecutory nature. He harbored the belief that the departmental recommendation had been the first step in a plot to distract his progress. He reasoned that he was probably nearing a major scientific discovery which, if publicized, would revolutionize science and make all current scientific theories, from Darwinism to nuclear theory, obsolete. The psychology faculty were simply pawns given the task of preventing him from [making] his imminent contribution. As he pondered his insight, he felt he more clearly understood his undergraduate career. He had been "guided" toward the particular college by those who had recognized his potential genius and who had hoped even then to sidetrack him by subtle brainwashing. Magazine solicitations through the mail were attempts to direct him towards the "right" kind of reading. He believed that it was even possible that his parents were part of the scheme and, with this in mind, he spent long hours in retracing the places they had taken him as a child with the hopes of finding a pattern. He was beside himself with satisfaction when he recognized the telephone repairman coming out of the department chairman's office as the same one who had installed his telephone in his apartment. This link proved his suspicion that his telephone wires had been tapped. He was henceforth careful to listen for telltale sounds during his telephone conversations; when he was unable to detect any, he became even more impressed by the technical skills of the wiretappers. Since he was still enrolled in school, his draft board renewed his deferment. This event was taken by the patient to mean that the federal government was deeply involved in the attempt to keep him in a location where he could continue to be surveyed. In a shrewd maneuver, he decided to "play the game" and not reveal his new found knowledge. Instead, he became the model student and impressed the faculty in his more controlled, seemingly attentive, and mild manner. He continued to apply his above average intellect to his schoolwork and was doing relatively well. In an attempt to impress the department and to "lull them into a false sense of confidence," he joined in a group psychotherapy program. During the fourth meeting, he became excited by the "revelations" he thought he detected in another member's comments and announced in a tone of mixed anger and pride that he could no longer be treated as a fool and that he would expose the whole plot and work on his scientific discovery besides! (Suinn, 1975, p. 423, italics added)

Paranoid State

The paranoid state differs from the other paranoid disorders primarily in that its onset is relatively sudden, the condition rarely becomes chronic, and a significant life change often precedes the development of the behavior. Its most common form is seen in individuals who must deal with a life change such as emigration to a new land, induction into the military, menopause, separation from family for the first time, major disasters, and failing health. The following case illustrates a paranoid state that developed subsequent to the stressful relocation of a federal government employee:

> A 28-year-old American engineer was sent by a government agency on a three-week inspection tour of several African countries. Though thoroughly competent professionally, he was culturally and personally unprepared for the experience. Indeed, when he moved to Washington from the Midwest only the year before, he had experienced more than average anxiety and brief feelings of depersonalization.
>
> On arrival in East Africa he became panicky at the sight of so many black faces and soon began to fear for his life. He had some insight into his feelings but he could not control his frightened thinking. By the time he reached Zaire, he was filled with thoughts of imminent annihilation by the Africans and compensatory thoughts of omnipotence and union with God, and was no longer able to do his job. He began to act [disturbed] and waded into the crocodile-infested waters of the Congo River. When brought to the U.S. Embassy, he disrobed completely in order "to offer testimony."
>
> Immediate air evacuation to Washington and admission to our unit led to [a reduction of symptoms] within a few days. We have frequently observed this rapid recovery in cases of . . . paranoid thought disorder as the individual leaves the unfamiliar overseas scene of his fears and approaches his home country. This patient's pre- and postmorbid personality was of a somewhat [withdrawn] type, but we felt that without the trauma of his overseas mission he might never have become psychotic. (Barnes, 1980, p. 757)

The sudden onset and rapid recovery described above are typical of the paranoid state when the stressful circumstances develop and then are decreased.

ETIOLOGY OF PARANOID DISORDERS

How do delusions develop? Swanson, Bohnert, and Smith (1970) have described a style of thinking which they believe summarizes the development of delusions in people who become paranoid. The individual mistrusts others, fears being taken advantage of, and becomes constantly alert (hypervigilant) to possible threat. (LaRusso, 1978, has demonstrated convincingly that persons diagnosed as manifesting paranoid symptoms are significantly more sensitive to nonverbal cues than normal persons.) Swanson et al. suggest that the person then selectively perceives the actions of others (i.e., focuses on the slights and affronts of others, and ignores their positive behaviors). At this point, individuals use projection to blame others for their own failures and respond to perceived injustice with anger and hostility, becoming even more suspicious of the others' motives. Finally, everything falls into place when the individuals' figure out what is happening. In other words, they conceptualize a false belief (delusion) which explains their perception.

Along these same lines, Maher (1974) has suggested that the frequent experience of having perceptions not shared by others can lead one to a sense of being unique and very special, and the feeling of persecution may arise when one's perceptions are repeatedly rejected by others. However, not all individuals whose life-style consists of rigidity, arrogance, suspiciousness, oversensitivity to criticism, and unwillingness to accept blame develop a paranoid disorder. Thus, theorists have attempted to conceptualize the specific factors involved in the development of the paranoid disorders.

Freud's Psychoanalytic Theory

Freud developed a theory of paranoid behavior which today is held by a variety of mental health professionals. Of particular importance to this theory are the concepts of the defense mechanisms of denial, reaction formation, and projection: the denial of unacceptable impulses, their conversion by reaction formation into the opposite emotion, and their subsequent projection onto the motivation of others. Freud applied these concepts to an analysis of Daniel Schreber, a judge who at the age of 42 developed paranoid schizophrenic behavior which varied from severe to mild until his death at the age of 69. Although Freud never saw Schreber, his analysis was based on Schreber's autobiography, and is a tour de force of psychoanalytic reasoning.

A more recent analysis of Schreber's life by Schatzman (1973) indicates that as a child Schreber was treated in a persecutory manner by his father, and that his delusional system related more to this relationship than to the unconscious processes Freud proposed. (see Fig-

Figure 14.2.
Freud attributed Daniel Paul Schreber's paranoid delusions to unconscious, unacceptable homosexual impulses. More recently, Schatzman has found that as a child, Schreber was treated in a persecutory manner by his father. Schreber's father used the belt illustrated to keep Daniel lying straight and flat while asleep. What might Daniel learn about the world from such treatment?

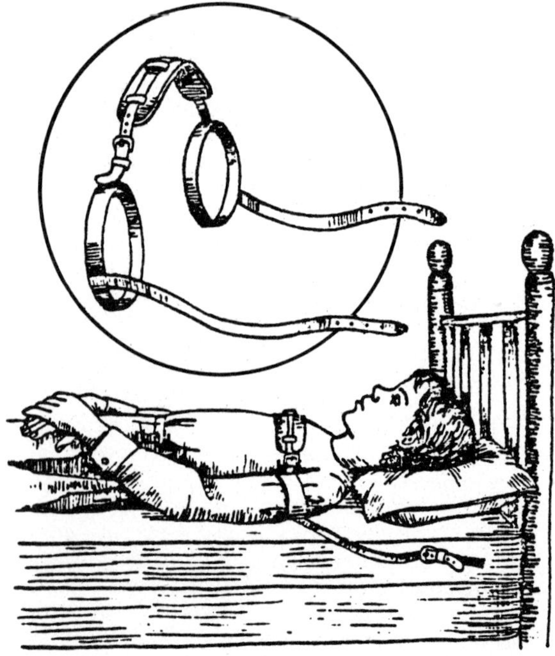

ure 14.2). However, Freud's formulation of paranoia remains widely accepted. In essence, Freud concluded from his studies of Daniel Schreber's autobiography that paranoid projection was a function of unacceptable homosexual impulses. These impulses are denied, converted to hostility and hate, and these emotions are projected onto others.

In effect the paranoid behaviors are explained by the following inferred internal sequences of events. The male subject begins with an unconscious homosexual impulse: "I love a man." This unacceptable homosexual feeling generates anxiety and is defensively denied and converted into "I hate a man"; however, "hate" is also unacceptable and is defended against by projecting it upon another, "He hates me." The nonpersecutory delusions develop according to the sequences shown in Table 14.3.

The usual criticisms of psychoanalytic theory have been leveled at Freud's theory of paranoid behavior: Freud reasoned from limited data, the generalizations are too encompassing, and little methodologically sound evidence exists to support the concepts. In addition, while some people might become paranoid from the threat of "latent" homosexuality, it seems unreasonable to suggest that *all* paranoid behavior must by definition be a function of this etiology (Ullmann & Krasner, 1975). The generalizability of the theory is also compromised by the existence of people with both paranoid *and* overt homosexual behavior (Colby, 1977). If paranoid behavior is a defense against homosexuality, then we would not expect to see much homosexual behavior in paranoids. Indeed, more recent conceptions of paranoid behavior have focused on the projection of unacceptable impulses such as rage and hostility without the need for the intervening concept of homosexuality.

Cameron's Theory of Pseudocommunity

Cameron (1967) focuses on a major issue in paranoid behavior: a deficiency in basic trust. He suggests that people who become paranoid were unable in early childhood to develop a trusting relationship with significant figures. Most children when frustrated to an intolerable degree find someone who will relieve the frustration and restore equilibrium. When such equilibrium is not restored, or when the frustration is increased by significant figures like parents, trust cannot develop. The children develop a basic mistrustful stance towards life, combined with a strong tendency to deny their own hostility.

Cameron suggests that mistrustful persons who later become paranoid experience a *preliminary threat*. In the face of environmental or interpersonal stress, they experience an upsurge of overwhelming fear *in reaction* to their own hostile response to the threat. The *onset* of paranoid behavior follows the threat and compounds these persons' estrangement and isolation from others. The increase in severity of symptoms may give the appearance of sudden onset, when in fact the problem has been brewing for a lifetime. The early phases after onset are characterized by continuing isolation and reconstruction of the environment so as to reaffirm its threatening nature in what appears to be a maneuver to maintain self-esteem (e.g., "My feelings of rage and hostility are acceptable because I am being threatened"). Selective perception of threat arouses high levels of anxiety and confirms the false beliefs. The para-

Table 14.3
The development of nonpersecutory delusions according to psychoanalytic theory

Delusion	*Sequence of development* IMPULSE	→	DENIAL	→	PROJECTION
Erotic delusion, or erotomania	"I love a man"		"I do not love him, I love her"		"She loves me"
Delusion of jealousy	"I love a man"		"I do not love him"		"She loves him"
Grandiose delusion	"I love a man" (a man cannot be lovable by another man)		"He is not lovable"		"Only I am lovable"

noid individual is then likely to conclude that "something is going on."

The stage of *preliminary crystalization* involves an attempt to find meaning in what the paranoid person perceives to be happening. Inevitably, he or she communicates these concerns and suspicions to others. However, the already persecutory concerns almost always receive negative responses from others, including confrontation. Thus, the listeners are soon included in the persecutory concerns in order to make sense of their negative reactions. The final step for the paranoid is the final crystalization: the **paranoid pseudocommunity.**

The paranoid pseudocommunity is the group of real and imagined people or agencies who the paranoid person perceives as united in a determination to destroy the person's reputation or life. It is a pseudocommunity, since these people, real and imagined, are not actually united against the paranoid. The paranoid individual experiences this final crystalization as a sudden enlightenment. Everything is figured out: who the persecutors are (the FBI, Ford Motor Company, etc.), what their motives are (to prevent world peace, keep the subject from inventing something), and what the individual must do (go to the United Nations and expose the plot, report the problem to the police). The paranoid person's actions at this point almost always lead to responses by others which strongly support the persecutory premise. People reject paranoids, avoid them, and at times react to them with hostility.

Lemert's Exclusionary Hypothesis

Lemert (1967) has suggested that many paranoid behaviors are to some extent realistic responses to real situations. People *are* "against" the paranoid individual.

An individual who exhibits paranoid behaviors is likely to be cold, aloof, suspicious, hostile, accusatory, and blaming—such a person sounds thoroughly unlikable! It is quite understandable that people might avoid such an individual or be angered by such behavior. They might, indeed, talk about the person behind his or her back, report the disliked behaviors to a work supervisor, or confront the individual directly in an effort to induce change. If the behavior continues, they might apply the label of "paranoid." This labeling, in effect, allows others to ignore the "paranoid" person's complaints of injustice, and may lead to the person's exclusion from further interactions. The exclusionary response of the environment precipitates more persecutory feelings in the subject, so that the intensity of the "paranoid" behaviors is likely to increase, further escalating the interpersonal avoidance.

Lemert's notion fits in well with the latter stages of Cameron's theory. Its major significance, however, is its implicit demand that paranoid behavior not be treated simply as a problem of individual pathology. The paranoid's "delusions" of persecution may not *all* be delusions.

Paranoid Disorders as Learned Behavior

Ullmann and Krasner (1975) view paranoia as learned behavior. They suggest that since people's responses alter their environment, and the environment in turn reinforces or extinguishes behavior, behaviors that appear irrational to the majority may be learned. If, for example, one learns from one's parents (through a process of modeling) that the world is a dangerous place, and behaves accordingly, one may well avoid being "hurt." If such behavior *is* reinforced, one may become even more sensitive to environmental stimuli that are signals of impending danger. One becomes sensitive to stimuli such as people staring at one, people abruptly stopping conversation when one walks into the room, and people following one on the street.

The paranoid person may be one who "thinks straight about a biased sample of information." The basic problem may be one of information processing. Once set in motion, this process appears to be so self-reinforcing that the false belief becomes very ingrained and resistant to change. In addition, the process of labeling people "paranoid" undoubtedly influences how others react to them. No doubt, paranoids are reinforced for their beliefs on an intermittent reinforcement schedule; at times they will find that their suspicions are true (people really are talking about them behind their backs). As many investigators have indicated, an intermittent reinforcement schedule is a powerful one which leads to behavior that is very resistant to extinction.

Shame-Humiliation Theory

Colby (1975, 1976, 1977) has focused on the notion of shame and humiliation as an important issue in the development of paranoid behavior. He proposes that when people are threatened with a possible humiliating experience, they feel shame. This experience of shame occurs in anticipation of the possibly humiliating event, and serves as a signal to defend against the humiliation by blaming others: "It is not me who is inadequate, but they who are wronging me." Through the use of a computer simulation model, Colby (1975) has demonstrated that many aspects of paranoid behavior can be simulated using this theory. He sees other theoretical formulations which focus on the issue of defense against homosexuality or projection of unacceptable hostile impulses as special cases of the shame-humiliation issue.

At this early stage of theoretical development, the shame-humiliation theory has many unanswered questions. Do all people react paranoidally when experiencing shame? Apparently not. Colby (1976) suggests that parental use of intense shaming techniques during child rearing is an important factor; and treatment of adult paranoid behavior should focus on developing a sense of personal adequacy and desensitization to threats of humiliation. However, many people who are not paranoid feel inadequate and react to threatened humiliation with shame. Future research may clarify these issues.

Additional Etiological Factors

Unlike the evidence for some of the other major psychotic disorders, genetic or biochemcial explanations of paranoid behavior remain weak. Little research has been completed in this area. However, biochemical disturbances can be associated with paranoid behavior. For example, the individual who abuses amphetamines (speed) may develop paranoid-like delusions, stereotypic behavior, and visual and auditory hallucinations (Snyder, 1972). This amphetamine psychosis resembles both paranoia and schizophrenia.

Organic issues sometimes can be involved in the development of paranoia (Manschreck & Petri, 1978). In the following case, paranoid symptoms developed subsequent to hypothyroidism (underactivity of the thyroid gland):

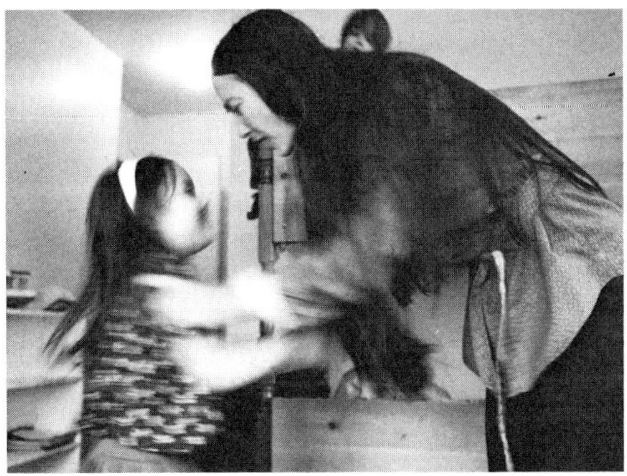

Frequent, intense scolding may lead to feelings of shame and humiliation which, according to one theoretical viewpoint, *may* be a factor in the development of adult paranoid behavior.

> The integration of endocrine, psychological and environmental factors is illustrated in the case of a 46-year-old saleswoman. She and her husband were upwardly mobile and had moved into an upper-class neighborhood three months before. She was worried about the cost of their new home and the expense of having a daughter and a son in college. She felt uncomfortable with her neighbors and told her husband that they looked down on her "as a nouveau riche." She returned to work both for financial reasons and because she did not feel accepted in the new neighborhood.
>
> She became very fatigued, gained 12 pounds and developed menorrhagia [abnormally heavy blood flow during menstruation] with anemia. These symptoms grew worse, and she suffered from ankle [swelling] as well. One night she could not sleep because she felt someone was planning to break into her home. She became more agitated and awoke her husband at 1:30 A.M., because she was convinced that "people were walking outside the house planning to hurt the children and steal our money." She heard a voice telling her to "get out of this dangerous neighborhood." She was taken to the hospital, where she appeared confused and sluggish; she was suspicious and afraid to confide in any of the staff. Physical examination revealed that she was obese, had

dry skin, and talked slowly. Her hair was coarse and she was generally pale. . . .

She was clinically hypothyroid, but her paranoid symptoms were also determined by feelings of inadequacy in the new neighborhood. Anxiety about her financial situation was translated via projection into a delusion that others were trying to harm her and steal her money. She was given three grains of thyroid initially; this dosage was later tapered off. Both her physical and psychiatric symptoms gradually disappeared, and she was able to return to work in five weeks. (Swanson et al., 1970, p. 116)

Sensory losses, such as deafness, seem at times to be precipitating factors for paranoid ideation. Other forms of changes in sensory input, such as sensory overload or sensory deprivation, are also sometimes associated with paranoid ideation (Busse & Pfeiffer, 1977). The operative factor in these situations (and perhaps in amphetamine psychosis) appears to be the loss of coherent information from the environment. Individuals who develop paranoid ideation under these conditions rely on their own thinking without being able or inclined to check their conclusions with other people.

Paranoia is common in the sensorily deprived elderly. It is a behavior second only to depression as a problem for senior citizens (K. Berger & Zarit, 1978). Elderly people often have sensory losses; losses of physical function due to aging; and losses of friends, spouse, and financial resources. Perhaps these losses are so threatening that the elderly person protects against them by becoming hypervigilant and suspicious.

Mrs. X, a 72-year-old Jewish woman living alone, requested help from a family service agency. She complained that her neighbor was putting gas in her cupboards, ripping her curtains, and doing other damage. She wanted a caseworker to come out and prove that she was right, since others did not believe her.

Mrs. X had two children. . . . When she came to the U.S.A., she lived with her single son in his little house until two years before this contact, when he moved out. She expressed anger that she used to work and be her own boss and now her children were bossing her around. . . . She apparently had not had any paranoid symptomatology while her son lived with her. Her relationship with her son had been poor since he left the house, and she was not seeing much of him. . . . Mrs. X was both friendly and aloof. She would offer the caseworker tea and food, but would always express relief when only the tea was accepted. On numerous occasions, she would indicate that she preferred not to feed visitors.

Mrs. X did not see herself as sick. She would not have anything to do with her daughter's insistence that she see a psychiatrist. The consultant for the family service agency felt she should be placed in a "nice" locked facility where she would get good treatment and care. The caseworker, however, decided to disregard this advice and attempt instead to develop a trusting relationship and to maintain her in her own home. She listened to Mrs. X's stories, and never told her that she did not believe them. Mrs. X sensed that her stories were not fully believed, but was able to accept the caseworker anyway, perhaps because she was such a willing listener.

Mrs. X was visited in her home every two weeks for five or six months. During that time, she continued having her paranoid symptomatology, but became calmer and more willing to go out occasionally. When the caseworker was leaving the family service agency, she proposed that Mrs. X see another worker or a volunteer. Mrs. X declined, stating that she had enjoyed these visits but was aware that the worker did not believe her stories. Though ending prematurely, this supportive therapy appeared to have enhanced Mrs. X's abilities to continue to function in her home. (K. Berger & Zarit, 1978, pp. 533–534)

This case illustrates the circumscribed nature of the delusions, the absence of other thought disorder, the sudden onset, and the absence of affective disturbance identified as characteristic of the late-life paranoid state by Verwoerdt (1976).

Some Conclusions about Etiology

Much remains to be learned about paranoid behavior, but some conclusions can be drawn about how such behavior comes about. It seems likely that as a child, the individual who later becomes paranoid was unable to develop a trusting relationship. The parents may have communicated that the world is a dangerous place and people are not trustworthy. This parental communication could be made either verbally or through a process of demonstrating their own lack of trustworthiness to the child. The parents may reinforce the child in obvious and subtle ways for being vigilant and suspicious of others, and for blaming others for the child's own errors.

If parents treat the child in ways that lead to intense shame, the child could learn to defend against the experience by becoming even more vigilant and by blaming others. Although appearing very self-centered and rejecting of criticism, the child would feel very inadequate at a deeper level. The individual could go through life defending against the recognition of his or her own vulnerability and low self-esteem by behaving as if blameless. A life-long pattern of such behavior would predispose the individual to react to threats, disorganization, or crisis by blaming others for the upset. The paranoidal reactions of the individual would compound the problem by driving others to behave in an exclusionary manner which would confirm the paranoid's beliefs. Many events could provide the threatening stimulus that might precipitate the disorganization: unacceptable homosexual feelings; sensory changes caused by drugs or metabolic disturbances; stressors such as emigration to strange lands; intolerable self-doubts about failures such as poor performance in college or in work; physical disability; and so on.

KEY TREATMENTS

Paranoid disorders are considered among the least amenable to treatment (Cameron, 1967). An important factor in this regard is the poor motivation of paranoids for treatment. When you believe that the problem is outside yourself, it makes little sense to want to change. Paranoid persons would prefer that something be done to make their persecutors stop, or their spouses stop "fooling around." They want the mysterious voices and visions to be stopped by shutting off the machine that is making them happen. When treatment is offered, paranoids usually see it as one more ploy to gain control over them. The therapist may be seen as a member of the conspiracy or pseudocommunity.

Paranoids become involved in treatment usually at the insistence of some other person or agency—a spouse, child, parent, a court, or some other social agency. Therapists may also encounter paranoid individuals in treatment for another issue (e.g., in couples' therapy or family therapy). When therapists begin to treat a paranoid individual, they find that they have a reluctant, probably suspiciously resistant involuntary patient whose attitude complicates even the simplest therapeutic tasks. Tranquilizers may be prescribed to reduce anxiety, but the paranoid person may refuse tham because of suspicions that they are poison. Psychotherapy, which requires trust building, is particularly difficult.

Psychotherapy

The basic lack of trust of the paranoid person requires that a psychotherapist approach the therapy session with great skill. The patient has had years of experience in which others have fulfilled the paranoid expectations. To have even a chance of being effective, the therapist must be nonthreatening, permissive, and extremely truthful and honest. The slightest hint of manipulation or dishonesty will only confirm the patient's paranoid suspicions. Criticism, confrontation, and argumentation will drive the patient away from a potentially helpful relationship. Delusions can be neither argued against nor agreed with; instead the therapist must listen openly, acknowledge the patient's right to the belief, and point out that there may be a different viewpoint.

Cameron (1967) suggests that the reduction of anxiety is the first step in this trust-building process. The environmental sources of the paranoid anxiety and stress must be reduced. For example, if current employment or co-workers are contributing to the person's anger, fear, or humiliation, a job change may be required. Once the upset is reduced, the therapist can concentrate on being the detached but interested listener who the paranoid requires. The therapist can listen without judging or arguing, and can provide feedback without unintentionally demeaning the patient's beliefs. As trust develops, the therapist can begin to suggest that other viewpoints about the events that have transpired are different from the paranoid's beliefs. Even when these conditions are met, the treatment of paranoid patients requires the therapist to engage in a difficult balancing act: On one side is acceptance, on the other, presentation of more re-

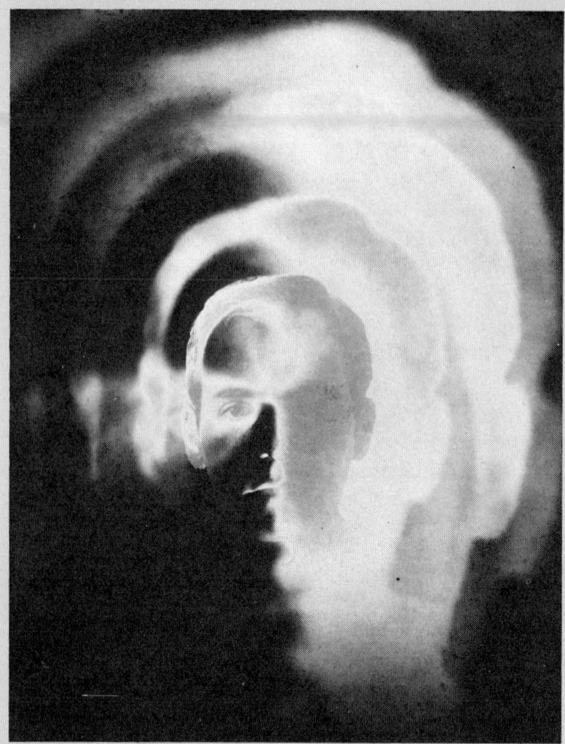

The paranoid's distrust of others may lead to a preoccupation with his or her own bodily sensations or unrealistic beliefs.

alistic views. The utility of this approach is dependent on many factors. For example, the longer the paranoid beliefs have been present, and the more gradual their onset, the less likely significant gains are to occur.

Approaches Based on Learning Theory

Ullmann and Krasner (1975) report successful attempts to modify paranoid behavior using approaches based on learning theory, including systematic desensitization and verbal conditioning. Davison (1966) used a verbal labeling process successfully, in which the subject learned relaxation techniques and renamed his experiences from "pressure points" to "sensations." In the process of this individual's treatment, major changes seem to have occurred sponaneously:

> Mr. B. had been diagnosed by one psychiatrist as a paranoid state, and by another as a paranoid schizophrenic. [He] had been hospitalized at his wife's insistence, rather than because he wanted treatment on his own motivation.
>
> Mr. B's personal concerns were over physical sensations of pressure around his right eye, heart, and abdomen. These sensations (and his paranoid behavior) started four years before, after the suicide of his brother. Mr. B. described the sensations of pressure as "pressure points" and he believed they were caused by a spirit which helped him make decisions. Over the years he had obtained tranquilizers and even surgery in order to get rid of the sensations, but neither had much effect.
>
> Behavioral treatment began with the therapist determining what led to the experience of "pressure." A number of tension-producing situations were identified which had that effect. During eight sessions over a nine-week period the therapist taught Mr. B. simple relaxation procedures which could be used to reduce tension. Games were created and introduced which were tension provoking so that on the spot relaxation training could be experienced. The therapist taught Mr. B. to relabel his behavior, and after one month Mr. B. described the pressure points as sensations. He no longer spoke of a spirit as causing the sensations. After nine weeks Mr. B. was more appropriately assertive and his relationship with his wife was better than it had been for years. (Adapted from Davison, 1966.)

The approach used in this case embodies some of the factors that Cameron describes as important in the psychotherapy of paranoids: reduction of anxiety (through the relaxation technique), a detached but interested therapist, an absence of argumentation about the folly of the belief, presentation of a differing viewpoint about reality (the process of relabeling "pressure points" as "sensations"), and probably the development of a trusting relationship. Such an approach also seems likely to appeal to the cognitive-intellectual side of a paranoid individual who is searching for an answer to why he is having these "unusual" physical experiences.

In a somewhat similar approach, W. G. Johnson, Ross, and Mastria (1977) used **attribution theory** to develop a treatment strategy for delusional behavior. Attribution theory proposes that persons form causal impressions or explanations for their own and others' behavior. That is, they "attribute" a cause to what they experience or observe. At times, because of a lack of knowledge, data, or experience, events are attributed to unrealistic or irrational causes. The following case is adapted from Johnson and colleagues' report:

> A 37-year-old man voluntarily admitted himself to a hospital with an isolated delusion. He was extremely frightened by his belief that he was having sexual intercourse with an invisible "warm form." The sexual experience was unpre-

> dictable and "involuntary," and included penile erection and ejaculation. By the time of admission, he was attributing other circumstantial events to the presence of this "warm form." During hospitalization, it was observed that when he believed the form was present, he had been moving his legs in a manner sufficient to create penile stimulation. In an earlier clinical assessment, the subject had indicated that he felt shameful about the sexual effects of the "warm form's visits." He also said that he believed masturbation was wrongful and would not do it. When told about the leg movements, which occurred when he believed the warm form was present, he stated that he was unaware of them. His penile erection and the associated tactile feelings were then reattributed by the therapist to the *natural* buildup of sexual tension and his *inadvertent* leg movements. He was very accepting of this explanation and of the notion that, from lack of information, he had created an irrational explanation of the experience. He was shortly thereafter discharged, and followed up for six months. Several spontaneous erections during this time were interpreted by him as due to the buildup of sexual tension, rather than as a visitation by the "warm form," and he no longer manifested the "delusion."

Taken with caution, this case demonstrates the promise of reattribution techniques in treating delusional beliefs. However, the authors were dealing with a delusion that had only recently been formed. The technique may not be as effective with persons whose delusional beliefs are of a long-standing, insidious onset, In addition, W. G. Johnson et al. emphasize that they use veridical (truthful) manipulations rather than deceptive ones; they feel that deception does not allow a lasting learning experience. As Kopel and Arkowitz (1975) have pointed out, deceptive manipulations have the potential of undermining the therapeutic relationship. Furthermore, reattribution is quite different from confrontation. To attempt to argue the paranoid out of a delusional belief appears useless. Swanson et al. (1970) present an apocryphal story which indicates the failure of an argumentative, confrontative approach:

> An ambitious first-year psychiatric resident—by fable—decided to show a patient the illogic of his delusion that he was dead. Eager to establish a first premise, the resident asked, "Do dead men walk?" "Definitely," the patient replied. Thwarted, the doctor said, "Do dead men eat?" "Yes," came the calm reply. Becoming desperate the resident spotted a pin on his desk and got an inspiration. "Do dead men bleed?" "Of course not," was the patient's answer. Quickly the resident grabbed the pin, jabbed it into the startled patient's leg, and triumphantly said, "See that?" The patient looked at his bleeding leg, then back at the resident, and made his final conclusion, "My God, dead men do bleed!" (p. 405)

For the individual who manifests a paranoid approach to life, the pressure to maintain the behavior seems extremely strong. As Zentner (1980) has suggested, even in people who do not manifest the major symptoms of the disorder, treatment is hampered by the behaviors which one intends to change: rigidity; self-centered, distorted perspectives; rejection of change; projection; and the need to be dominant in relationships.

Summary

1. Two major patterns of psychotic paranoid behavior have been described in this chapter: 1. paranoia and 2. the paranoid state. They share several major characteristics with 3. a less frequent subtype called shared paranoid disorder. Although the reported frequency of all three disorders is low, we have reason to believe that the incidence in the general population is significant.

2. Paranoid personality disorder, the psychotic paranoid disorders, and paranoid schizophrenia are believed by some clinicians to be degrees of severity on a continum of schizophrenic disorganization. Recent evidence tentatively supports the view that the paranoid disorders are entities distinct from schizophrenia, the position taken in this chapter.

3. The major characteristics common to paranoia, shared paranoid disorder, and paranoid state are: 1. organized delusions of persecution, jealousy, or grandeur; 2. appropriate orientation and affect; 3. adequate judgment except in the areas of delusional beliefs; 4. absence of bizarre fragmentation of thinking processes; 5. hallucinations may be present, but are not a prominent feature.

4. In paranoia the primary feature is an insidious development of a lasting, relatively unmodifiable system of false beliefs. Paranoids relate to others in an angry, often arrogant, suspicious, distant manner which hides an underlying fear and anxiety about the threats they experience.

5. The paranoid state differs from paranoia in that

the former usually has a sudden onset, is rarely chronic, and is often preceded by stressful events, such as emigration or migration, major disasters, major life-style changes, or threatened failure of important life goals.

6. Shared paranoid disorder is an unusual phenomenon in which two or more people share a system of delusional beliefs. When two people have the shared paranoid disorder, one is usually more paranoid and is the dominant member of this duo. The submissive member often loses the symptoms if separated from the dominant partner.

7. The premorbid personality of paranoids often fits a particular life pattern. They may be overly sensitive, rigid, suspicious, cold, and distant. Magical thinking is sometimes seen, in which the individuals have a sense of having special knowledge (e.g., extrasensory perception) or power. Premorbid paranoids tend to be arrogant, self-important, and unable to accept blame.

8. Paranoids progress through a process of mistrust, fear, and hypervigilance to threats. They then selectively perceive events which signify threats and do not perceive positive nonthreatening occurrences. Next they project blame and relate angrily to others who are driven away by these behaviors. The events finally become organized into a delusional belief system in order to make sense out of the paranoid's perceptions.

9. Freud proposed that paranoid behavior is a defense against unacceptable homosexual impulses. The mechanisms of denial, reaction formation, and projection are used to change homosexual love into hate, and the hate is projected onto others as their motivation for behavior. There is little support for the generalization that all paranoids are defending against homosexual impulses.

10. The concept of pseudocommunity has been advanced by Cameron to explain paranoid behavior. Basic trust has not developed in childhood, so that the mistrustful adult who experiences a major stressful threat reacts first with rage, and then with fear of this rage. The paranoid's perception of others as dangerous allows him or her to experience rage as justified. Selective perceptions of danger confirm the false beliefs, and the delusions become crystalized. Finally, the pseudocommunity develops, in which the paranoid now perceives real and imagined people united as persecutors.

11. Lemert's exclusionary hypothesis emphasizes that there is some truth in the paranoid's beliefs. The paranoid probably is being talked about, reported to employers, excluded from relationships, primarily because of the unpleasant qualities of paranoid behaviors.

12. Behaviorists have suggested that people may be reinforced for behaving as if the environment is threatening, and for shifting blame onto others. Behavior thus may be shaped into what we call paranoia. People may learn to "think straight about biased information."

13. Colby proposes that the paranoid behavior of blaming others occurs to avoid humiliation, and that the experience of shame is the signal that a humiliating situation is impending. He further suggests that people who become paranoid experienced intense shame as a primary parental child-rearing approach.

14. Organic factors contribute to paranoid behavior in some individuals. Examples include amphetamine abuse; sensory losses such as deafness; sensory isolation and overstimulation; and hypothyroidism.

15. Paranoid ideation is second only to depression as a behavioral problem in the elderly. The elderly may be particularly vulnerable to beliefs of persecution and threat, and especially likely to blame others because they have experienced so many emotional and physical losses in our culture.

16. Paranoids are particularly difficult to treat. Their unwillingness to find fault (problems) within themselves makes them resistant to treatment. In addition, they are usually suspicious of the therapist's motives.

17. Effective therapy with paranoid disorders requires the building of trust, a difficult task. Therapists must be open, honest, nonconfrontative, if they are to maintain a relationship with the client. The anxieties and fears of the paranoid person must first be reduced, so that alternative viewpoints about the delusional perceptions can be offered by the therapist without arousing the paranoid suspicions of the client.

18. Some cases of successful modification of paranoid behavior using anxiety reduction procedures such as relaxation training and verbal relabeling have been reported. In the case provided, the approach embodied many of the factors identified as necessary for successful verbal psychotherapy with paranoid clients.

19. The application of attribution theory to the treatment of delusional beliefs seems to hold promise. The paranoid perceptions are attributed to more realistic causes. This enables the client to interpret events in a more acceptable manner which avoids delusional concepts.

20. The therapies described all emphasize truthfulness and avoidance of confrontation and argumentation. While the therapies can be successful with some paranoids, treatment is hampered by the behaviors that need to be modified: rigidity; self-centered, distorted perspectives; rejection of the need to change; projection; and the need to be dominant in relationships.

KEY TERMS

Insidious. A gradual, relatively unnoticeable progression of a disorder.

Magical thinking. Thinking characterized by a simple or primitive perception of cause and effect, such as belief in superstitions.

Preliminary crystalization. The individuals' experience of forming their often mistaken perceptions into a paranoid belief system which makes sense to them.

Projection. The externalization of one's feelings, beliefs, and motivations onto other people.

Paranoid pseudocommunity. The group of unrelated people or agencies which a paranoid person mistakenly believes are in a conspiracy against him or her.

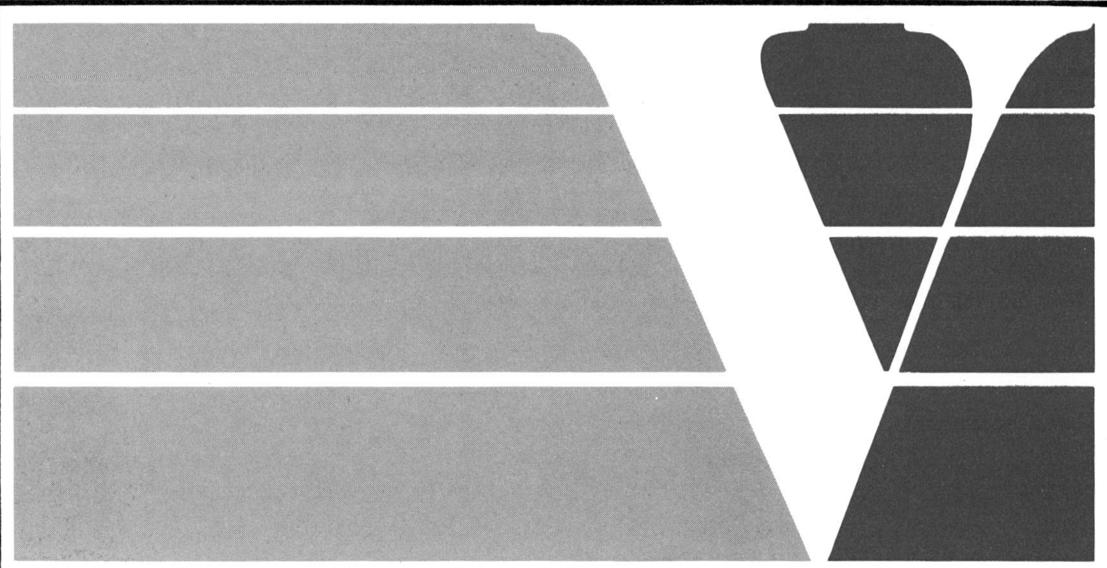

AFFECTIVE DISORDERS

- **Chapter 15 Affective disorders I: phenomenology**
- **Chapter 16 Affective disorders II: theories, research, and treatment**

Affective disorders range from mild depression to moods extreme enough to be associated with hallucinations and delusions. The mild and moderate levels of depression are often called neurotic depression, while those characterized by hallucinations and delusions are often called psychotic depression. The mild and moderate levels of mood disorder seem quite familiar to most of us. Many of our friends and relatives, perhaps even ourselves, have had firsthand experience of mild depression. Certainly, we all know feelings of sadness, guilt, and pessimism. The intense feelings of severe depression and, at the other extreme, the elation, excitement, or irritability of mania are probably less familiar to us.

In Chapter 15, the clinical features of depression and mania are presented. In addition, unipolar depression is differentiated from bipolar affective disorder; the latter involves major mood swings between mania and depression. The chapter closes with a section on suicide, a behavior often associated with depression. Chapter 16 focuses on etiological theories of the affective (mood) disorders, relevant research, and key treatment approaches for these disorders.

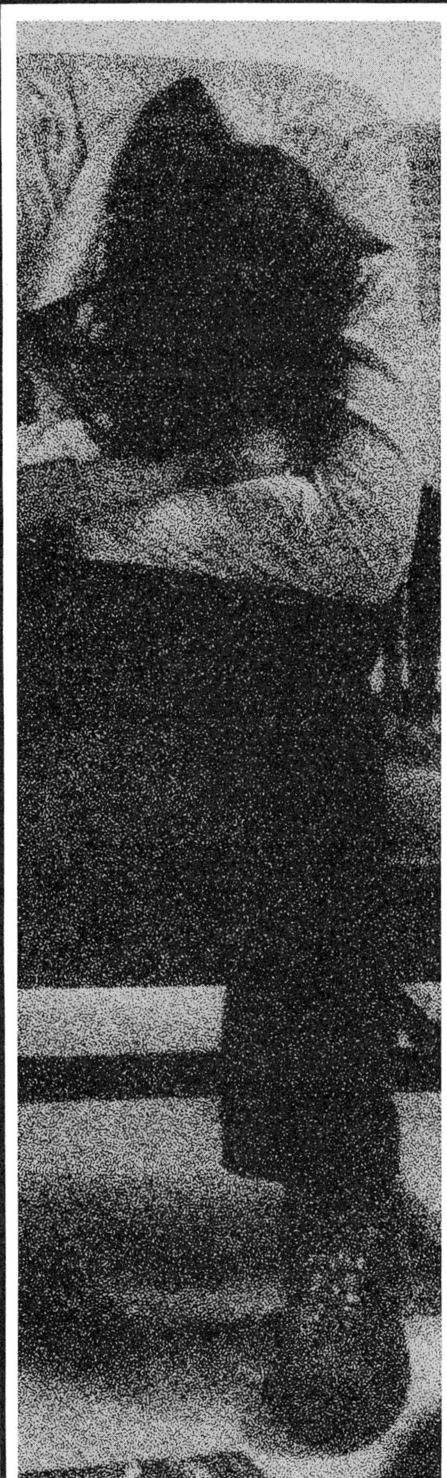

5

Affective disorders I: phenomenology

- Characteristics of the depressive disorders
- Mania and the bipolar affective disorders
- Suicide
- Summary
- Key terms

Do you recall the last time you had the Monday morning blues? Remember that fatigued feeling, the sense of being drained of energy, the lack of interest in doing much more than lying around, the distaste you felt about going to work or class? Multiply the intensity of these feelings by perhaps 10 or 100 times and you may begin to get some idea of what a clinical **depression** feels like. On the other hand, think back to a time when you felt exuberant, joyous, and elated. Perhaps you got an "A" on an extremely difficult test, or you first experienced romantic love. You may have made sweeping plans during the rush of feeling, only to be prevented from carrying them through. Did your elation turn to irritability and anger? Such mood swings, when multiplied to an extreme degree, are part of what we call **mania,** another of the affective disorders.

Each of us has some variability in our **mood.** Mood is a prolonged emotion that colors our psychic life. It affects how we perceive things, how we behave, and how others behave toward us. In this chapter, we will consider the **affective disorders,** which are disorders of mood. In the affective disorders, people experience extremes of mood which are either subjectively very unpleasant or which interfere with their usual day-to-day functioning. People may experience depression so deep that they become virtually immobile and may even take their own lives. When a depression becomes very severe, the individual may have hallucinations and delusions. These depressions are called **psychotic depression.** Some people may experience emotional highs or mania of such intensity and length that the emotion interferes with their ability to relate to others, to support themselves, and to maintain rational behavior. Some individuals swing from one extreme to the other: from normal mood to mania, and then into a numbing depression. The most severe of the major depressions is often described as **melancholia,** a term used by Hippocrates. Many different patterns of mood swings are possible. Figure 15.1 illustrates four patterns which might occur in a day. When an individual has an affective disorder, however, the disturbance of mood typically endures for long periods, not just a day.

We will examine the symptoms of **unipolar depression** and mania, and the characteristics of individuals with **bipolar affective disorder,** who swing between these extremes. The chapter will end with a discussion of suicide, a behavior of special concern in people with depressive disorders. Theories and related research about the etiology of the affective disorders will be presented in Chapter 16, which will examine the key therapies used in the treatment of these disorders.

CHARACTERISTICS OF THE DEPRESSIVE DISORDERS

General Features of Unipolar Depression

We have already seen that the symptoms of depression are more intense than the "Monday morning blues." Yet even among people whom we would describe as depressed, the symptoms' intensity ranges from mild to severe. If we count only people with clinically significant depressions, it has been estimated that 15 percent of the population experience an affective disorder at one time or another. Mendels (1970) notes that while the symptoms may vary among individuals, some are common.

Mood and Thought. The typical mood of the depressed individual is one of sadness and misery, as if all pleasure has gone out of life. Pessimism about oneself and one's chances are common, as are ideas of guilt. The depressed individual is likely to be self-critical. There is a loss of interest in previously valued pursuits, and even when the interest remains (as in a hobby), the individual lacks the motivation to engage in the behavior. The efficiency of thinking and concentration also decreases. Working out problems (such as balancing a checkbook) becomes difficult, and the individual may have concentration difficulties (such as having to read a paragraph over and over before being aware of what it says).

Behavior. The physical movements of individuals may be affected. Some persons mani-

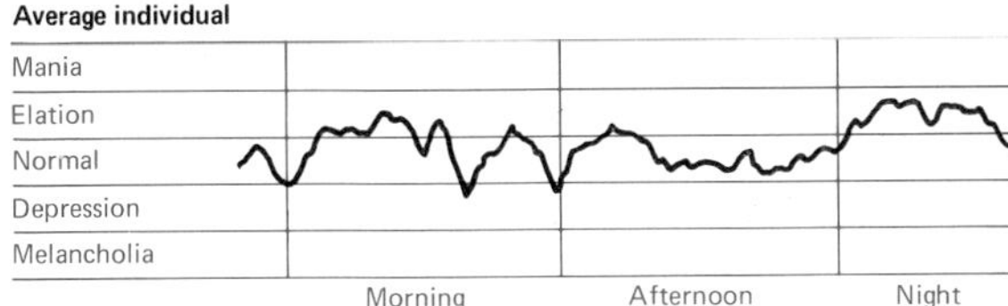

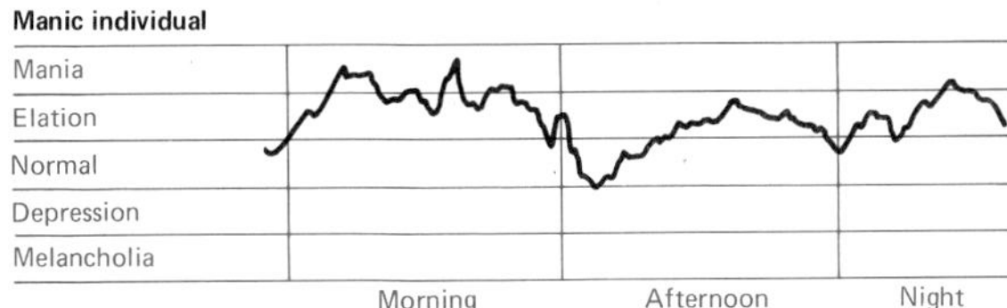

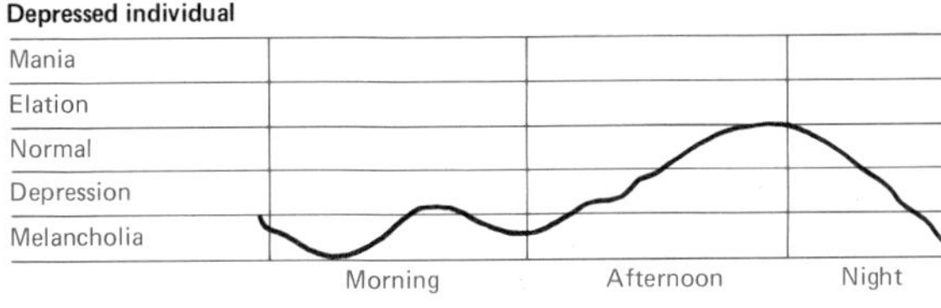

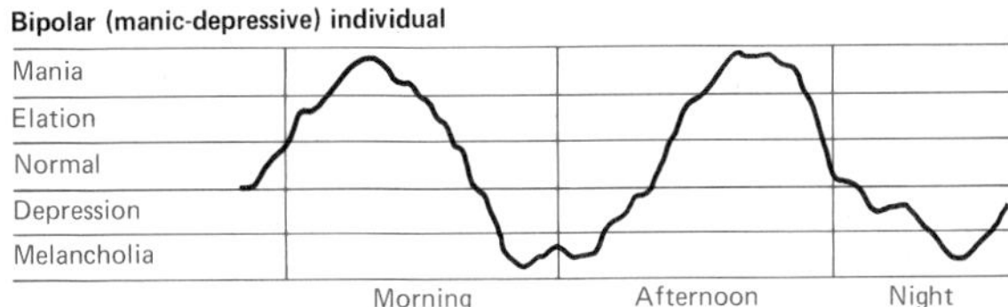

Figure 15.1. Hypothetical changes in mood during one day for an average individual, manic individual, depressed individual, and manic-depressive individual.

From Vetter (1972, pp. 349–350).

fest **psychomotor retardation,** in which movements become slow and deliberate, with a reduction in spontaneous movements; they may move as if encased in glue. In contrast, other individuals show an agitated depression; their behaviors may be jerky and rapid, with hand wringing and pacing. Agitated individuals appear to be anxious as well as depressed.

The outward appearance of the individual may manifest depression in a variety of ways. The facial features may be dejected and saddened, and eye contact with others may decrease. Posture may appear stooped, as if one is carrying the world on one's shoulders. When depressions are deep, the individual may lose interest in personal appearance and become sloppy or even dirty. Men may stop shaving and bathing; women may give up the use of cosmetics, and neglect the care of hair and clothing.

Physical, or Somatic, Changes. Changes in bodily functioning have been noted in many individuals who become seriously depressed. These changes may be due to both psychological and physiological factors in depression. Frequently, there is a loss of appetite and a subsequent loss of weight from lowered food consumption. Since some people eat in order to feel better, there also may be weight increases. Constipation may be a problem, particularly when the depression is severe. Many depressed individuals develop difficulties in

Sometimes depression is clearly visible in a person's posture.

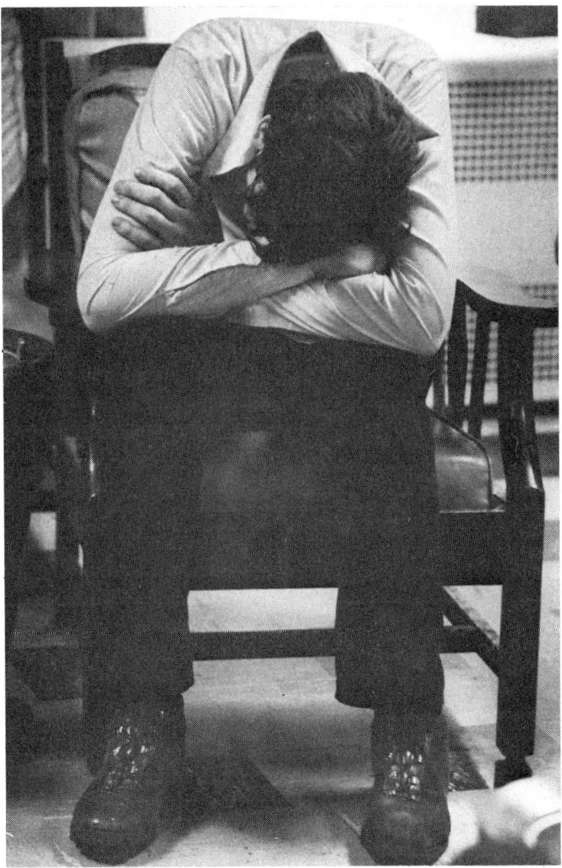

Table 15.1
Frequency of clinical features among 486 patients with varying depths of depression

Clinical feature	*Depth of depression (percent)*			
	NONE	MILD	MODERATE	SEVERE
Sad face	18	72	94	98
Stooped posture	6	32	70	87
Crying in interview	3	11	29	28
Speech: slow, etc.	25	53	72	75
Low mood	16	72	94	94
Daily variation of mood	6	13	37	37
Suicidal wishes	13	47	73	94
Indecisiveness	18	42	68	83
Hopelessness	14	58	85	86
Feeling inadequate	25	56	75	90
Conscious guilt	27	46	64	60
Loss of interest	14	56	83	92
Loss of motivation	23	54	88	88
Fatigability	39	62	89	84
Sleep disturbance	31	55	73	88
Loss of appetite	17	33	61	88
Constipation	19	26	38	52

Adapted from A. T. Beck (1967, p. 40).

sleeping. They may have trouble falling asleep, or they may wake up in the middle of the night and have difficulty returning to sleep. When they do sleep, they often awaken in the morning feeling just as fatigued as the night before. In cases of milder depression, the individual may sleep more deeply and for longer periods of time than normal. Depressed individuals, preoccupied with themselves, may experience an increase in aches and pains. Depressed women often have disruptions in their menstrual cycles. Both sexes may experience a marked decrease in sexual desire.

The signs of depression in an individual vary to some degree with the depth of depression, and sometimes are seen in individuals who are not depressed (see Table 15.1).

Depression: A Continuum?

Is depression one disorder that varies from person to person in severity? While this notion might seem reasonable, for many years clinicians and researchers have suspected that this may not be the case. Depression has, for example, often been subclassified into exogenous and endogenous types.

Exogenous depressions appear to have an external precipitant such as a loss. Losses identified as important in depression include the death of a loved one (see Highlight 15.1), loss of employment, divorce, and symbolic losses. As an example of a symbolic loss, consider the loss of a job. A "normal" reaction to a job loss would be to seek other employment. However, if the individual becomes very depressed, we might infer that the loss of the job symbolized a deeper loss from childhood, such as the absence of parental love. Thus, the job loss becomes emotionally much more significant for the individual. This notion about depression is a cornerstone of the psychoanalytic theory, as we shall see in Chapter 16. When an environmental precipitant such as a loss is identifiable in the life of a depressed individual, the term "reactive depression" has also been applied. Many clinical and research studies have indicated that the loss of a parent during childhood predisposes an adult to depression. However, Lloyd (1980a), in a major review of the literature, found that only 20–40 percent of adults who were depressed had experienced such a loss. She concludes that while childhood losses may be important in some cases, other factors must also be operating. Lloyd (1980b) also reviewed the evidence for immediate losses as precipitating events in depression. The issue was whether events such as job losses, divorce, or death of a loved one had occurred in the immediate period (six months to one year) prior to the depressive episode. For this factor, much more evidence existed. Several controlled studies indicated that depressed people had three to four times as many losses or stress events prior to their episode than did nondepressives in the same time period. But once again Lloyd was forced to conclude that the studies did not prove causality. It is quite likely that other factors operate in the presence of an immediate loss. Many people experience such losses, but do not become depressed. Others do *not* experience any such identifiable loss, but manifest severe depressions.

The existence of the latter group has led to the concept of **endogenous depression.** This term refers to relatively severe depressive behavior that is neither preceded by a predisposing or precipitating environmental stress, nor influenced by subsequent changes in the environment. For example, the depression does not lessen even when major positive events occur in the individual's life. In addition, many studies have suggested that endogenous depressions are primarily due to dysfunctions of physiology and biochemistry (Winoker, 1979). When we examine the various theories of depression, we will cover this research in greater detail. J. C. Nelson and Charney (1981) have identified symptoms which they believe are most characteristic of the endogenous type of depression (see Table 15.2). This type of depression is by definition severe and often involves psychotic behavior. In DSM-III (1980), it is called "melancholia" in its most severe form.

Unfortunately, in real life, things are not always clear-cut. It would be convenient if mild depressions were always related to environmental or exogenous factors, and major depressions were always endogenous. This does

HIGHLIGHT 15.1
UNCOMPLICATED BEREAVEMENT

If you have lived through the death of someone you loved—a grandparent, parent, spouse, child, or sibling—you have probably experienced many of the symptoms of depression. Yet your feelings probably were significantly different from depression. First, you were probably more concerned for the person you lost than for yourself. This lack of self-centeredness does not characterize clinical depression. Second, you probably "worked through" the bereavement within a few months and went on with the business of living. The process which most people normally go through after the death of a loved one is called **uncomplicated bereavement.** When the process goes awry, it becomes complicated.

Normal, or uncomplicated, bereavement involves a series of reactions and processes beginning with expressions of shock, sadness, tears, and grief. This is usually followed rapidly by a mild social withdrawal. Resolution of this affective reaction proceeds through a slow and initially painful process of recollecting memories of the lost person. The opportunity to talk and share these memories with others helps. These initially painful memories become less painful after the feelings associated with them have been expressed. The resurrection of the memories becomes less frequent as time passes and the pain of the loss becomes less acute. Finally, the deceased can be remembered, the memories shared, and the feelings are primarily positive. Usually, the process takes from a few to six months.

This normal bereavement process can go wrong in a number of ways. In some cases, total emotional denial may occur. While the individual may admit that the loved one has died, the deceased's possessions (e.g., bedroom and clothing) may be maintained as a shrine. The survivor lives on, but does not go about the business of *living*. In other cases, the bereavement may turn to self-centered depression. Rather than mourning the loss, the individual seems to focus on being left behind, being abandoned. The reaction seems to involve buried anger at the deceased for no longer being there to take care of the survivor.

The similarity of uncomplicated bereavement to depression, and the complications of bereavement just noted, have stimulated many theorists to conceptualize emotional loss as an important factor in the development of most affective disorders.

Table 15.2
Degree to which specific symptoms are characteristic of endogenous depression (melancholia)

Degree	*Symptoms*
Strongly characteristic	Retardation (motor) Agitation Lack of reactivity Severe depressed mood Depressive delusions Self-reproach Loss of interest
Mildly characteristic	Distinct quality of mood Decreased concentration Depression worse in morning
Weakly characteristic	Weight loss Early morning awakening Midnight awakening Suicidal thoughts, attempts Difficulty falling asleep

Adapted from J. C. Nelson and Charney (1981, p. 10).

not appear to be the case. Some very severe depressions appear to be related to predisposing stresses, while some mild depressions do not; and vice versa. There do not appear to be two discrete types of depression—one of psychosocial origin and one of biochemical origin. Rather, depressive behavior appears to fall on a continuum from psychosocial to biochemical, which is only partially related to the severity of symptoms. In the following section, we will provide examples of two types of depressive disorders, **dysthymic disorder** and major depressive disorder. Although the adjective "major" may seem to imply that the depth of depression is greater in the latter, this is only partially true.

Dysthymic Disorder

The rather obscure term "dysthymic disorder" has been introduced in DSM-III (1980) to label depressions that used to be called "depressive neurosis." The latter term has been dropped, since it originated from one theoretical framework, the psychoanalytic. We might best consider the dysthymic disorder as depression of moderate symptomatology. Psychotic symptoms are not present, and there is little likelihood of other severe symptoms such as motor retardation and psychomotor agitation. Although we describe this disorder as a moderate depression, the disorder can be extremely distressing in terms of the individual's subjective experience. People who have this type of depression are very unhappy and emotionally pained, and some may become distraught enough to commit suicide. The following case illustrates a dysthymic disorder severe enough to require hospitalization:

> In his mid-thirties, John and his wife had decided that their marriage was no longer satisfactory and obtained a basically uncontested divorce. Approximately eight months later, John developed a fairly serious depression. He no longer took pleasure from the things he had done before (work, racquetball, golf, etc.). He felt saddened and alone, believed his friends really did not care for him, and felt guilty for not trying harder in his marriage. Knowing that his wife was quite happy in her new single life accentuated his unhappiness. He began having difficulty sleeping, and it became a major effort to drag himself to work every day. He spent most of his nonwork time at home and stopped seeing many of his friends. It was just too much effort for him to go out and pretend that he was "happy." He believed that he would not get anywhere in his job, and that he would feel "lousy" the rest of his life. Nothing seemed to cheer him up for more than a few hours. Life seemed to be bleak and painful, and he began to think of "getting away from it all." A supervisor finally confronted him about the deteriorating quality of his work due to his apparent inability to concentrate. In this supervisory session, he opened up with the supervisor (a former racquetball partner) about his feelings and suicidal thoughts. The supervisor brought him to a local hospital where he was admitted for 10 days and treated with mood-elevating drugs. At discharge, he contacted a psychologist and was treated for his depression with psychotherapy for 14 months on an outpatient basis. During the following 15 years, there has been no recurrence of the depression.

Depressions like the above have been considered the "common cold" of mental health (Seligman, 1973). They are among the most frequently seen disorders in private practice and clinics. It has been estimated that 5 percent of men and 10 percent of women are clinically depressed at least once in their lives (Woodruff, Goodwin, & Guze, 1974).

Major Depressive Episode

When the depressive symptoms include the full range of depressive behaviors—especially psychomotor retardation or agitation—and the symptomatology is severe, we diagnose the individual as suffering from a major depressive disorder. As these symptoms become more and more severe, psychotic symptoms of hallucinations and delusions may be seen. Depressions of this severity almost always require hospitalization. In this disorder, the delusions and hallucinations are often **mood congruent;** that is, a delusion may consist of a guilty belief that the person's sins led to the end of the world, and now the world does not exist. Hallucinations are often auditory, in which voices accuse the person of committing sinful acts or of being worthless and disgusting. Kolb (1968) presents the following case:

> E. D., aged sixty, was admitted to the hospital because he was depressed, ate insufficiently, and believed that his stomach was "rotting away." The patient was described as a friendly, sociable individual, not quarrelsome, jealous, or critical and with a sense of humor. He was considered even-tempered, slow to anger, tenderhearted, and emotional. At fifty-one the patient suffered from a depression when he was obliged to resign his position. This depression continued for about nine months, after which he apparently fully recovered. He resumed his work but after two years suffered from a second depression. Again he recovered after several months and returned to a similar position which he held until two months before his admission. At this time he began to worry lest he was not doing his work well, talked much of his lack of fitness for his duties, and finally resigned. He spent Thanksgiving Day at his son's in a neighboring city but while there he was sure that the water pipes in his own house would freeze during his absence and that he and his family would be "turned out into the street." A few days later he was found standing by a pond, evidently contemplating suicide. He soon began to remain in bed and would sometimes wrap his head in the bed clothing to shut out the external world. He declared that he was "rotting away inside," and that if he ate, the food would kill him. He urged the family not to touch the glasses or towels he used lest they become contaminated.
>
> On arrival at the hospital he appeared older than his years. He was pale, poorly nourished, dehydrated, with his lips dry, cracked and covered with sores. His facial expression and general bearing suggested a feeling of utter hopelessness. He was self-absorbed and manifested no interest in his environment. When urged to answer questions there would be a long delay before attempting to reply but he would finally speak briefly, hesitatingly, and in a low tone. He occasionally became agitated and would repeatedly say, "Oh, Doctor, why did I ever get into anything like this? Doctor, I am all filled up. I can't get anything through me—what am I going to do? Oh, dear! Oh, dear!" In explaining his presence in the hospital he said he realized he had been sent by his family because they believed he would be benefited by the treatment, but added, "I don't know how they sent me here when they had not the means. My wife cannot pay for me and by this time she must have been put out of the house."

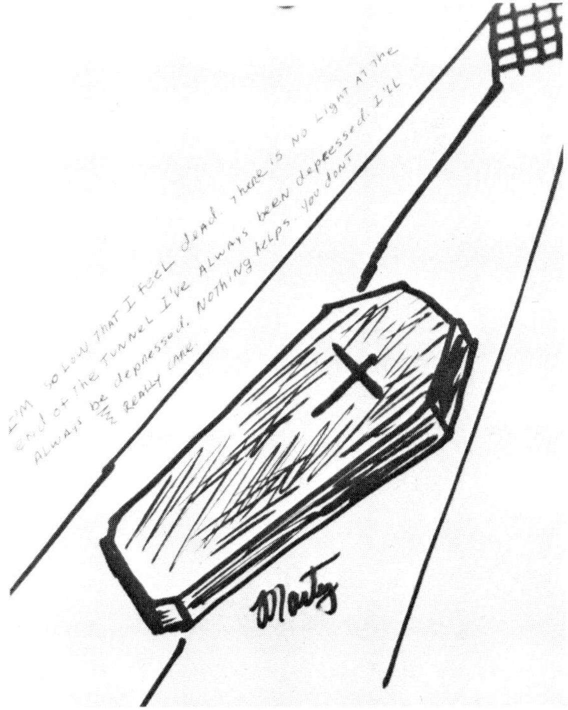

This drawing and comment illustrate the despair of the person with severe unipolar depression.

After several months the patient began to improve, although hypochondriacal ideas persisted for a considerable period. Finally when the matter of freedom of the hospital grounds was considered he seemed in a normal mood and indicated that he was beginning to think somewhat differently concerning his gastrointestinal tract. At that time he commented, "There's a good deal of life in the old horse yet." (pp. 343–344)

MANIA AND THE BIPOLAR AFFECTIVE DISORDERS

In this section, we will examine the symptoms of disturbed affect which lie at the opposite pole from depression: mania. Before considering the symptoms of mania, we must point out that few individuals who experience mania seem to avoid depression. While unipolar mania exists, it is unusual (Abrams & Taylor, 1974). Much more frequently an episode (or episodes) of mania is associated with one or more episodes of severe depression. Because of this, when one or more episodes of mania are manifested but no depressions have been present, the individual is still given a diagnosis of bipolar affective disorder. A presumption is made that at some time in the *future* a major depressive episode will occur. That such a depressive episode will *always* occur has not been demonstrated through controlled research, but is based on clinical inference. The diagnosis of bipolar affective disorder seems warranted, since there appears to be little difference between unipolar manics who have not had a depressive episode and bipolar manics who have (Abrams & Taylor, 1974).

Figure 15.2. Phases of a manic episode based on behavior ratings of a hospitalized patient.

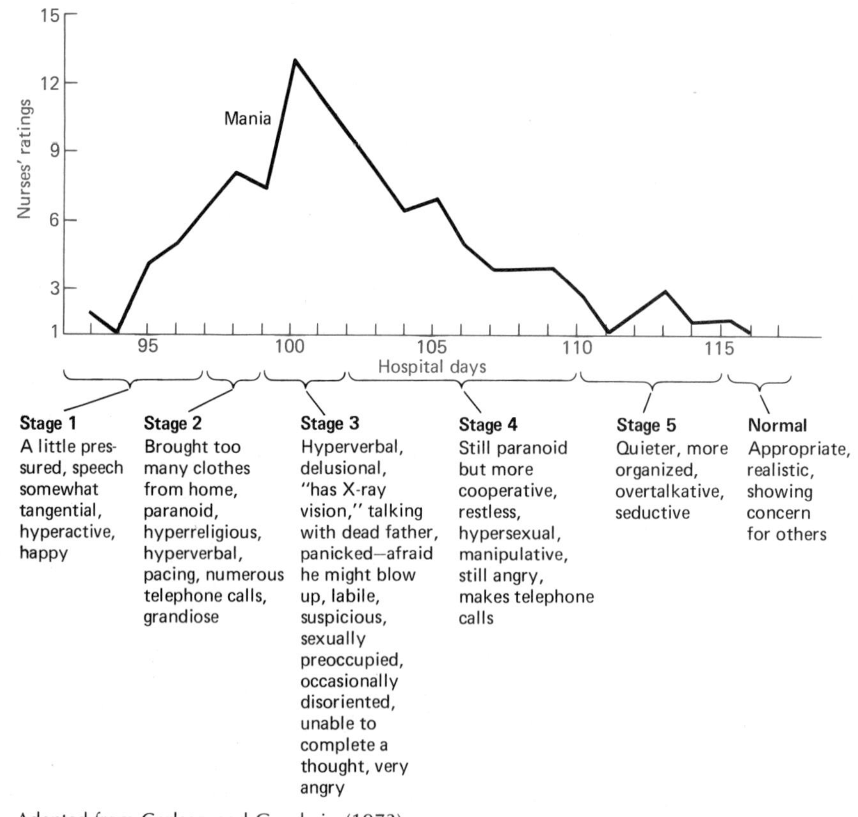

Adapted from Carlson and Goodwin (1973).

Manic Behavior

The typical signs of mania involve a period when an individual is unusually elated and expansive, and often irritable when frustrated. The manic mood usually fluctuates over time (see Figure 15.2).

Mood. The manic has been described as on a natural high. Mood is euphoric and cheerful. The person often feels that anything is possible if only one puts one's mind to the task. Great plans are often made, and if these plans are disrupted by external frustration, the mood may change to one of anger and irritability.

Thought. In a manic phase, the individual has an overwhelmingly positive self-image. Belief in one's own abilities is boundless, and expectations of success are unrealistic. Failure is blamed on others; problems are denied; and manics often insist they have never felt better, thought clearer, or been more powerful. As the mania becomes more pronounced, there may be delusions of grandiosity: beliefs that one has special powers or talents. Hallucinations may occur, and usually consist of voices (such as God's) telling the person that he or she has a special mission or ability.

Behavior. In a manic episode, the individual's energy seems boundless. Often only a few hours' sleep are required per night. The individual may be very active planning many events, taking on new duties, developing new relationships. Vacations may be started only to be broken off so that the individual can return to work. There may be buying sprees, high risk money investments, and hypersexuality. Behaviorally, the individual appears "supercharged." Judgment is often impaired. Dress may become bizarre, and women may apply their makeup in unusual and odd ways, using strange colors that make them appear to be wearing warpaint. A notable characteristic of manic behavior is speech that is loud and rapid, as if spewing out under some internal pressure. The manic may manifest "flight of ideas," a continuous stream of speech in which one idea tumbles after another. In severe cases, the manic's speech may become disorganized, and the individual may be extremely distractible by environmental stimuli. The following example of manic behavior is given by Cameron and Magaret (1957); the second paragraph includes **clang associations,** a type of speech characterized by a rhyming quality.

> A thirty-five-year-old biochemist was brought to the clinic by his frightened wife. To his psychiatrist, the patient explained, "I discovered that I had been drifting, broke the bonds and suddenly found myself doing things and doing them by telegraph. I was dead tired, and decided to go on a vacation; but even there it wasn't long before I was sending more telegrams. I got into high gear and started to buzz. Then a gentle hint from a friend took effect and I decided to come here and see if the changes in my personality were real." He entered the ward in high spirits, went about greeting the patients, insisted that the place was "swell," and made quick puns on the names of doctors to whom he was introduced. Meanwhile his wife said she was "scared to death." "His friends used to call him 'Crazy Charley,' " she said, "but I haven't seen this streak in him for years."
>
> When his wife had left, the patient soon demonstrated what he meant by "high gear." He bounded down the hall, threw his medication on the floor, leaped on a window ledge and dared any one to get him down. When he was put in a room alone where he could be free, he promptly dismantled the bed, pounded on the walls, yelled and sang. He made a sudden sally into the hall and did a kind of hula-hula dance before he could be returned to his room. His shouting continued throughout the night, and betrayed in its content the ambivalent attitudes which the patient maintained toward his hospitalization: "What the hell kind of a place is this? A swell place? I'm not staying here. I'm having a hell of a good time. Oh, I'm so happy. I have to get going. My gray suit please, my gray coat please, my gray socks, all gray on their way, going to be gay. I'm going out as fast as I came in, only faster, I'm happier than I have ever been in my life. I'm 100 per cent better than normal." (p. 332)

Bipolar Affective Disorders

Cyclothymic Disorder. When the mood swings of the bipolar disorder are mild, the behavior is called **cyclothymic disorder.** Even in this milder form of affective disorder, many problems appear—as the following case study reveals:

> A 29-year-old man was referred by his ex-wife for psychiatric evaluation. After 7 years of marriage they had just been divorced for the second time as a result of his many extramarital affairs. During their second marriage, he had undergone 2 years of outpatient analytical treatment to alter his "narcissistic personality makeup." Shortly after the second divorce, the wife went to graduate school to train as a social worker; there she became acquainted with descriptions of manic-depressive illness. She started experiencing guilt feelings because she felt that her husband might have been sick rather than "simply refusing to grow up." After many months of persistent effort, she finally succeeded in getting her ex-husband to go to the psychiatrist who had lectured to her class.
>
> The patient had 3–4 day periods of "hypersexuality" during which he would sleep 4–5 hours a night and demand frequent intercourse. This was enjoyable to his wife during the first year of their marriage, but then she started experiencing discomfort. . . . He then started frequenting bars in order to satisfy his "satyriacal needs." At other times he was intermittently lethargic or irritable, indulged in alcohol, slept 8–9 hours a day, and neglected his wife sexually. He was employed as an architect and during his "up" periods he would sometimes go to his office at 4:00 A.M. on weekends; during his "down" periods he would accomplish very little and resort to the use of amphetamines to keep going. He felt that what he termed his "naturally occurring up periods" were superior to "artificial speeding."
>
> His employer valued him because he developed outstanding and creative projects at certain times of the year, even though his overall yearly output was considerably less than that of his colleagues. He was quite unpredictable in many areas; for instance, during a vacation, while his wife slept in a motel he took off from Miami to New York and returned the following afternoon. The patient denied subjectively experiencing mood swings; he was only aware of being "active and up" or "lazy and down." He stated that during his "up" periods he felt driven to do "crazy things, such as reading Time magazine from cover to cover, including all the ads." He was known to be generous and showered his wife and lovers with expensive jewelry. . . . (Akiskal et al., 1977, p. 1230)

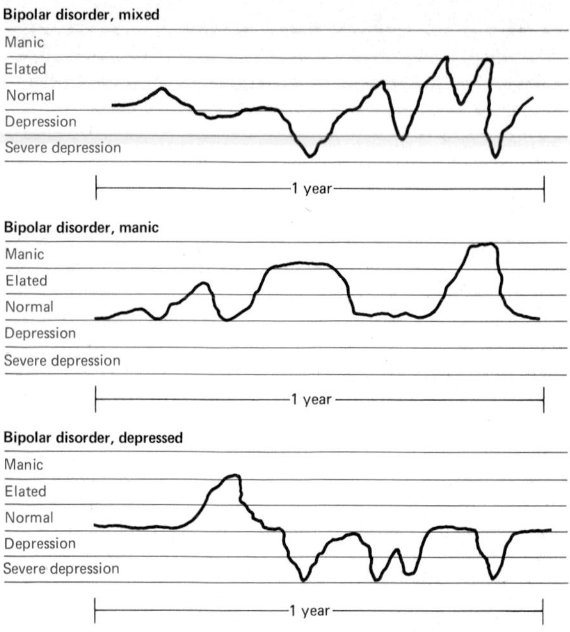

Figure 15.3. Variants of the major bipolar disorders.

Major Bipolar Affective Disorder. The more severe bipolar affective disorders are represented in Figure 15.3. In bipolar disorder, mixed, the manic and depressive mood and behaviors alternate. The individual goes from one extreme to the other with periods of normal mood in between. In the bipolar disorder, mixed, depicted in Figure 15.3 the individual would have been first diagnosed as having a major depressive episode. The diagnosis would be changed after the occurrence of the first manic episode. In the bipolar disorder, manic (see Figure 15.3), the individual swings between normal moods and mania. If at some point the individual manifests a depressive episode, however, the diagnosis could be changed to bipolar disorder, mixed. In the final example in Figure 15.3, the diagnosis is bipolar disorder, depressed. For this diagnosis to be made, rather than a diagnosis of major depressive disorder, at least one manic episode must have occurred, as Figure 15.3 illustrates. The three specific patterns in Figure 15.3 are only a few of the many mood swing variants which could lead to these three diagnoses.

In the following case, the subject first had three episodes of depression before manifesting the bipolar, mixed, disorder. Note that even in his mania, he almost immediately reverted to a severe depressive mood during an interview, and then returned to mania. This rapid mood fluctuation, where episodes last for moments or sometimes for a few days, is more common in bipolar disorder, mixed, than are fluctuations over periods of months.

> At ages 35, 41, and 47, the patient suffered from depressed episodes, each attack being from four to six months in duration. In January [at age 54] he became restless and talkative. Early in February he began to send checks to friends, sometimes even to strangers who, he said, might be in need. Ten days later he was sent home from the office where he was employed with the explanation that he was becoming overwrought. A few days after his suspension from work he was admitted to a private institution for mental disorders where he pretended to commit suicide by mercury poisoning. He then drew a skull and cross bones on the wall of his room. After three weeks he was taken home, but a few days later he was committed to a public institution where he bustled about the ward, giving the impression that he had important business to which he must attend.
>
> Occasionally he was seen lying on a bench, pretending to sleep, but in a few minutes he resumed his usual activity. He talked quickly, loudly, and nearly constantly. He was interested in everything and everyone around him. He talked familiarly to patients, attendants, nurses, and physicians. He took a fancy to the woman physician on duty in the admission building, calling her by her first name and annoying her with letters and with his familiar, ill-mannered, and obtrusive attentions. On his arrival he gave five dollars to one patient and one dollar to another. He made many comments and asked many questions about other patients and promised that he would secure their discharge. He interfered with their affairs and soon received a blow on the jaw from one patient and a black eye from another. He wrote letters demanding his release, also letters to friends describing in a circumstantial, inaccurate, and facetious way conditions in the hospital. His letters were interlarded with trite Latin phrases. He drew caricatures of the physicians and the nurses and wrote music on toilet paper. He drew pictures on his arms; on one occasion he secured a bottle of mercurochrome and painted the face of another manic patient. When permitted to play the ward piano, he played piece after piece without stopping, improvising a great deal. A doctor rarely passed through the ward without being called by the patient, who would slap the physician on the back or shake hands effusively and talk until the door closed. At times during an interview his voice became tremulous, tears came to his eyes, and he sobbed audibly with his face buried in his arms. A moment later, however, he was laughing—a manifestation of the bipolarity of emotion so markedly illustrated in this disease. (Kolb, 1968, p. 340)

By now, it is obvious that a major feature of the bipolar disorder is the change from one mood extreme to another. What could account for such a change? Could the process be similar to what occurs when normal mood changes to depression? Such questions raise the issue of the factors involved in the development and maintenance of the affective disorders. In the next chapter, theories regarding the development of the affective disorders will be presented, along with the relevant research.

SUICIDE

Suicide is one of the more obvious and dramatic complications of depression in unipolar and bipolar affective disorder. When an individual takes one's own life, we frequently think that person *must* have been depressed. However, not all people who kill themselves are depressed. Some may commit suicide to escape the severe and unending pain of an incurable disease. Others may kill themselves for altruistic reasons: A Buddhist monk burns himself to death as a protest against a war, for the greater good of his fellows. While most people who are depressed do not kill themselves, some do; and these depressed individuals compose the greater proportion of those who do kill themselves.

Approximately 30,000 people kill themselves each year in the United States, but the rate of attempted suicide is approximately 20–30 times higher (Wexler, Weissman, & Kasl, 1978). Among these suicide attempters are more women than men, but more men actually succeed and kill themselves than women. Violent methods are more likely to be used by men than women. Men are more likely to use guns, knives, and jumping; women are more likely to use poisons, especially barbiturates (Frederick,

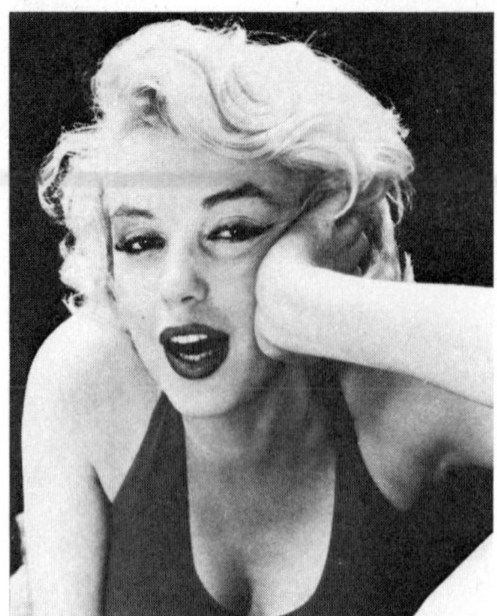

Did Marilyn Monroe intend to die? This film star of the 1950s and 1960s had taken barbiturates and alcohol on several previous occasions. She had always called someone for help, and they had always responded. On the day she died, she had tried to reach several people (including her psychiatrist) after she had taken an overdose. No one was available. Marilyn Monroe was a suicide victim. Perhaps unintentionally.

1978). Accurate statistics on suicide are difficult to obtain. It has often been pointed out that many suicides may be thought to be accidental deaths. One study (C. W. Schmidt et al., 1977) found that at least 1.5 percent of fatal auto "accidents" in one county during a seven-year period could have been suicides. In addition, many suicidal deaths are listed as accidental by physicians or coroners because of the stigma of the suicide label.

A relatively recent problem is the increase in the suicide rate of young people between the ages of 15 to 24. Figure 15.4 presents the suicide rates per 100,000 persons during two decades. The rates for this age group have more than doubled since 1955. In one affluent Chicago suburb, the suicide rate for teens from 15 to 19 increased by 20 percent in 1977 alone ("Suicide Belt," 1980). For this age group, suicide is the third most common cause of death, after accidents and homicide. The concern is legitimate, but most suicides still occur among older people. The typical suicide is an adult male. Litman (1970) gives the following case:

> Mr. A, age 51, shot himself with a rifle through his heart, while sitting in his automobile, at approximately 8 A.M. He had been a real estate salesman who led a conventional life, ambitiously oriented toward financial success, which, to him, was especially important, since he felt inadequate at times because he lacked a college education. During a short period, about four months before his death, he lost three important business transactions that he had counted on, and following this loss he became morose, depressed, irritable, and despondent, and he began to drink, mostly beer, rather heavily. He became indecisive and began to talk about changing to some different type of work.
>
> This disturbed his wife. Although there was no obvious marital disharmony, in recent years they had grown apart. The children were grown, and her main interest was religious. There had been almost no sexual intercourse for several years. The wife had Mr. A examined by a physician, who diagnosed high blood pressure and prescribed an antihypertensive drug. She tried to interest Mr. A in church affairs, but he did not attend regularly.
>
> One week prior to Mr. A's death his wife, concerned about his lethargy, sleeplessness, lack of appetite, and hopeless attitude, telephoned the physician, who said that the patient should have more activity. Two days be-

Figure 15.4. Age-specific suicide rates by five-year age groups, 1955, 1965, 1975.

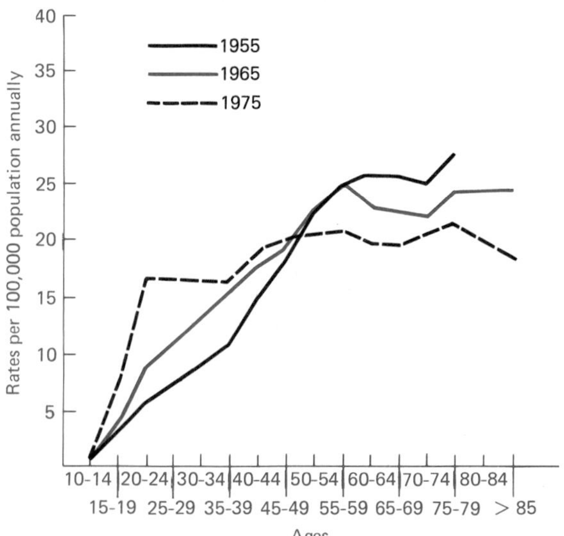

From Frederick (1978, p. 180).

fore his death Mr. A went to a department store and bought a rifle, which he left in his car. The night before his death he talked to a clergyman for several hours, mostly about his failure and anxiety. He woke around 5 A.M. and went for a walk, during which he unwrapped the gun and loaded it. Then he returned for breakfast. At his wife's request, they prayed. Then he went for another walk, again to his automobile, and this time he shot himself.

Later, his wife found several notes, torn up in small pieces in the wastebasket. Apparently he wrote the notes before going for a walk at 5 A.M. and tore them up when he returned for breakfast at 7. When reassembled, the notes read, "Honey, I am unable to take this any longer. God have mercy on my soul. I'm sorry, but I am unable to go on living in the condition I am in. Please be brave. Sorry that life turned out this way. I hope you can find a better life without me. I know I must be nuts. Life isn't worth living, and I have to go through hell every day that I have been through."

After the death Mrs. A wondered if she had been in some way responsible. She herself had been feeling let down and depressed. She said they had no financial problems. Mr. A's father had died in an accident on the thirteenth of the month, which was the date Mr. A committed suicide.

We infer that the main internal conflict concerned Mr. A's feeling that he could not live up to the demands of his conscience, of God, and of his wife. There might have been an identification with his dead father involved in choosing the exact day of his death. He had evidently considered suicide for some time, gradually moving toward the final act. (pp. 296–297)

Popular Misconceptions about Suicide

It's likely that you have heard a number of statements about suicide that may sound quite reasonable, but are false. Here are a few:

1. *If people talk about committing suicide, they will not do it.* Most people who kill themselves do talk about it beforehand with someone. Many people who talk about suicide do not try it, but others are making a cry for help.
2. *When depressed people begin to feel better, the risk that they will kill themselves decreases.* In fact, just the opposite is true. In the depths of a depression, a person may be too immobilized to attempt suicide. A person who is getting better may have enough energy to actually attempt the act.
3. *People have to be psychotic to kill themselves.* Some psychotics do commit suicide. But most people who commit suicide are emotionally disturbed, *not* psychotic. They are in good contact with reality and are neither hallucinating or delusional.
4. *Suicides occur much more frequently at certain times of the year such as Christmas, during stormy weather, or during the full moon.* No *consistent* data have been found to indicate that seasonal or other similar factors influence suicidal behavior.
5. *Suicide is inherited.* Although some families have had multiple suicides, there is no evidence that this behavior is genetically transmitted. The fact that major affective disorders may be genetically transmitted might increase the risk for depression, and therefore for suicide, but the relationship is unlikely. Multiple suicides in families even with affective disorders are rare.
6. *If you think about committing suicide, you are likely to do it.* In fact, probably 1 (or more) out of 10 people has thought about committing suicide, at least briefly (Paykel et al., 1974). Thoughts and fantasies about suicide are especially common among adolescents who feel unloved and unaccepted, but most youths do not act on these thoughts. Rather, they grow, mature, and find that their lives are really worthwhile.

Why Do People Commit Suicide?

We have already noted that a few people commit suicide for altruistic motives. Most others attempt suicide to escape a situation that they perceive as intolerable (Baechler, 1979). In some cases, this motive may make sense even on superficial examination, such as the individual who commits suicide to escape the agony of a slow and painful death from bone cancer. In other cases, the intolerable situation may be less obvious: Individuals may not see any resolution to family agony or economic failure (see Highlight 15.2). Escape may be perceived as the only resolution to a setting filled with shame, guilt, fear, and humiliation. We cannot be much more specific: People who commit suicide compose a population that is very difficult to study. All studies must be retrospective, since the subject is no longer alive. While

HIGHLIGHT 15.2
SUICIDE NOTES

Most people who commit suicide do not leave notes. Schneidman and Farbérow (1970) provide the following notes, which are typical of those that are left:

> Mary:
>
> Here is the note you wanted giving you power of attorney for the house and everything else (including all of *your* bills.)
>
> I hope that my insurance will get you out of the whole mess that you got us both in.
>
> This isn't hard for me to do because it's probably the only way I'll ever get rid of you, we both know how the California courts only see the women's side.
>
> My only hope is that you can raise Junior to be as honest and as good as he is right now.
>
> I think that Junior and Betty and George are really the only things in the world that I'll miss. Please take good care of them.
>
> Good luck, Bill
>
> P.S. I love you Junior, and thank you Betty for all you've done for me and Junior. Love Daddy. (p. 242)

> To Whom It May Concern: I live at 100 Main Street, Los Angeles, California. In case of extreme emergency, please notify my daughter, Mary B. Jones, Box 100, San Diego, California. In my apartment there is a letter to her giving all necessary instructions about what to do with my affairs. I have a checking account with the National Bank, 1st Street Branch, Los Angeles. It is my wish that all of my friends listed in my address book be notified. I am a Protestant. Belong to no lodges now. My apartment rent is paid to the 15th of next month. William B. Smith (p. 244)

we can study suicide attempters, there is general agreement that they are significantly different from those who do successfully commit the act (Lester, 1972). Those who have made a serious suicide attempt and who have been saved by chance (rather than by their own efforts to get help) are a relatively small group for study. We have yet to find out what differentiates individuals who feel that life is intolerable but do not commit suicide, from people who feel the same and take their own lives.

Helping the Suicidal Individual

During the past few decades, more effort has been invested in suicide prevention than ever before. Much of the focus has been on suicide "hot lines," or "crisis lines." These are 24-hour telephone numbers staffed by volunteers and professionals who take emergency calls from people contemplating suicide. When a call is received, the person who answers tries to determine the seriousness of the problem, and tries to get the caller to seek help before doing anything rash. Often the phone contact is successful. However, many researchers have questioned whether this approach really helps *serious* suicides (Lester, 1972). These hot lines help people who are in crisis, but in major cities where they have been established, less than 2 percent of the people who kill themselves try to call such a center. Do they, though, *prevent* people from reaching a point where they would commit suicide? Perhaps, but we have no way of telling with any accuracy.

What can we do if we encounter a person who is a serious suicidal risk? The following case from J. Miller (1980) illustrates what we might try to achieve:

> After a few counseling sessions with a staff worker in which he complained of feelings of depression, a 21-year-old self-referred young man announced to her that he intended to kill himself in two weeks and had a specific plan, developed over the previous weeks, as to time, place, and means. The worker immediately called in senior clinical staff. The client was judged to be seriously depressed, withdrawn, hopeless as to future improvement; he expressed feelings of worthlessness and had recently been abandoned by a girlfriend to whom he was very attached. There was a history of poor impulse control. The confluence of these factors made the risk of a suicide attempt extremely high. On the other hand, the client was continuing to hold down a job, was

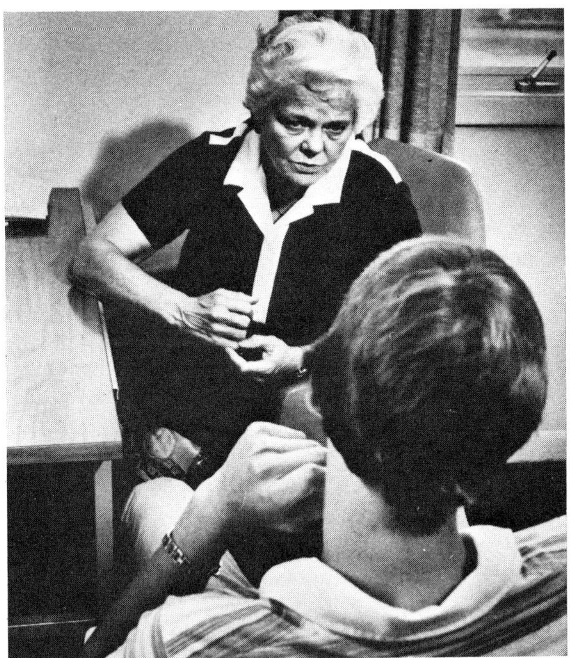

Mary Giffin, a psychiatrist, counsels depressed teenagers who are at high risk for suicide.

very willing to come for treatment sessions, and reliably kept his appointments; he was also in regular contact with friends. He was not psychotic, had adequate reality-testing and capacity to form relationships. On the basis of the latter factors, we decided to go ahead with treatment on an out-patient basis even in the context of high suicidal risk.

During the assessment-oriented conversation with the client, we decided and communicated to him that it was essential that his parents be informed of the critical situation he was in and that we arrange to meet with him and them to discuss it. Over the client's both strenuous and half-hearted objections, we called his parents (he gave us the number). The client's family were living in another state a considerable distance away but readily agreed to come to New York immediately to see their son and meet with us in a family session within a few days. The client was evaluated as well by the clinic psychiatrist and given a small supply of anti-anxiety and anti-depressant medication. The parents indeed arrived and two family sessions were held on successive days. Although the client was fairly withdrawn during the meetings, yet expressing some important feelings, and though he disparaged the worth of having his parents come, it seemed clear that the parents' response and their expression of caring and concern had real positive impact on the client. Since that time, about four months ago, the client has been in individual therapy twice weekly and the suicidal intentions have steadily receded and are not currently manifested. The client has maintained his job and has resumed a relationship with the girl who had left him. It should be stressed that this case is not accurately viewed as an instance of mere attention-getting behavior which receded when attention was provided but is seen by the several professional clinic personnel involved as one in which suicide might well have occurred were it not for the active interventionist treatment approach that was followed. (p. 100)

An important aspect in resolving the crisis for this young man consisted of involving others who cared about him. In this case, an issue is raised regarding his objections to the involvement of his parents. The therapists insisted that the parents be involved. Some people might argue that the young man had the right to keep his parents out of the situation. If he had, and the therapists were convinced he would follow through on his suicidal plans, they probably would have had him hospitalized, even against his will, to protect him "from himself." Most clinicians believe that their duty is to keep people from killing themselves. What do you think?

Summary

1. Mood is a prolonged emotion that colors our psychic life. It influences how we perceive things, the manner in which we behave, and how others react toward us.

2. In the affective disorders, people experience extremes of mood which are either subjectively very unpleasant or which interfere with their day-to-day functioning. The extremes of mood may vary from deep depression to mania.

3. Unipolar depression is a disorder characterized by a mood of sadness and misery. The individual has self-critical and pessimistic thoughts, and may be so depressed that physical movements are slowed. Others may become agitated. Depression may be so severe that bodily functions including appetite, sleeping, and elimination may be disturbed.

4. Depression has been separated into exogenous and endogenous types. Exogenous depression seems to be related to losses and stresses in life, while endogenous depression usually is not related to external stresses or losses. Many researchers believe that endogenous depression is primarily physiological or biochemical in origin.

5. Two categories of unipolar depression have been identified. "Dysthymic disorder" is the term used for the type of depression which is usually associated with external stressors such as losses, and which does not show the signs of major depressive disorder. Major depressive disorder involves depression associated with signs such as psychomotor retardation or agitation. Major depressive disorder may become so severe that psychotic symptoms such as hallucinations and delusions appear.

6. Bipolar affective disorders are diagnosed when individuals manifest mood swings from mania or depression to the opposite end of the affective spectrum. The symptoms of depression in bipolar affective disorder are identical to unipolar depression. Mania is characterized by an elated and expansive or irritable mood. The individual has an unrealisti cally positive self-appraisal and seemingly boundless energy. Mania may be so severe that it is associated with grandiose delusions and hallucinations. Milder degrees of mood swings are diagnosed as cyclothymic disorder.

7. Individuals who commit suicide are often depressed. However, not all individuals are depressed when they commit suicide.

8. Suicide is the known cause of 30,000 deaths per year, but many deaths that are labeled accidental are probably suicides. In recent years, suicidal deaths in the 15–24 -year-old age group have more than doubled.

9. People who commit suicide often talk about it beforehand. Suicides rarely occur in the depths of depression, but are more likely when the person feels slightly better and has the energy to act. Few individuals who kill themselves are psychotic; most are in contact with reality. Suicide is not consistently more frequent at certain times of the year such as at Christmas or in the spring. Nor is suicide an "inherited" trait. Many people think about suicide at some time in their lives, but do not act on these thoughts.

10. It is difficult to study successful suicides, since we must rely on a retrospective analysis of their lives. However, most suicides seem to be an attempt to escape from a situation that appears intolerable and for which no other solutions appear workable.

11. Many large metropolitan communities have developed crisis phone lines for people who are contemplating suicide. Unfortunately, less than 2 percent of successful suicides try to call such a program before they take their lives. Such crisis hot lines may prevent people from reaching the point of actually trying to kill themselves.

KEY TERMS

Bipolar affective disorder. A severe disorder of mood which involves episodes of elation and depression.

Cyclothymic disorder. A bipolar affective disorder which consists of mild swings in mood.

Dysthymic disorder. Mild to moderate depression which does not have the severe symptoms of major depressive disorder. Sometimes called "neurotic" depression.

Endogenous depression. A depression that is not due to an external stressor such as a loss of job or divorce.

Exogenous depression. A depression that seems to be related to external precipitants such as the loss of a loved one.

Mood congruent. A term used to refer to behavior or thoughts which are congruent with the individual's feelings.

Unipolar affective disorder. A disorder of mood which involves only one extreme—only depression or only mania.

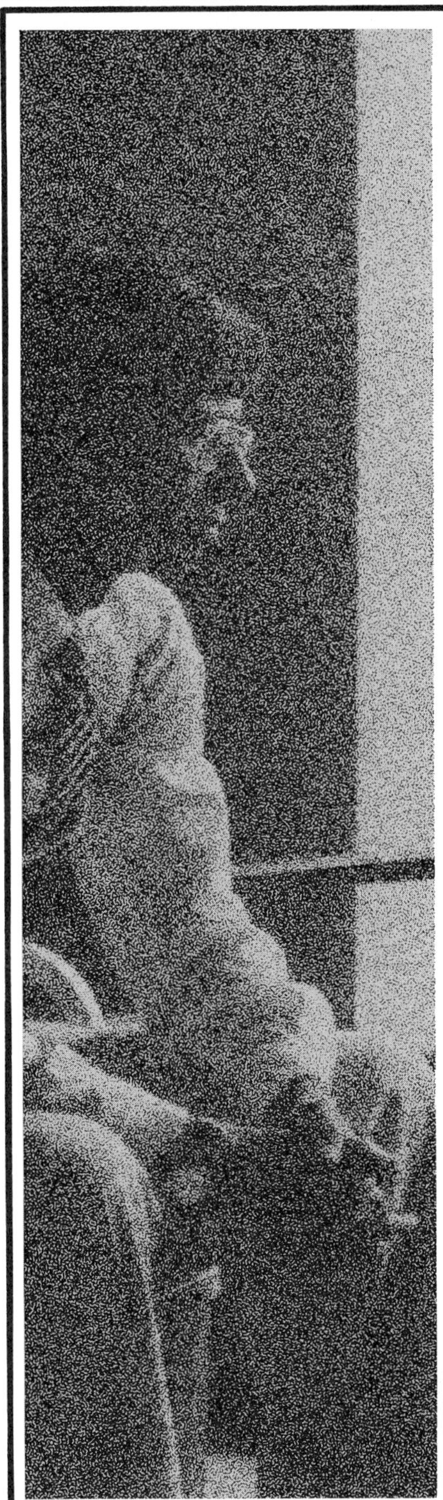

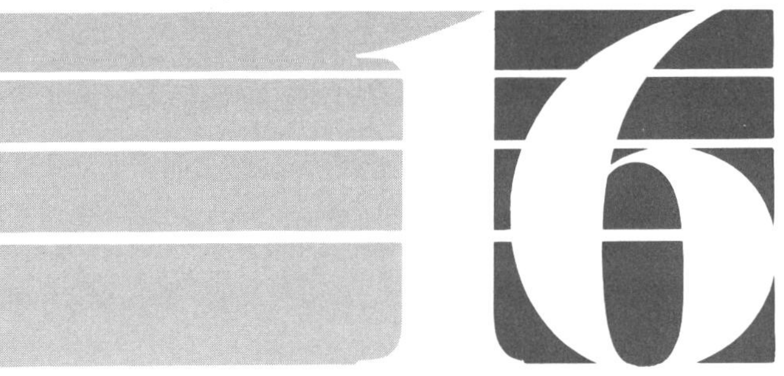

16 Affective disorders II: theories, research, and treatment

Unipolar depression and the bipolar affective disorders together affect more than 15 percent of the population of the United States. The high incidence of affective disorder is one reason why research and the development of etiological theories are extremely important. Each major theoretical framework has made contributions to the understanding of this area of abnormal behavior. Research on unipolar and bipolar disorders continues to add to the data available for theory development and the development of treatment approaches. Although much remains to be learned about these disorders, several treatment approaches are currently in use.

In this chapter we will first look at various theories of the affective disorders and at some research relevant to these theoretical formulations. The first theoretical framework considered will be the psychoanalytic. This will be followed by the contribution of learning theory, the concept of learned helplessness, cognitive theories, research on genetic factors, and the biochemistry of affective disorders. Then the key treatments of affective disorders will be examined. The biological treatments discussed are electroconvulsive therapy and drug therapy; the psychological approaches are dynamic psychotherapy, behavior therapy, and cognitive therapy. Finally, the merits of using a combination of biologically and psychologically based approaches are considered.

THEORIES AND RESEARCH ON THE AFFECTIVE DISORDERS

Psychoanalytic Theory

Sigmund Freud compared clinical depression to the process of mourning or grieving which all of us go through when someone we love dies. Our normal reaction to such loss is so similar to depression that many clinicians have inferred that some type of loss must be associated with the depressive disorder. Freud contended that depressive behavior is rooted in early childhood relationships.

Freud believed that infants develop depressive predispositions because of relationships with their mothers. The mother is extraordinarily important to the infant, whom she has the all-powerful capacity to satisfy or to frustrate at will. Infants experience both a good mother and a bad mother, since even the best mother must sometimes frustrate the child. Freud theorized that during the "oral stage" of development, infants cope with the external world by taking it into themselves through the process of introjection; and, since the mother is the most important aspect of the environment, the infant introjects the image of the mother. Of course, this image includes both the good and the bad. If the infant's feelings of love for the good mother and hate for the bad mother are unusually strong, the way is paved for a later predisposition to depression.

In adulthood such an individual handles losses in a peculiar way. For example, if a young man is rejected by his love, we might expect him to be angry at the young woman who rejected him. Instead, he becomes depressed and self-accusatory; he blames himself, and comes to see himself as not worth her love. In regard to such a situation, Freud noted:

> If one listens patiently to a melancholic's many various self-accusations, one cannot in the end avoid the impression that often the most violent of them are hardly at all applicable to the patient himself, but that with insignificant modifications they do fit someone else, someone whom the patient loves or has loved or should love. . . . We perceive that the self-reproaches are reproaches against a loved object which have been shifted away from it on [to] the patient's own ego. (Mendelson, 1975, p. 30)

Thus, the loss of his girlfriend has resulted in the young man's regression to the oral stage; the loss has reactivated his feelings toward the introjected maternal image of goodness and badness. The anger toward the bad mother is reactivated by the anger toward the lost love object, but this anger is not directed outward; instead, it is turned inward, toward the introject within the person. Anger toward the lost object is turned against the self, resulting in depression. This turning against the self is seen partly as a function of a dominant and punitive superego. This superego development occurs because of the individual's introjection of the maternal and paternal authority figures.

Later psychoanalytic writers have greatly modified Freud's early conceptions. Many have stressed the concept of self-esteem. These later psychoanalytic theorists have conceptualized depressives as individuals who have not fully differentiated themselves from **introjected objects** (parents) and who cannot maintain their self-esteem unless it is continually bolstered from outside sources (symbolic of the support of the parent in childhood). When these external sources of self-esteem are lost, the individual no longer has a source of value and becomes depressed. From this perspective, current losses are symbolic of a loss of parental support experienced in regard to the "bad" mother.

What of mania? Analysts have focused on the etiology of depression, and have much less to say about the development of mania. However, a few points can be made. Many analysts view mania as a *defense* against depression. Mania is seen as a denial of the underlying introjection of the bad mother, and a denial of the current losses. B. I. Lewin (1950) suggests that in mania the individual derives a sense of "reality" from reliving a primary feeling experienced during nursing at the breast. The elation and euphoria of this feeling is displaced onto fantasies that help to contradict and deny the unhappiness and frustrations of the current loss of a real or symbolic love object.

As noted in the discussion of other disorders, the metaphorical and inferential concepts of psychoanalytic theory are virtually impossible to prove or disprove. In the case of the affective disorders, how can one measure or directly study the degree to which an approximately 1-year-old infant "introjects" an ambivalent image of a good/bad mother? In fact, we cannot. The evidence for the psychoanalytic theory consists primarily of retrospective recollections by psychoanalysts' clients. In terms of issues that can be measured—for example, whether precipitating or predisposing losses exist in the lives of those who develop depression—the evidence is not very supportive of the psychoanalytic concept (Lloyd, 1980a, 1980b). In spite of the lack of supporting research, the psychoanalytic conception of the affective disorders—particularly for the dysthymic and cyclothymic disorders—remains influential in the thinking of many clinicians.

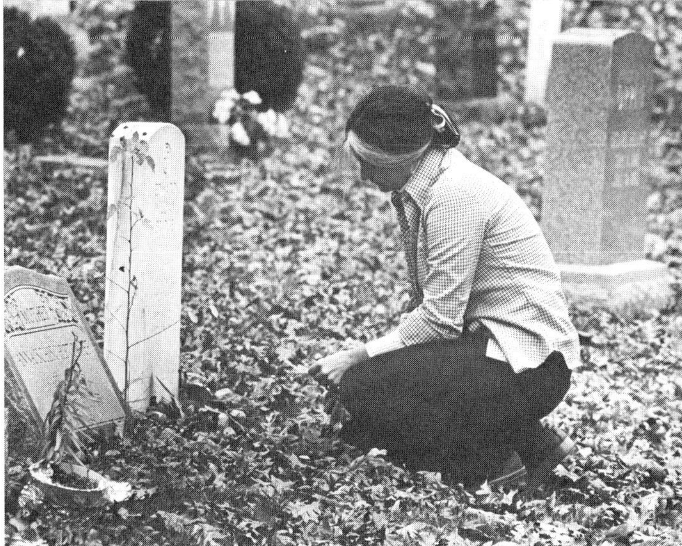

Loss of a loved one may trigger depression. In psychoanalytic theory, this type of loss is thought to resurrect repressed feelings about losses in childhood.

Learning Theory and Affective Disorder

An alternative psychological theory of depression has been proposed by operant learning theorists. In this theory, the symptoms of depression are seen as due to low rates of reinforcement for normal affective behavior (Lewinsohn, 1974). This approach can explain depression with or without a precipitating loss. If no precipitating loss is present, we would presume that the individual is in a situation with a reduced likelihood of positive reinforcement for social behavior. Some examples of such a situation are leaving family and friends to go away to school, entering the military, moving away from friends to a new town. We can also include here the individuals who were not positively reinforced when growing up to develop social competence (i.e., skill in performing behaviors that gain positive social reinforcement).

The situation where there is a loss is even clearer: Death of a loved one results in less availability of positive reinforcement, as do divorce, job loss, and so on. In either situation, where there is a loss or where the environment is low in positive reinforcement the lower rate of positive reinforcement for normal affectivity would lead to a reduction in frequency of those behaviors and symptoms of depression may appear. Positive reinforcement of the depressive behavior may result when it appears, so that the individual is likely to gain attention and sympathy. This reinforcement makes the depressive behaviors likely to be more frequent, and the nondepressive behaviors less frequent. As the depressive behaviors increase, they are likely to become less attractive to those who were sympathetic in the beginning. These sympathizers may attend less to the depressed person, further reducing positive reinforcement. A vicious cycle develops, which results in a deepening of the depression. Although this type of theory has been proposed by several theorists, most research has focused on Lewinsohn's (1974) conceptualization.

Blaney (1977) has reviewed the research on Lewinsohn's theory and concluded that the supportive research is primarily correlation. For example, Coyne (1976) had normal subjects carry on a phone conversation with depressed or nondepressed subjects. After the conversations, normal subjects who talked to depressives were more depressed, anxious, hostile, and rejecting of those they talked to than normal subjects who talked to nondepressed subjects. The data suggest that depressives are less likely to receive positive social reinforcement from their contacts with others, and more likely to receive hostility and rejection. Blaney (1977) also notes that some experimental studies that attempted to manipulate depression by increasing positive reinforcing activity failed to find results supportive of this theory. Further research should seek to determine the specific influences of positive reinforcement on depressive moods.

Perhaps these negative results led to Lewinsohn's work on another possible factor in depression (Lewinsohn et al., 1980). A frequent criticism has been that the operant approach to depression fails to take into account the self-perceptions of the depressed individual. Lewinsohn and colleagues became interested in individuals' self-perceptions of their social competence compared to others' assessment of their level of social competence. Lewinsohn et al. obtained some remarkable results. In their study, they examined self-ratings and ratings by observers of social competence in depressed patients, psychiatric patient controls, and normal controls. They expected that depressed patients would have lower levels of social competence (remember Lewinsohn's original theory). The three groups rated themselves and were rated by observers on social competence several times during treatment. As expected, the depressed patients saw themselves as less socially competent and desirable than normals, and the observers saw them in a similar way. However, the normals and the psychiatric controls saw themselves as *more* socially competent and desirable than the observers rated them. These latter two groups had the illusion that they were more socially competent than they really were. Perhaps to avoid depression we need to be unrealistic about ourselves! This "warm glow" may allow us to pay greater attention to and better remember our positive, as opposed to our negative, attributes.

The effects of treatment on these groups was also interesting (see Figure 16.1). Treatment of the depressed patients increased the degree to

Figure 16.1. Discrepancy between self-ratings and observer ratings on social competence during treatment.

Discrepancy was obtained by subtracting the observer rating from the self-rating.

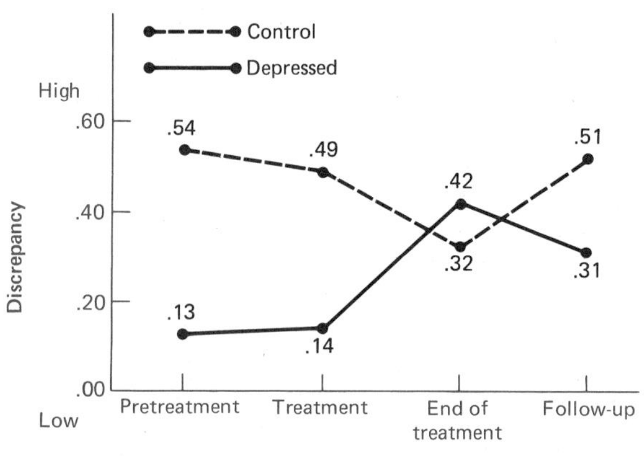

From Lewinsohn et al. (1980, p. 208).

which they rated themselves as socially competent and desirable, but the *discrepancy* between their self-ratings and the observers' ratings of them also increased. That is, while the observers rated the depressives as more socially competent, the observers did not rate the change to be as great as the patients did. The depressed patients became more unrealistic about themselves as treatment progressed. Lewinsohn and colleagues (1980) conclude that to feel good about ourselves, we may have to judge ourselves more kindly than others judge us.

Lewinsohn's provocative research may result in heightened interest in the self-perceptions of depressed patients. Meanwhile, the study of the relationship of cognitions to depressed affect has been ongoing. One theorist prominent in this area is Martin Seligman (1975).

Seligman: Depression and Learned Helplessness

A fairly consistent observation of depressed individuals has been that they feel helpless. In clinical situations, one often hears depressed individuals make statements such as "I can't do it" or "No matter what I do, it doesn't help." Could this sense of helplessness cause the depressive affect? Could this helplessness be learned?

Seligman's theory that **learned helplessness** leads to depression originated from animal learning experiments. He and his colleagues were studying conditioned fear and instrumental learning when an unexpected event occurred. In their study, dogs were being trained to make an avoidance response to electric shock. Most dogs quickly learned to jump over a barrier when the shock was presented, a result the experimenters expected. By leaping the barrier, the dogs could avoid the onset of the painful shock, and they quickly learned to escape as soon as they received a preparatory signal. The unexpected result occurred when the experimenters took some dogs and presented them with an unavoidable shock, which the dogs were helpless to escape. Seligman (1975) describes the results:

> A dog that had first been given inescapable shock showed a strikingly different pattern. This dog's first reactions to shock in the shuttle box were much the same as those of a naive dog: It ran around frantically for about thirty seconds. But then it stopped moving; to our surprise, it lay down and quietly whined. After one minute of this we turned the shock off; the dog had failed to cross the barrier and had not escaped from shock. On the next trial, the dog did it again; at first it struggled a bit, and then, after a few seconds, it seemed to give up and to accept the shock passively.
>
> On all succeeding trials, the dog failed to escape. (p. 22)

Further work demonstrated that laboratory animals exposed to aversive situations that they are unable to avoid show many of the signs of depression seen in humans. The animals were passive in the face of stress; their ability to learn to deal with stress was hampered; they developed eating disturbances; and, perhaps most interestingly, they manifested a depletion of norepinephrine, one of the neurotransmitters implicated in depression in humans (this relationship will be examined in a later section).

The application of the learned helplessness model of depression to human subjects has received considerable experimental support (Abramson, Seligman, & Teasdale, 1978). However, in response to some critics (e.g., Costello, 1978), Seligman has broadened his theory considerably. The original formulation was that persons become depressed because they learn that they are helpless. They find that nothing they do improves their situation. Such individuals may learn helplessness even when they really could do something to improve a situation. The sense of helplessness becomes a *belief* in self-powerlessness which leads to powerless behavior that confirms the belief. Seligman (1978) has reformulated his theory to include the concept of attribution of causality: Learned helplessness develops when the individual attributes failures to himself or herself. When individuals who fail, attribute the failure to factors *outside* their control, then the sense of helplessness is less likely to develop.

Golin et al. (1979) have demonstrated these factors in a study of depressed patients. If they feel more helpless than normals, depressed patients should have lower expectations of suc-

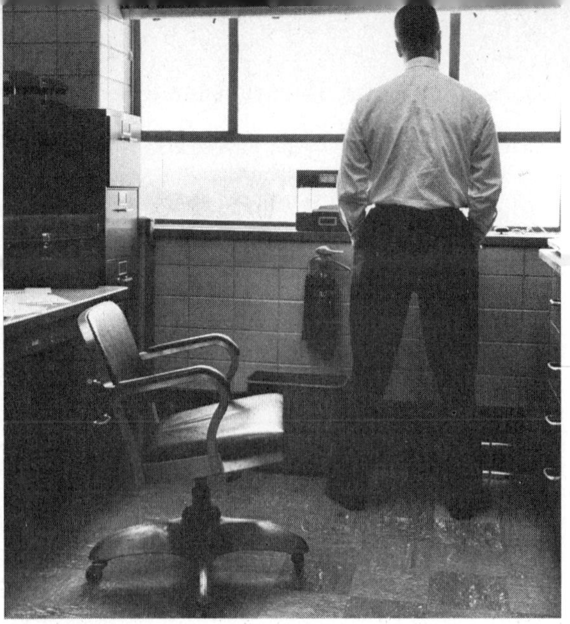

According to Seligman, several symptoms of learned helplessness are similar to those of depression. People who develop feelings of helplessness come to believe that they have no efficacy or control over their environment. They may become passive and withdrawn and may feel incapable of functioning on their jobs. They believe that their actions will not have any positive effect on the tasks in front of them. Even if they succeed at a task, they do not feel it is due to their efforts.

cess when they believe the outcome of a task is under their control, not the control of an outside agent. Golin and colleagues subjected depressed patients and normal controls to a gambling game with two conditions. In one condition, the results appeared to be under the control of the subject; in the second condition, the results appeared to be under the control of an external agent (a "croupier" who ran the game). Figure 16.2 indicates the difference in expectation of success for the two groups under the two conditions. When depressed subjects thought they had some control over the results, they expected to do worse than when they had no control. When normal subjects had the illusion of control over the results, they expected to do better than when they perceived that control was out of their hands. These results would be expected if depressed subjects attribute their helplessness to themselves, not to an external agent. In fact, in both conditions, the results of the gambling game were due to the probability of the roll of a die, not to the subjects' manipulation.

The learned helplessness model cannot be applied to all depressive disorders. Seligman (1978) has indicated that his model applies only to some individuals who are depressed. He notes that most evidence for this model comes from studies of mild depression, and the model seems eminently applicable to this group. What of the major depressive disorders? Seligman believes that the learned helplessness model may apply to some severe depressions, but he notes that when the disorder is bipolar (involving mania) the application is less likely.

In conclusion, let us return to the major depressive disorder. Porsolt, LePichon, and Jalfre (1977) have demonstrated that situations closely allied to the learned helplessness model result in passivity in rats under stress. This passivity disappears in rats who are treated with electroconvulsive therapy, chemical mood elevators, major tranquilizers, and other approaches used with humans who have major depression. Remember also Seligman's (1975) early finding of the depletion of the neurotransmitter norepinephrine in dogs subjected to a helpless, no-escape situation. We have seen that one concept views major depression as endogenous, or due to an internal physiological state. We will soon see that a major theory of depression centers on the concept of a physiological cause. However, the findings just described suggest that the physiological distur-

Figure 16.2. Mean expectancy of success of depressed and nondepressed patients under personal, (player) control and external (croupier) control conditions.

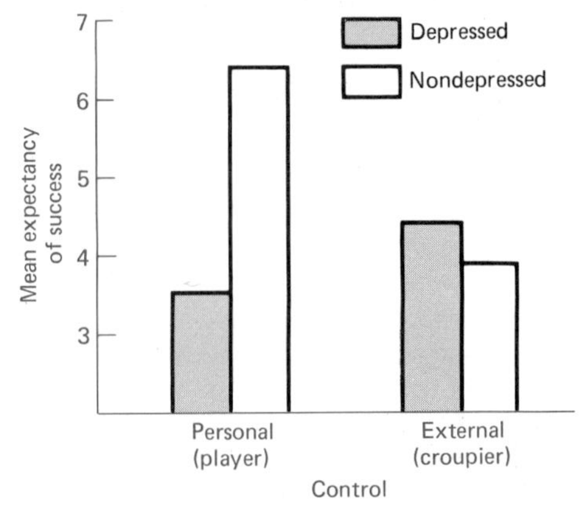

From Golin et al. (1979, p. 455).

bances of major depression may be a result of learned helplessness. This notion is an intriguing one, which is sure to be subjected to much more research.

Beck's Cognitive Theory of Depression

An alternative view of depressive affect is that it results from negative cognitions or thoughts. Several theorists have espoused this position (e.g., Albert Ellis, 1962; Valins & Nisbett, 1971), but one of the better known is Aaron T. Beck. Beck (1967, 1976), a psychiatrist, had used the psychoanalytic treatment approach of free association to study 50 depressed patients (16 men, 34 women). He saw these patients approximately three hours per week for about two years each. During the course of the study, Beck became increasingly aware that the subjects' depressive feelings were associated with consistent logical errors in their thinking.

The thoughts of these depressed individuals had particular themes: low self-regard; ideas of deprivation, self-criticism, and blame; a sense of being overwhelmed by problems and responsibilities; and self-commands that one "should" or "must" fulfill obligations. In addition, there were thoughts centered on a desire to escape (sometimes by suicide) from what the individuals perceived as an untenable situation. The depressive individual interprets events and experiences in a distorted manner that leads to a self-blaming, devalued perception of the self. Beck observed that the errors in logic committed by the depressive person are of five types:

1. Arbitrary inference. Conclusions are drawn without supporting evidence or in the face of evidence to the contrary. A student receives a "B" on an exam and concludes that "I'll never get an 'A.' "
2. Selective abstraction. A detail is taken out of context while more important features are ignored, and the whole experience is conceptualized on the basis of the detail. For example, someone gives a stirring speech at a political rally, but stumbles over the name of a prominent politician. The speaker focuses on her "stupidity" and "lack of poise," and feels "mortified" at how "poor" her performance was.
3. Overgeneralization. A general conclusion is drawn about one's ability, performance, or worth on the basis of a single incident. Someone who asked for a date and was turned down concluded that he was not attractive to women.
4. Magnification and minimization. Strengths are minimized, weaknesses are magnified. When praised, the person responds: "Oh, anyone could have done as well." Someone has a minor car accident and thinks, "I'm the world's worst driver, they should take my license away."
5. Inexact labeling. Depressives tend to label events or experiences in exaggerated terms: "I'm the 'worst,' 'weakest,' 'lousiest,' or 'biggest' failure."

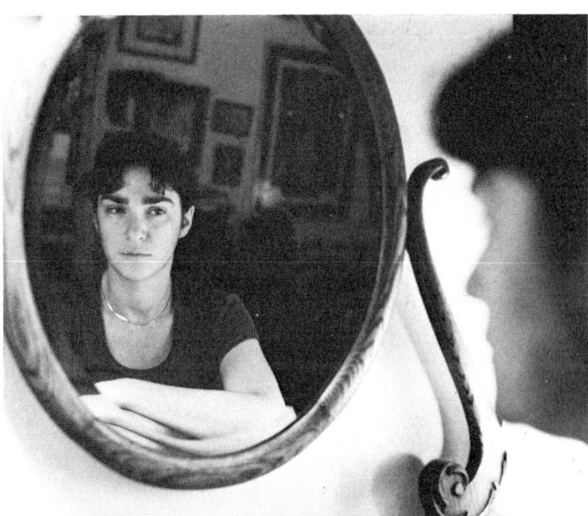

The way people perceive themselves may lead to depressogenic ways of thinking.

A. T. Beck suggests that the illogical, erroneous cognitions of the depressive comprise **depressogenic schemata.** These are enduring cognitive structures (ways of thinking) that code or organize information about life situations. The schemata are based on the individual's basic premises, which make excessive use of directives such as "should," "ought," and "must." For example, an individual may hold the premise that "I should be smart and capable all the time." These premises are often inflexible and absolute rules of conduct that virtually no one could successfully comply with. The premises and depressogenic schemata probably develop early in life, perhaps when a critical event such as the death of a loved one occurs. They may also develop when a parent holds similar premises and communicates them to the child. Once the schemata develop, they are self-perpetuating, since they color the individual's perceptions of new experiences.

The illogical cognitions of depressives have been described by Beck as automatic, involuntary, and (to the depressive) plausible. In addition, they are perseverative; this means that the cognitions occur without reflection or evaluation, they occur even when the subject tries to ward them off, they seem justified, and they are repetitive. The individual who reaches such a negative self-evaluation in this illogical manner ends up thinking about himself or herself in depression-generating terms: "If I'm not important, I can't go on living"; "No one loves me"; "I'm no good at anything."

Most of the supportive evidence for Beck's approach is correlational (A. T. Beck, 1974; Blaney, 1977). Many studies have consistently demonstrated that depressives conceptualize their experiences and themselves in these illogical ways. However, few studies have demonstrated that these types of cognitions *induce* depressive affect. One notable exception is a study by Ludwig (1975), which found that some depression could be induced in college women by presenting feedback (false psychological test results) that the individual was immature and uncreative. The theory proposed by Beck continues to be extensively researched. Specific treatment strategies for depression have been developed and organized around the modification of the illogical concepts held by depressives (A. T. Beck, 1976), and will be considered later in this chapter.

Genetic Factors in Depression and Mania

The affective disorders appear to run in families (Weitkamp, Pardue, & Huntzinger, 1980). This means that the incidence of unipolar and bipolar affective disorder is greater among the close relatives (e.g., parents, children, and siblings) of people diagnosed as having these disorders than it is among the general population. An increased incidence of affective disorders among biological relatives does not separate genetic factors from psychosocial factors. Depressed or manic relatives may well share similar symptom-producing psychosocial environments. In order to further clarify this issue in relation to the affective disorders, researchers have applied methodologies similar to those used to study genetic factors in schizophrenia. Several twin studies of affective disorder have found higher rates of concordance for affective disorder in identical twins than in fraternal twins (see Table 16.1). Remember, identical (monozygotic) twins share an identical genetic makeup, while fraternal (dizygotic) twins are no more genetically similar than ordinary brothers and sisters.

Genetic studies have generally focused on severe affective disorders in the index cases. The differences in concordance rates are much less when mild to moderate cases of depression are studied. In addition, the twin studies have generally lumped together the unipolar and bipolar affective disorders. One that did not is the Bertelson, Harvald, and Hauge (1977) study, completed in Denmark. This study used the same Danish psychiatric register as the studies of children at high risk for schizophrenia described in Chapter 13. Bertelson et al. found a concordance rate of 74 percent for bipolar disorder in identical twins. For unipolar disorder (depression only), the identical twin concordance rate was 43 percent. The data suggest that genetic factors are more important in

Table 16.1
Concordance rates for affective disorder in identical and fraternal twin pairs

Study	*Number of pairs*		*Percent of concordance*[1]	
	IDENTICAL	FRATERNAL	IDENTICAL	FRATERNAL
Kallmann (1953)	27	55	93	24
E. Slater (1953)	7	17	57	24
Kringlen (1967)	6	20	33	0
Bertelson et al. (1977)	55	52	58	17

[1]Percentages reported are within ± .5 percent of those reported.

the bipolar affective disorders than in the unipolar affective disorders.

Although this evidence is impressive, the family's psychosocial environment remains a complicating factor. Recently, researchers have begun to do adoption studies to control for this factor. In the United States, Remi Cadoret (1978) screened midwestern adoption records and selected 83 adults who had been adopted as children and who had biological parents who manifested psychopathology of some sort. These experimental subjects were matched with 43 adopted control subjects whose biological parents were free of symptoms. Out of 8 adoptees from the experimental group whose biological parents showed symptoms of affective disorder, 3 had developed an affective disorder. Only 4 of the remaining 75 in the experimental group had also developed an affective disorder. In the control group, 4 adoptees of biological parents who had no psychiatric disorder had an affective disorder. Cadoret's results indicated that having a biologic parent who manifested an affective disorder vastly increased the offspring's risk of developing an affective disorder. The risk was especially high when the mother manifested the disturbance. Unfortunately, the size of the sample was so small that we must be cautious about our interpretations. Helzer and Winoker (1974) made similar observations in a retrospective study of males with bipolar disorder. In their study, the risk was eight times as high when the mother had an affective disorder as when the father did. Such data suggest that this possibly inherited predisposition may be sex linked, which may partly explain why women seem to have a higher incidence of affective disorders than men.

The genetic studies completed to date strongly suggest that a genetic factor is operating in the major affective disorders. The influence of inheritance appears to be more significant in the bipolar (manic-depressive) disorder than in the unipolar (depressive) disorder, and more significant in severe disorders than in mild disorders. However, as is the case with schizophrenia, the concordance rates are not great enough to rule out environmental factors. With the severe affective disorders also, we appear to be dealing with an inherited predisposition or vulnerability similar to that discussed in Chapter 13, on schizophrenia. The evidence for a genetic factor in mild to moderate depression has yet to be demonstrated. Perhaps these levels of affective disorder may be primarily psychosocially determined.

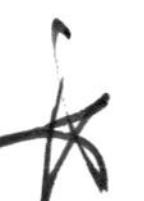

Biochemical Factors in Affective Disorder

A very significant theory of affective disorders hypothesizes that physiological or biochemical disturbances in the brain result in the observed symptoms of depression and mania. Tremendous impetus has been given to this idea by the discovery that certain chemicals administered to human subjects can reduce or increase depressive or manic symptomatology.

In the late 1940s, J. F. Cade, an Australian physician-researcher, found that administration of a lithium salt to manic patients reduced their exaggerated mood. At about the same time, the drug reserpine was noted to sometimes induce depressive features among patients using it to reduce high blood pressure. A third drug, iproniazid, used in the treatment of tuberculosis, was found in the early 1950s to produce a mild euphoric mood in some patients. It became clear that these chemicals were somehow influencing neural processes to result in mood changes.

Further research, primarily on animals, led to the following discoveries:

1. Reserpine decreases the availability of the neurotransmitters norepinephrine and serotonin in the brain. This finding raised the suspicion that clinically depressed individuals may not have enough of these substances available in their neural tissue.
2. In 1952, it was found that iproniazid increased the levels of the neurotransmitters norepinephrine and serotonin in the brain by blocking a chemical enzyme called monoamine oxidase (MAO), which is involved in the chemical process by which these neurotransmitters are broken down (rendered ineffective) in the brain. Additional drugs were found to inhibit MAO and reduce depression.
3. A lithium salt (lithium carbonate) was found to decrease levels of norepinephrine in the brains of laboratory animals.

Subsequent research has dramatically supported and expanded upon these findings (e.g., see F. K. Goodwin & Athanasios, 1979; Prange, 1973). The findings of such research have resulted in three basic conceptions of biochemical influence in depression. The first is the possibility that depression results from an insufficiency of the neurotransmitter; the second is that depression results from a deficiency in norepinephrine, and mania results from an excess of norepinephrine; and the third is that affective disorder is due to a "carburation effect," a mixture of various levels of neurotransmitters including norepinephrine, serotonin, dopamine, and possibly others (Mendels et al., 1975).

In Chapter 13, we reviewed the action of neurotransmitters in the brain (see Figure 13.2) and the relationship of the neurotransmitter dopamine to schizophrenia. The action of the neurotransmitters norepinephrine and serotonin may be quite similar. If in the neural synaptic clefts (or "synapses") a deficiency of either or both neurotransmitters exists, transmission of neural impulses will be less frequent, with an associated slowing of mental and behavioral processes. An excess of neurotransmitters may well increase the frequency of neural transmission, resulting in behavioral and mental overactivity like those in mania. In fact, we know that the processes are more complex; but to understand the process to any

HIGHLIGHT 16.1

HOW CAN BIOCHEMICAL ACTIONS AFFECT NEURAL TRANSMISSION?

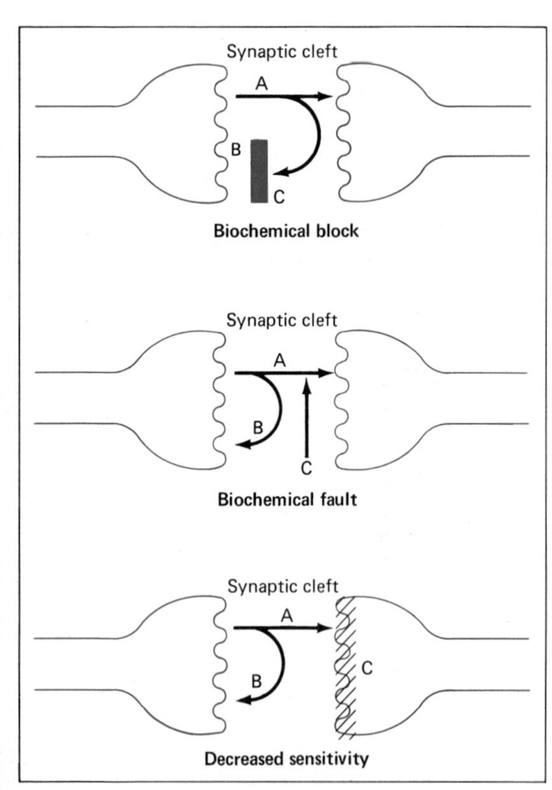

Neurons release a neurotransmitter (A) such as norepinephrine or serotonin, biochemical messengers, which tell the next neuron to fire. Neurons have a re-uptake mechanism (B) which takes up some of the released neurotransmitter. If a biochemical substance were to block (C) the re-uptake mechanism, too much neurotransmitter would remain in the synaptic cleft. The neurons would fire too frequently and mania might result. Some evidence exists that sodium may act to block the re-uptake mechanism in mania (F. K. Goodwin & Athanasios, 1979).

Another possibility is that a biochemical fault (C) in the metabolism of the neurotransmitter (A) results in a process through which the neurotransmitter breaks down into other biochemicals too quickly, resulting in lower levels of the effective neurotransmitting chemical in the synaptic cleft. Excessive levels of MAO appear to have this effect. The lower levels of neurotransmitter would result in a lowered frequency of neural impulses, and depressive behavior.

A third possibility may be that there is no fault in either the neurotransmitter biochemistry (A) or in the re-uptake mechanism (B). Rather, the problem may be a decreased sensitivity of the neural receptor (C) to the neurotransmitter (Montigny & Aghajanian, 1978).

At our current stage of knowledge, we do not know if one of these actions is the culprit, if all three possibilities occur, or if some other biochemical action is the primary factor in the major affective disorders.

greater degree requires a strong basis in biochemistry. For our purposes, this simplified understanding will suffice (see Highlight 16.1).

Before we leave the topic of brain biochemistry, one further interesting finding can be noted in regard to the bipolar disorder. Norepinephrine appears to be implicated in the switch mechanism involved in the change of mood from depression to mania and mania to depression. Some researchers (Bunney et al., 1972) have studied the biochemistry of individuals in the process of mood swings from depression to mania and back to depression. One finding in these studies has been that as an individual goes from depression to mania, there is a significant increase in the levels of some biochemicals in the individual's urine which are related to the levels of brain norepinephrine. As the person returns from mania to depression, the levels of the measured biochemicals return to normal, then appears to decrease. Bunney et al. (1972) found that the levels of norepinephrine seemed to rise prior to the onset of the behavior change from depression to mania, suggesting that these differences were not a *result* of the behavior change, but may have been its cause. The presence of increased levels of brain norepinephrine in mania is supported by the fact that manic behavior is effectively treated with lithium carbonate, which reduces the level of norepinephrine in the brain.

Questions about the Etiology of the Affective Disorders

The preceding sections have presented several theories of depression and mania which contribute to our understanding of the unipolar and bipolar affective disorders. Many questions remain, however. Mild to moderate depressions appear to be caused primarily by psychosocial factors. The major affective disorders seem to have an inherited component and significant biochemical factors. Do the biochemical factors lead to the mood change? Or does the mood change result in biochemical disturbance in the brain? Most research seems to favor the former etiology over the latter. However, remember Martin Seligman's (1975) early finding with laboratory dogs who had to face a painful electric shock that they were helpless to escape. After they had "learned to be helpless," the dogs manifested a depletion of the neurotransmitter norepinephrine. We do not yet have a conclusive answer to the question of what comes first: the biochemical change leading to behavior change or behavior change leading to biochemical changes.

KEY TREATMENTS

Biological treatments

Electroconvulsive therapy. Chapter 13 described the specific procedures of electroconvulsive therapy (ECT or EST) when used with schizophrenic disorders. The same procedures are used to treat the affective disorders. An electrical current is applied to the patient's brain in order to induce seizures. The manifestations of the seizures are "softened" by the use of muscle-relaxant drugs; and the patient is also given a drug which results in unconsciousness to avoid the unpleasant and often frightening experience of the treatment.

ECT was often applied indiscriminately to psychotic disorders until the mid 1960s. Its use has declined, but it still has popularity, particularly in treatment of major depressive disorders when the depression is so severe that it reaches psychotic levels. ECT appears to be effective with major depressions (Avery & Winoker, 1977). It seems to have an advantage over other approaches in that in many cases the depression lifts rapidly, within days or weeks. This rapid improvement is especially advantageous when there is danger of suicide. The risk of suicide occurring is much greater if one has to wait for mood-elevating drugs to take effect, and even greater if one tries to use psychotherapy alone to treat the problem. The efficacy of ECT with suicidal patients has often been demonstrated (Avery & Winoker, 1978). Because of its adverse side effects, ECT is much less likely to be used to treat nonsuicidal, nonpsychotic depression. These effects (discussed in Chapter 13) include significant memory impairment, which may be long lasting. In addition, the evidence indicates that the beneficial effects of ECT lessen over time, and depression may recur. ECT is definitely not a cure for most depressions, and its possibly cumulative side effects make its frequent use with one individual in the treatment of recurrent depressive episodes a less than desirable approach.

Drug therapy. The use of chemical compounds to treat the affective disorders is very common. The unipolar disorders are typically treated with drugs of the tricyclic class (antidepressants), which increase the availability of norepinephrine in the synaptic cleft. A commonly used tricyclic is named Elavil. Bipolar disorders are often treated with both tricyclics and lithium, depending upon whether the individual is in a depressed or manic phase. Once the individual's mood has been changed by the chemical, the drug may continue to be taken for maintenance purposes.

In addition to the tricyclics, drugs which are monoamine oxidase (MAO) inhibitors are sometimes used to treat depression. One such drug is called Nardil. By preventing the breakdown of norepinephrine, they also increase its availability in the synaptic cleft. However, the tricyclics are preferred, since their toxic effects are less dangerous than those of the MAO inhibitors (see Table 16.2). Numerous studies have demonstrated that the tricyclics are more effective in the relief of depressive symptomatology than placebo treatment, and more effective than psychotherapy alone (e.g., see Akiskal & McKinney, 1975; Prange, 1973). While drug therapy for depressives works fairly well, ECT, when effective, works more quickly. Once drug therapy begins to be successful (usually after about five days to three weeks), individuals are usually kept on the drug for one month after full remission of symptoms and on half-dosages for six months thereafter (Prange, 1973). Although a valuable treatment, the antidepressant drugs do not work in all cases. About 15–30 percent of severely depressed individuals do not respond to these drugs, and their value in milder depressions is questionable (Appleton & Davis, 1973).

When an individual manifests a bipolar affective disorder and is in a depressive episode, the antidepressant drugs are sometimes used to lift the mood, but this sometimes precipitates a manic episode. The bipolar disorder is most commonly treated today through the administration of lithium carbonate. Many studies indicate that this lithium salt is highly effective in reducing the exaggerated mood of mania in about 80 percent of the persons who take it (Fieve, 1971). Once the manic mood is reduced to normal approximation by lithium, a maintenance dosage is continued. Once again, we can see that the drug does not "cure" mania in the sense of rectifying a basic, causal factor. If the medication is stopped, the periodic manic behavior is likely to recur. J. G. Small, Small, and Moore (1971) demonstrated in an early study that substitution of a placebo (inert substance) for lithium resulted in a return of symptoms, and restarting the lithium again reduced the symptoms. In the following example from their study, the symptoms appeared from two to three weeks after the placebo was substituted for the lithium:

> Both the patient and his wife were in touch with the institution before the time of the next scheduled appointment. This was the first time that they had initiated any such unplanned contact. The patient stated spontaneously to the research nurse and to others that he was afraid he was "going high." At the same time his wife, without his knowledge, contacted the social worker with similar concerns. An interim clinic visit was scheduled and reexamination by separate raters confirmed indications of hypomania with increased rate and quantity of speech, expressions of excitement and exhilaration, and increased irritability. At that point the patient was restarted on his regular dosage of lithium carbonate (300 mg. four times a day) and his symptoms subsided within seven to ten days; he and his wife reported this to the social worker and it was confirmed on reexamination. (J. G. Small et al., 1971, p. 1557)

After having been used for mania, lithium was discovered to have some utility for the depressive

Table 16.2
Toxic side effects

Tricyclics	*MAO inhibitors*
Dry mouth	Constipation
Constipation	Gastrointestinal disturbance
Dizziness	Blurred vision
Weight gain	Dizziness
Headaches	Weight gain
Insomnia	Sexual disturbance
Gastrointestinal disturbance	Drowsiness
Agitation	Insomnia
Parkinsonism reaction (involuntary tremor)	Confusion
	Possible fatality

episodes in bipolar disorders and in recurrent unipolar disorders. The data, however, are contradictory. Fieve et al. (1975) found in a double-blind study that lithium reduced the frequency and depth of depression in unipolar depressives. But in another double-blind study, Dunner, Stallone, and Fieve (1976) found that lithium did not significantly affect depressive episodes in bipolar disorders. Both studies were equally well designed. Perhaps further research will clarify this issue.

The effectiveness of lithium in moderating manic behavior has been so dramatic that lithium has become the treatment of choice for the bipolar disorder. Many amazing recoveries have occurred. One well-known individual who has not hesitated to talk about his experience with the treatment is a Broadway musical producer. When mildly "high," he could produce major musicals; but when manic, he would squander his money and alienate family and friends. After years of fruitless therapies, he was given lithium. Its effects were profound. He was able to retain his creative abilities, and maintenance doses of lithium have enabled him to avoid the disastrous mania of the bipolar disorder. Unfortunately, lithium, like many other drugs, has its drawbacks. Effective lithium therapy depends on patient compliance. That is, the patient must remember to take the prescribed dose of lithium at the prescribed time. Many patients do not—and as the manic episode begins, they are even less likely to take the lithium, since the mania often involve a positive sense of energy and grandiosity in its early stages. Some patients stop taking lithium because of its negative side effects (see Table 16.3). When properly monitored, however, lithium's effects may be very beneficial.

Psychological approaches

Psychological approaches to the affective disorders, including traditional psychotherapy and the cognitive and behavioral therapies, have focused on the unipolar depressions and especially on the nonpsychotic depressions. Reports of the treatment of mania with psychodynamically oriented therapy have been mainly single case studies. It is difficult to tell in these studies if the psychotherapy was useful, or if the improvement was due to the cyclical nature of the disorder. Because of the treatment focus on depression in these techniques, this discussion will be limited to that problem.

Dynamic psychotherapy. Treating severe depression with psychotherapy is a difficult task. Such patients rarely have enough energy to participate actively in an interpersonal interchange with a therapist. However, as with schizophrenia, some therapists have tried to deal with severely depressed individuals on an interpersonal basis. Silvano Arieti (1977) is such a therapist. He focuses on the inferred loss that such individuals are thought to have experienced. In his approach, the therapist is an active, intrusive agent, and must become a significant factor in the life of the client. Arieti (1977) describes the process as follows:

> The first task of the therapist is not that of interpreting to the patient the inappropriateness of his patterns of living or the maladaptive quality of his endless sorrow, but that of entering into his life with a strong and significant impact.
>
> The therapist assumes an active role. He is a firm person who makes clear and sure statements. He is compassionate, but not in a way that can be interpreted as acknowledgment of helplessness. He tells the patient that he knows how deep his anguish can be, but that he also knows that depression does not come from nothing. There is always a reason, which the patient, alone, cannot find. In other words, the patient is invited to lean on the therapist.
>
> When the therapist succeeds in establishing rapport and proves his genuine desire to help, to reach, to nourish, to offer more clarity about certain issues and hope about others, he will often be accepted by the patient. . . . Immediate relief may be obtained because the patient sees in the therapist a new and reliable love object. The therapeutic approach must [then] proceed toward a more advanced stage, in which the therapist [becomes even more significant . . . a] person who, with this firm, sincere, and unambiguous type of personality, wants to help the patient without making threatening demands or requesting a continuation of the patient's pathogenetic pattern of living.

Table 16.3
Some side effects of lithium, from mild to severe

Range	*Effect*
Mild	Nausea
	Tremor of hands
Moderate	Vomiting
	Diarrhea
	Stomachache
	Weakness
	Major tremors
Severe	Impairment of consciousness
	Seizures
	Coma
	Death

> Once the therapist has been able to gather enough information, the [patient's] relation with [important people] must be interpreted. The patient must come to the conscious realization that he did not know how to live for himself. He never listened to himself; in situations of great affective significance he was never able to assert himself. He cared only about obtaining the approval, affection, love, admiration, or care of [others]. . . .
>
> When the patient has somewhat improved and is able either by himself or with the help of the therapist to realize that alternative ways of living are available to him, he may state that he is afraid to embark upon them, even though the depression has lifted and the motor retardation is no longer present. . . . Again the therapist must help the patient gradually to develop the lacking motivation for different paths of living. . . . The therapist must guide the patient so that he can catch himself in the act of having these ideas or in an attitude in which he expects to be or to become depressed. If he becomes aware of these ideas and of expecting to be consequently depressed, he may be able to intercept the process and avert the depression. He will become more and more receptive to alternative ways of living. (pp. 866–867)

When depression is not severe enough to be called psychotic, the psychodynamic approach is similar, though possibly less difficult and more likely to be successful.

Behavior therapy. In spite of its high incidence, depression has received little attention from behavioral clinicians. However, if depression is due to a reduction in reinforcement, one approach to the problem would be to teach a patient to engage in more self-reinforcing activities (Lewinsohn, 1975). Another approach is to train the individual to behave in ways that maximize the likelihood of reinforcement. Lewinsohn's social competence approach follows this direction. Reinforcement of the manifestation of appropriate social skills results in an increased likelihood that the individual will receive positive reinforcement from others and, thus, feel better.

Depressive feelings are not even the issue for some behavioral approaches. The overt behaviors that we label depressed may be changed directly. In some studies, behaviors such as crying, withdrawal, immobility, and low rate of speech have been extinguished (not given reinforcement); and behaviors such as smiling, social interaction, physical activity, and talking have been increased by positive reinforcement (Rehm & Kornblith, 1979). This approach has often been used in token economy programs in residential institutions.

A simple focus on behavior, however, is considered incomplete by most behaviorally oriented clinicians (Goldfried & Davison, 1976). Many clinicians favor a more comprehensive approach, and include the concept of "learned helplessness" in their treatment (Seligman, 1975). To combat learned helplessness, most therapists focus on teaching the depressed client that the world is controllable to a greater extent than the client believes. One approach is to provide training in areas in which the client is, in fact, helpless. For example, the client may have behavioral deficits in social skills which prevent adequate social interaction with others. Effective behaviorally reinforced training in social skills would reduce the individual's perception of helplessness and, thus, reduce depression. In addition to the modification of behavioral deficits, we might consider restructuring

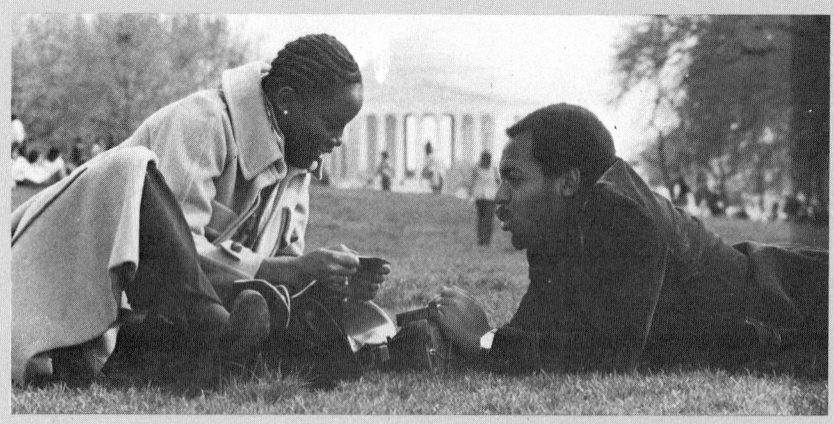

The simple social skills of verbal and physical communication can be reinforced to increase their probability of occurence. If the social skills increase, then positive reinforcement from others is more likely.

the client's environment or helping the client to restructure it. In this case, we might be concerned that the client is living in an unresponsive environment. By creating a more rewarding environment, the individual should feel less depressed.

Cognitive therapy. The behavior therapies mentioned above often involve the modification of cognitions (e.g., the belief that one is helpless to change oneself or to control the environment). These cognitions are seen as a result of reinforcement contingencies in the environment. A somewhat broader and less behaviorally oriented cognitive therapy approach to the treatment of depression has been developed by Aaron Beck (A. T. Beck et al., 1980). Cognitive therapy focuses on modifying the erroneous, irrational cognitions held by depressed individuals. These persons have a predominately negative view of themselves: They are self-blaming, exaggerate external problems, devalue themselves, and are pessimistic about their future. Beck describes this outlook as a "depressogenic schemata," a schemata which is relatively enduring and which acts to color the individual's perceptions.

Cognitive therapy intervenes in these schemata through a variety of techniques. Therapy is structured and directive, and usually short-term. The therapist uses behavioral techniques, which include planning productive activities and scheduling potentially enjoyable events, to break the depressive cycle. However, the core of the approach consists of sessions in which the therapist questions the illogical assumptions and premises held by the client as they talk about the client's life and current experiences. In the therapy session, the client reaches a point where he or she can ultimately question the assumptions he or she holds without the help of the therapist. Kovacs and Beck (1978) provide the following example of the premises, assumptions, and negative cognitions discovered in the therapy of a middle-aged married scientist:

> Mr. D. had a 10 year history of chronic depression with periodic exacerbations. His current depressive episode coincided with a promotion and was reinforced by long-standing marital problems.
>
> In the first phase of treatment the patient learned to monitor and record his negative automatic thoughts associated with dysphoria. The following three self-observations were typical: "I'm unable to respond to my wife emotionally," "I'm alienated from my family," "I'm responsible for my wife's depression." In the next phase of treatment these kinds of negative thoughts were grouped in order to abstract general cognitive themes. As the cognitions cited above reflect, one theme concerned Mr. D.'s self-perceived inadequacy in the roles of husband and father. As therapy progressed the therapist sought to elicit the meaning of Mr. D.'s presumed inadequate performance in the family. According to the patient, the above observations indicated that he was "emotionally empty" and a miserable person who had "nothing to give." The theme of interpersonal self-derogation was subsequently also abstracted from his distorted cognitive responses to his relationships with other people in various settings. To be interpersonally incompetent meant that he was "unworthy." Underlying all of the patient's depressive cognitions was the basic formula that if he did not live up to his own idiosyncratic expectations of perfection (which he unquestioningly believed everyone shared), other people "would not approve" of him.
>
> After considerable questioning and trial-and-error "fitting," the therapist and patient were able to derive a meaningful chain of assumptions and premises. . . .
>
> The patient's underlying belief that he did not have "the right to exist" was apparently related to his discovery, about age 10, that he was an unplanned child. Mr. D.'s highly negative interpretation of this information and its concomitant affective impact was conveyed by the fact that even at 55, he was able to state with conviction, "I *am* an unwanted baby." This basic belief seemed to underlie Mr. D.'s other assumptions, e.g., "I need the approval of others to justify my existence."
>
> The assumptions relevant to interpersonal disapproval could also be used to explain the preponderance of negative depressive cognitions in response to different stimulus conditions. For example, at work Mr. D. was preoccupied with the recurrent negative cognitions "I have no opinion on anything," "My mind is sluggish . . . I can't speak up at meetings." The possibility of being called upon at a meeting activated Mr. D.'s interpersonal schema concerned with disapproval, which led, in turn, to the cognition that if he did speak up, he would make a fool of himself. Subsequent to the uncovering of Mr. D.'s depressogenic schemata, treatment focused on questioning their relevance and plausibility and having Mr. D. test out new, alternative behaviors and interpretations.
>
> By testing and modifying the dysfunctional premises, the patient was helped to process, in a more realistic way, information regarding other people's reactions to him. One technique that demonstrated the inappropriateness of his system of assumptions consisted of Mr. D.'s adopting

> behaviors that were contrary to his dysfunctional beliefs, for example, behaving as if the assumption that he needed the approval of other people were untrue. The consequences of such "new" behaviors led to an increase in more reality—oriented adaptive cognitions. (p. 531).

Cognitive therapy, like traditional psychodynamic or interpersonal psychotherapy and behavior therapy, has been used most successfully with mild to moderate depressive disorders. There have been occasional reports of reasonable levels of effectiveness with the more severe unipolar depressions (Kovacs, 1980). When depression is severe enough to have psychotic manifestations, drug treatment is typically used to reduce the depressive symptomatology; and at that point, one of the psychological therapies may also be used.

Treatment of depression: drugs, psychotherapy, or both?

For some time, a debate has raged over which treatment is most effective. The prevailing opinion has been that for mild to moderate levels of depression, psychotherapy, behavior therapy, or cognitive therapy are most useful; while for the severe depressive disorder, chemotherapy is essential. A recent study by Rounsaville, Klerman, and Weissman (1981) has substantiated this opinion. They studied three groups of patients: One group was treated with chemotherapy alone, one with psychotherapy alone, and one with chemotherapy and psychotherapy at the same time. Rounsaville et al. found that the combined treatment group experienced more relief of symptoms and maintained a better adjustment at a four-month followup. In addition, Rounsaville et al. (1981) explored common beliefs held by some therapists about negative interactions of drug treatment and psychotherapy and reached the following conclusions:

1. In regard to the belief that "The use of medication implies to a patient that he or she does not need to work on interpersonal problems." No evidence was found that this occurred.
2. "Symptom reduction from medication would reduce the patient's motivation for psychotherapy." No evidence for this was found.
3. "Relief from symptoms by medication reduces the likelihood that the patient will work on the "core" problem and symptom substitution may occur." No evidence for this was found in the drug/psychotherapy group.
4. "Use of drugs in combination with psychotherapy makes the patient dependent on a chemical crutch." No evidence was found for this.
5. "Psychotherapy may upset the patient and reduce the effectiveness of the medication." No evidence was found for this.
6. "Psychotherapy is ineffective, and patients who are treated with it do not receive the "best" treatment (i.e., medication)." The group obtaining only medication did less well on follow-up (medication alone is not the "best" treatment).

Studies such as this clearly suggest that psychotherapy and chemotherapy can be effectively combined to treat major depression. In addition, interpersonal psychotherapy appears to have long-term positive effects on the social functioning of depressives which drug treatment alone does not have (Weissman et al., 1981), and drug treatment may work more quickly than psychotherapy alone. Many studies of the effects of psychotherapy on depression do not define what the psychotherapy consists of; often a general interpersonal approach is used.

A recent study of the relative effectiveness of cognitive therapy vs. chemotherapy found that this specific type of psychotherapy was more effective than drug treatment (Kovacs et al., 1981). In this study, 44 nonpsychotic unipolar depressives, who were at least moderately depressed, were split into

Figure 16.3. Short-term and long-term results of cognitive therapy and chemotherapy for depression.

Cognitive therapy group $n = 18$, chemotherapy group $n = 17$.

From Kovacs et al. (1981, p. 35).

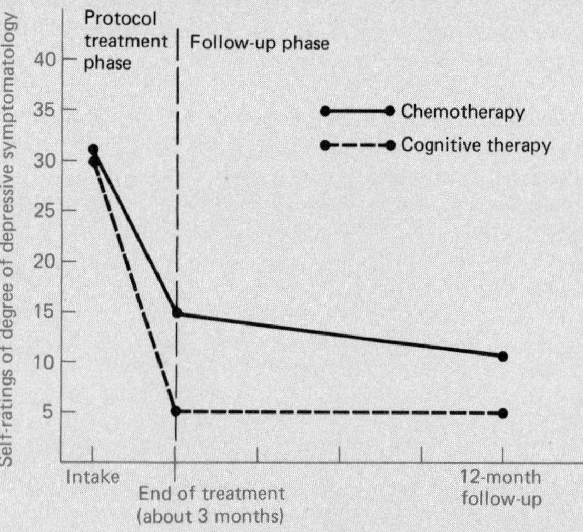

two treatment groups. One group received an antidepressant medication, imipramine hydrochloride, while the other received 12 weeks of cognitive therapy. In the total sample, 76 percent of the subjects had had previous depressions, 22 percent had been hospitalized for depression in the past, and 72 percent reported suicidal ideation. They were definitely depressed to a clinical degree, although none had been so depressed as to be considered psychotic. Patients were assigned to the treatment group on a random basis. During the study, nine subjects dropped out. The results of the study of the remaining thirty-five people are illustrated in Figure 16.3, which shows that cognitive therapy worked more rapidly and resulted in greater reduction of self-reported depression than chemotherapy. Furthermore, the results persisted at a one-year follow-up. These interesting results must be tempered by our awareness that the study was conducted by proponents of cognitive therapy, and was not double or even single blind. Perhaps future research may confirm that particular psychological treatment approaches are more effective than chemotherapy for many depressives.

Several generalizations about the treatment of affective disorder, can be made. The most severe unipolar and bipolar disorders are most effectively treated through pharmacology: antidepressants for unipolar disorder and lithium for bipolar disorder. After symptom reduction in these cases, psychological approaches can contribute to the individual's adjustment, but maintenance chemotherapy is often necessary. Moderate to severe depression seems best treated by a combination of medication and psychological approaches. The milder levels of depressive disorder (which are still very painful and unpleasant to the subject) can be effectively treated with the psychological approaches alone. This may be a distinct advantage, since the chemotherapies have rather unpleasant, sometimes dangerous, side effects.

Summary

1. Why do people develop an affective disorder? The psychoanalytic theory basically proposes that depression is a manifestation of aggression turned toward the self. The loss of a real or symbolic object leads one to direct aggression to the "bad mother," who was introjected by one during infancy. From the psychoanalytic perspective, mania is seen as a defense against depression and a denial of the introjected "bad mother."

2. Later psychoanalytic theorists included the concept of poor self-esteem as an important factor in depression. They suggested that the depressive cannot maintain sufficient self-esteem unless continually bolstered from outside sources. When the outside sources are lost, the individual's self-esteem drops and depression results. Little evidence, other than clinical inference, exists for either psychoanalytic conception of depression.

3. Some learning theory conceptions of depression have been presented. One school of thought suggests that depression is due to a low rate of positive reinforcement. Manifestation of depressive behavior may then be reinforced by sympathy from others. This notion has been augmented by the concept that an individual's perception of social competence is important in depression. Some studies have demonstrated that an unrealistically positive evaluation of one's self-competence may be necessary to avoid depression. Perhaps depression results from the lack of this illusion.

4. Another theory involves learned helplessness. Depression seems to result when people learn (or believe) that they are helpless to modify their fate. This factor appears to be especially relevant in mild and moderate depression, the types of depression most frequently seen. It is probably less useful for major depressive disorder and bipolar affective disorder.

5. Cognitions may be very important in the development of depression. Some theorists believe that depression is a result of illogical ways of thinking. Self-perceptions and assumptions may lead to self-blame, pessimism, and negativism, which result in depressive feelings and giving up.

6. Cognitive errors that depressives seem to make include arbitrary inference, selective abstraction, overgeneralization, magnification and minimization, and inexact labeling.

7. Genetic research has demonstrated that at least some types of depression run in families, and adoptee studies suggest that severe affective disorders of both the unipolar and bipolar type have an inherited component. The genetic component appears stronger in bipolar affective disorder than in unipolar depression.

8. Research has implicated disturbed biochemical functioning in the affective disorders. Depression may be due to a malfunction in neurotransmitter effectiveness. Mania may be due to excess norepinephrine or oversensitivity to this neurotransmitter. The evidence is strong for these possibilities, but conclusive evidence that these malfunctions are the cause rather than the result of major affective disorders must still be found.

9. Electroconvulsive therapy (ECT or EST) is an effective treatment for some major depressive disorders. Because of its controversial side effects, ECT is usually limited to use with people who present a serious suicidal risk. The frequency of its use has declined significantly since the discovery of antidepressant drugs.

10. Treatment of the major affective disorders has focused on chemotherapy and psychotherapy. When symptoms are severe, chemotherapy is usually necessary to allow the process of psychotherapy to begin. The antidepressants and lithium have been valuable in treating the unipolar and bipolar disorders, respectively. However, some individuals do not respond to these treatments.

11. Dynamic psychotherapy involves taking an active, intrusive role in the patient's life. The therapist becomes dominant in the life of the patient. This important role allows the therapist to interpret the patient's behavior so that the depressed individual can see alternatives and try them.

12. Behavior therapy may focus on teaching depressives to engage in activities that provide more social reinforcement. At times a reduction in depression occurs when specific behaviors such as crying or depressive verbalizations are extinguished (not reinforced), while positive behaviors such as smiling, social interaction, and physical activity are reinforced.

13. Social skills training approaches have been utilized in an attempt to combat learned helplessness. An increase in relevant social competence may reduce the individual's sense of helplessness and, thus, depression.

14. The cognitive therapy of Aaron Beck focuses on modifying the irrational cognitions characteristic of depressed people. Cognitive therapy utilizes directive techniques such as planning productive, enjoyable activities that the client can perform. More importantly, the cognitive therapist elicits and questions the irrational cognitions of the depressed person during counseling sessions. The questioning of the irrational cognitions helps the client to become aware of their irrationality, and then to begin to change them.

15. Psychological treatments are often effective with mild to moderate depression, and are useful in conjunction with chemotherapy in the treatment of even severe affective disorders. The prevailing belief, supported by experimental data, indicates that for severe affective disorders a combined treatment of chemotherapy and psychological approaches is more effective than either alone. This appears to be especially true in regard to the long-term adjustment of people who have had an affective disorder. Further research on various specific psychological treatments may determine that one is more effective than others in treating depression, but we can expect the use of chemotherapy to continue to be necessary in the treatment of the most severe forms of the unipolar and bipolar affective disorders.

KEY TERMS

Depressogenic schemata. Enduring cognitive structures (ways of thinking) that make excessive use of directives such as "should," "ought," and "must" when individuals think about themselves and their behavior.

Introjected object. An "object" (such as a parental figure) whose qualities or values are incorporated into a person's own ego structure. Aspects of the parent are taken in by the child and become part of her or him.

Social competence. The degree to which a person is competent at positively reinforced social skills such as joining groups, talking and being assertive with others.

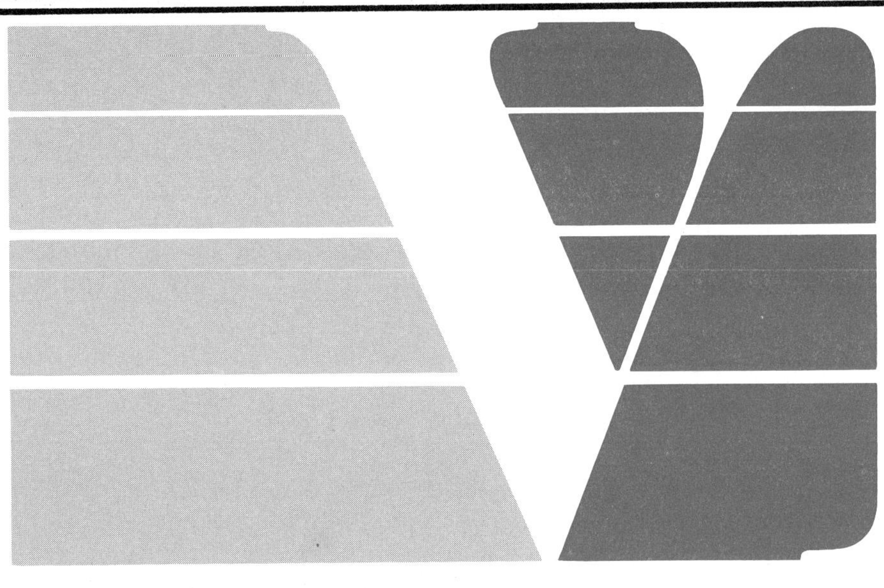

DISORDERS OF CHILDHOOD, MENTAL RETARDATION, AND ORGANIC MENTAL DISORDER

Infancy and childhood are periods during which many learning tasks must be accomplished. Even children whose development is normal may have problems. Some children, however, have major problems in achieving a satisfactory adjustment to the demands of home, school, and community. They may engage in unacceptable behavior; or their social, emotional, and intellectual development may be slower than that of other children. Chapter 17 presents some representative disorders of childhood; the disorders covered include problems of anxiety, depression, and activity level. The chapter also covers infantile autism and childhood psychosis, two rare disorders which are extremely disabling. Chapter 18 is devoted to mental retardation; an estimated 6 million people in the United States have significantly subaverage intellectual abilities. Most people who are mentally retarded are identified during their first few years of school. The most serious category of mental retardation is usually due to organic damage.

Chapter 19 covers mental disorder caused by the occurrence of organic damage in adulthood. A broad range of problems in thinking, emotion, and behavior may be due to organic brain damage or dysfunction. Such problems are of special concern for the elderly, since aging seems to be associated with an increased incidence of at least one form of organic mental disorder.

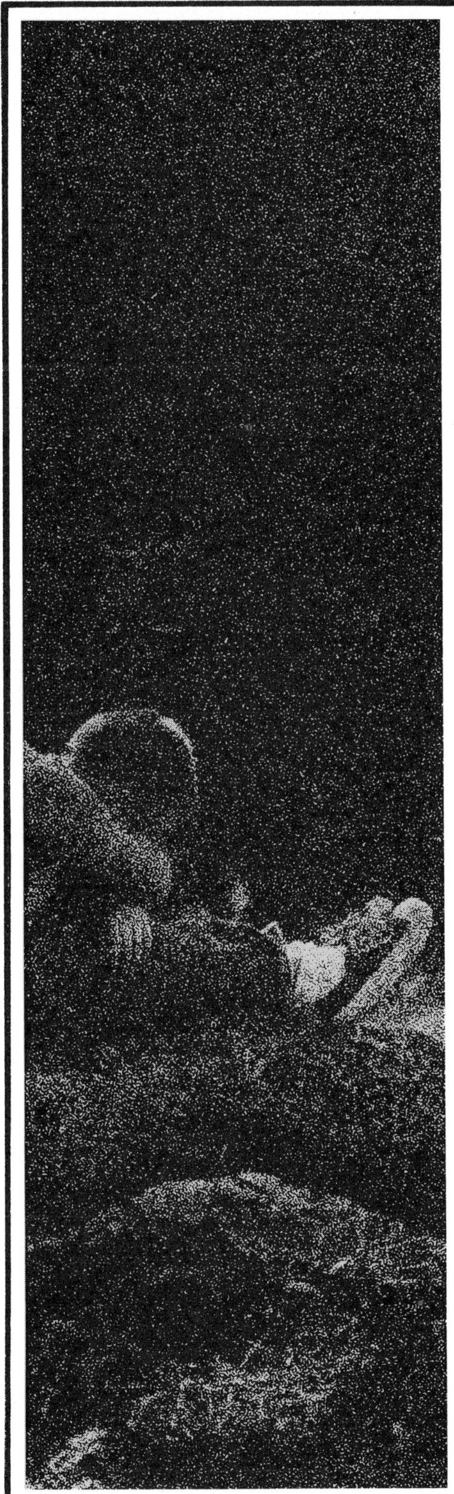

17

Disorders of childhood

- Behavior within a developmental perspective
- DSM-III and disorders of childhood
- Problems of anxiety, depression, and enuresis
- Hyperactivity/hyperkinetic syndrome
- Pervasive developmental disorders
- Key treatments
- Summary
- Key terms

Childhood has been celebrated in myth and fiction as a time of joy, with few pressures and demands. Was your childhood carefree and happy? While you can probably remember good times, you can probably remember times of unhappiness and stress, too. Perhaps you recall childhood fears and doubts and periods of insecurity, along with unpleasant feelings about the kind of person you were. If so, your recollections are not unusual. Contrary to the romanticized version of childhood as a carefree time, many problems may arise in this period. A truly carefree childhood is rare, if not impossible. In spite of the problems that children face, and the troubled behaviors that they may manifest, most children do not become identified as "problem children." In this chapter, we will examine some "problem" childhood behaviors considered to be manifestations of disordered functioning. Causal factors will be presented for each disorder, and treatments will be covered in the "Key Treatments" section.

BEHAVIOR WITHIN A DEVELOPMENTAL PERSPECTIVE

Factors involved in the identification of abnormality have been discussed in Chapter 1. When we consider the problem of abnormal behavior in children, we must remember an additional variable: Children are ever changing. Ideally, they develop from "primitive organisms" to mature, stable adults. During the course of development, some behaviors may frequently be bothersome to others, or may cause psychological pain for the child. Fortunately, these behaviors often disappear with time; the child "grows out" of them.

In Chapter 3, we saw that many theorists view life as a series of developmental periods through which children progress. During this progression, many tasks must be completed if the child is to become a reasonably well-functioning human being. How well each of us resolves these developmental tasks depends on many factors, including our genetic endowment, physical environment, and the psychosocial support we receive from those raising us. Rather than review the developmental stages presented by one theorist, we will look more generally at what faces a child.

Early Childhood

Through the age of 3, a person changes from a relatively undifferentiated infant to a little person. By the age of 3, the brain has developed to over 75 percent of its adult size, and the child is more than half its adult height. Children differ from each other at very early ages in regard to temperament: Some are quiet and calm, others noisy and active. Some are good sleepers, others are not. The characteristics of the child do not develop in a vacuum; the parents profoundly influence behavior. For example, one couple had a son who was a poor sleeper. Initially, the child woke every 30–45 minutes each night with colic (stomach pains from intestinal gas). Sleepless and distraught, the parents tried to ignore the child's crying, but could not. As the colickiness decreased, the infant's nighttime waking increased, since the parents' attentiveness was apparently reinforcing for the infant. The couple accommodated themselves to a disturbing routine in which they took turns rising and rocking the infant to sleep 12 to 14 times each night! At the age of 2½ years, the child spontaneously began sleeping through the night, resolving the sleep problem. Who had the problem? The parents or the child?

Preschool and School Years

The ages 3–6 are marked by significant developments in social behavior, language, and thinking. Children begin to turn outward from the family, and begin to become more independent. During this time, many children's behaviors may be of concern to parents: shyness, incomplete toilet training, temper tantrums, dependency, and aggression.

Entry into the formal world of school leads to many changes in children's lives. There are new expectations, new demands, and people outside the family begin to formally evaluate the child. Children are expected to conform, to be obedient, and to achieve intellectually. Many childhood problems center on success or failure in school. The school system is often the primary source for the identification of many behaviors that are considered problems: poor academic achievement, overactivity, fearfulness, shyness, withdrawal, aggression, impulsivity, rebellion against authority.

A business executive and his schoolteacher wife got a divorce. After the divorce, one of their daughters became very shy, appeared anxious, and began to do very poorly in school. The school authorities called the mother in for many conferences about Annie's "problems." Nothing seemed to help for three years. When her mother finally remarried a warm, thoughtful man whom the children were very fond of, Annie seemed like a new person in school. She became more outgoing, was no longer frightened, and had a better academic performance. Was Annie's problem inside Annie? Was it inside the whole family? Perhaps Annie's difficulty was a part of "normal growing up" in a society where divorce is common.

Each of us can recall some behavior which we engaged in as children that could have been symptomatic of disturbed functioning. Perhaps it was painful shyness, anxiety about school, bedwetting, feelings of loneliness, a sense of being unloved, nail biting, or bullying. As we developed, these problems probably passed. Such transient behavioral problems are quite common in children. In Table 17.1, the incidence of several problem behaviors in a sample of rural United States 3-year-olds is compared to a sample of 3-year-olds in London, England. Problem behaviors were common in both groups of normal children (Earls, 1980). Future reports by Earls will examine the degree to which these problems are transient or long-term. If many problem behaviors of children are temporary and intimately involved in the usual developmental process, how do we decide which are "normal" problems and which are "abnormal" problems?

Table 17.1
Frequency of behavior in two samples of 3-year-olds (percent)

Behavior items	*London study (n = 705)*	*Rural U.S. study (n = 100)*
Eating problem	17.2	4.9
Sleeping problem	14.3	25.7
Encopresis	12.6	11.9
Overactivity	13.7	1.9
Poor concentration	5.3	5.9
High dependency	9.6	10.9
Unhappy mood	3.9	7.9
Several worries	2.6	7.9
Several fears	12.8	13.9
Poor relationships with sibs or peers	10.7	6.9
Frequent temper tantrums	5.5	6.9
Difficult to manage	11.1	8.9
Nocturnal enuresis, ≥ 3/week	36.8	33.7
Diurnal enuresis, ≥ 3/week	16.9	8.9

From Earls (1980, p. 1156).

Defining Disordered Behavior

Many criteria have been suggested for distinguishing whether the behavior of a child is disordered (see, e.g., Rutter, 1975). A child's behavior may not meet all these criteria, or even most of them, and still be of concern to a parent. For example, a child who is fearful about school might not be diagnosed as suffering from a disorder, but the child would benefit from parental understanding and assistance in resolving this fear. One commonly used set of criteria for determining whether a childhood problem can be given a diagnostic label is included in DSM-III.

DSM-III AND DISORDERS OF CHILDHOOD

DSM-III (1980) lists over 40 specific disorders of childhood, a twofold increase over DSM-II (1968). As frequently noted, DSM-III descriptions of disorders are much more concrete and specific than those in DSM-II and DSM-I, the previous editions of this manual (see Highlight 17.1). The increase in specificity of criteria may strengthen the reliability and validity of these diagnoses. However, many clinicians feel that the broadening of DSM-III to include many

HIGHLIGHT 17.1
CONTRASTING CRITERIA FOR HYPERKINETIC OR HYPERACTIVE BEHAVIOR IN DSM-II AND DSM-III

DSM-II Hyperkinetic reaction of childhood (or adolescence)

This disorder is characterized by overactivity, restlessness, distractibility, and short attention span, especially in young children; the behavior usually diminishes in adolescence.

If this behavior is caused by organic brain damage, it should be diagnosed under the appropriate non-psychotic *organic brain syndrome*. (DSM-II, 1968, p. 50)

DSM-III Diagnostic criteria for Attention Deficit Disorder with Hyperactivity

The child displays, for his or her mental and chronological age, signs of developmentally inappropriate inattention, impulsivity, and hyperactivity. The signs must be reported by adults in the child's environment, such as parents and teachers. Because the symptoms are typically variable, they may not be observed directly by the clinician. When the reports of teachers and parents conflict, primary consideration should be given to the teacher reports because of greater familiarity with age-appropriate norms. Symptoms typically worsen in situations that require self-application, as in the classroom. Signs of the disorder may be absent when the child is in a new or a one-to-one situation.

The number of symptoms specified is for children between the ages of eight and ten, the peak age range for referral. In younger children, more severe forms of the symptoms and a greater number of symptoms are usually present. The opposite is true of older children.

A. Inattention. At least three of the following:
   (1) often fails to finish things he or she starts
   (2) often doesn't seem to listen
   (3) easily distracted
   (4) has difficulty concentrating on schoolwork or other tasks requiring sustained attention
   (5) has difficulty sticking to a play activity

B. Impulsivity. At least three of the following:
   (1) often acts before thinking
   (2) shifts excessively from one activity to another
   (3) has difficulty organizing work (this not being due to cognitive impairment)
   (4) needs a lot of supervision
   (5) frequently calls out in class
   (6) has difficulty awaiting turn in games or group situations

C. Hyperactivity. At least two of the following:
   (1) runs about or climbs on things excessively
   (2) has difficulty sitting still or fidgets excessively
   (3) has difficulty staying seated
   (4) moves about excessively during sleep
   (5) is always "on the go" or acts as if "driven by a motor"

D. Onset before the age of seven.

E. Duration of at least six months. (DSM-III, 1980, pp. 43–44)

new behaviors will do a disservice to many children.

The application of a formal diagnosis to many childhood problems may result in negative labeling effects for many diagnosed children, who are likely to carry the stigma of diagnosis throughout their school career. The more severe labels may correctly or incorrectly influence teachers' perceptions of the assets and deficits of children. If a child is *expected* to be a problem student because of a diagnostic label, the teacher may well behave in a way that elicits problem behavior from the child. The label may lead to a self-fulfilling prophecy.

The problem of labeling is not a small one. Some 6 million children in the United States have problems severe enough to be diagnosed. The issue of labeling is highlighted by the discovery that one-third of the children in a kindergarten class could have been diagnosed as having brain dysfunction on the basis of neurological evaluations. However, during the second grade only 10 percent of this group of children continued to have signs of irregular patterns of neural development (Siegl, 1979). What if one-third of the kindergarten children had been diagnosed as having a brain dysfunction, and the information had been given to their teachers? Two years later, would the teachers still have perceived the now "normal" children as "abnormal"? Perhaps. Such a perception may have significantly influenced how the teachers reacted to the children, and how the children perceived themselves. Diagnosis of pathological behavior in children is not a task to be taken lightly, since the labeling effect of the diagnosis may outlast the behavior for a long time.

PROBLEMS OF ANXIETY, DEPRESSION, AND ENURESIS

Separation Anxiety

The acute and severe anxiety a child experiences upon being removed from a parental figure (usually the mother) is called **separation anxiety.** You may have seen families in which a mother and child are inseparable. If the parents arrange for a babysitter, the child is inconsolable when they depart. The child often cries, trembles, and may hang onto the mother's clothing or body with amazing tenacity to prevent her departure. Parents may be so upset by this behavior that they do not go out. But other situations may result in similar occurrences, for example, when the parent must leave the child alone in a dentist's office. If even these possibilities can be avoided, there is one which cannot: school. Few schools will allow a parent to sit beside the child each day in order to avoid separation.

Causal Factors. How might such anxious behavior come about? Bowlby (1960) reviewed many studies and concluded that some degree of separation anxiety is "built in," or innate; it is seen not only in human infants but also in primates and lower animals. Many studies have described how human infants "bond" to an attachment figure, usually the mother. Bonding occurs when mothers (or other caretakers) give particular, appropriate cues to an infant. Such cues appear to include cuddling, holding, cooing, touching, and other affectionate responses. When the bonding occurs, the infant becomes anxious when removed from the bonded attachment figure. Pathological separation anxiety, according to Bowlby, occurs when the infant or child becomes excessively sensitive to separation or loss of love and nurture through the actual experience of such a loss, or when the parent uses separation or loss of love as a threat. The child's anxiety occurs when separated because *this time* the separation may, in fact, be abandonment.

Research by Ainsworth et al. (1978) has suggested that specific maternal behaviors may lead to separation anxiety. Observation of mother-child interactions indicated that children who were excessively attached to their mothers had experienced a style of maternal responding in which the mothers were inconsistent in their responses. At times the mothers responded playfully and affectionately toward the children; but at other times, the mothers ignored the children or directly interfered with childish exploratory behavior. The behavior of the children was not only overattached but also ambivalent (the children sometimes resisted their mothers' contact).

A third factor that may promote overdependence and anxiety is rather obvious. Many investigators have noted that the mothers of children who manifest separation anxiety are overprotective (e.g., Eisenberg, 1958). In behavioral terms, the mothers reinforced the children for being fearful of separation. As children first begin to explore their world, there are many opportunities for frightening experiences and minor hurts. The overprotective mother may teach the child directly that there are many things to fear, or may do it more indirectly. A slight bump may become a crisis which mother responds to with overconcern and anxiety. The child is smothered with comfort and warned of other dangers. Mother's presence may become a guarantee of safety, and her absence a signal of danger. For the mother, the process may be just as reinforcing. The sense of being critical to a "helpless" child's well-being may be very important to the mother.

School Phobia

You will recall that adults may manifest irrational fears called phobias. While irrational fears are not uncommon in children (e.g., fear of thunderstorms), the fear of school is one that causes particular difficulty. Most childhood fears diminish as the child matures and time passes (Gray, 1971; Mussen, Conger, & Kagan, 1974). **School phobias,** however, must be resolved, or the child suffers the consequence of possible academic setbacks. Such phobias occur in roughly 17 out of 1000 students (W. A. Kennedy, 1965).

Some researchers have called this behavior "school refusal." However, this term fails to capture the magnitude of the problem: Children who are phobic *dread* school. When forced to go (as they often are by parents), they may experience acute anxiety attacks, headaches, panic, nausea, and dizziness. The behavior appears to the parents to have begun suddenly and is usually so severe that the parents often capitulate and let the child stay home after a few episodes. At home, the symptoms are not present, and the child is comfortable.

Causal Factors. Psychoanalytic writers such as Jarvis (1964) have focused on the unconscious dynamics of the relationship between the child and school personnel as a causal factor in school phobia. Such dynamics would require extensive psychoanalytic treatment for resolution, but even psychoanalysts recommend that the child be returned to school immediately. A somewhat simpler explanation seems possible.

Waldron et al. (1975) studied 35 school-phobic children and their parents. Most of the mothers had difficulty separating from their child, and most felt that the relationship with their child was more important than with their husband. At the same time, both parents were rated as being resentful of their child's demands on them. In many cases, this conflicted family situation is linked with some traumatic event, such as an illness in a family member some time before the onset of the symptoms. A. O. Ross (1980) suggests that in most cases, the traumatic event is directly involved with the school setting (poor grades, being bullied, etc.). Hersen (1971) proposes a simple learning theory approach: School phobia is a conditioned fear-and-avoidance response which is amenable to an extinction or counterconditioning process. The child has been reinforced for avoidance of an unpleasant situation (school) by anxiety reduction.

Depression

Depression is not listed in DSM-III (1980) as a childhood disorder. The implication is not that children do not become depressed, but that the category of affective disorder, used for adults, can be applied to children. This position seems misleading, since major depression and bipolar affective disorders are extremely rare in children (Welner, 1978). If we were to apply one of the affective disorder labels to childhood depression, it would most likely be dysthymic disorder, a moderate variant of depressive syndrome.

A surprisingly large number of children have one or more symptoms usually associated with depression. Albert (1973) administered a depression survey to seventh- and eighth-grade students in a parochial school and found that one-third would be classified as moderately or severely depressed. Table 17.2 indicates how the students from the total sample described themselves. The many children who apparently have one or more of these symptoms suggests that mild depression is common in children. Fortunately, studies show that these behaviors and feelings often improve with maturity (e.g., Chess & Thomas, 1972). Yet a significant number of children have clinical depressions and experience most of its symptoms for extended periods. In many cases, the depression is masked by another

Table 17.2
A. T. Beck depression inventory results for seventh- and eighth-grade students

Item	*Percent endorsing*
Self-dislike	60
Work difficulty	57
Dissatisfaction	56
Indecisiveness	51
Sense of failure	48
Fatigability	44
Self-image change	41
Guilt	38
Loss of appetite	37
Social withdrawal	35
Self-harm	33
Pessimism	32
Sadness	29

Adapted from Albert (1973, p. 13).

presenting problem such as anger and aggression. Poor self-esteem, guilt, and loss of appetite are also found in the disorder of anorexia (see Highlight 17.2). I. Philips (1979) cites several cases in which an underlying depression was diagnosed after referral for another behavior problem. In the following example, the child was referred for encopresis (defecation in unacceptable circumstances):

> George, an 8-year-old, was referred because of encopresis. When George entered the office the psychiatrist's pinched nose reflected the symptoms. George remarked, "Doctor, I have troubles. I stink inside and out." His mother had been repeatedly hospitalized for psychotic depression since his birth, and his father was a chronic alcoholic. George was a highly intelligent youngster who was failing in school because of daydreaming and isolating behavior. His teacher remarked that she had never known a sadder youngster. When barely scolded, he broke into tears. (I. Philips, 1979, pp. 512–513)

Causal Factors. In the discussion of adult depression, it was noted that depressives were often more likely to have experienced the loss of a loved object (parent) as a child. A well-known study by R. A. Spitz (1945, 1946) indicated that separation from nurturant figures

HIGHLIGHT 17.2
A STRANGE DISORDER: ANOREXIA NERVOSA

Anorexia nervosa has received a great deal of attention in the popular media in recent years. This disorder is listed under the category of disorders of childhood or adolescence in DSM-III (1980). Anorexia consists of extreme weight loss due to a reduction in eating. It occurs most frequently in female adolescents; only about 1 in 10 people with anorexia is male. The disorder is believed to be rare, but one study found an incidence of 1 case out of 200 adolescent girls.

Anorexia begins when the adolescent starts to diet. The person often has major problems in self-esteem and concerns about physical appearance. Weight reduction may be one way for the person to feel in control of her or his behavior, and to improve self-esteem. However, for anorexics, dieting gets out of hand. They develop an unreasonable fear of eating, and often surpress hunger by engaging in repetitive activity such as frequent exercising. When anorexics must eat because others (e.g., parents) demand it, they often will induce vomiting after meals to get rid of the food ingested.

Even though the anorexic begins to waste away and develops such physical problems as cessation of menstruation (for girls), constipation, and imbalances in body chemistry, she or he is often unconcerned about the life-threatening aspect of the behavior. Anorexics continue to perceive themselves as heavier than they really are, and some continue to avoid eating until they die from starvation. Death may occur in up to 15 percent of anorexics.

Anorexia is a puzzling disorder. Why would an otherwise healthy young person starve to death? Although some explanations of anorexia have focused on biological causes (a possible malfunction of the hypothalamus which could lead to a lack of desire for food), current views focus on problems in the family which may lead to anorexic behavior. The parents of anorexic adolescents are often very controlling and attempt to order their children's lives to a greater extent than do parents of nonanorexics. Furthermore, the families are often filled with conflict between family members. Anorexic behavior may be an extreme, distorted attempt by the adolescent to control at least one aspect of her or his own behavior.

Treatment of anorexia usually involves several different emphases. If the weight loss is life threatening, medical intervention (e.g., intravenous feeding) is necessary. The reinstitution of eating behavior and immediate weight gain has been successfully achieved using behavioral approaches; however, these gains are often short-lived. Most treatment programs for anorexia have a major emphasis on individual psychotherapy and **family therapy.** Some treatment programs report success rates as high as 86 percent. However, anorexia still results in death for some individuals. Further information on this disorder is available in *The Golden Cage: The Enigma of Anorexia Nervosa* by Hilde Bruch (1978).

during infancy resulted in what he called **anaclitic depression,** a syndrome marked by apathy, withdrawal, retardation in development, and unresponsiveness. Similar results were found by H. F. Harlow and Harlow (1969) when they separated rhesus monkey infants from their mothers. Bowlby (1973) has pointed out that the separation need not be physical. The loss may be psychological if the parent is emotionally absent or unresponsive to the child's need for affection and nurturance. Ainsworth et al. (1978), in their study of mother-infant interaction styles, found that mothers who were insensitive, rejecting, and ignoring had infants who responded with a lack of interest in their mothers (and presumably in other stimuli). Depression in children may be due to the physical or emotional loss of nurturant parenting. However, other factors may also be important.

Clinically depressed children often are found to have depressed mothers (I. Philips, 1979). It is quite conceivable that the children have modeled the depressed behavior of the mothers, as a social learning theory might propose. In addition, cognitive factors such as those proposed by Aaron Beck are likely to be important. It seems likely that these cognitive factors become most salient after the age of 6 or 7, when cognitive processes become more formalized (Piaget, 1954). In fact, the depressive behaviors of children become most similar to those of depressed adults at 6 or 7.

Functional Enuresis

Bedwetting (or other occasions of bladder incontinence) is normal in young infants. However, once a child achieves moderate daytime toilet training, parents very quickly expect rapid progress toward total continence. Bedwetting, however, occurs in about 20 percent of 3-year-olds, 15 percent of 6-year-olds, and about 3 percent of 14-year-olds (Azrin & Thienes, 1978). **Enuresis** may be due to an organic problem. When it is not, parents are often embarrassed by its presence, and the child often feels guilty and ashamed of the behavior. The enuretic child's problem is not so much that the behavior occurs (most children *do* gain nighttime continence eventually), but that our culture views it so negatively. The school-age bedwetter, in particular, suffers much anxiety, shame, and embarrassment when others find out.

Causal Factors. Psychoanalytically oriented theorists have viewed enuresis as a symptom of an underlying unconscious problem (often hostility directed towards the parent), that the child has not been able to resolve. However, a complex inferential theory such as this does not seem to be necessary to explain bedwet-

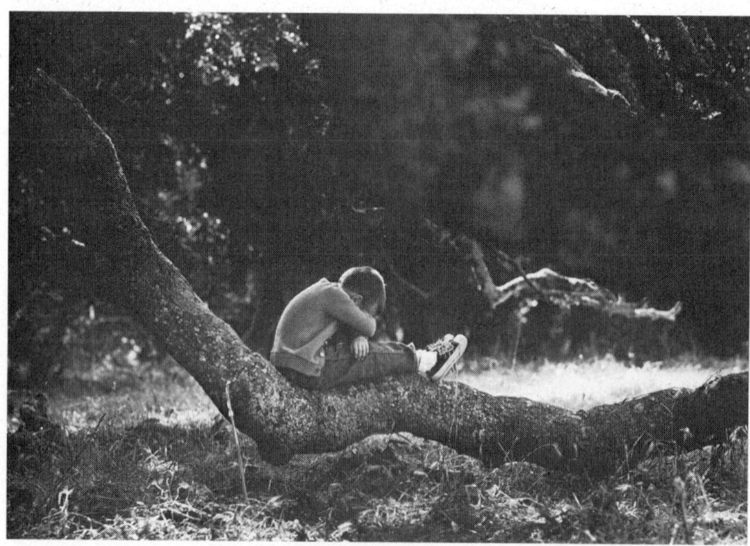

Feeling depressed is not an unusual experience for children.

ting. Enuresis seems to be a function of faulty learning, possibly combined with inadequate neural development in the child. Urination is a reflex which we learn to inhibit. A slightly delayed neural maturation at the time of toilet training may interfere with adequate learning, at least initially. After the start of enuretic behavior, the enuresis may be actually reinforced and maintained by parental attention, long after the child has developed the neurological capability for bladder control. Since reinforcement is important in the maintenance of this behavior, enuresis has been successfully treated with approaches based on learning theory.

HYPERACTIVITY/HYPERKINETIC SYNDROME

> Johnny wouldn't go to sleep. Instead, he spent most of the night tearing around the house. When he was tall enough to unhook the screen door, he began to explore the neighborhood, and his frantic parents once found him wandering down the middle of the street in his diapers. On another occasion, he turned on the clothes dryer and climbed inside. At the age of 2, he was expelled from nursery school.
>
> One-year-old Hugh had to be strapped into his highchair, but he still managed to fall over the side. When he began to talk, the words came out so fast no one could understand him. He was a mass of bruises from bumping into anything that stood in his frenetic path. By the time he was 7, he had dislocated his thumb, broken his wrist, and fractured his collarbone twice. "He looked like an abused child," his mother recalls.
>
> Steven was the terror of the neighborhood. Once, he went after the boy next door with a golf club. Another time, he tried to strangle a little girl with a jump rope. By the age of 9, he had been expelled from three schools. "We couldn't leave him alone," says his mother. "I thought I was going crazy." ("The Curse of Hyperactivity," 1980, p. 59)

Children like the three described above manifest behavior commonly called **hyperactivity,** or the **hyperkinetic syndrome.** In DSM-III (1980) this syndrome is categorized as a specific developmental disorder called "attention deficit disorder, with hyperactivity." Extremely active behavior, impulsiveness, poor motor coordination, and low frustration tolerance are associated with this label. Although in the examples above the behaviors were obvious early, many children are identified as having this disorder only when they enter school. Many children who receive this label are not distinguishable from typical children in unstructured free-play situations (Schleifer et al., 1975). However, when hyperkinetic children are in a structured schoolroom, teachers perceive them as creating havoc. The hyperactive behavior is associated with difficulty in learning the academic materials in the schoolroom. Hyperactive children get poor grades, and are often held back to repeat classes. It is one of several learning disabilities seen in some children.

In today's classrooms, there is an unfortunate tendency to mislabel many active, rambunctious male children as hyperactive. Some teachers may believe that as many as one-third of the children in their classroom are "hyperactive." In fact, most of these children are simply energetic and slightly unruly. True hyperactivity appears to affect only about 5–10 percent of children, mostly males (Lambert, Sandoval, & Sassone, 1978). However, this means that 2.5–5.0 million children in the United States manifest these behaviors to a degree that interferes with their functioning.

A hyperactive child can drive parents to distraction and alienate the most dedicated teacher. The teacher is trying to teach a child who appears extremely distractible: The child cannot read more than a few words or do more than a few math problems before squirming in his seat, tapping feet, whispering, getting out of his seat, throwing spit balls, or stumbling over other children's feet. The child is constantly moving, chattering, as if supercharged. Only during recess or gym does he or she seem to be content. The child's grades are poor and achievement is low. Often the teacher is doubly frustrated because the child appears to have average intelligence or even to be bright. The child's presence is like an unspoken dare: Teach me if you can. Without help, most teachers cannot teach such an "impossible" child.

A century ago, hyperactive behavior was seen as being due to "naughtiness." Today, it is primarily conceptualized as a function of insufficiently focused attention (Hiscock et al., 1979). But why does this inability to focus attention exist?

Neurological Factors

Many theorists have proposed that hyperactive behavior is due to damage to the brain from birth trauma such as oxygen starvation or infection. This concept has resulted from frequent findings that these children show mild or "soft" signs of neurological disorder (Wikler, Dixon, & Parker, 1970). One finding consists of abnormal electroencephalogram (EEG) brain wave patterns. However, Satterfield et al. (1974) studied 120 hyperactive children and found that only 18.5 percent had an abnormal EEG, 29 percent a borderline EEG, and 52.5 percent a normal EEG. In addition, Satterfield et al. found that the children who had abnormal EEG tracings scored *highest* on intelligence tests, had greater academic achievement, could cooperate better with classroom routines, and could concentrate better than hyperactive children who had normal EEGs. Another compromising factor for this concept is that many children with no behavioral difficulties also show soft signs of neurological disorder. Satterfield et al. (1974) conclude that one *subgroup* of hyperactive children can be distinguished by neurological problems such as delayed reflexes, motor incoordination, or abnormal EEGs. This group responded the best to stimulant medications in the treatment of their disorder. We cannot generalize and say that hyperactivity is due to mild brain damage.

Many other theories about the cause of neurological dysfunction have been proposed, and have resulted in popularized treatments. For example, one physician (Feingold, 1975) has proposed that hyperactivity is due to an allergy to certain food additives (dyes, flavorings, etc.). The Feingold diet is being used with some 200,000 children to control their hyperactivity, but no well-controlled studies of this theory have been completed.

Heredity

Could a predisposition to hyperactivity be inherited? The evidence seems to suggest so, at least in some cases. Safer (1973) studied adopted full and half-siblings of hyperactive children and found concordance rates of almost 50 percent for full siblings and 9 percent for half-siblings. Willerman (1973) studied 93 sets of same-sex twins and derived a heritability estimate of 71 percent for hyperactivity. In a study of biological and adoptive parents of adopted hyperactive children by Cantwell (1972), a higher percentage of biological parents reported that as children they had been hyperactive. What may be inherited could be a defect that results in lowered levels of neurotransmitters norepinephrine and dopamine (R. H. Rosenthal & Allen, 1978). Drugs that increase the levels of these neurotransmitters reduce hyperactivity in about 70 percent of the children who take them.

Psychosocial Factors

Hardly any direct evidence exists for the influence of psychological causes in hyperactivity. However, some psychosocial treatments result in decreases in hyperactive behavior. Some clinicians therefore have sought psychosocial factors which could *lead* to hyperactive behavior. It seems likely that the parents of hyperactive children may unknowingly have shaped the children's behavior in the direction of hyperactivity. Modeling may also be a factor. P. T. Ackerman, Dykman, and Peters (1977) found that fathers of hyperactive children (mostly boys) led more "active" and less contemplative lives than did fathers of a matched normal control group. Another interesting finding from this four-year, long-term study of 29 hyperactive children was that maternal discipline was more lax in the families of hyperactives.

Long-term Outcomes

Hyperactive children are likely to have problems as long as they are in school. Ackerman et al. (1977) followed up 23 adolescents identified in grade school as hyperactive. Sixteen had tried medications for varying periods. On the average, this sample was almost three grade levels behind in academic achievement, compared to a normal control group. Fifteen of the boys continued to have behavior problems in school. Hyperactive behavior remained a problem for most, and academic deficits were problems for all by the age of 14. The majority had not "outgrown" the problem.

More favorable outcomes were found by G. Weiss, Hechtman, and Perlman (1978) in a 10-year follow-up of 75 hyperactive children who had reached young adulthood. The subjects' ages ranged from 17 to 24. Their teachers from their last year of school were surveyed along with their current employers. The data were compared to those of a matched control group of 44 nonhyperactive young adults. Even in the last year of school, the hyperactive group was rated as performing less adequately than the controls, and as being more troublesome. However, employers' rating of adults diagnosed (when children) as nonhyperactive or hyperactive were not significantly different! As a group, the adults who had been hyperactive as children were just as punctual and competent as the control group. The former hyperactives got along as well with supervisors and co-workers, completed their tasks as well, and were just as likely to be hired again if the opportunity arose. As young adults, the hyperactive children found jobs in which their school behaviors (capacity for physical work, high energy level, etc.) were no longer problems, but assets. Unfortunately, the study did not note the kind of jobs involved. We can speculate, however, that the jobs did not involve behaviors expected in school (sitting, detailed mathematical work, etc.). It is unlikely that any were bookkeepers or bank tellers.

PERVASIVE DEVELOPMENTAL DISORDERS

Some children have problems of development which pervade multiple psychological functions. They have serious distortions in relationships with others; in language, attention, reality testing, and perception. Their behavior is so disturbed that they have frequently been considered to be suffering from a form of schizophrenia. Yet, as we will see, these children's functioning is not really a direct equivalent of adult schizophrenia. In Chapter 18, the major developmental disorder of intellectual retardation will be discussed. It too may have a pervasive impact on a child's functioning. However, in the two disorders to be discussed here, intellectual retardation is often not seen. These disorders are called **infantile autism** and **childhood-onset pervasive developmental disorder** in DSM-III. The latter disorder has been typically called "childhood psychosis," and this less awkward term will be used in the following discussion.

Childhood Psychosis

Until the present, childhood psychosis has been defined in so many different ways that it is difficult to find overall estimates of its incidence (Werry, 1979). It is rare, being much less frequent in children than schizophrenia is in adults, but it is more common than infantile autism, the other pervasive developmental disorder. An educated guess is that almost 150,000 children have psychoses in the United States. Although the problem is rare, when it appears it is extraordinarily disabling.

The disorder appears usually between the ages of 2½ to 12 years. The pre-onset development of the child is fairly normal. Much like schizophrenia, the symptoms often appear slowly, gathering magnitude. The child's behavior disorganizes from a previously higher level of functioning. There may be withdrawal, inappropriate affect (e.g., unpredictable rage), extreme dependency, and bizarre behavior. The child may engage in ritualistic behavior, singsong speech, or may be mute or babbling. Sudden "spells" of excessive anxiety are often present. The child may exhibit extreme emotional reactions and resistance to changes in home routine. A frequent behavior that is extremely disturbing to parents and other observers is **self-mutilation.** These children may pick, scratch, or bite themselves; try to pluck out their own eyes; or repeatedly and monotonously bang their heads or limbs against objects with such force that serious, even fatal injuries may occur. Unlike adult psychoses, there is an absence of hallucinations and delusions in this childhood disorder. The following individual, first seen as an adult, manifested this syndrome as a child:

> Joan is a 34-year-old female resident of a state hospital. As a child, her development and behavior were relatively normal, within a chaotic family, until she entered school. In the first grade, her teacher described her as of average intelligence, but "odd." The teacher noted that during the course of the year, Joan had become more and more withdrawn. A few months into second grade, her behavior became more disturbed. She was unresponsive and withdrawn, occasionally whiney and crying, and temper tantrums became frequent. Joan was fearful of strangers and fearful of going to the toilet anywhere but at home.
>
> Joan became preoccupied with fantasies. She began drawing pictures of animals (mainly reptiles) and gave them her own name, insisting that she be called "Becky." Her walk became peculiar and ritualistic. Joan walked with a bobbing, jerky movement that was repeated in a series of stereotyped patterns. She began talking to herself and imaginary friends. This resulted in a great deal of teasing by classmates. She developed tic-like movements and began to stare and smile inappropriately, while flapping her arms like wings. The arm flapping resulted in severe bruising of her arms when she would hit objects (including other children). When she was finally kept home from school, her bizarre behavior increased rapidly. Joan openly masturbated while talking to herself, and began to destroy the household furnishings. She then became extremely withdrawn, retreated to her room, and would not speak to anyone. She would not eat, and continuously moaned or repeated in a singsong voice, "Beck's a doll, Beck's a doll, Beck's a doll. . . ."
>
> Joan has never substantially recovered from this disorder. Although discharged from hospitals a number of times during adolescence, she was always rehospitalized due to recurrence of very bizarre behavior. Since the age of 22 she has been hospitalized continuously for 12 years.

The outcome for Joan is not unusual for children who have this disorder. Eggers (1978) followed up a group of 57 people diagnosed as having a childhood psychosis between the ages of 7 to 13. Children who had been diagnosed as autistic, retarded, or as having a clear organic psychosis were not included. At an average 15-year follow-up, about half of the study group showed improvement; 20 percent were believed to be fully recovered. The other half showed fair to poor improvement. An interesting finding was that all those whose disorder had begun prior to the age of 10 had a poor outcome. In later life, they were much like Joan. Their symptoms had become much like chronic schizophrenia, and hallucinations and delusions had become prominent.

Early Infantile Autism

Child psychiatrist Leo Kanner (1943) proposed the existence of a syndrome different from the other childhood psychoses. He had intensively studied 11 children who had this newly identified syndrome, which we now call early infantile autism. Highlight 17.3 includes the complete list of characteristics that Kanner observed. Kanner indicated that the primary difference between these children and children who manifested other psychoses include: 1. onset of the "aloneness" at the beginning of life (these children seem unusually unresponsive to others almost from birth, rather than manifesting this disorganization at some later time); 2. relating to objects, not to people; 3. extreme desire for sameness and extraordinary memory of how objects had been arranged.

The sample of 11 children which Kanner studied was so small that one might expect many of his findings to be later disproved. However, most of his findings are considered to be accurately descriptive of children with infantile autism. There are two notable exceptions. First, the onset of this disorder is now considered possible up to the age of 30 months, with reasonably normal developmental behavior preceding the occurrence of symptoms. Kanner had thought that the autistic behaviors were usually apparent very soon after birth. When onset is after 30 months, similar symptoms are called childhood psychosis, a rather arbitrary division. The second exception concerns intellectual level. Kanner believed that children with infantile autism were usually of average or above-average intelligence. It is now recognized that only about 30 percent of autistic children have an IQ of 70 or over. Even children who have low functional IQs may, however, perform at a superior level on some measures such as memory tasks.

Excerpts from the case of Donald, one of

HIGHLIGHT 17.3
CHARACTERISTICS OF INFANTILE AUTISM IDENTIFIED BY LEO KANNER

The 11 children studied by Kanner (1943) manifested the following characteristics:

1. *Inability to relate* to people present from the beginning of life.
2. *Extreme autistic aloneness.* They ignored and shut out stimuli by treating them as if they were not there unless the stimuli reached painful proportions.
3. *Failure to assume an anticipatory posture* in preparation for being picked up. When picked up, these children do not mold to the holder's body, usually they arch away.
4. *Failure to use speech to convey meaning to others.* The 8 autistic children who did speak used language primarily to name objects and to repeat phrases, rhymes, songs, and so on.
5. *Excellent rote memory.* The children could remember names, pictures, tunes, and so on.
6. *The literal repetition of phrases the child has heard.* This "parroting" is known as **echolalia.**
7. *Extreme literalness in the use of words.* For example, a child who learned to say "yes" when his father promised to put the child on his shoulders used the word "yes" *only* to ask to be placed on his father's shoulders.
8. *Reversal of personal pronouns.* The children referred to themselves as "you," "he," or "she," and to other people as "I."
9. *Eating difficulties,* including vomiting and food refusal.
10. *Extreme fear of certain loud noises and moving objects* such as vacuum cleaners, egg beaters, tricycles, elevators.
11. *Monotonously repetitious noises and motions by the child.*
12. *Anxious desire for sameness.* The children became upset when furniture, clothing, and other objects are changed.
13. *Minimal variety in spontaneous activity.*
14. *A good relation to objects.* The children could play happily with objects for hours, ignoring all living creatures.
15. *Apparently good intellectual potential.* The children's potential was suggested by average or better performance on some items of intelligence tests and by intelligent facial expressions.
16. *Serious facial expressions.* Their facial expressions were typically serious, but the children showed tenseness in the presence of others and placid smiles when alone with objects.
17. *Normal physical condition.*

Kanner's original subjects, illustrate many of the behaviors of the autistic child:

> At the age of 1 year he could hum and sing many tunes accurately. Before he was 2 years old, he had an unusual memory for faces and names. . . . He was encouraged by the family in learning and reciting short poems. . . . The parents observed that he was not learning to ask questions or to answer questions unless they pertained to rhymes or things of this nature, . . .
>
> It was observed at an early time that he was happiest when left alone, almost never cried to go with his mother, did not seem to notice his father's homecomings, and was indifferent to visiting relatives. . . . Donald even failed to pay the slightest attention to Santa Claus in full regalia.
>
> The parents said: "He seems to be so self-satisfied. He has no apparent affection when petted. He does not observe the fact that anyone comes or goes, and never seems glad to see father or mother or any playmate. . . .
>
> In his second year, he developed a mania for spinning blocks and pans and other round objects. At the same time he had a dislike for self-propelling vehicles . . . tricycles and swings. He is still fearful of tricycles and seems to have almost a horror of them when he is forced to ride. . . . This summer we bought him a playground slide and on the first afternoon when other children were sliding on it he would not get about it, and when we put him up to slide down it he seemed horror-struck. The next morning when nobody was present, however, he walked out, climbed the ladder, and slid down, and he has slid on it frequently since, but slides only when no other child is present. . . ."
>
> When interfered with, he had temper tantrums, during which he was destructive. He was dreadfully fearful of being spanked or

switched but could not associate his misconduct with his punishment. (Kanner, 1943, pp. 217–218)

The long-term outlook for the 80,000 or more children who have the disorder is not especially good, but some make a reasonable adult adjustment. Donald was one of these. Donald (Kanner, 1971) was placed on a rural farm by his parents, where he lived under the warm, caring, firm supervision of the farmer and his wife. Donald attended a small country school where his unusual behavior was accepted. As he grew older, many of his more peculiar behaviors ceased. Donald was able to attend college and graduate, and at the age of 36 worked as a bank teller. He enjoyed several hobbies and remained a quiet, aloof person who had little interest in social relationships or the opposite sex.

Donald had the advantages of the apparently positive farm placement and his own reasonably high intelligence. In addition, his early language skills were good. This latter factor seems very important in the prognosis for autistic children. Kanner, Rodriguez, and Alexander (1972) followed up 96 autistic children and found only 11 who made an adjustment like Donald's. In this study, children who had developed useful speech by age 5 had the best prognosis. In a review of eight follow-up studies, Lotter (1978) found that 61–74 percent of autistic children were reported to have had poor outcomes, and half were living in institutions. The autistic disorder has profoundly negative long-term effects on most children.

Etiology of Pervasive Developmental Disorders

Although the pervasive developmental disorders are low in incidence, much emphasis has been placed on attempting to determine their causes. However, much of the research has mixed together children with different disorders in the study groups. This is especially true of the study of childhood psychosis or schizophrenia, and makes uncritical acceptance of the results difficult.

Heredity. Findings from the study of schizophrenia (Chapter 13) in twin and adoptee studies and in the high risk studies of children of schizophrenics suggest that there may be an inherited predisposition toward childhood psychosis. However, no strong studies of childhood schizophrenia (psychosis) show direct evidence for this. While children with psychoses have a higher incidence of schizophrenic parents (Bender, 1974), the studies have not controlled for the environmental effects of living in a disturbed household.

In the case of autism, the early onset of strange behaviors (in some cases, within weeks or months of birth) suggest an inherited problem. Of course, this onset can also suggest some problem during pregnancy or the birth process. However, a recent twin study (Folstein & Rutter, 1977) found a concordance rate for autism of 36 percent in identical twins and 0 percent in fraternal twins. Concordance rates for identical twins were even higher when the degree of cognitive or speech impairment, rather than obvious autism, was the variable measured. Identical twins were found to be 86 percent concordant on this measure, while for fraternal twins the concordance was only 10 percent. Perhaps what is inherited is a predisposition for a cognitive deficit that involves speech utilization. It is unlikely that many twin or adoptee studies of these disorders will be done, or that they will have large numbers of subjects. The population to be studied is so small that subjects with twins are hard to find.

Biological Factors. The early onset of pervasive developmental disorders has suggested to some researchers that the behaviors might be due to brain damage, possibly occurring during pregnancy or birth. Some evidence exists that pregnancy and birth complications are more frequent in both disorders (Piggott, 1979; see also Chapter 13). However, the incidence of complications such as delayed labor or oxygen starvation is not sufficiently high to be convincing. The possible presence of brain defects continues to be an area of research in these disorders, and current research continues to hint that defects of some type (e.g., abnormalities in brain structure) are present (Delong, 1978; Lotter, 1974).

Psychosocial Factors. Could psychosocial factors be prominent in the pervasive developmental disorders? Several theorists think so. In

Chapter 13, we saw that many psychosocial theories have attempted to account for the development of adult schizophrenia. Bruno Bettelheim, a well-known psychoanalyst, has studied childhood psychoses and infantile autism extensively at the Orthogenic School of the University of Chicago. His view of these disorders implicates a rejecting attitude on the part of the child's parents as a causal factor. In his formulation, the child responds to the rejection with frustration and a sense of helplessness. Rather than express these feelings (because expression would not help), the child withdraws from the real world (Bettelheim, 1967).

The early studies of characteristics of parents of adult schizophrenics were taken to support this theory, as were early clinical impressions of the parents of autistic children. These early studies described the parents of autistic children as cold, intellectual, distant, and aloof; but these studies have not been supported by later studies of the parents of autistic children (Cantwell, Baker, & Rutter, 1978). In contrast to the findings on autistic children's parents, studies of the parents of schizophrenic children continue to reveal parenting defects (Bender, 1974; Massie, 1978). These studies indicate that the parents are often psychotic, inadequate, perplexed, anxious, or unresponsive to their infants and children. Yet these same parents respond similarly to some of their other children who do not become psychotic. As we noted in Chapter 13 in regard to parents of adult schizophrenics, impoverished, disturbed parenting seems important in the development of psychotic behavior; but these parenting problems alone do not seem sufficient for the development of psychosis.

Can a pervasive developmental disorder be learned? Ferster (1961) proposed that the childhood psychoses develop because the parents do not become reinforcers for the child. If parental attention is not reinforcing, then the responses and behaviors of other humans will not be reinforcing either. The child is not reinforced for emitting socially appropriate behavior. Ferster's theory has received little support, but has stimulated much study of the application of behavioral treatment techniques to these two disorders. The treatment approaches have had moderate success, but this fact does not necessarily support Ferster's theory of the etiology of the disorder.

Which cause is most important? Once again we are in the unenviable position of living with ambiguity. We cannot conclude that one causal factor is the primary factor in pervasive developmental disorders. The vulnerability model outlined in Chapter 13 again makes a great deal of sense. The early onset of these disorders makes it seem that some biophysiological factor acts as a predisposition for the development of the disorders. The importance of a predisposition seems greatest in autism. Unfortunately, such conclusions must await further research; we are still trying to determine the basic deficits in these disorders. It is still not certain if these disorders are basically perceptual (Lovaas, Koegel, & Schreibman, 1979), cognitive-communicative (Rutter, 1974), or due to over- or underarousal (Rimland, 1964).

KEY TREATMENTS

Children, especially when very young, have little idea that they can be helped in formal ways; thus, they rarely seek professional assistance. If a child is in psychological pain, (e.g., depressed or anxious), one or both parents may seek therapeutic help for the child. With many of the behavior disorders, parents bring children to a therapist because the child's behavior does not fit their model of what the child "should be like." In other instances, the child is brought for treatment because some social agent (school system, juvenile court, etc.) has pressured or ordered the parents to get the child treated. Thus, when a child is seen in therapy, a very real question for the therapist is "Who is the client?" the parent? a school system? society? the child? Most therapists would see the child as the client, no matter who is paying for the therapy, and no matter who wants the behavior to change. The therapist must walk a tightrope between meeting the child's best interests, changing the child's behavior, and satisfying the caretakers (such as parents) so that they will keep the child in therapy long enough for the child to feel better and get better. At times, the impact of therapy on a child may be the development of behavior that the parents find objectionable, such as more assertiveness or greater independence.

When children are seen for therapeutic purposes, the process may require a vehicle different from the traditional therapy process. Adults usually understand the purpose of therapy; young children often do not. Since children may not be able to participate in the traditional therapeutic exchange, play is often used as the vehicle for the process. The use of play techniques creates an intrinsically interesting experience for the child, which a therapist can use for therapeutic purposes.

Medication and psychotherapy

Medication. Medications have been widely used with many disorders of childhood. Anxiety and depression have been treated with tranquilizers and antidepressants, respectively. The treatment of enuresis with imipramine (Tofranil), an antidepressant drug, has resulted in relief of symptoms in 70–80 percent of enuretic children. The imipramine may help mainly because it enlarges bladder capacity, not because it is an antidepressant. When the medication is stopped, about two-thirds relapse (Kolb, 1968). As noted in Chapter 13, the phenothiazines (antipsychotic drugs) are commonly used with psychotic disorders, and these include infantile autism and childhood psychosis. (Chapter 13 provides further information on the effectiveness of antipsychotic medications.)

Medication has been a primary treatment approach for hyperactivity since the 1930s and provides a good example of the effectiveness of this approach. The drugs used to treat hyperactivity are central nervous system stimulants, since there is some evidence that hyperkinetic children have lower than normal levels of some neurotransmitters. These drugs (Ritalin and Dexedrine) raise the levels of norepinephrine and may allow the subsequently more aroused nervous system to screen out distracting stimuli and, thus, focus on relevant tasks. Approximately 75 percent of hyperactive children benefit from these medications (Barkley, 1977). Although overall motor behavior may increase, the behavior becomes more focused and attention span improves (see Figure 17.1). However, some long-term studies have indicated that medicated children do no better than unmedicated children when assessed on a variety of measures of emotional adjustment and academic progress (G. Weiss et al., 1974, 1978). In spite of their short-term effectiveness, the use of stimulating drugs with hyperactive children has been harshly criticized. The drugs have significant side effects; they may decrease appetite, increase irritability, and temporarily slow physical growth rates and, at high levels, interfere with learning. Most physicians prescribe dosages at high levels in order to decrease disruptive behavior, but at high levels, academic performance suffers. Thus, academic benefits are sometimes sacrificed for an increase in compliant behavior.

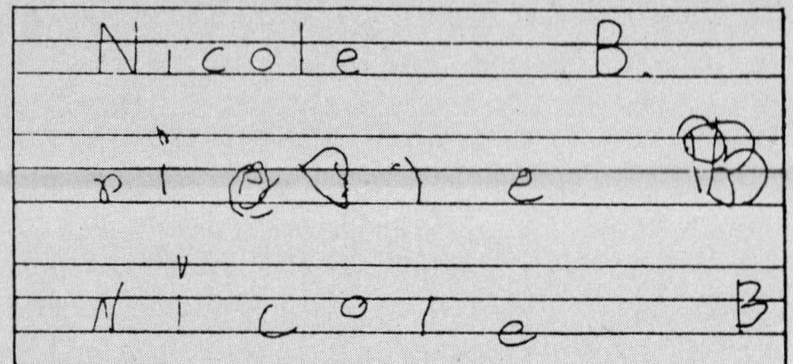

Figure 17.1. Short-term effects of stimulant drugs on hyperactivity.

These handwriting samples show how stimulants can help a hyperactive child. The teacher wrote the top line, the child the middle one before taking a stimulant. After drug treatment the child wrote the bottom line—an obvious improvement.

From "The Curse of Hyperactivity" (1980, p. 60).

Individual psychotherapy. While traditional one-to-one verbal psychotherapy may be used with older children, play therapy is one of the commonest forms of psychological treatment for children. Play is a normal mode of expression for children. The child is presented with a variety of toys and allowed to play freely. The therapist observes the child's interaction, games, fantasies, and often joins in the play. During the course of play, the child often acts out conflicts, behaviors, and emotions important to the therapeutic contact. A child playing with a doll family may have the parent doll spank and abuse a child doll. The child may be role-playing events that have occurred in the child's own family. These play behaviors, observed by the therapist, can form the subjects of interaction with the child which are designed to explore and resolve feelings and conflicts about the child's relationship with the parent. The therapist's exact approach depends upon his or her theoretical orientation. The client-centered therapist will focus on creating an accepting climate, in which the child can express feelings and grow more comfortable with the self; the psychoanalyst will focus on symbolic meanings of the play and on interpreting these meanings to the child in such a way that the child gains insight into the behavior.

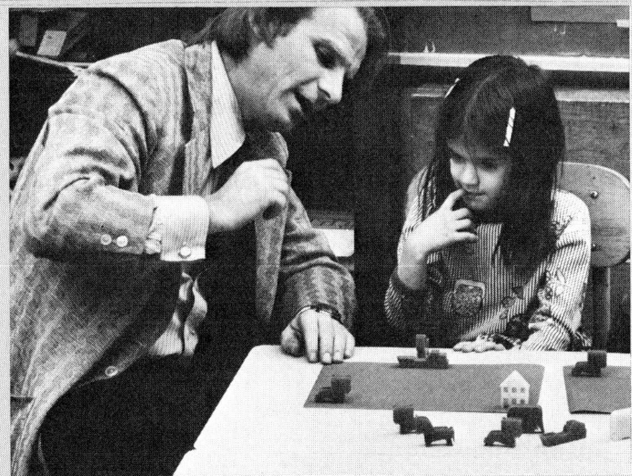

In play therapy, typical children's toys and other activities are the vehicles for therapy.

Play therapy has been used with a broad spectrum of disorders, including the pervasive developmental disorders. These more severe disorders are often treated in residential settings. One well-known setting which treats such children is the Orthogenic School in Chicago. The school takes a primarily psychoanalytic approach to these disorders. In this program, the total environment is geared to be therapeutic. Counselors well trained in the psychoanalytic approach provide large amounts of support, affection, and limit setting (when necessary). The child has little "down time" in such a program, since it is well staffed, and all activities—whether academic schoolwork, eating, or playing—are considered a vehicle for therapy. Bettelheim (1973) has reported that 85 percent of the children who completed his program achieved a reasonably well-adjusted level of functioning. This is a remarkable success rate, considering the usual prognosis of these disorders—so remarkable that we wonder about his criteria for "adjustment." Since control group comparisons have not been made, it is difficult to tell exactly how accurate the data are.

Family therapy. The recognition that childhood disorders occur in the context of a family interaction system has resulted in the therapy of whole families becoming a major modality of treatment. This approach is used not only when a child is having difficulty but also when the identified patient is an adult. In the context of this chapter, the focus is on family therapy's widespread application in the treatment of children.

In family therapy, the child is not considered the patient. Rather the behavior of the child is seen as a symptom of a disorder in the family (Ferber, Mendelsohn, & Napier, 1972). Thus, the whole family is seen as the "patient." The particular techniques of the family therapist depend upon her or his orientation. A psychoanalytic therapist will be concerned with unconscious conflict and the transference of buried childhood emotions not only in the problem child but also in the parents. A client-centered, Rogerian therapist will be more concerned with here-and-now relationships and the creation of an accepting atmosphere in which conflict can be explored and resolved. A behavior therapist will focus on changing reinforcement strategies to alter behaviors in the family. Other family therapists are less identified with one school of thought and use a variety of techniques and concepts in their work with families. Most share the following principles: 1. All family members must be involved (except very small children who are so young that the process would be meaningless to them); 2. a family member's problems are a result of, or maintained by, problematic interactions in the family; and 3. changing the individual child is relatively ineffective if the family also does not change.

Does family therapy work? Certainly, the subjective experience of family therapists is that this therapy works—and it works better, generally, than individual treatment. However, few controlled large-scale studies of family therapy have compared its effectiveness to other approaches and to untreated controls.

Behavior therapy for specific disorders

The behavioral therapies have become an important approach to treating the variety of problem behaviors which some children develop. In order to illustrate the wide applicability of these approaches, several examples of their utility with specific childhood disorders are included here.

School phobia. Virtually all treatment techniques for school phobias, including long-term psychoanalytic psychotherapy, attempt to get the child back into the classroom as quickly as possible. The behavior therapies make this the main goal of treatment. One carefully documented approach used by Ayllon, Smith, and Rogers (1970) is summarized by Hersen (1971) as a prime example of this approach:

> Their [client] was an 8-year-old Negro girl whose school phobic tendencies were first manifested in the second grade, and intensified in the third grade to the extent that she only attended 4 days of school. A most thorough behavioral assessment of the case was conducted in which the child was observed at home with her mother, at the neighbor's house during school hours, in ad-

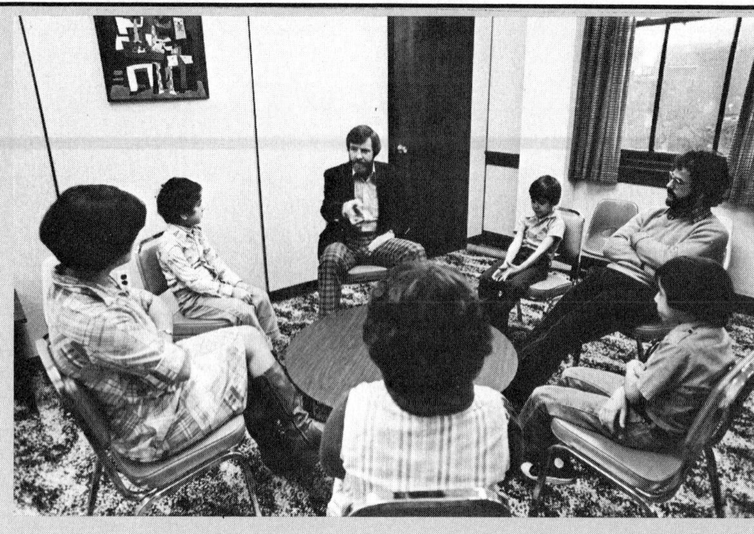

In family therapy, there often are two therapists, a male and a female. The family is treated as a total unit.

dition to obtaining reports from relevant school personnel. School attendance was reinstated by [1. reinforcing small steps towards returning to school, 2. withdrawing rewarding social consequences at home upon failure to attend school, and 3. setting up contingencies in order that the child's remaining at home produced aversive consequences in the mother.] Prior to the application of the [third] step school attendance had been reinstated, but the [early] procedures failed to bring about the girl's voluntary attendance. Indeed, it is pointed out that "only when . . . refusal to go to school resulted in her mother's having to walk from the school back home and then again back to school that the aversive properties of the procedure led to the mother finding a 'natural' way of putting an end to such inconveniences" [Ayllon et al., 1970] (pp. 137–138). In short, a method for dealing with the mother's resistance (continued reinforcement of the girl's [problem] behavior) was effectively put into practice.

Forty-five days were needed to bring about the child's full-time return to school. Follow-up studies conducted with the parents and child's teachers 6 and 9 months following behavioral treatment revealed that her grades had increased from C's to B's and A's, normal school attendance was reported, and the girl's cooperation at home was said to have improved considerably. Social skills were also listed as being much improved. (Hersen, 1971, p. 105)

Other studies have reported similarly positive results for behavioral approaches with school phobia. W. A. Kennedy (1965) has reported on the treatment and follow-up of 50 cases. Symptoms disappeared and remained in remission in all cases over a several-year follow-up.

Enuresis. A standard early behavioral treatment of functional enuresis was developed by Mowrer and Mowrer (1938). In this approach, a moisture-sensitive pad is placed under the child's bed linen. Urination causes an electrical circuit to be completed, which rings an alarm bell. The child is awakened and can attempt urinary control in the presence of bladder distention. The response associated with bladder control becomes conditioned to the stimuli of a full bladder, and continence is learned after a number of pairings of these stimuli and the bladder control response. The procedure, when properly supervised, was found in at least one study to be effective in about 80 percent of cases when followed up four years later (DeLeon & Sacks, 1972).

Problems with the electrical paraphernalia and the 20–35 percent relapse rate reported in some studies led Azrin and Thienes (1978) to develop a training technique based on operant procedures and active training interventions. In this approach, counselors spent one day reinforcing children for inhibiting urination, practicing appropriate urination, and trained them in bladder awareness. They had the children rehearse (during the daytime) the toileting behavior to be used at night. Positive reinforcement was provided when the child remained dry at night, and the children were required to clean themselves and put dry bedding on their beds if they wet. 55 enuretic children, 41 boys and 14 girls, were trained in this manner. The children ranged in age from 3 to 14 years. Figure 17.2 presents the results during training and at a 12-month follow-up for the children on whom data were available. Ninety-two percent of the children achieved 14 days of consecutive dryness (91 percent had been wetting every night prior to training). The procedure is simple enough to be taught to parents, who can then implement it without the need for a counselor.

Pervasive developmental disorders. Behavioral therapies are very important in the treatment and management of the disturbing behaviors of psychotic and autistic children. A bizarre behavior sometimes seen in such children is self-mutilation. It is extremely difficult to stand by and see children (or adults) frequently and severely injure their bodies. Psychotic children may bite chunks from their flesh, bang their heads until their skulls fracture, and pluck out their eyes. You can imagine the torment such behavior causes the child, the parents, and the staff responsible for the child's care. These behaviors have sometimes been thought to be a function of the lack of caring and attention these children were thought to have received. However, when people tried to respond to such behaviors with sympathy, concern, and affection for the child, the behaviors increased in frequency (Lovaas, Schriebman, & Koegel, 1974). Apparently, attention reinforces even these self-damaging behaviors. On the other hand, punishment (usually the application of a painful electric shock) reduces the frequency and intensity of such behaviors (Bucher & Lovaas, 1968). Many people (including psychologists), however, find moral and ethical problems in punishing a child who is self-mutilating. Because of this concern psychologists have searched for approaches to eliminate this behavior without the use of a painful stimulus.

Azrin and colleagues (1975) have developed such a method. In their approach, clients who self-mutilate are positively reinforced for engaging in activities incompatible with the self-mutilation. The clients are reinforced for combing their hair, playing with objects, playing educational games, and so on. If they become agitated, they are guided through a relaxation procedure for 10 minutes. A very important part of the approach is the implementation of "hand control." When the subject begins a movement, such as making a fist and swinging it toward his or her head, which ends with self-mutilation, he or she is guided in a series of hand exercises incompatible with the hitting. These exercises continue for 20 minutes each time a self-mutilation occurs. Before treatment, the subjects engaged in such self-mutilating behaviors as self-biting, face slapping, head banging, finger biting, and ear punching. All subjects had visible damage, and some had open wounds from the behavior. The frequency of the self-assaults ranged from 6 per day in 1 case to over 3000 times per day in 2 cases. The decrease in behavior was rapid and dramatic. In Figure 17.3, the change in behavior for

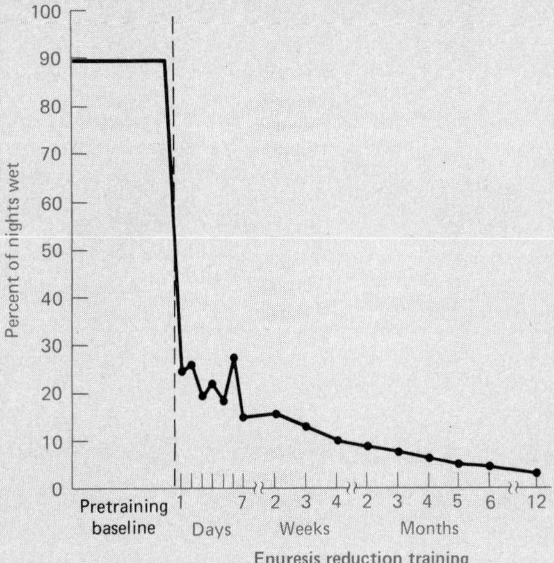

Figure 17.2. Rapid elimination of enuresis.
From Azrin and Thienes (1978, p. 351).

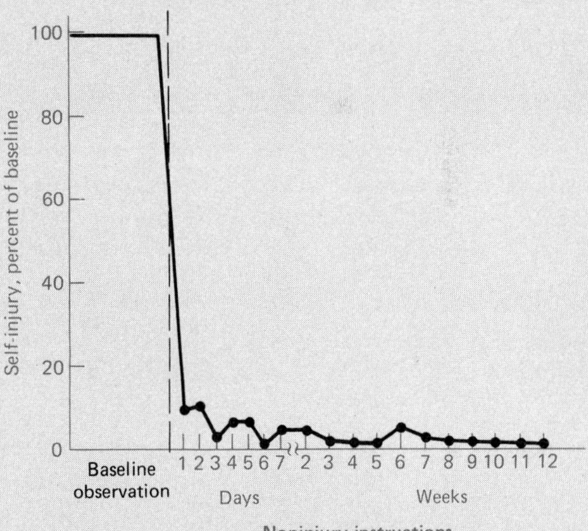

Figure 17.3. Reduction in self-mutilation with a nonaversive behavioral program.
Self-injuries were observed and recorded during the baseline. Treatment was implemented at dashed line. Group $n = 11$; 2 clients reached zero frequency at the third week, 3 by the fourth week, and 5 by the eighth week.
From Azrin et al. (1975, p. 109).

the 11 subjects is presented. The behavioral techniques have been similarly effective with other types of behaviors seen in autistic and psychotic children.

Ivar Lovaas, a psychologist, has become well known for his work on speech deficit, a more general problem for autistic children. The lack of functional, communicative speech has been widely cited as a major problem for autistic children; and the absence of functional speech in autistic children under the age of 5 is an indicator that they will have a poor outcome.

Lovaas et al. (1966, 1974) developed an approach for teaching functional speech by taking children through the following process:

1. The child's vocalizations (noises, grunts, etc.) are increased by reinforcement (usually with bits of food, juice, candy, etc.).
2. The child is reinforced for making a sound in response to (or soon after) a sound the therapist makes.
3. The reinforcement becomes contingent on the child's vocal response imitating the therapist.
4. The procedure is repeated again and again, until the child is imitating many sounds and words. This speech (echolalia) is like a parrot's. It has no meaning.
5. The parroted words are then reinforced when they occur in relation to the object. For example, the word "water" is reinforced only when the child points to a glass of water.
6. The process continues until the child can both express personal needs and wants verbally and understand the basic communications of others.

This approach has been fairly successful in teaching some communicative speech skills to psychotic children. Although none of the behavioral techniques cure autism or childhood psychoses, they are impressive in their utility in modifying disruptive psychotic behavior.

Autistic behavior can be modified to some extent by structured social approval and affection **(left)**, speech can be shaped by food reinforcers **(top right)**, as can social interaction **(bottom right)**.

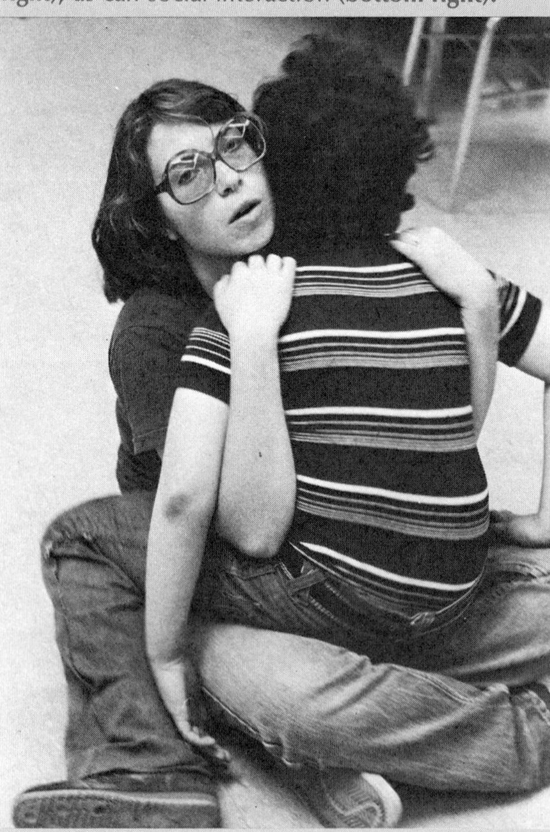

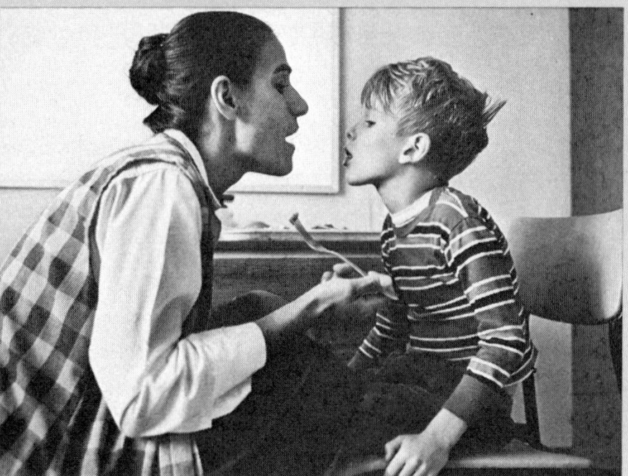

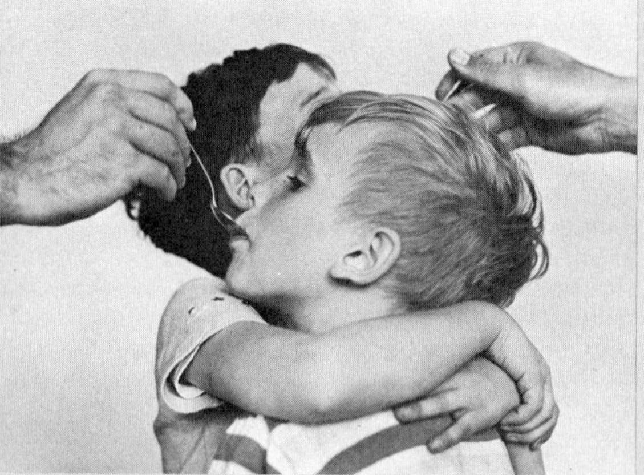

Summary

1. The disorders of childhood must be viewed from the perspective of occurring within a developing, maturing organism. Many of the problems of childhood will, in fact, dissipate with time. Some are so severe that they will remain life-long problems.

2. DSM-III lists and describes over 40 specific disorders of childhood. In this chapter, we have studied some disorders representative of those listed in DSM-III.

3. The disorders covered in this chapter include the following:

1. Separation Anxiety
2. School Phobia
3. Depression
4. Functional Enuresis
5. Hyperactivity
6. Childhood Psychosis
7. Early Infantile Autism.

4. Hyperactivity is a disorder with profound effects on children's functioning in academic settings. The 2.5–5.0 million United States children who have this disorder must struggle with academic expectations, rules, and requirements for many years. Fortunately, outcome studies indicate that after they leave school, their hyperactivity is less often perceived as a problem.

5. Childhood psychosis and early infantile autism are profound disorders which affect far fewer children than hyperactivity. The causes of these disorders are poorly understood. While treatment techniques have been developed for them, the typical outcome is quite poor.

6. Although the treatment of childhood disorders is similar to the treatment of adults, children are typically brought into treatment by parents or other social agencies, rather than through their own initiative.

7. The approach of therapists to children is often through play therapy, a process that has intrinsic interest for the child.

8. Since the behavior problems of children almost always occur within the context of the family, many therapists treat the whole family unit. Specific techniques of family therapy depend to some extent on the theoretical perspective of the therapist.

9. Virtually all family therapists would agree that the whole family must be involved in treatment, the disturbed member's problems are due to or maintained by problematic family interactions, and treatment of the family is necessary if the disturbed member is to maintain improved functioning after treatment.

10. The superiority of family therapy over individual therapy has not been conclusively demonstrated in controlled outcome studies. However, the clinical opinion of family therapists is strongly supportive of the position that family therapy is usually more effective than individual therapy with children.

11. The behavioral therapy approaches have found wide applicability for the clinical disorders of childhood. The techniques have been quite effective in eliminating or decreasing problem behaviors. Even these powerful approaches, however, are not a cure for the pervasive developmental disorders of infantile autism and childhood psychosis.

KEY TERMS

Anaclitic depression. A syndrome sometimes seen in children who are separated from nurturing figures. It includes apathy, withdrawal, and unresponsiveness.

Echolalia. A behavior in which the speech of another is echoed without meaning.

Enuresis. Lack of bladder control.

Family therapy. A treatment approach that involves all family members, under the presumption that a person's disturbed behavior is a result of problems in family interactions.

Self-mutilation. Repetitive harming of one's own body. Includes behaviors such as head banging, picking at sores, biting one's limbs.

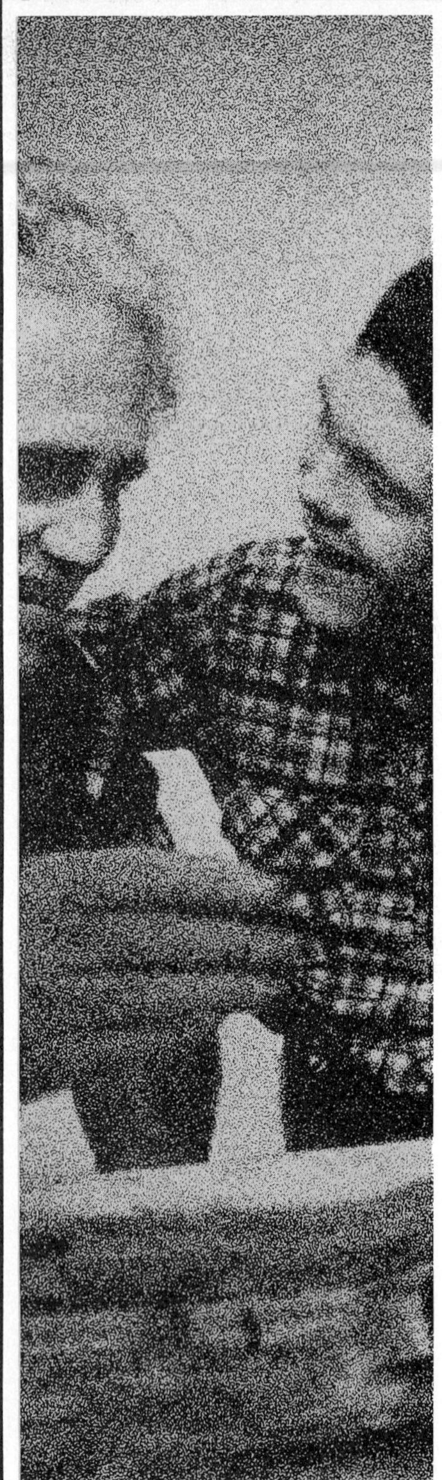

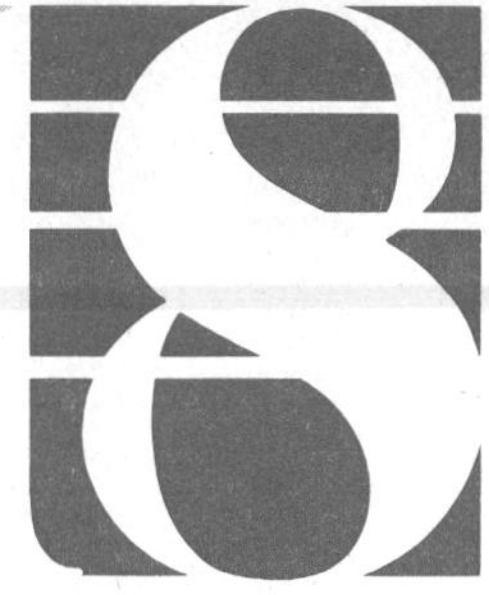

Mental retardation

- Age of onset
- Intellectual deficit and intelligence quotient
- Social adaptation
- Levels of mental retardation
- Mental retardation: developmental delay, defect, or both?
- Etiology of mental retardation: organic causes
- Etiology of cultural-familial retardation
- Key treatments
- Summary
- Key terms

As the tractor roared by, Bud waved and gave one of his usual wide smiles. At the age of 47, he was as friendly a man as I had ever met. Bud's easygoing manner was particularly noticeable with children. He was one of the few adults that local kids considered a real friend. The ability to relate to children carried over into his relationship with his own offspring, who were now young adults.

Bud was not a very good disciplinarian, but his wife adequately filled that role. Bud's parents had a very similar relationship when he was a child; an easygoing father and a mother who ran the household strictly, but with love and warmth. Bud's childhood was a happy one, but he had at least one major problem. He was academically "slow."

During Bud's school years, from 1941 to 1948, it was pretty much sink or swim for students in small rural grade schools. Bud sank. He had plenty of extra help from his teachers, but he simply could not seem to grasp most of the material he needed to learn. After failing many grades and being held back more than he was promoted, Bud left school at the age of 13.

The year he left school, Bud was hired by a local farmer to be the "hired hand" on a large farm. Bud loved his work. It became his major interest and he slowly learned to handle the farm animals, to plow, disk, and harvest. By 16, he could operate all the equipment and was an accomplished truck and auto driver. With help and many long nights of study, he just barely passed his written driver's licensing exam, and received his operator's license. It was the last written test he ever had to pass.

In his twenties, Bud married Marie and within a few years became the father of two children. He and his family lived in a small house, rent free, on the farm owner's property. Bud's wages have always been low, but the free housing is supplemented by a free vegetable garden. His employer provides meat, at cost, from the farm's cattle and pigs. Marie works in town, and between the two of them, they have enough money to live a simple but good life. Marie runs the household and does the budgeting, since Bud "just doesn't have the time." He works 10 hours most days except Sundays. Bud and Marie like to socialize with their church friends, and watch television together. She sometimes reads while he putters around the house. Bud probably has not read anything more complicated than a church service program since he took his driver's exam.

Bud is well liked and respected as a good family man and a good worker. The farmer who has employed him since Bud was 13 says Bud is the best hired hand he ever had. Bud needs direction, but once he is told what to do, he does it well—at least when it is a familiar task. His employer knows that Bud needs a lot of experience and training on new, different tasks before he feels comfortable with them.

When asked if he would like his own farm, Bud says, "Nah, my folks didn't have any land to leave me. 'Sides, too durn much trouble."

Bud can illustrate a number of things for us about the concept of **mental retardation.** Bud has an IQ of 67. His intellectual ability as measured by a standard individual intelligence scale falls in the range of mild mental retardation. Yet Bud has never been diagnosed as being retarded and probably never will be. Why? There are a number of probable reasons. Bud grew up in a rural area and went to a school which had no formal program for the assessment of learning problems. Even if such an assessment had been made, there were no special programs into which Bud could have been placed. Also Bud caused no other trouble in school. He was a pleasant, friendly boy who never misbehaved. A point of major significance for Bud was finding a job with few demands on his intellectual abilities. He became a "productive member of society" in a job which provided a flexible accepting atmosphere. Bud's wife is also very important in terms of her acceptance of his limitations, *and* in terms of her willingness to take responsibility for the things Bud either cannot or will not do. She handles most of the decision making in the family, including budgeting, major purchases and family savings. She creates a situation in which Bud can lead a relatively uncomplicated life.

Bud's case demonstrates that the concept of mental retardation involves more than just intellectual deficit. According to the American Association on Mental Deficiency (AAMD, 1977) an individual must meet three criteria before being diagnosed as retarded: 1. significantly subaverage general intellectual functioning, 2. deficits in **adaptive behavior,** 3. deficits manifested in the developmental period (prior to age 18).

Bud's intellectual deficits obviously were present during childhood, the developmental period. His estimated IQ of 67 is significantly subaverage. Yet Bud has been very socially adaptive: He works, supports a family, and maintains close personal relationships. Bud has found ways to compensate for his deficits, and does not meet the criteria for a diagnosis of mental retardation.

AGE OF ONSET

The criterion of onset of mental retardation in the developmental years is fairly clear. A wide variety of signs may be used to identify whether the intellectual deficit developed before or after the age of 18. A child's normal developmental pattern may be obviously delayed in areas such as learning to walk or talk. At milder levels of retardation, these developmental tasks of early childhood may occur within the expected age period. The individual's retardation may not become apparent until the child enters the academically oriented school system. Even very mild levels of retardation usually become apparent in the early grades.

If a person functions at a normal intellectual level through childhood and adolescence, but has major intellectual deficits in adulthood, the problem is something other than mental retardation. The individual might appear to be mentally retarded because of a disorder such as schizophrenia or a major depression. The apparent intellectual deficit might also be due to actual brain injury or disease that occurred in adulthood. In this case, the disorder would be diagnosed as **dementia,** an organic brain syndrome (see Chapter 19). These types of intellectual deficits would not be diagnosed as mental retardation because they have occurred after normal adult intellectual development had been attained.

INTELLECTUAL DEFICIT AND INTELLIGENCE QUOTIENT

To say that mental retardation involves "significantly subaverage general intellectual functioning" sounds straightforward. Yet the definition of intelligence remains controversial. Is intelligence a quality of the mind? Is it a set of behaviors? Is it an aspect of how thoughts are organized? Does it include traits such as drive and motivation? Is it a single general capacity or the composite of many differing abilities? If many different experts on intellectual functioning were asked these questions, we would get a variety of answers.

David Wechsler, one well-known authority, has suggested that intelligence is composed of separate abilities which combine to form a global capacity to act purposefully, think rationally, and *deal effectively with the environment* (Wechsler, 1971). When we speak of intelligence, we must remember that people learn skills that are embedded in a cultural context. If one is native to the jungles of the Amazon River basin, then intelligence is likely to involve the ability to track and kill game animals for food. In academically oriented societies, intelligence is assessed by measuring behaviors considered important in dealing with that way of life, for example, verbal skills, arithmetical skills, concept-forming ability, and various motor tasks. Measurements are actually a means to an end. They provide some estimate of an individual's capacity to understand the world, and of the person's intellectual resources available to cope with it (Wechsler, 1975).

In Chapter 4, one test of intelligence, the Wechsler Adult Intelligence Scale-Revised (WAIS-R) was described in detail. Along with the Wechsler Intelligence Scale for Children-Revised (WISC-R) and other tests such as the Stanford-Binet intelligence scale, the WAIS-R yields a score called the **intelligence quotient** (IQ). This score tells us the degree to which the individual varies from the average of his or her age group. For these and most other tests of intelligence, the average has been arbitrarily set at the number 100.

In using the intelligence quotient, we presume that intelligence is distributed in the population in a bell-shaped curve (see Figure 18.1). Most individuals fall in the central area of the curve, around the mean of 100. The numbers of people who deviate from the mean become smaller as one moves away from the central portion of the distribution. The convention has been to set the beginning of what we call mental retardation at a point equivalent to an IQ of

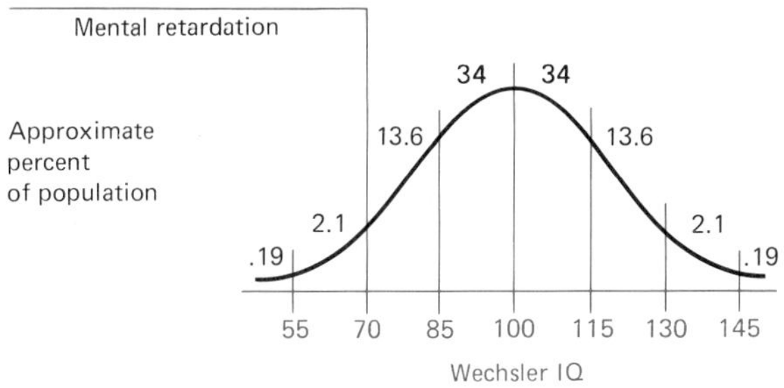

Figure 18.1. Normal probability curve with Wechsler IQ equivalents.

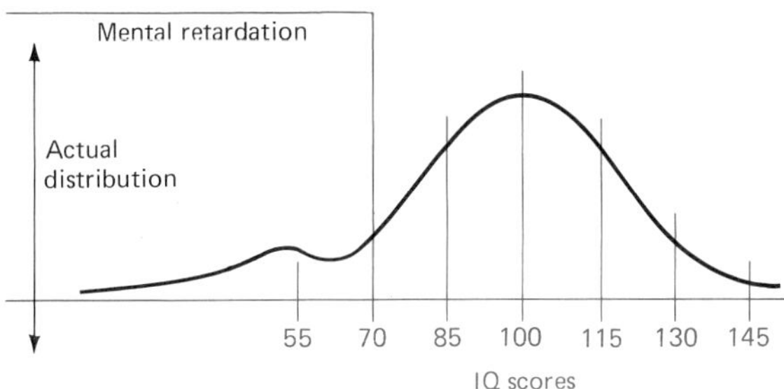

Figure 18.2. Actual distribution of IQ scores in large-scale studies.

about 70. By doing this, we arbitrarily place about 2.5 percent of the population in the category of mental retardation.

Is this an accurate reflection of the real distribution of IQs in the population? It seems to be, with one important difference. Large-scale studies of the actual distribution of IQ scores indicate that the frequency of IQ scores below 50 is higher than this curve would predict (e.g., see Zigler, 1967). Figure 18.2 illustrates this finding. The "bump" in the curve appears to be due to retardation that is a function of clear physiological etiology. If these retarded people had not suffered some physiological deficit, their IQs probably would have been distributed throughout the curve. In spite of this slight departure from the actual data, the normal probability curve (or bell-shaped curve) remains the standard for assessing mental retardation. If an individual obtains an IQ of 70 or below, we know that at least 97 percent of the population would do better on that test of intelligence.

Before leaving the discussion of IQ, we need to consider how much confidence we can have in such a score. We must remember that many factors influence test-taking behavior. A test is a sample of performance. The skill of the examiner, the physical surroundings, the motivation of the subject, are only a few of the factors which may facilitate or hamper an individual's performance on an intelligence test. A subject might obtain an IQ of 69 on one day, and if the testing had occurred on a different day or under different circumstances, might obtain an IQ of 65 or 74. It is much less probable that an individual's score would be 69 one day and 50 or 88 under different circumstances. The intelligence quotient is an *estimate* of intellectual functioning which can be used with other evidence to categorize an individual relative to the general population.

SOCIAL ADAPTATION

Early in this chapter, the example of Bud was given to illustrate that mental retardation is not simply a question of having an IQ below a particular cut-off point. Although Bud would do poorly on many of the abilities measured by standard intelligence scales, he has what we might call social adaptability, social maturity, or social intelligence. Bud is as independent as most other people, and he meets our culture's demands of social responsibility.

Adaptive behavior consists of many skills and abilities. It includes sensorimotor development, the ability to communicate, the ability to engage in self-care tasks such as washing and dressing, and more complex self-care skills such as eating properly and avoiding dangerous situations. It also involves the ability to socialize, to follow rules, to handle leisure, to handle money responsibly, and to care for others. The domain of abilities which falls into the category of adaptive behavior is very broad.

The development of adaptive behavior involves a complex learning process, and requires some of the learning abilities needed for formalized education. It is therefore not surprising that there is a positive correlation between intelligence, as measured by standard intelligence scales, and ratings of individual adaptive behavior. However, adaptive behavior is not perfectly correlated with IQ, as Bud's case shows.

The measurement of adaptive behavior is much more subjective than the measurement of intelligence. To assess the range of adaptive behavior, one must observe an individual engaging in many activities in many settings, and compare the observed behaviors with some standard. To assist in this process, several rating scales have been developed and administered to fairly sizable samples of the general population and to large numbers of individuals diagnosed as mentally retarded. In terms of reliability, these scales leave something to be desired. Since they are based on observers' judgments, there is much room for subjectivity in the assessments.

Two of the most commonly used scales for rating social adaptation are the Adaptive Behavior Scale (AAMD, 1977) and the Vineland Social Maturity Scale (Doll, 1953). Both scales provide an estimate of adaptive functioning which can be compared to an individual's functioning on one of the standard intelligence scales. If the individual manifests significant deficits on both the adaptive and IQ assessments, and has a history of deficits in the developmental years, a diagnosis of mental retardation can be made with some confidence. Highlight 18.1 presents a retarded individual's reactions to this diagnosis.

LEVELS OF MENTAL RETARDATION

Within the range of IQs that fall into the category of mental retardation, tremendous differences exist in intellectual and adaptive deficits. A generally accepted convention breaks the range of deficits into four levels: mild, moderate, severe, and profound. This terminology is linked to scores on standardized intelligence tests and assessments of levels of adaptive be-

HIGHLIGHT 18.1
BEING CALLED RETARDED

In talking about mental retardation, we can often lose sight of the individual. There is also a tendency to focus on the deficits and problems of the retarded, rather than on their similarities to those of normal intelligence. Bogdan and Taylor (1976) have provided excerpts from their discussions with a 26-year-old man who tells what it was like to be found mentally retarded. The following selections from Bogdan and Taylor (1976) demonstrate that this man is an individual in his own right, and suggest that the label of mental retardation has many negative social consequences:

> When I was born the doctors didn't give me six months to live. My mother told them that she could keep me alive, but they didn't believe it. It took a hell of a lot of work, but she showed with love and determination that she could be the mother to a handicapped child. I don't know for a fact what I had, but they thought it was severe retardation and cerebral palsy. They thought I would never walk. I still have seizures. Maybe that has something to do with it too. (p. 47)
>
> Right before they sent me and my sister to the State School, they had six psychologists examine us to determine how intelligent we were. . . . (p. 48)
>
> If you're going to do something with a person's life you don't have to pay all that money to be testing them. I had no place else to go. I mean here I am pretty intelligent and here are six psychologists testing me and sending me to the State School. How would you feel if you were examined by all those people and then wound up where I did? (p. 48)
>
> I guess the State School wasn't all that bad. It was tough to leave though. You had all your needs taken care of there. You didn't have to worry about where your next meal was coming from or where you were going to sleep. (p. 49)
>
> What is retardation? It's hard to say. I guess it's having problems thinking. Some people think that you can tell if a person is retarded by looking at them. If you think that way you don't give people the benefit of the doubt. You judge a person by how they look or how they talk or what the tests show, but you can never really tell what is inside the person. (p. 51)

havior. However, the specific IQ score range for each level varies slightly with the particular intelligence scale used to test the individual. In addition, an individual's test scores are only an approximation of intellectual functioning and may vary from time to time. The IQ cut-off points between levels are thus not as absolute as they may appear. The relationship between IQ level and expected level of adaptive behavior is summarized in Table 18.1.

Mild Retardation

It has been estimated that 75–90 percent of the approximately 6.5 million retarded people in the United States are in the category of mild retardation. As young children, their development may seem somewhat slower than normal, but this delay is often not noticeable. Their intellectual impairment usually becomes most noticeable in their academic studies. In school, they have difficulty learning at the same rate and to the same depth as their age-mates, fall behind in their studies, and are likely to be held back from grade level promotions. Through social promotions, they may graduate from the primary grades and enter high school. However, as adults, their academic skills may reach only about the sixth-grade level.

As adults, most of these individuals can function at unskilled or semiskilled occupations, but some require sheltered work settings with supervision. Mildly retarded people are able to live fairly independently, yet may require assistance with social and financial problems when under stress. Most requirements of day-to-day living are handled fairly well; and once past school age, these people are often no longer formally labeled as retarded. As Figure

Table 18.1
Level of adaptive behavior expected at various ages according to degree of retardation

Degree of mental retardation	*Preschool age 0–5 maturation and development*	*School age 6–20 training and education*	*Adult 21 and over social and vocational adequacy*
Profound (IQ 0–19)[1]	Gross retardation; minimal capacity for functioning in sensorimotor areas; needs nursing care	Some motor development present; may respond to minimal or limited training in self-help	Some motor and speech development; may achieve very limited self-care; needs nursing care
Severe (IQ 20–34)	Poor motor development; speech minimal; generally unable to profit from training in self-help; little or no communication skills	Can talk or learn to communicate; can be trained in elemental health habits; profits from systematic habit training	May contribute partially to self-maintenance under complete supervision; can develop self-protection skills to a minimally useful level in controlled environment
Moderate (IQ 35–49)	Can talk or learn to communicate; poor social awareness; fair motor development; profits from training in self-help; can be managed with moderate supervision	Can profit from training in social and occupational skills; unlikely to progress beyond second-grade level in academic subjects; may learn to travel alone in familiar places	May achieve self-maintenance in unskilled or semiskilled work under sheltered conditions; needs supervision and guidance when under mild social or economic stress
Mild (IQ 50–70)	Can develop social and communication skills; minimal retardation in sensorimotor areas; often not distinguished from normal until later age	Can learn academic skills up to approximately sixth-grade level by late teens; can be guided toward social conformity	Can usually achieve social and vocational skills adequate to minimum self-support, but may need guidance and assistance when under unusual social or economic stress

Adapted from *Mental Retardation Activities of the U.S. Dept. of Health, Education and Welfare,* (1963, p. 2).
[1]Based on DSM-III (1980) IQ ranges.

18.3 indicates, the incidence of *identified* retardation peaks in the adolescent years, and then declines. This may be due to the "blending" of many mildly retarded individuals into the general population when they reach adulthood. Significant problems for people in this group are often characterized by social inappropriateness, rather than by the intellectual deficit. For a variety of reasons, some individuals in this group are so unable to conform their conduct to minimal social expectations that they continue to be seen as social problems. The following case provides an illustration:

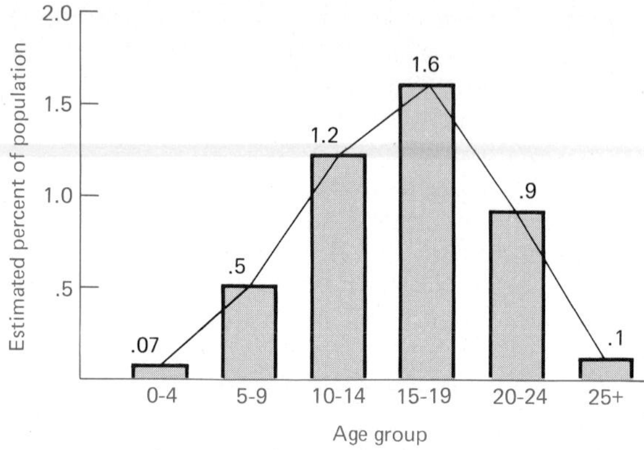

Figure 18.3. Identified mental retardation in various age groups based on a survey of a sample of a medium-sized city.
Based on data from Mercer (1973).

Mark is a pleasant-looking 22-year-old currently hospitalized at a state mental hospital for the second time. Unlike his brothers and sisters, Mark did not begin to walk and talk until he was about 2 years of age. Except for this, Mark's parents noticed nothing unusual about him.

By the second grade, the teachers at Mark's school had several conferences with his parents. Mark just was not doing as well as the other children. The parents were encouraged to work extra hard at home with Mark so that he could keep up. Their efforts were of little help; Mark was not promoted and had to repeat the second grade. When he was finally promoted to third grade, Mark's troubles continued.

In his third-grade class, Mark had many of the same problems as in earlier grades. He was the slowest child in the class, and he rarely completed his assignments. While most other children listened to the instructor's teachings, Mark daydreamed or stared out the window. Sometimes he dozed on his desk. When called upon to answer the teacher's questions, Mark never had a ready answer. His classmates teased him unmercifully for being "stupid" and "lazy." Mark was finding that school was one of life's most unpleasant experiences, full of failure, humiliation, and shame.

Mark was finally referred to a psychologist for an intellectual assessment. The psychologist administered an individual test of intelligence and found that Mark's IQ was 64. The psychologist's report noted that while Mark could read simple words, he was unable to read complex sentences. Mark's memory was below average, and his ability to concentrate and attend was impaired. Although Mark was almost 10 years old, his intellectual development or mental age was about that of a 6½-year-old boy. Mark was mentally retarded.

Mark spent the next 10 years in special education classes in both grade school and high school. These years were characterized by exceedingly slow academic progress. By the age of 19, Mark could read at a fifth-grade level, spell at a fourth-grade level, and do math at a third-grade level. Mark's academic performance was similar to that of many mildly retarded people. Psychological testing at the age of 19 indicated that Mark's IQ was 72.

But Mark had developed a much more significant problem. Like a small proportion of other mildly retarded people, Mark got into trouble over his behavior. Around the age of 10, not long after he started special education classes, Mark began to engage in inappropriate touching behavior. He would rub the girls in his class and his female teachers on the breast and buttocks. The behavior started infrequently, then became more common, much to the distress and then anger of the teachers. Their many attempts to deal with the behavior met with little success. Except for this touching behavior, Mark remained a loner, shy and withdrawn.

Mark finally left school, but was unable to hold a job. The few jobs he tried lasted less than a day. With time on his hands, Mark's problem behavior extended outside the home. He began to loiter in local stores; soon he was inappropriately grabbing female customers and clerks, and stealing items. He often was bodily thrown out of stores. During a one-year period, Mark was arrested and charged on three occasions with theft or disorderly conduct. He was never convicted in court because everyone knew he was "retarded." On the last occasion, Mark was committed to a state hospital by a judge, on the grounds that the behavior was "dangerous."

Mark's life illustrates certain features of mild mental retardation:

1. Early preschool development was not dramatically different from that of many children of normal intelligence.
2. Intellectual deficits were first noticeable during the structured academic learning experiences of the primary grades.
3. The most significant problem for some mildly retarded individuals (as it was for Mark) may be the avoidance of socially inappropriate behavior.

Mark's problems in early adulthood are characteristic of one extreme in mild retardation. At the other extreme are a small proportion of mildly retarded people who do remarkably well as adults, like Bud whose case opened this chapter.

Moderate Retardation

Individuals who attain IQ scores of approximately 35–49 are categorized as moderately retarded. Roughly 6 percent of retarded individuals fall into this category. Intellectual impairment in these individuals is great enough to noticeably slow their preschool development. They walk and talk at a significantly later age than normal children, and their childhood motor coordination is poor. By the usual school age (around 5 or 6 years of age), the moderately retarded child has progressed to a level more similar to a normal 2- or 3-year-old. Moderately retarded 5- or 6-year-olds feed themselves (but are messy), have a difficult time dressing unassisted, and may have problems in toileting. Moderately retarded children at age 6 talk in two- or three-word sentences ("Mommy go store"), name simple objects, and understand simple directions.

These children are unable to benefit from the regular school curriculum. In special education classes, they generally receive training in self-help skills, rather than a traditional academic curriculum. In later years, the focus of their training is on occupational skills. As adults, moderately retarded individuals can live semi-independently. They can usually perform self-care skills, and most are reasonably well coordinated. Their speech has developed and they are able to use complex sentences. With training, they can read at about the level of a child in the early grades, and are able to read street signs, comic books, and other simple prose material. Most arithmetical computation is beyond them, but they can count, make change, and do simple shopping. Some moderately retarded persons have unusual mathematical or artistic abilities (see Highlight 18.2).

Many moderately retarded adults manage quite well in supervised living settings or group homes in the community. Often they are employed in sheltered work settings, where they are paid for relatively simple assembly-type tasks. Behavior problems, however, are more common at this level of retardation than among those who are mildly retarded. When such problems do occur, the individual is likely to be hospitalized or placed in a state institution for the retarded. Bonnie is a typical case:

Bonnie is 31 years old. Her mother reported that Bonnie's birth was difficult. As her childhood years passed, Bonnie was obviously slow in development. At the age of 6, she was diagnosed as moderately retarded.

At the age of 9, Bonnie functioned at about the level of a normal 4- to 5-year-old child. She was soon placed in a class for the trainable mentally retarded. In this class, Bonnie was taught such basic self-care skills as dressing, washing, and eating properly. The class also focused on group social interaction. In later classes, Bonnie learned to read simple words such as "stop" and "walk." As she progressed, more emphasis was placed on following directions, counting, and making change. These were all skills she would need to live a marginally independent life. The classes continued into adolescence, a period with new problems.

At the age of 18, Bonnie was a physically mature woman who had the intellectual and emotional development of a 9-year-old. She went to live in a group home. There she could continue her training and begin doing very simple work a few hours each day in a vocational training program. Not long after this placement, Bonnie began to engage in sexual behavior. For several years, Bonnie's adjustment in the group home was stormy. Her impulsive sexual behavior was a serious problem in the minds of the staff.

In addition to the sexual problems, her other behaviors also caused difficulty. She was often

HIGHLIGHT 18.2
UNUSUAL ABILITIES IN THE MENTALLY RETARDED

Some retarded individuals have what appear to be unusually superior abilities in a narrow area of functioning. These individuals have been described by the term **idiot savant.** Some examples of these abilities in otherwise retarded individuals include the ability to calculate the day of the week on which any date in recorded history falls; the ability to play on the piano any tune the individual ever heard (even if heard only once); and the ability to engage in complicated mathematical computations. Most of these unusual abilities have been explained as due to channeling all energy into rote memorization and practice of the one skill (E. Hoffman & Reeves, 1979; Morishima & Brown, 1976, 1977).

One very unusual case has been found by the Japanese psychologist Akira Morishima (1975). The subject is now a renowned prize-winning Japanese artist, although his measured IQ is in the moderate range of retardation. (Most retarded individuals with these unusual talents are moderately retarded.) The artist, Yoshihiko Yamamoto, entered special education classes at the age of 12, with a measured IQ of 23. A dedicated teacher, Tahashi Kowasaki, noticed that Yoshihiko liked to draw, and painstakingly trained him in the process of print making. Yamamoto is now in his thirties, and has lived an unvarying schedule of a life dedicated to art. At the age of 26, he had never scored above 47 on an IQ scale, but his visual perception and memory skills were above average. His verbal and other intellectual skills are far below normal. Morishima thinks that other mentally retarded individuals may have similar hidden talents. If they could be found and encouraged, Morishima thinks that they, too, could support themselves well and contribute to the arts.

moody, and periodically became loud and abusive when rules interfered with her impulses. She seemed to cause major disturbances when she felt neglected. Around the age of 25, Bonnie went through a period of increasing physical aggressiveness when frustrated.

In the five years since that time Bonnie has adjusted fairly well to the group home. She continues to receive daily training and education. She now functions at a second-grade level in reading and arithmetic, but her social and work skills are more advanced. She is a likable woman who can sometimes be irritatingly stubborn and demanding. A major problem that Bonnie, her parents, and the staff of the group home now face is that Bonnie and her boyfriend of two years want to get married and "make babies like everyone else." No one is sure how to handle this issue.

Bonnie is very typical of the moderately retarded person. Her case illustrates several likely characteristics:

1. An increased probability of suspected organic etiology. In Bonnie's case, there was the likelihood of anoxia (oxygen deprivation) at birth.
2. Obviously slowed development during the preschool years.
3. Inability to gain from academic education, but able to learn basic self-help skills, habits, and minimal vocational skills.
4. Can live as adults in a protected environment, but independent functioning is not possible.
5. Behavior problems are more common in this group than in the mildly retarded.
6. The expectation to be like "everyone else" is unrealistic for almost all people at this level, since they lack the capacity to responsibly manage their lives without supervision.

Severe Retardation

Approximately 3 percent of retarded people have IQs between 20 and 34. The intellectual deficit present at this level is so disabling that almost all these individuals spend most of their lives in institutions. Almost all severely retarded individuals are retarded because of genetic problems or major organic damage before, during, or shortly after birth. Those with genetic defects often have obvious physical abnormalities. Visual-motor coordination is often very poor. Speech may not develop until late childhood, and even adults' vocabulary is limited. As adults, these individuals communicate only at a simple concrete level, even after many years of training. The severely retarded are extremely dependent upon others, since they can usually acquire only the most basic self-help skills, and require frequent reminders and supervision to maintain what they have learned. Alberta's case follows:

> Alberta is severely retarded. The highest score she has ever attained on an intelligence scale is an IQ of 27 on the Stanford-Binet. Now 47 years old, she has been a resident of a state school for the retarded since the age of 11. She was institutionalized when her mother became ill and could no longer care for her at home. Her mother died when Alberta was 12, and she has not seen her father since she was 13, and he remarried.
>
> Alberta was born with a disorder called phenylketonuria. This defect of recessive genes results in mental retardation unless the child is provided with a special diet. The disorder was first identified in 1934, but by the time it was widely known, it was too late to treat Alberta. Intensive training since childhood has enabled Alberta to talk in simple sentences and to make her wants known. Continuing supervision ensures that Alberta washes and bathes regularly and, with some help, dresses herself. She now enjoys watching television, particularly action-filled cartoons. Alberta has tried doing simple tasks in the school's workshop, but she cannot attend to a single task long enough to be productive. A major current problem for Alberta is that she is self-mutilative. She hits herself in the head rapidly with her closed fist and picks and scratches at her arms and legs. She may go months at a time with open sores from the picking and scratching.

The following features of Alberta's case are typical of a severely retarded individual:

1. Clearly impaired development in infancy or early childhood.
2. Usually a genetic or other obvious organic cause such as physical injury, infection, or metabolic disorder is found.
3. Usually these individuals can only profit from lengthy training in self-care skills and habit training.
4. Parents have major difficulty managing the individual in the home, and usually must place the child in an organized institutional setting where almost constant supervision is available.
5. Social adaptation skills are minimal even in adulthood, and major behavior problems may occur.

Profound Retardation

The most disabling level of retardation occurs when measured IQs fall in the range of 20 and below. Only about 1 percent of retarded individuals fall into the profound category. During early childhood (to age 6), these children are extremely limited physically, with very poor sensorimotor skills and coordination. They need almost total custodial nursing care during this time. Their physical handicaps are often complicated by physical deformities. From later childhood to early adulthood, some speech skills may develop, but only rarely does the person learn more than a few words for naming objects. The damage to the physical organism results in a high death rate among these children.

Individuals who survive to adulthood may develop some very limited self-care skills such as the ability to comb their hair or use a wet soaped cloth to wash their face. However, even these simple activities usually require assistance or supervision. At the profound level of retardation, learning to walk, to speak simple phrases, and to attain toileting skills are major accomplishments.

> Bobby, at age 23, is so retarded that he cannot be tested with either the Wechsler or the Stanford-Binet intelligence scales. He spends his life in a hospital bed in the infirmary of a state school. Bobby does not talk, cannot walk, and has little motor coordination in his arms and hands. He is not toilet trained and must be fed by an attendant. He responds only to major changes in his environment, mainly to the presence of human figures around his bed.
>
> The most striking thing about Bobby is his grotesquely enlarged head. Although his lower face is normal in size, his upper skull is almost the size of a basketball. The contrast between his enlarged head and the wasted musculature of his body is dramatic. Bobby has hydrocephalus. In this condition, the enlarged head is due to the increased pressure of intracranial fluid which is not reabsorbed by the individual's body, as it is in most other people. The increased pressure has destroyed much of Bobby's brain tissue.
>
> Bobby has lived unusually long. His attendants take great pride in having provided such good care that he has lived much longer than expected. Unfortunately, Bobby was never strong enough to survive an operation in which a shunt (a plastic tube) would have

been inserted in his head, and from there into his abdomen, to provide a route for the excess fluid to be drained. If this could have been done in infancy or early childhood, his retardation would probably have been less severe. He is unlikely to survive for many more years in his present condition.

Bobby's case is only slightly more extreme than many of the individuals who are profoundly retarded. As a group, they share many characteristics:

1. Almost no development of self-care skills, even if they survive into adulthood. At higher levels, they may be able to feed themselves and dress with assistance.
2. Rudimentary speech, but at higher levels they may have a vocabulary of around 300 simple words.
3. Most have major problems in motor skills; but some can hop, skip, and play games.
4. A high incidence of physical deformity, although not all the profoundly retarded manifest this.
5. Nursing care or supervision in most aspects of living is required throughout their lives.

MENTAL RETARDATION: DEVELOPMENTAL DELAY, DEFECT, OR BOTH?

The mentally retarded are different from the intellectually normal. But just how do these groups differ? Some investigators propose that the retarded suffer from one or more specific cognitive defects that interfere with learning. Others take the position that the retarded learn just as normals do, but at a slower rate and with a lower upper limit.

N. A. Milgram (1973) proposes that the mentally retarded suffer from specific cognitive defects. He emphasizes that the retarded fail to use mediators to associate words or concepts. Normal children who need or want to associate two words such as "table" and "book" usually use a cognitive mediator such as "the book is on the table." Retarded children fail to do this, and thus do poorly on such memory tasks. Milgram has demonstrated that when retarded children are provided with the mediators, their performance improves. Many other specific cognitive deficits have been investigated in the hope that some basic defect could be identified as a primary problem in mental retardation.

Some researchers have recently focused on a deficit of memory (Saccuzzo et al., 1979). Memorization, according to most researchers, occurs in several steps. First, a stimulus is perceived, and for a very short period is represented on a neural network in the brain. This phase is called **iconic storage** or sensory memory. After this step, information is processed and stored in what is called the short-term memory. Saccuzzo and colleagues have demonstrated that at least for visual stimuli, retarded individuals need a longer period of time to accurately put information into iconic storage, and take longer to get it into short-term memory, than nonretarded people. This finding was consistent even when retarded individuals were compared to nonretarded individuals of the same *mental* age, but different chronological ages. That is, a 20-year-old mentally retarded individual with an IQ of 70 would have a *mental* age of 14, and would manifest more difficulty with these tasks than a 14-year-old with an IQ of 100, whose *mental* age is also 14.

What does the Saccuzzo et al. (1979) study mean? It does not prove that a defect exists in iconic memory storage, yet it does support the possibility of such a deficiency (Saccuzzo, 1981). The results of Saccuzzo et al.'s study could have been influenced by variables such as attention and motivation (Stanovich & Purcell, 1981). Further studies will have to be completed before we can say that the Saccuzzo et al. study identified a primary defect in the mentally retarded. Their line of research is promising, in spite of the difficulty in controlling the many extraneous factors that influence the cognitive performance of retarded individuals.

An alternative formulation to the proposal that mental retardation is due to specific cognitive defects states that the retarded develop through the same basic stages of cognitive processes as the intellectually normal, but do so at a slower rate and with a lower upper limit. Zigler (1966) is a major advocate of this position. He and a colleague (Weisz & Zigler, 1979) reviewed more than 30 studies and concluded that the bulk of the evidence favors this formulation.

The process of cognitive development which might be delayed in the retarded is often described according to the theories of Jean Piaget, a brilliant Swiss theorist who studied the development of intelligence and problem solving in children during his career of over 60 years. Piaget (1970) proposed that cognitive development occurs in stages. His position is that intellectual development is not simply the accumulation of information; but at each stage, cognition is qualitatively different from the preceding stage. According to Piaget, normal intellectual development has at least the four following distinct stages:

1. Sensorimotor Intelligence. From birth to the age of about 2 years, the child learns to perceive the environment, organize these perceptions, and manipulate objects in the environment. The child has little interest in why things occur, only that they do. Learning occurs by doing.
2. Preoperational Thought. From ages 2–7, children develop the ability for internal symbolization. As language becomes more complicated, it reflects the child's increasing ability to think symbolically, although thought remains primarily egocentric.
3. Concrete Operations. From ages 7–11, children think more logically. They develop ideas about time and space and number concepts, and come to understand transformations that change the appearance of things, but not their essential qualities.
4. Formal Operations. From the age of 11 onward, the cognitive processes involve the application of concrete operations to hypothetical situations. The abstract thinking required for this is characteristic of normal adults. Questions that begin "What if . . . ?" can be answered, and increasingly complex reasoning can be used.

How might these stages of cognitive development relate to mental retardation? Barbel Inhelder (1968), a student of Piaget's, has studied the mentally retarded and found that the severely and profoundly retarded function at the sensorimotor stage, moderately retarded adults function at the stage of preoperational thought, and the mildly retarded function at the stage of concrete operations. Inhelder's findings have been supported by others. Stephens and her associates studied performances on a large variety of reasoning tasks by groups of retarded and nonretarded people over a two-year period (B. Stephens, 1974; B. Stephens, Mahoney, & McLaughlin, 1972). They found that while both groups developed increased reasoning abilities in a developmental sequence consistent with Piaget's stages, the mentally retarded mastered the reasoning tasks more slowly than the nonretarded people. They also found that the more severely retarded people were less likely to follow the same sequence as the more mildly retarded and nonretarded individuals.

Evidence supports both the developmental delay and the developmental defect positions. Are these positions necessarily exclusive? The work of Stephens and her colleagues gives some clues that both these positions may be partially correct. To begin with, Piaget's developmental theory focuses on differences in cognitive functioning during different stages of development, an idea that is not necessarily inconsistent with defect theories such as Milgram's. Even more important is the finding that the more severely retarded individuals are less likely to move through a sequence of cognitive development shared by the mildly retarded and nonretarded individuals.

Perhaps there are two overlapping groups of mentally retarded individuals. One group may be composed primarily of the more moderately and mildly retarded individuals, who do go through the same sequence of developmental stages as nonretarded individuals. The other group may consist mainly of the severely and profoundly retarded, who do not go through a similar sequence of cognitive development. This latter group may differ from others because one or more cognitive defects prevents its progression through a normal developmental sequence.

The hypothesized difference between these two overlapping groups is fairly well supported by indirect evidence. Figure 18.2 illustrates that the frequency of lower levels of retardation is greater than we would expect. Zigler (1967) suggests that these increased frequencies are due to people who would have fallen elsewhere on the distribution if they did not have an organic defect. The estimated 10–20 percent of retarded persons who have experienced damage to their brain seem likely to have a specific cognitive defect from the organic damage (Heber, 1970).

The differentiation between these two groups of retarded individuals is further supported by studies of prevalence across socioeconomic groups. Retarded individuals with IQs below 50 (who are most likely to have organic damage and thus more likely to have a specific cognitive defect) are distributed more equally across socioeconomic classes than are retarded persons with IQs above 60. Figure 18.4 illustrates the distribution of three levels of retardation across socioeconomic classes. The relative stability in frequency of lower-level retardation (IQ below 50) across socioeconomic classes suggests that the organic damage that this group has suffered is relatively insensitive to social class differences. On the other hand, individuals who are retarded without evidence of organic damage are much more prevalent in the lowest socioeconomic classes. Their retardation appears not to be due primarily to specific cognitive defects, but to cultural, psychosocial, and environmental factors more common in the lowest socioeconomic groups (N. M. Robinson & Robinson, 1976).

Organic damage and psychosocial factors are the two broad areas of etiology which are important in mental retardation. "Mental retardation" is a term applied to a grouping of behaviors regardless of etiology (AAMD, 1977). The many possible etiologies of mental retardation can be grouped into two broad categories: organic causes and cultural-familial causes.

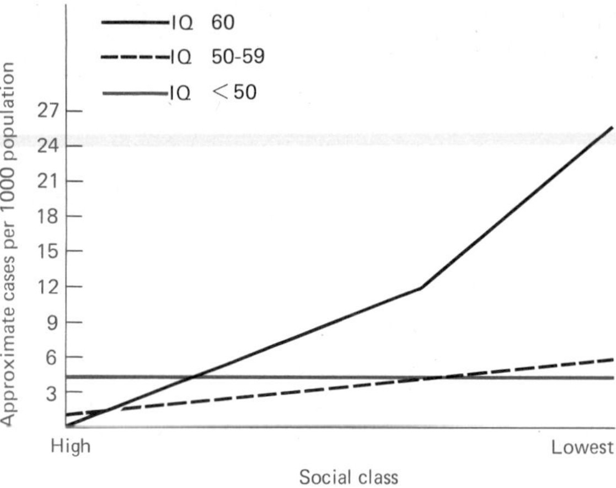

Figure 18.4. Distribution of IQ levels of individuals with mental retardation across socioeconomic classes.
Based on data from Birch et al. (1970).

ETIOLOGY OF MENTAL RETARDATION: ORGANIC CAUSES

The lower levels of retardation are usually associated with signs of organic damage to the brain. Verville (1967) has estimated that there are at least 200 distinct organic causes of mental retardation. We cannot discuss each, but the organic causes of mental retardation can be presented in general categories with examples of the more common types of disorders. In this context, the term "common" is used relative to the other types of organically caused retardation.

Genetic Causes

Mental retardation may be due to the transmission of recessive genes from parents, or to other abnormalities of the chromosomes of the child. Mental retardation is rarely transmitted by dominant genes, since in such cases the individual is usually sterile and unable to transmit the genetic makeup.

Chromosome Abnormalities. A small percentage of infants show chromosomal abnormalities. One of the best known chromosomal defects is called "trisomy 21," or **Down's syndrome.** In the past, this disorder was known as mongolism because such individuals were thought to resemble members of the "Mongol race." The disorder is due to the presence of 47 chromosomes, rather than the normal complement of 46. The twenty-first pair of chromosomes has three chromosomes, not the usual two.

The risk of Down's syndrome increases with the age of the mother. Under the maternal age of 30, the risk is one in 1500 births. The risk doubles after the age of 30, is more than 10 times as great after the age of 40; and after a mother reaches 45, the incidence of such births is 1 in 65 (D. W. Smith & Wilson, 1973).

As in most cases of retardation caused by genetic transmission or chromosomal abnormalities, the Down's syndrome child has many

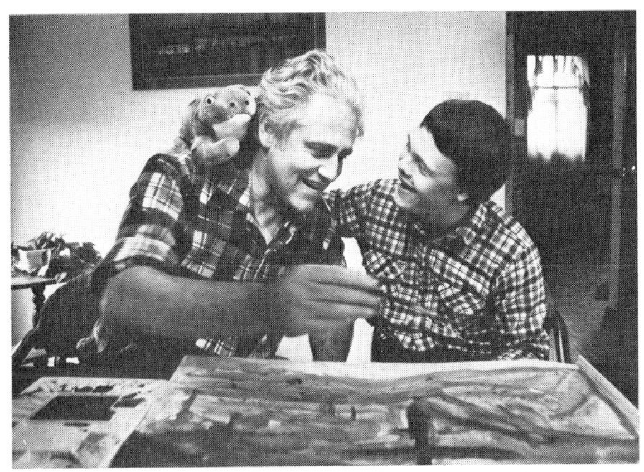

This Down's Syndrome child is being raised in a stimulating, loving family environment. Such children are likely to develop higher IQs when raised in a loving home rather than in an institution.

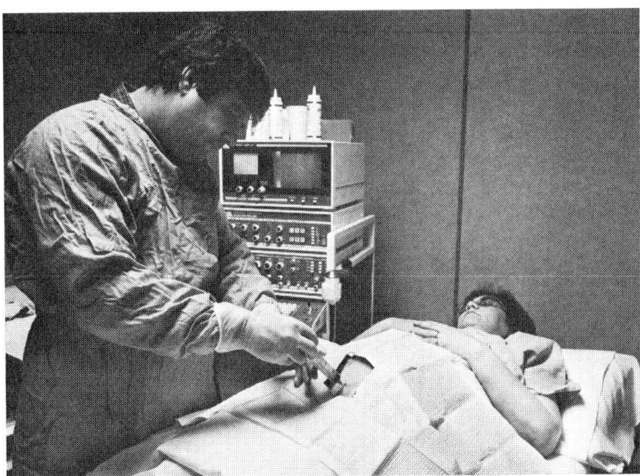

In the prenatal testing procedure known as amniocentesis, a hollow needle is inserted through the mother's abdomen and into the uterus. The needle is used to withdraw a small amount of amniotic fluid, which contains some loose cells cast off from the developing fetus. These cells are then examined for chromosomal damage or defect.

physical abnormalities. Some features that identify the Down's syndrome child include eyes that appear to be slanted upward, a flat face and nose, a large fissured tongue, stubby fingers, small skull, and short stature. Defects in the heart and other internal organs also occur. The life expectancy of people with Down's syndrome is shorter than the norm. Some do not survive childhood; and after middle age, the death rate is very high.

The measured intelligence of the Down's child usually does not exceed an IQ of 50, yet a small proportion (about 5 percent) may have IQs above 70 (Connolly, 1978). Organic defects do not always result in more extreme degrees of retardation. Down's children raised in a warm, loving, and stimulating home environment may be more likely to do better on intellectual and adaptive tasks than Down's children who are placed in an impersonal, unstimulating institution because they have an organic defect. Down's syndrome is but one of a number of syndromes caused by chromosomal abnormalities.

The heartache of having a child who becomes retarded due to a chromosomal abnormality like Down's syndrome is to some extent avoidable. A technique called **amniocentesis** can be used to identify such defects after conception, but before the child is born. In this test, amniotic fluid is removed from the uterus of the pregnant woman and examined microscopically and biochemically. This fluid contains cast-off cells from the fetus, and a chromosomal analysis sometimes reveals defects. If a defect is found, the parents have the option of a therapeutic abortion, which they may reject on religious or other grounds. In this case, a mentally retarded child will be born.

Recessive Genes. Not all recessive genes combine to result in mental retardation. However, some recessive gene combinations cause problems of enzyme production and metabolism which lead to deficits in intellectual processes. A prime example is **phenylketonuria** (PKU). In this disorder, each parent contributes a recessive gene which leads to a deficiency of a liver enzyme (phenylalanine hydroxylase) in their infant. Without this enzyme, the amino acid phenylalanine and phenylpyruvic acid build up in the infant's body and interfere in the development of neural tissue. The brain damage is particularly extensive in the frontal lobes. The damage is progressive, so that the affected infant may appear normal at birth, with retardation first becoming apparent around 6 months of age. A blood test for abnormal amounts of phenylalanine is available and required by law in all states. If PKU is detected, the use of a diet low in phenylalanine from birth to 6 years allows greater cognitive development, often to the normal level. However, the test for phenylalanine is not totally accurate, and some children still are not tested (Engel, 1977). Thus, PKU develops and is untreated in some children.

In many of the recessive gene disorders, infants are so damaged biologically that they rarely survive. In Tay-Sachs disease, a rare disorder seen most commonly in Jews whose ancestors lived in a particular area of Europe, the child rarely survives beyond the age of 3 or 4. In Maple Syrup Urine disease (named because of the urine's distinctive odor), the child's life expectancy is usually less than 1 year. These and the other recessive gene disorders are individually rare. However, when combined in a group, they contribute significantly to the number of children who are severely and profoundly retarded.

The Prenatal Environment

At the moment of conception, when the father's sperm cell and mother's egg cell unite, the development of a new organism begins in a highly protected environment. This organism, first called an embryo and later a fetus, is protected from external dangers by the mother's body. For approximately nine months, the embryo or fetus makes gigantic strides in development while in this protected, controlled **prenatal** environment. However, events that can endanger the health and development of the organism may occur during this time.

Maternal Infections. Many infectious illnesses of the mother do not cross the placenta into the blood supply of the fetus. However, some diseases do, and present a serious danger to normal development. One of the best known is the rubella virus, or German measles. The danger is particularly great during the first three months of pregnancy. About half the infants of mothers who have German measles during the first trimester (three months) of pregnancy become infected, and about one-third of them are born retarded (Chess, 1978). The rubella virus also may cause physical abnormalities such as blindness, deafness, and congenital heart disease. Today there are vaccines to prevent German measles, and the incidence of this cause of retardation is much lower than in the past.

Other maternal infections which can cause fetal retardation and other congenital abnormalities include untreated syphilis, herpes simplex, and a protozoan infection called toxoplasmosis. The dangers which such infections present to the fetuses of pregnant women illustrate the importance of good prenatal care and regular visits to an obstetrician during pregnancy.

Blood RH Factors. If substances are present in the blood of a fetus which are not present in the mother's blood, problems may result. For example, a fetus may inherit a substance from the father called an **RH factor.** The fetus then has RH-positive (RH+) blood. A mother who does not have this factor has RH-negative (RH−) blood. In such cases, the mother will develop antibodies against the RH factor in the fetus's blood. This usually does not cause a problem for the mother's first child. However, a second pregnancy can be complicated by the antibodies that remain in the mother's blood when the second conception occurs. In some cases, the mother's antibodies enter the bloodstream of the fetus and destroy its red blood cells. The fetus then suffers oxygen deprivation and destruction of brain cells. Babies born with this condition are known as "blue babies," because of the bluish cast to their complexion from the lack of oxygenation of the blood. If the damage at birth is relatively mild, a complete blood transfusion can save the infant's life and reduce the likelihood of mental retardation. A new medical treatment should lessen the incidence of RH-factor retardation. Within 72 hours of a birth, abortion, or miscarriage, RH-negative women can receive a RhoGAM injection to prevent the threat of RH antibodies to future pregnancies.

Drugs. Many prescription drugs can have serious developmental effects on a fetus. Physicians must weigh these risks when prescribing such drugs for an expectant mother. In addition, the use of many illegal drugs such as marihuana and LSD is suspected to result in an increased incidence of birth defect, although this evidence remains controversial. Fetal alcohol syndrome, a recently identified disorder, has been discussed in Chapter 11. About 40 percent of the children born to women who are chronic alcoholics have serious physical abnormalities, including mental retardation (K. L. Jones & Smith, 1973).

Specific maternal illnesses, the RH factor, and drug use are only a few of the factors that can disrupt the prenatal environment and may result in mental retardation of the child. Other complicating factors may be as specific as exposure to radiation during the first months of pregnancy or as general as diet (N. M. Robinson & Robinson, 1976). For example, before iodine was used as a common table salt additive, more children were born with the type of mental retardation known as cretinism. This retardation was often due to a lack of development of the thyroid gland because of an iodine-deficient diet. A well-balanced diet, containing sufficient proteins, carbohydrates, vitamins, and trace elements is believed to be extremely important in assuring that a child has the best possible prenatal and **postnatal** environments (Winick, 1970).

Birth Complications. Two of the many complications that can occur during an infant's delivery are particularly associated with retarded intellectual functioning: prematurity and anoxia (oxygen deprivation). Studies have indicated that people who are born prematurely have lower than normal IQs and a generally higher incidence of mental retardation (e.g., see Drillien, 1967). Infants who suffered oxygen deprivation at birth have also been found to have a higher incidence of mental retardation (F. V. Graham et al., 1963).

Does prematurity cause mental retardation? N. M. Robinson and Robinson (1976) conclude that it does not. The mothers of premature infants tend to be older, tend to have had poorer diets and poor medical care, and more problems during pregnancy than mothers of full-term babies. Prematurity and mental retardation, when they occur in the same infant, may well be due to a third causal factor which has not been adequately identified.

Heber (1970) questions the easy conclusion that anoxia at birth leads to mental retardation. While prolonged anoxia results in the destruction of brain cells and ultimately death, Heber has found that most studies implicating anoxia in mental retardation are retrospective. We have generally looked at the histories of retarded people, found some "clue" that they suffered anoxia at birth, and concluded that the anoxia "caused" the retardation. In fact, we do not know how many intellectually normal people suffered anoxia at birth. Was the number fewer? more? the same? Without such a study, we cannot be certain whether the cause of some individuals' retardation is anoxia at birth or some other factor. At the same time, studies have not shown that anoxia does not cause mental retardation.

Postnatal Factors

After a child is born, many factors can lead to damage of the brain tissue and mental retardation. Three major postnatal factors are infections, head trauma, and poisoning.

Infections. Any infection that leads to prolonged fever may result in damage to the neural tissue of the brain and subsequent mental retardation. For this reason, it is critical that infants and young children be treated rapidly when they have high fevers. Direct infections of the brain (encephalitis) or of the tissues surrounding the brain (meningitis) are even more likely to result in mental retardation than high fevers from other causes.

Head Trauma. Damage to the brain may occur in childhood from a number of sources. Children may fall and hit their heads on sharp objects; they may be in automobile accidents; or they may even be injured by abusive parents. Injuries to the head may directly destroy tissue by penetration; or the brain tissue may be damaged from swelling, bleeding, or lack of oxygen. All these types of damage may result in lifetime mental retardation. Unlike other tissues, brain tissue does not regenerate.

Poisons. The average home contains many poisons in the form of cleaning agents and other household supplies. In many older homes, some layers of old paint contain large proportions of lead. Many cases of mental retardation have resulted from **lead encephalitis,** a complication of lead poisoning. Many children living in substandard housing developed lead poisoning from eating paint flakes from this old type of paint (Lin-fu, 1972). Today, lead-based paints can no longer be sold for interior use, and the incidence of this cause of retardation has decreased.

In addition to poisons present in the home such as arsenic (in some rat poisons) and lead, industrial pollutants may result in children's brain damage. Although numerous governmental regulations now control the dumping of hazardous wastes, occasional scandals have resulted from the discovery of the effects of industrial pollutants on unsuspecting citizens. In Japan, for example, large numbers of adults and children died from mercury poisoning, and many surviving children became mentally retarded.

Organic Disorders of Unknown Etiology

Several known organic causes of retardation have been described above as illustrations of the organic etiology of mental retardation. Disorders such as brain tumor, congenital syphilis, or hypoglycemia could also have been used as examples of known organic causes of mental retardation. The fact that so many known organic causes of mental retardation have been identified should not suggest that we know the etiology of all the organic conditions that lead to mental retardation (AAMD, 1977). Many organic conditions that result in mental retardation remain mysteries.

Some children, for example, manifest a progressive destruction of white matter of the brain, for no known reason. We know that their retardation is due to destruction of the brain tissue, but we do not know the cause of this destruction. Another example is anencephaly. In this condition, an infant is born without most of the important structures of the brain and the flat bones of the skull. We do not know if this condition is due to genetic or to other biological causes. Again we know that the disorder is organic, but we do not know its exact etiology. These are just two of many types of organic mental retardation with an unclear etiology.

ETIOLOGY OF CULTURAL-FAMILIAL RETARDATION

The vast majority of individuals who fall into the range of mental retardation function at the mildly retarded level. Individuals in this category rarely have an identifiable organic cause of retardation. To a lesser extent, some individuals in the moderate range of functioning also have no identifiable physiological etiology associated with their retarded intellectual functioning. However, a large proportion (though not all) of retarded people who have no identifiable organic etiology come from disadvantaged families and have parents or siblings who are also mildly retarded. When conditions

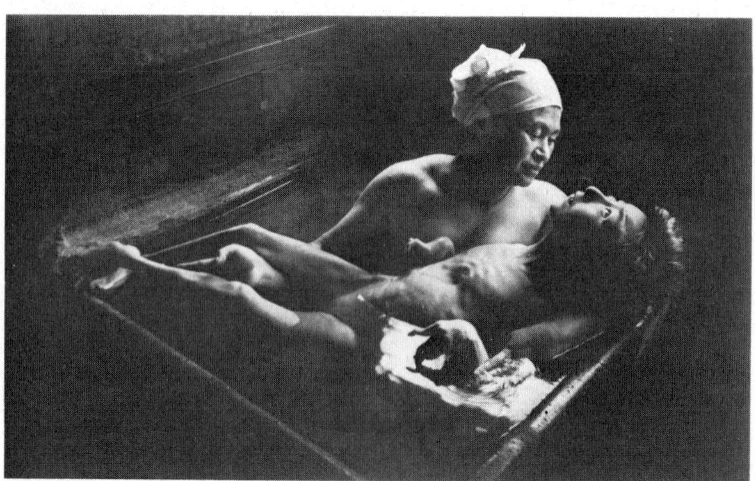

A mother holds her brain-damaged child who was poisoned by industrial wastes, including mercury, over a long period of time. As many as 10,000 people were affected by such toxins in Minamata, Japan.

of mild (or sometimes moderate) retardation, no physiological pathology, and, evidence of retardation in one or more family members exist, we conclude that the cause is **cultural-familial retardation.** In other words, the functional intellectual level of the individual is due to an interaction of environment and heredity.

Heredity

There is an ongoing debate in psychology over the degree of influence that heredity has over level of intelligence. Some psychologists believe that intelligence is not limited by heredity, while others believe that heredity is far more important than environment in determining intellectual level. This debate cannot be resolved here. We can safely say, however, that most evidence indicates some genetic contribution to intelligence (Scarr, 1975; Scarr & Weinberg, 1978; Horn, Loehlin, & Willerman, 1979).

When we say that heredity is an important factor in the intellectual level of an offspring, we do not mean that retarded people always give birth to retarded children. E. W. Reed and Reed (1965) have obtained data on 50 families over several generations (a total of 18,730 family members) which demonstrate that this is not so. Table 18.2 illustrates the range of IQs Reed and Reed found when they studied children of couples in which the mother, the father, or both parents were known to be retarded. Notice that many of the children of these parents were normal or well above normal in intelligence.

While heredity appears quite important in determining levels of intellectual functioning, the effects of environment cannot be discounted. Munzinger (1975) found a correlation of .48 between the average of biological parents' intelligence and the intelligence of their adopted-away offspring. That still leaves about 75 percent of the variability in the children's intelligence unaccounted for. Something other than heredity appears to have an important influence on level of intellectual functioning. Intellectual ability is a function of both heredity and environment.

Environment

How might environment and heredity interact to produce mild retardation? Assume that a man and a woman each have IQs of approximately 80–85, and these IQ estimates accurately reflect their intellectual functioning. The man and woman also have little interest in intellectual pursuits such as reading, problem-solving games, the theater, or the arts. Assume that the man and woman produce an infant who inherits an intellectual potential the equivalent of the parents. In one hypothetical situation, the child is raised by the parents in an environment with no emphasis on cognitive development, education, or problem solving. The family meets the minimal physical needs of the child, but little else. The environment is intellectually sterile. The home has no books, no games, and no stimulating interactions between parents or between parents and child. We later find that the child has difficulty in school and obtains an IQ of 65, in the mildly retarded range.

With the same basic scenario, let's hypothesize a different possibility: At birth the child described above is adopted by a family of average or above-average intelligence. Their

Table 18.2
IQ range of tested children of retarded parents

Parents	*IQ range of children*							*Average IQ*	*Percent retarded*
	0–49	50–69	70–89	90–100	111–130	131+	*Total*		
Both retarded	6	29	36	17	1	0	89	74	39.4
Retarded father, normal mother	0	12	31	75	24	1	153	95	7.8
Retarded mother, normal father	6	15	32	43	10	1	107	87	19.6

Adapted from E. W. Reed and Reed (1965, pp. 238–239).

home has an abundance of cognitive stimulation. The parents read to the young child, play interactive games, and encourage the child to begin the struggle of learning to read even before school age. The parents enroll the child in preschool classes where creative play is encouraged and intellectual curiosity is rewarded. Later, during the school years, the child has no major problems, and performs at a low average level. The child's measured IQ is found to be 90, at the low end of the average range. In both hypothetical cases, the child's intellectual ability is dramatically affected by the environment. In both examples, the hypothetical child has the identical genetic makeup, but the resulting levels of intellectual functioning are very different.

The evidence that a deprived environment can interact with hereditary potential to result in mild retardation is primarily indirect. We know that the incidence of mild retardation is much higher in the lower socioeconomic classes (see Figure 18.4) We also know that families at this socioeconomic level are less likely to value education and intellectual pursuits (N. M. Robinson & Robinson, 1976). In addition, a study of poor rural Appalachian families found that poor intellectual ability in children correlated with an attitude of apathy and futility in the children's mothers (Polansky, Borgman, & DeSaix, 1972). The greater the mother's attitude of apathy and futility, the lower the intellectual competence of the child.

The many adverse consequences of poverty on family interactions, family stability, and individual health sometimes appear to combine to lead to cultural-familial retardation. The consequences are both organic and environmental. Poor mothers are more likely to have poor nutrition and less medical care while pregnant. They are more likely to feel defeated and helpless, and thus are more likely to communicate these attitudes to their children. The children are more likely to be exposed to health hazards such as poor nutrition and poor hygiene, and to receive less medical care while growing up. Schools in poverty areas are less likely to be as good as those in middle-class areas, and the education of the poor child suffers.

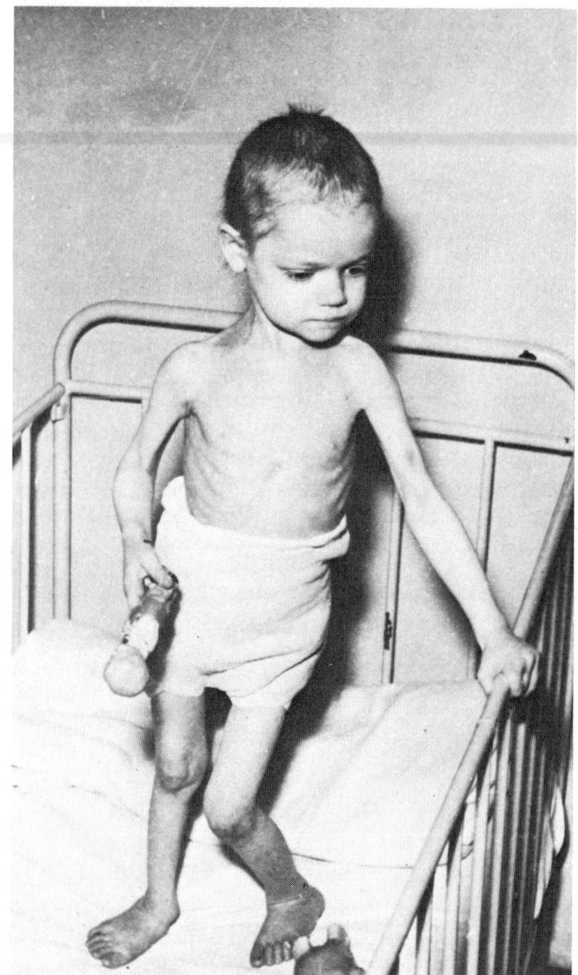

Extreme poverty, abandonment, or extremely poor parenting skills may lead to the degree of malnutrition shown in this photo. Some investigators believe that malnutrition can lead to mental retardation due to reduction in the number of brain cells (Winick, Rosso, & Waterlow, 1970).

The importance of a lack of cognitive stimulation in poor families for the development of lower levels of intellectual functioning has been more directly demonstrated. If intellectual level is depressed by the futility and lack of cognitive stimulation common to a poverty existence, then we would expect the intellectual levels of disadvantaged children to increase if they are provided with cognitive stimulation, and if their mothers are trained in positive child-rearing techniques. Several studies have demonstrated that this does indeed happen (e.g., Madden, Levenstein, & Levenstein, 1976).

In one major effort, Garber and Heber (1977; Heber & Garber, 1980) and their staff successfully raised the IQ levels of children at risk for mild retardation. From a black ghetto of Milwaukee, they selected mothers with IQs of less than 75. The mothers and their children were randomly assigned to a control or experimental group. From the ages of 3 months until 6 years, the 20 children in the experimental group received a special enrichment program five days a week, every week of the year. The 20 control children did not receive the program. The experimental children were given cognitive stimulation, language training, perceptual-motor training, and positive social-emotional experiences. Their mothers were trained in homemaking, child rearing, remedial academic training, and vocational education. From the ages of 2 to 10, both the experimental group of children and the controls were assessed on many measures of intellectual functioning. After the training, the children in the experimental group averaged more than 20 IQ points higher than the children who had not had the enrichment program. At age 10, four years after the program ended, the average IQ of the children in the experimental group was 105, while the average IQ of the control children was 85. The mothers also were different after the active intervention was completed. Mothers of children in the experimental group had more positive self-concepts and used more verbal responses with their children. They were more likely to be employed, and their average income was greater than employed mothers of the children from the control group.

Studies such as Garber and Heber's Milwaukee project may give the impression that cultural-familial retardation can be wiped out, given enough resources. Before we can draw such a conclusion, we need much more information on the long-term effectiveness of such programs. What, for example, will the IQs of these two groups of children be when they are adults? Will the differences continue to be as marked as they are now? If so, do we have the financial and human resources to mount such intensive programs for all children who are at risk for mild retardation, rather than for just a few pilot programs?

KEY TREATMENTS

Although the mentally retarded have been with us throughout recorded history, treatment approaches are a relatively recent development. The major social response to the retarded has been to isolate them in large, often rural institutions, and often to use psychotropic medication to control their behavior (Tu, 1979). However, since the 1930s the application of new psychological and medical knowledge to mental retardation has offered some promise (Crissey, 1975). Broadly defined, the treatments of mental retardation can be grouped into several areas: prenatal prevention, early intervention, and skills training.

Prenatal prevention

Prenatal prevention consists of efforts to decrease the likelihood of children being born who are at high risk for mental retardation. Although not a "treatment" per se, this approach may reduce the need for later intervention.

One important aspect of prenatal prevention is **genetic counseling.** If families have a history of retardation, such counseling can provide them with information about the risk of retardation in future pregnancies. For example, when parents are known to carry a recessive gene for retardation, the risk of retardation in their offspring is one in four. If the gene were dominant (a less likely occurrence), the risk for the infant would be one in two. Genetic counseling allows parents to make informed decisions about whether to risk pregnancy. Similar counseling is important when other chromosomal defects (such as Down's syndrome) are probable. When pregnancies are already in progress, the technique of amniocentesis may provide needed information. In one study of more than

10,000 risky pregnancies, more than 600 fetuses were found through amniocentesis to have chromosomal defects (C. J. Epstein & Golbus, 1977). The parents of these fetuses could use this information to make informed decisions about their course of action.

Prenatal prevention can also be used for mental retardation that is not due to genetic problems. Parents can be trained in proper childbearing and child-rearing techniques if these skills are absent. Parents of the cultural-familial retarded often have significant deficits in these areas. Such training emphasizes proper maternal nutrition, medical care, and avoidance of drugs during pregnancy. In addition, programs can train expectant parents in appropriate parent-child interactions. These types of programs appear to be particularly relevant for parents who are mildly retarded, since they are more likely than nonretarded parents to have a retarded child (Baroff, 1974).

Early intervention

Infants require a safe, secure, and stimulating environment for maximum development. It may seem obvious that we need to protect young children from household poisons, falls, auto traffic, and other dangers. However, people learn about this necessity in a variety of ways. Some may model other parents, read a child-care book while they are expecting a child, or discuss child safety with a family physician. Other parents are unaware that cleaning agents should be locked away, well-balanced meals should be provided, and children should be played with in a stimulating manner. Garber and Heber's Milwaukee project on cultural-familial retardation, which trained mothers and provided cognitive stimulation for their children, was an early intervention program that tried to deal with some of these issues. Wide-scale enrichment programs, such as Head Start in the 1960s, attempted to do this for disadvantaged preschool children on a national level. Unfortunately, the gains made by Head Start were generally short-term (Bronfenbrenner, 1974). Apparently, the Head Start program did not start early enough with the children, was not intense enough, and did not last long enough (N. M. Robinson & Robinson, 1976).

Skills training

The great majority of the mentally retarded live at home and are educated in the public school system. However, approximately 200,000 people are in residential schools for the mentally retarded. Those living in state schools are predominantly in the lower levels (severe and profound categories) of mental retardation. Whether at home, in the public schools, or in a residential institution, a major focus in the treatment of the mentally retarded is the training of behavioral skills.

Depending on the individual's age and level of retardation, the skills to be trained may vary greatly in complexity. A severely retarded adult may require special training to learn a task as simple as hand washing. A mildly retarded child may learn hygiene skills with relative ease, but needs special training for more complex academic tasks.

Whether the needed skills are simple or complex, behavioral approaches have been quite effective in training the mentally retarded. These approaches have become very important in the training of the mentally retarded in recent years. As an example of the application of a behavioral approach to a simple skill, consider toothbrushing. Brushing one's teeth has cosmetic, hygienic, and health-related goals. It seems to be a simple behavior, yet many severely retarded individuals have difficulty learning such a simple skill. A simple behavior like toothbrushing can be taught to a severely retarded individual by breaking it down into a series of component steps and shaping each desired behavioral step with a reinforcer. For example the substeps of toothbrushing in such a program might be 1: turning on the water; 2. opening the tube of paste; 3. picking up the toothbrush; 4. wetting the brush; 5. placing paste on brush; and so on. Each step is either verbally instructed, modeled, or physically guided; reinforced when successfully completed; then the next step is taken. The end result is the chaining of many steps of behavior into the total behavior of toothbrushing, with reinforcement given only for the successful completion of the whole series of behaviors. Such programs have often been implemented in institutional settings to train a broad variety of skills in severely retarded people. Figure 18.5 illustrates the improvement in one individual's frequency of toothbrushing. This person was a resident of a large ward, which instituted a hygiene program for its residents as one part of a broad behavioral treatment program. For many of the profoundly and severely retarded, such changes are very significant, but constant supervision and continued intermittent reinforcement are needed to maintain the changes.

Self-care and social and academic skills are important training areas for the mentally retarded. In recent years there has also been an increasing emphasis on the training of vocational skills. We live in a culture which values productivity and self-support, and in which a significant portion of our self-identity may come not only from who we are but from what we do. Many organized systems of care for the mentally retarded include programs that teach vocational skills.

Many retarded persons are fully employable in normal jobs of an unskilled nature, such as routine janitorial work. Some retarded need ongoing training and supervision, but are able to work and earn money in sheltered workshops. In these settings, real work is performed for companies on a contract, piecework basis. Large companies such as Western Electric (manufacturer of telephones) farm out work to such sheltered workshops just as to any other small company. The jobs range from simple (such as placing items in boxes) to complex.

In the sheltered workshop setting, the emphasis is on the development of good work habits (e.g., getting to work on time, focusing on the task) and also on producing a quality product for the contractor. The application of simple reinforcement contingencies in such settings not only trains retarded individuals to work well on surprisingly complex tasks (Eilbracht & Thompson, 1977; Gold, 1972) but also allows them to earn wages and be productive members of society. In such ways the self-concept and self-satisfaction of a retarded individual can be enhanced (Gold, 1973).

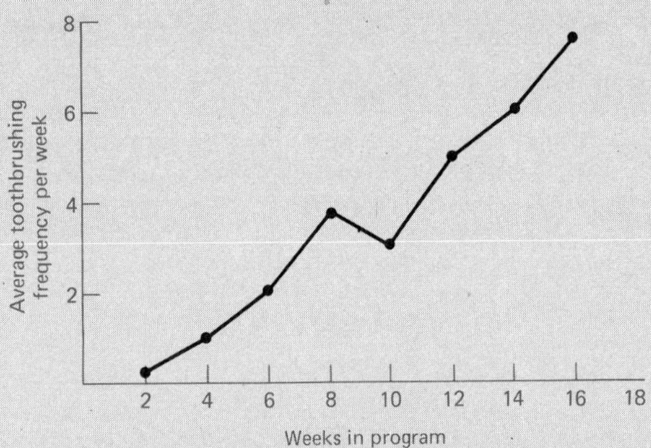

Figure 18.5. Improvement of a severely retarded woman in an oral hygiene training program.
Adapted from Bigelow and Griffiths (1977, p. 129).

Summary

1. Mental retardation has been defined as a condition in which an individual manifests: 1. significantly subaverage general intellectual functioning, 2. deficits in adaptive behavior, 3. onset of the condition during the developmental (childhood) years.

2. Although intelligence has been defined in a variety of ways, Wechsler's definition is fairly well accepted. He describes intelligence as composed of separate abilities which combine to form a global capacity to act purposefully, think rationally, and deal effectively with the environment. We do recognize that the abilities thought to compose intelligence may vary somewhat from culture to culture.

3. It has become a convention to use a numerical "intelligence quotient" (or IQ) to designate the level of intelligence. An IQ of 70 is considered to be the top range of mental retardation, and approximately 97 percent of the population would be expected to achieve a higher quotient than 70.

4. The range of retardation is broken into four levels. In descending order, these levels are mild, moderate, severe, and profound. The great majority of the retarded are in the mild range.

5. Theorists disagree on the basic nature of retardation. Some favor the position that retardation consists of a slowed development in which the individual passes through the same stages as a person of normal intelligence, but reaches a lower upper limit.

6. Other theorists take the position that retardation is due to one or more specific cognitive defects. Current research provides some support for both positions.

7. There is speculation that more mildly retarded individuals conform more to the developmental model; while the more extremely retarded, who also tend to have more organic signs, have one or more specific cognitive defects which account for their retardation. The two groups are not distinct, however, and further research may integrate the two theoretical positions.

8. The etiology of mental retardation may be either organic or cultural-familial. Organic causes of mental retardation include transmission by recessive genes, or chromosomal abnormalities. Other organic causes are maternal infections which can be transmitted to the fetus, RH factors, the use or abuse of drugs, and possibly poor nutrition of the pregnant mother. Organic damage that results in mental retardation may also occur during or after birth.

9. For many years, prematurity and oxygen deprivation at birth have been thought to lead to mental retardation. However, some researchers believe that retardation in such cases may be due to another unknown factor.

10. Even though an infant may be born normal, later events such as childhood fevers or infections, poisons, or direct head trauma may lead to retarded intellectual development. In this chapter, we have not reviewed all known specific organic causes of retardation, but have examined representative examples of the approximately 200 known causes.

11. Individuals who fall in the mildly retarded range, and some who fall in the moderate range, are considered to have retardation with a cultural-familial cause. The incidence of mild retardation is much higher in lower socioeconomic, poverty-level families than it is in middle- and upper-class families. In contrast, extreme retardation from organic causes is almost equally distributed across socioeconomic classes.

12. Epidemiological evidence supports the idea that the psychosocially deprived environment of poor families interacts with hereditary risk to produce mild retardation. This indirect evidence is bolstered by studies which demonstrate that the enrichment of the poverty family environment results in significant IQ increases in the family's children.

13. The treatment of mental retardation includes three broad areas: prenatal prevention, early intervention, and skills training. Prenatal prevention consists of counseling and educating parents who are at risk of having retarded children. Parents can be counseled and educated regarding the likelihood of genetic defects, the importance of good maternal health and nutrition, and perhaps even trained in parenting techniques before a child is born.

14. After cultural-familial retardation occurs, early intervention efforts can focus on further parental training and on organized efforts to provide the child with compensatory enrichment experiences (e.g., cognitive stimulation). Structured programs can occur both in the home and in other settings, such as a preschool. These types of interventions can significantly raise the IQs of psychosocially deprived children. However, questions remain regarding their long-term effectiveness.

15. A focus of programs for all levels of retarded children is skills training. The use of behaviorally oriented treatment programs with the retarded has proven very effective in training skills as simple as dressing, eating, and personal hygiene. More complex behaviors can also be trained using a behavioral approach. The application of these skills-training techniques to complex activities such as work skills, social interaction, and homemaking skills assists the retarded individual to reach a level of functioning closer to his or her maximum potential.

KEY TERMS

Adaptive behavior. Behavior that assists the individual in adapting to the stresses and problems of everyday living.

Cultural-familial retardation. Retardation which is presumed to be influenced by a possible genetic vulnerability but most importantly is influenced by a deprived psychosocial environment.

Developmental task. A task which a child must confront that is an important aspect of development, for example, learning to talk or walk.

IQ. The intelligence quotient. A standard way of expressing level of intelligence, in which an IQ of 90–110 is considered to be average.

Postnatal. The period after the infant is born.

Prenatal. The period from conception to birth.

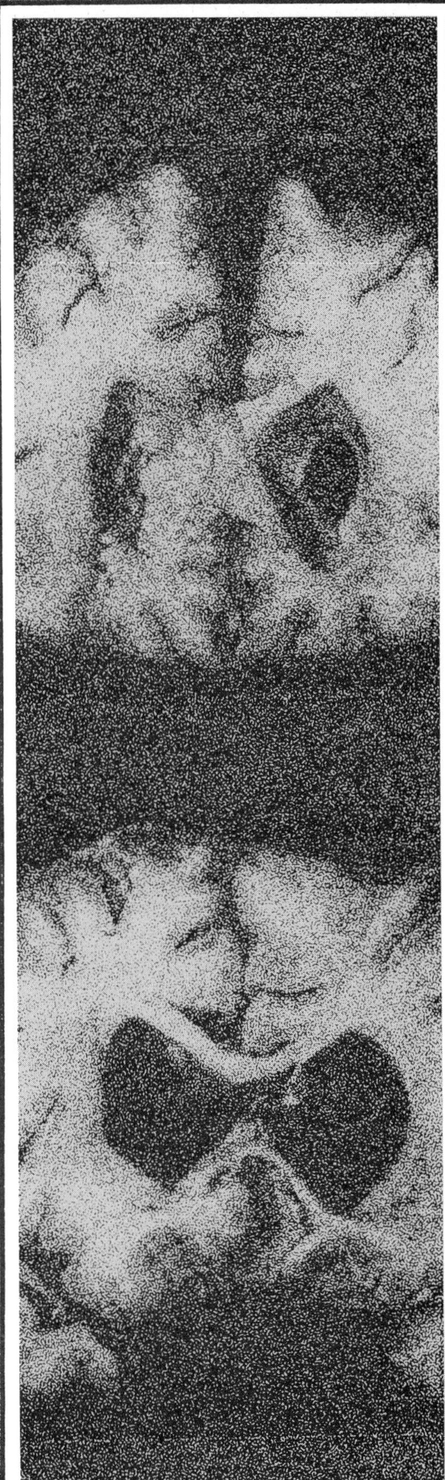

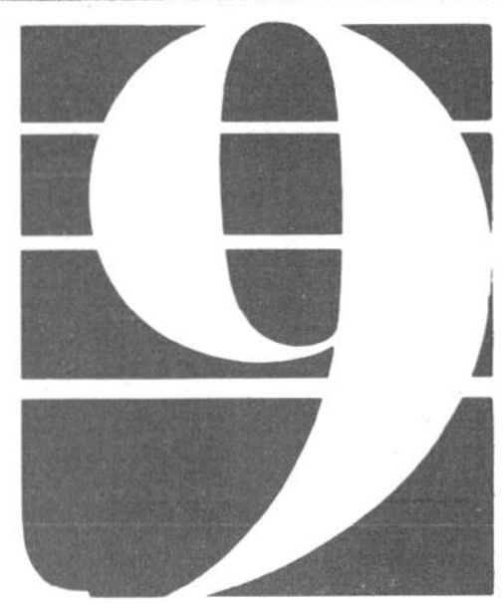

19

Organic mental disorder

- General features of organic mental disorder
- Factors associated with degree of symptomatology
- Categories of organic brain syndromes
- Causal factors of brain injury and damage
- Age-associated degenerative disorders
- Epilepsy: a very special group of brain disorders
- Key treatments
- Summary
- Key terms

The discussions of the many disorders in previous chapters have shown that disturbed behavior may be a function of both organic and nonorganic factors. In this chapter, the focus is on adult disorders of thinking, feeling, and behaving which we are fairly certain have organic factors as primary causal agents. In these conditions, some structural or physiological disorder in brain tissue can account for the disturbances we observe. Even in these conditions, we will see again that the effects of environment and personality are important variables which affect human behavior.

The exact incidence of **organic mental disorder** is not known. However, about one-fourth of the people in public mental hospitals have this type of diagnosis. In addition, 10–20 percent of elderly people are estimated to show signs of organic mental disorder (Fisch, Goldfarb, & Shahinian, 1968). Based on this latter estimate, 2.3–4.6 million elderly have this type of disorder in the United States. The total number of persons who have an organic mental disorder is even higher. For example, **delirium** is a form of organic mental disorder. It has been estimated that one out of five individuals who receives surgery under a general anesthetic has a postsurgical delirium (Morse, 1970); and three out of ten acutely ill patients in medical hospitals experience delirium (Hofling, 1975). Any physician or nurse can confirm that delirium is a common (but fortunately short-term) organic mental disorder.

"Organic mental disorder" sounds chilling in its finality. However, we have just seen that delirium is a short-term disturbance. People often mistakenly think that all disorders which are due to disruption of organic brain function are irreversible. This is not necessarily the case, although the damage to brain tissue may sometimes be progressive or so extensive that the disruption in functioning is chronic or even fatal.

GENERAL FEATURES OF ORGANIC MENTAL DISORDER

"Organic mental disorder" is the term used for a great variety of symptoms or behaviors which may be due to any number of specific internal or external organic causes. The symptoms, behaviors, or deficits seen in organic mental disorder can be grouped into the following seven general areas:

1. Disorders of Orientation. The individual may be confused or mistaken about his location in time, geographic place, or even the identity of people. For example, an individual might think that she is in a hotel or at home, rather than in a hospital.
2. Disorders of Memory. Disordered memory or amnesia may be associated with disorientation, although persons can be disoriented when there is no memory loss, or vice versa. Two types of memory loss are common in organic mental disorder: retrograde and anterograde. In retrograde amnesia, the individual loses memories for a period of time preceding the brain disorder or injury. In anterograde amnesia, ongoing memory storage is disturbed. Mild retrograde amnesia, for example, often occurs after severe blows to the head are experienced. Anterograde amnesia is a sign that current or progressive brain damage exists and is interfering with the learning of new skills. When such memory loss occurs, old established memories are the strongest; but with progressive brain deterioration, even older memories may erode (M. Williams, 1979).
3. Disorders of Communication. Depending on the location and extent of the brain disorder, problems in both receptive and expressive communication may appear. Individuals may be unable to understand the words that they hear, yet they may be able to speak intelligibly. In other cases, people may be able to understand spoken language, but may be unable to say what they want. These speech disorders are called **aphasia.** Luria (1973) gives the following example of an aphasic's difficulty in finding the words to express his ideas. "Well now . . . I mean . . . so . . . we . . . now . . . went . . . went . . . suddenly . . . now this . . . like this . . . bang! . . . and then nothing . . . nothing . . . and since . . . little by little . . . better still . . . quite . . . and now . . . do you see?" (p. 140). Similar communication problems may appear in written language. The individual may be unable to recognize written or printed letters or words, and may be unable to read. Others may be able to read, but not to write; and some may be unable to do either. In these cases (called dyslexic or dysgraphic aphasia), as in problems with spoken communication, the individuals had these skills prior to the brain disorder. The problem is not one of motor coordination of hands and fin-

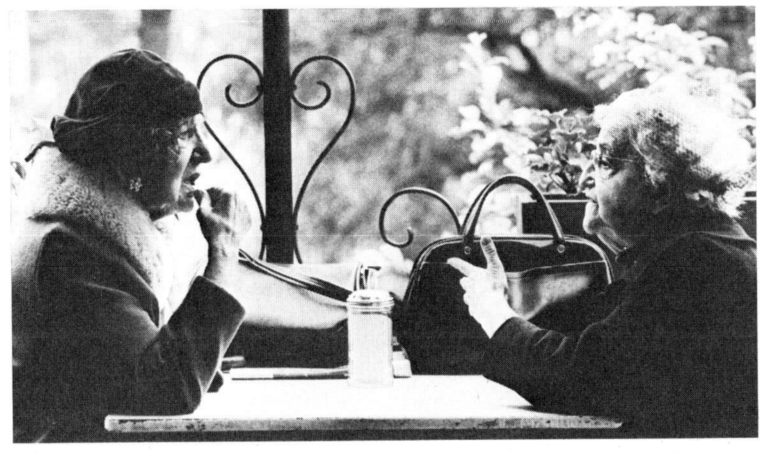

There may be an association between aging and difficulty in short term memory. Perhaps this is one reason why the elderly spend much time talking about events of years past—those older memories are likely to be clearer.

gers while writing, or of coordination of the tongue, larynx, or lips while speaking. Rather, the problem is one of recognition and use of symbols.

4. Disorders of Perception. Many perceptual problems may be present in organic brain disorder. Although the peripheral sensory apparatus (such as the eyes, ears, peripheral nervous system) may be intact, individuals may misinterpret sensory input. Some cases manifest hallucinations of the olfactory senses (such as vile smells), tactile hallucinations (e.g., bugs crawling on the skin), or hallucinations in any of the other sensory areas: sight, hearing, taste, or of body position or motion.
5. Disorders of Motor Behavior. Disturbances in movements of the voluntary musculature in organic mental disorder may range from mild defects in motor coordination to total paralysis. The defects depend on the site and extent of brain damage. Less obvious disorders of voluntary movement may also occur. For example, an individual whose motor coordination appears normal may suffer from **apraxia.** In this condition, the individual is unable to carry out one or more familiar sequential acts. When asked to touch the top of his head, a patient touches his nose, or if asked to comb her hair, she turns the comb over in her hands two or three times and lays it back down. Often these sequential acts can be completed if the individual is not thinking about doing them (M. Williams, 1979). Apraxia appears to be a disorder of cognitive intention which is reflected in motor behavior.
6. Disorders of Intellect. Organic mental disorders often include impairments of intellectual function. If the organic damage is mild or limited, impairments may be apparent only in a few specific intellectual abilities. With more severe or generalized damage or deterioration of brain tissue, the intellectual impairment may cut across many functions. If the impairment in intellectual functioning is limited to certain abilities, the individual may be able to compensate for the deficit by using unaffected abilities. For example, an individual with a memory disorder might compensate by leaving notes and reminders placed in strategic spots. When intellectual impairment is widespread, adequate compensation is less likely. The individual is likely then to have impaired comprehension and may be unable to make sound judgments, to reason, or to learn new information. This development of generalized defects in intellectual function is called **dementia.**
7. Disorders of Emotions. Organic damage to the structure, or changes in function, of brain tissue may result in dramatic impairment of the stability and character of an individual's emotions. Moods may fluctuate in a manner similar to bipolar affective disorder. Emotion or affect may sometimes be inappropriate, or affect may be blunted.

An individual who manifests an organic mental disorder may have impairments in all, several, or one of these general categories. The pattern of impairments which an individual manifests depends on several factors. These factors include the extent of damage, the site of the damage (whether localized in one area or generalized to all parts of the brain), and also the individual's vulnerability to the changes in brain function.

FACTORS ASSOCIATED WITH DEGREE OF SYMPTOMATOLOGY

Extent of Damage

The extent of brain tissue damage or tissue dysfunction which an individual suffers might seem to be the only important factor related to the extent and severity of symptoms manifested. However, an individual who has 20 percent of total brain cells damaged does not necessarily show twice the deficit of an individual who has 10 percent of brain cells damaged. The relationship between extent of damage and degree of impairment is not exact, yet studies have shown that in a gross sense, the amount of damage is important (Farmer, Peck, & Terry, 1976; Tomlinson, 1977).

Our understanding of the role of extent of damage is complicated by many factors. One important problem is the difficulty of measuring the actual extent of physiological tissue damage. The measures we use tend to be very rough: the gross size of a tumor, and estimate of percentage of brain tissue destroyed in a wound, or an estimate of the degree of atrophy (shrinkage) of brain tissue. Even microscopic analysis of brain cells provides only an estimate of the amount of tissue damage. It is not surprising, then, that all we can say is that the degree of tissue damage is one important factor, but not the only one, in determining the degree of impairment an individual suffers.

Location of Damage

For many years, investigators have tried to pinpoint the relationship between specific sites or parts of the brain and human behavior. One method has tried to correlate disordered behavior with the presence or absence of damage in different portions of the brain. For example, if individuals who have external wounds to the left side of the head with resulting brain damage are all found to have aphasia, we might speculate that the ability to use speech is centered on the left side of the brain. If we also find that individuals who have damage limited to the right side of the brain have no speech problems, we would be more confident of our speculation.

In the past century, many individuals whose brain tissue is damaged in specific limited areas have been studied. In both World Wars I and II, and in the increasing numbers of automobile and other types of accidents, many such individuals have been identified and studied. Neuropsychologists and neurologists (psycholgists and physicians who specialize in the study and treatment of neurologically damaged individuals) have been able to identify the location of some behavioral functions in the brain using this approach and more sophisticated methods of study.

Although locations in the brain have been determined for some types of behavior, these locations remain inexact. Many other behaviors cannot be localized (Lezak, 1976). There is no one site for "personality," for example. We cannot point to a place on the brain and say "This is where childhood memories are stored." While we know a great deal about the brain, we have much to learn.

The brain is a mass of about 10 billion neurons, surrounded by several membranes, and enclosed in a bony case (see Figure 19.1). It is divided into two interconnected hemispheres. The right hemisphere has motor control over the left side of the body, while the left hemisphere has control of the right side of the body. Each hemisphere is divided into four lobes; frontal, temporal, parietal, and occipital. The surface of the brain is convoluted, like a thick piece of foam with many folds. The creases are called **sulci,** and the areas of the lobes are often identified by the major creases that separate them. Beneath the outer layer of the brain (the cortex) are a number of identifiable structures. Within the brain there are several empty spaces or ventricles. The brain "floats" in cerebrospinal fluid which circulates around it and into these ventricles.

In Figure 19.1, the brain, its major divisions, and some of their functions are illustrated. The left hemisphere is shown as dominant, and contains the speech centers, as is the case in about 96 percent of right-handed people and 90 percent of left-handed people. About 4 percent of right-handed people and 10 percent of left-handed people, however, have either right hemisphere dominance or mixed dominance (E. Miller, 1972). Thus, their speech centers are located in the right hemisphere or appear to be split between hemispheres. These facts are contrary to a common misconception that

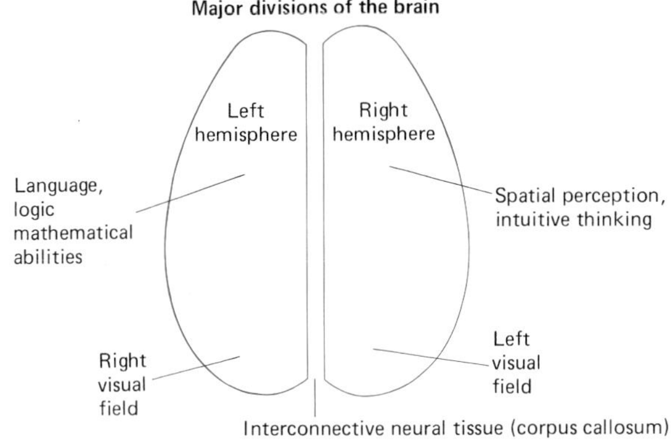

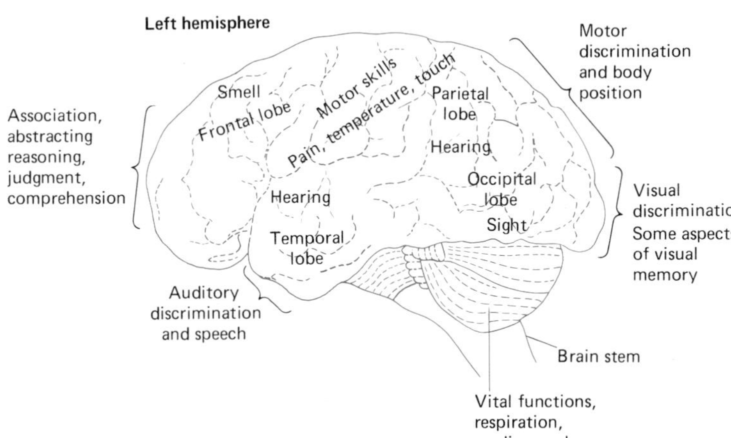

Figure 19.1. The major divisions of the brain and the left hemisphere.

handedness always indicates hemispheric dominance. It is important to remember that the localization of most functions in the brain remains fairly inexact. Most areas of the cortex do not have specific functions, but are involved in general associative processes. However, the general knowledge that we have is important in understanding the symptoms of organic mental disorder.

When brain tissue damage is localized to one site of the brain, an individual may have only limited deficits. For example, if the damage is limited to an area of the dominant left temporal lobe, called **Wernicke's area,** the individual may have difficulty with the comprehension of words, but no difficulty in expressive speech (Caramazza & Berndt, 1978). An individual with limited damage to the occipital lobe might manifest an inability to recognize objects visually, but could still recognize them using the senses of touch and taste (M. Williams, 1979). Damage to the motor area in the nondominant right hemisphere would result in paralysis of portions of the left side of the body, but no speech defect.

Isolated symptoms can provide a knowledgeable clinician with clues to the probable location of limited brain damage. However, cases where the damage is limited in scope and the symptoms are limited in expression are much less frequent than cases where the damage, whether limited or diffuse, results in deficits in many areas of functioning (Poeck, 1968; Williams, 1979). Even very localized tissue damage such as the growth of a brain tumor or a penetration wound from a projectile may lead to extensive behavior deficits from indirect effects on the whole brain. For example, a brain tumor in the left occipital lobe might cause an increase in intracranial pressure throughout the brain which could disrupt neural functions in the lobes of both hemispheres.

Other Factors

Both the extent of damage and location of damage influence the degree and type of impairment seen in organic mental disorder. Yet, different individuals with apparently very equivalent amounts of brain damage in the same parts of the brain do not necessarily have identical patterns or degree of impairment. The impairment exhibited by an individual depends to some extent on factors that are specific to the individual.

An individual's age is one important factor. Infants and children appear to be more sensitive to the effects of brain damage than adults. However, when brain damage occurs in the late teens and early adulthood, individuals seem to be more able to compensate for the deficits and even may regain most of the impaired functions through rehabilitation. Similarly damaged adults, who are past the age of 30, seem to have less resiliency and are less likely to regain functions to the same extent as a younger teen or adult (Williams, 1979).

A factor of major importance in degree of impairment is the premorbid personality of the individual (Lezak, 1976). Behavioral problems present prior to the brain damage are likely to be even more severe after the damage occurs. For example, tendencies toward antisocial behavior, irresponsibility, poor judgment, or impulsiveness are likely to become exaggerated after an individual experiences brain injury. Equivalent brain tissue damage usually results in less severe impairment in individuals who were stable and well adjusted before the injury than in individuals who had prior adjustment problems. Whether these differences are due to primarily organic factors, or are a function mainly of the individual's psychological ability to deal with catastrophic events and impairment, is still unclear.

CATEGORIES OF ORGANIC BRAIN SYNDROMES

So far, several general areas of functioning which can be impaired by organic damage to the brain have been described. In addition, we have considered specific deficits related to damage in different locations in the brain. When individuals experience brain damage, the impairments often include specific deficits (e.g., aphasia), which we can relate to particular locations in the brain, and also more generalized impairments in many areas of functioning. Clinical observations and research have resulted in the identification of a number of organic **syndromes** (commonly occurring groupings of psychological or behavioral manifestations) seen in individuals who have brain damage (DSM-III, 1980; Lipowski, 1975, 1980). An individual may develop one or more of these syndromes after suffering brain damage or deterioration. Two syndromes involve global impairment (delirium and dementia). The remainder are disorders in which impairment is limited to specific areas of functioning.

Delirium

Delirium is one of the most common organic brain syndromes. It is often seen in patients following surgery, in individuals who are ill with high temperatures, or in persons who have been exposed to toxic substances. Delirious individuals have clouded conciousness. They are disoriented and have difficulty distinguishing between real perceptions and dreams or hallucinations. The degree of confusion in delirium fluctuates. At times the person may be lucid and aware, at other times confused and agitated or lethargic. The maintenance of attention to environmental stimuli and goal-directed thinking are also impaired. At one moment, the individual may respond to questions accurately and, soon after, may appear to be overly distracted by other environmental events. Usually delirium begins rapidly (i.e., it has an acute onset) and is of short duration. Lipowski (1980) describes delirium as a manifestation of acute brain failure due to a widespread derangement of **cerebral metabolism** and disturbance of neurotransmission.

Dementia

Like delirium, dementia is a global disorder of cognition. In both syndromes, there is an impairment of acquisition, storage, and retrieval of information. Both feature deficits of memory, goal-oriented thinking, judgment, and intellectual performance. In contrast to delirium, dementia has a more stable, often progressively deteriorating course. The obvious fluctuations in levels of awareness seen in delirium are not present in dementia. Dementia is a chronic disorder, lasting months or years rather than days or weeks typical of delirium. Although dementia is a chronic disorder, it is not totally irreversible. Whether some recovery is possible depends largely on the underlying brain pathology, the degree of tissue damage, and the availability of treatment. We shall see that some forms of dementia are progressive and irreversible; for example, Alzheimer's disease. Other forms of dementia are not progressive, but so many brain cells are damaged that, even with treatment, prior levels of functioning cannot be regained. If an individual manifests dementia from a treatable cause, such as hypothyroidism (an underactive thyroid gland), treatment may reverse the dementia as long as the functioning of the brain cells were primarily disrupted, rather than destroyed. However, if brain cells have been destroyed, they cannot be regenerated, and the condition becomes chronic.

Amnestic Syndrome

When serious memory disorder occurs outside delirium or dementia, it is called an **amnestic syndrome.** In this case, long-term and short-term memory functions are disrupted due to an organic factor. Amnesia may also be due to psychological factors. But amnestic syndrome differs from this psychogenic amnesia because as long as the organic defect exists, the amnestic individual will have difficulty storing new memories. In this brain syndrome, individuals are often unable to store new memories for more than 25–30 minutes. For example, if you introduced yourself to an amnestic individual and repeated your name several times, then waited 30 minutes before asking the person to repeat your name, he/she would be unable to remember it. If you waited only 10 minutes, the individual would be more likely to respond accurately.

Long-term memory also suffers. Consider the 50-year-old who has had an amnestic syndrome for 20 years. For two decades, few or no events would be stored in this individual's memory. Memories would be limited to things that occurred up to the onset of the disorder. At best, the individual would remember things as they were 20 years ago. There would be no recollection of the person's children growing older, no knowledge of Presidents beyond John F. Kennedy, and no recollection of any personal events since that time. The individual's self perception would be that he or she was still 30 years old.

Organic Hallucinosis

The primary characteristic in organic hallucinosis is the presence of recurring hallucinations during a normal state of consciousness. There may occasionally be delusions, but they are related to the content of the hallucinations. Common organic causes of this condition are hallucinogenic drugs and chronic excessive use of alcohol (see Chapter 10 for additional information).

Organic Affective Syndrome

The organic affective syndrome is characterized by a major disturbance in mood which resembles either a manic or depressed state during a normal state of consciousness. The individual may be fearful, anxious, irritable, or grandiose and excitable. The diagnosis can be made most easily when some organic factor is definitely present, such as the use of a drug like reserpine, which is known to have side effects of mood disorder. Other known causes of this syndrome are endocrine disorders and cancer of the pancreas. If a serious mood disorder develops in an adult who has had a previously well-adjusted personality with no evidence of previous depressions or mania, no psychological losses, and no history of mood disorder in family members, an organic affective disorder is a distinct possibility.

Organic Personality Syndrome

Some individuals may manifest major personality changes because of brain damage. When these major changes occur in dementia or organic affective syndrome, these disorders are considered primary. A pattern that is often seen in organic personality syndrome consists of increased emotional variability—temper outbursts or hostility and belligerence alternating with tearfulness and remorse—in an individual who has become impulsive and manifests poor judgment and social control. Another common pattern is marked by apathy, withdrawal, and indifference. When these personality changes are clearly identified as having organic causes, the causes usually involve structural damage to the brain such as tumors, head wounds, vascular disease, and progressive dementia.

Intoxication and Withdrawal

In Chapter 10, both intoxication and withdrawal have been dealt with at length. The diagnosis of intoxication as an organic brain syndrome involves an assessment of the degree of maladaptative behavior. Social intoxication would not be diagnosed in this manner. If an individual engages in fighting, vandalism, or other behaviors that suggest significantly impaired impulse control, judgment, and social functioning, the organic diagnosis may be applied. Both intoxication and the syndrome of withdrawal vary with the substance regularly involved in the physiological state of intoxication.

CAUSAL FACTORS OF BRAIN INJURY AND DAMAGE

Brain Injuries

Brain tissue may be destroyed directly or indirectly by blows to the head, entry by projectiles, tumors, reduced blood supply, and other less obvious causes. These factors can be grouped into two categories—external and internal assaults.

External Assaults. If a projectile such as a bullet passes through the skull into the brain, brain tissue will be damaged. In addition, any severe blow to the head may damage brain function or tissue, with resulting short- or long-term effects.

A blow to the head may result in a **concussion,** a temporary disruption in the flow of blood to the brain. The individual may lose consciousness for several hours or longer, and may be dizzy, nauseous, and confused for a short period after consciousness is regained.

Although concussion and loss of consciousness have often been considered relatively mild brain injuries, longstanding deficits may appear after the initial medical recovery. The degree of impairment following concussion seems to be related to the length of unconsciousness or coma following the injury (Dye, Saxon, & Milby, 1981).

A severe blow may result in brain **contusion,** or bruising of the brain tissue. In such cases, the individual's confusion and disorientation are more severe and prolonged after consciousness is regained. Repeated contusions may result in a chronic condition. For example, boxers, who have received repeated severe blows to the head during long fighting careers may become "punch drunk." This chronic condition is characterized by slowness in speech, poor motor coordination, and confusion (A. H. Roberts, 1969).

Extremely severe blows to the head may cause tears in the brain tissue, as does the penetration of a projectile. These tears, or lacerations, may be complicated by the rupture of blood vessels and internal bleeding which results in hematomas (a mass of blood which infuses a section of the brain and causes a buildup of pressure). The increase in pressure and compression of brain tissue from the hematoma has short-term effects and, if severe enough, may destroy enough brain tissue for the effects to become chronic. The behavioral effects of this type of damage may be limited to functions specific to the site of damage, or may be generalized. If the direct damage is extensive, the hematoma is large or causes a major increase in intracranial pressure, or the brain swells from the damage, the individual may experience disordered functioning such as delirium or chronic dementia.

The general effects which may be seen in brain-injured individuals are illustrated in the following case, who developed an organic personality syndrome.

> Ron is a fairly average-looking 32-year-old man, but he has a striking six-inch scar which runs from above his hairline down across his forehead and ends on his nose. At the age of 20, Ron was in an automobile accident and received an injury to the left hemisphere from a piece of metal. The metal entered the center of his forehead destroying much of the left frontal lobe of his brain and portions of the left temporal and occipital lobes. During his hos-

pitalization, surgery was necessary to remove damaged and mutilated brain tissue from the left hemisphere. The damage has left him with surprisingly few obvious deficits. His speech is slurred and he speaks slowly. He is blind in the left eye because of damage to the optic nerve. Ron's gait, in addition, is uneven because of damage to the motor area of the left hemisphere.

While Ron's physical recovery has been excellent, considering the amount of brain damage he suffered, there have been serious personality changes which appear to be due to the damage. Before the accident, Ron was a stable, quiet, easygoing young man who had few problems. He had done well in school and was employed and self-sufficient. At the age of 20, he was living at home, but planning to obtain an apartment of his own. During and after his physical recovery, friends and relatives began to remark how different Ron had become. A common comment was that "He's just not like the Ron I used to know."

Ron became childlike and impulsive and had frequent temper outbursts. Three years after his accident, Ron was arrested and convicted of auto theft and was imprisoned for six months. In the nine years since that event, Ron has stolen four additional cars for "joy-rides," been in countless fights and violent arguments, and has committed at least one rape. He appears totally unconcerned with the consequences of his acts while he is engaged in them; but at other times, he becomes depressed, remorseful, and tearful about his inability to control his behavior. Because of his inability to control his impulses, his lack of judgment, and his temper outbursts, Ron is now living in a state mental hospital. There he can be provided with close supervision. Even in this setting, he is frequently aggressively and sexually assaultive. The association of marked changes in personality and behavior with the extensive brain damage has led to a general agreement that these problems are organic and unlikely to improve.

Internal Assaults. Events within the brain may cause structural damage just as surely as a blow to the head or a foreign projectile. The damage may be insidious, occurring slowly over time, as in a slow-growing brain tumor. It also may be sudden, as in the rupture of a major blood vessel.

Brain tumor. Brain tumors are new growths (neoplasms) in the brain. Like other structures in the brain, they are composed of cells, fibers, and blood vessels. Tumors are usually categorized as benign or malignant. A benign tumor tends to grow slowly, and if completely removed is not likely to recur. Malignant tumors grow more rapidly, and are likely to spread to other parts of the brain and body. Even if malignant tumors are completely removed, they are likely to grow again. This difference between benign and malignant tumors is important for the recovery of afflicted individuals; but even benign brain tumors are usually very disabling, depending on location and size. A benign tumor is often more easily removed through surgery. However, a benign tumor may be located in a vital area that cannot be reached. At times, surgery would cause so much brain damage that even benign tumors cannot be removed. A further complicating factor is the size of the tumor. A growing tumor displaces normal brain tissue and increases the pressure within the brain. The compression of brain tissue by the tumor and by the increased pressure can lead to neural tissue damage in all parts of the brain, which may lead to permanent damage even after the tumor is removed. The psychological and physical signs of a brain tumor can vary greatly depending upon its location and size.

Stroke. When a cerebral blood vessel becomes blocked by a blood clot or ruptures, the diminished blood flow no longer provides oxygen to the affected portions of the brain. Major strokes usually have a sudden onset and result in almost immediate symptoms, which may include dizziness, headache, confusion, memory deficits, aphasia, and partial motor paralysis.

For many years, it was presumed that a large portion of elderly people with organic brain syndrome developed the disorder by having several major strokes or many minor ones. In other words, it was believed that many of these people developed chronic dementia due to suffering many years of reduced blood supply to the brain. Most current studies indicate that only about 8–12 percent of chronic dementia is due to disturbance in cerebral blood flow from ruptures or blockages of blood vessels (Corsellis, 1977; Wells, 1978).

Brain Damage from Toxins and Infections

Toxins. Many substances in the environment can have adverse effects on brain functioning if they enter the body. Some substances, such as alcohol and other drugs, are used purposely to change brain functioning, and if used chronically or excessively, may cause irreversible brain damage. Certain substances may enter the body without the individual's awareness and result in similar damage. Lead or mercury may be ingested in food or may be inhaled in fumes. Even small amounts of these toxic substances may build up in the brain tissue and produce a delirium. Chronic effects such as changes in personality, memory loss, difficulty in concentration, and emotional lability may result from contact with toxic substances if brain tissue is destroyed, or if the toxic substances cannot be expelled by the body's metabolic processes.

Infections. Infections may influence brain functioning indirectly or directly. A bodily infection (such as pneumonia) may affect the brain when a high body temperature is produced. When an individual is feverish, brain cells need more oxygen to function; if the oxygen supply is not sufficient, a delirium will occur. Infections also may affect the brain more directly. The lining around the brain may become inflamed (meningitis) or the brain tissue may be infected by bacteria, viruses, or parasites (encephalitis).

One infectious disorder of the brain that has received a great deal of attention is **neurosyphilis.** It was recognized as a particular form of mental disorder and was called "general paresis" (generalized partial paralysis) in the early 1800s. By the late 1800s, there was considerable suspicion that the disorder was associated with syphilis. In the early 1900s, two researchers, Noguchi and Moore, discovered through postmortem examination that the brain tissue of those with general paresis had been destroyed by an invasion of the syphilis organism. Thus, neurosyphilis was the first mental disorder shown to be clearly due to organic causes.

Syphilis does not always lead to neurosyphilis. The discovery of powerful antibiotics has decreased the prevalence of syphilis. But syphilis is still a problem: About 1 million people in the United States have untreated syphilis. If not treated, syphilis becomes a secret killer which destroys any organs it invades. There are usually no obvious signs of this process for many years. If the syphilis enters the brain, years later the individual begins to manifest symptoms of neurosyphilis.

Brain tissue is attacked by syphilis in about 10 percent of the individuals with long-term untreated infections. Symptoms become apparent after 10–30 years of cumulative destruction by the syphilitic organism. The early signs of neurosyphilis include irritability, depression, fatigue, and impaired judgment and comprehension. As the damage progresses, cognitive and emotional functions deteriorate further, and grandiose delusions may appear. Later, memory loss becomes severe, and the individual enters a period of confusion. If treated at this late point, the individual's deterioration can be halted or postponed, but the damage to the brain tissue cannot be reversed. Without treatment, the individual may live for some years until the destruction of brain tissue is so great that death occurs after a period of advancing paralysis and total mental deterioration.

Nutritional Deficiencies and Endocrine Dysfunction

Effective functioning of brain cells depends on many factors, some of which are very subtle. The effects of blows to the head, tumors, poisons, and infections on the brain and behavior may seem obvious. However, some factors that disrupt brain function are much less apparent. As examples, we can consider nutrition and the endocrine system.

Nutrition. In addition to proteins and carbohydrates, the body requires vitamins and trace elements for proper functioning. When diets are insufficiently balanced or simply inadequate, individuals may develop disorders that affect psychological functioning. One such disorder is **pellagra,** which occurs when there is a serious deficiency in the B vitamin niacin.

Pellagra results in early mental symptoms of headaches, irritability, and poor concentration. As the disorder progresses, there may be memory deficits, confusion, disorientation, delirium, excitement, and delusions. In severe cases, stupor and convulsions occur.

Pellagra is a relatively uncommon disorder in well-fed societies, but is more frequent in economically disadvantaged parts of the world. In the United States, pellagra is sometimes seen in individuals who cannot or do not obtain adequate nutrition such as the very poor, some elderly, and occasionally in alcoholics who no longer eat enough appropriate foods. Early diagnosis is important, since the symptoms are usually reversible through vitamin therapy.

Endocrine Dysfunction. The endocrine glands secrete hormones directly into the bloodstream. These substances are carried to virtually every cell in the body and profoundly influence cellular functioning. Endocrine dysfunction occurs if an endocrine gland secretes too much or too little of its hormone; and behavioral and physical problems may result. The thyroid gland, for example, regulates the body's cellular metabolism, or rate at which the body produces and expends energy. An overactive thyroid gland may lead to Graves' disease, characterized by restlessness, agitation, and confusion. An underactive thyroid can lead to myxedema, in which thinking processes become slowed, affect is depressed, interest in one's surroundings is lost, and memory may be impaired.

AGE-ASSOCIATED DEGENERATIVE DISORDERS

Several degenerative disorders of the brain result in dementia. In these conditions, generalized destruction of brain tissue progresses until the damage is so great that the individual can no longer survive. The disorders have conventionally been separated into two groups: **presenile dementias,** which begin before the age of 65, and **senile dementias,** which begin at 65 or later. This differentiation has been made because many investigators believed that the dementia seen in elderly people probably had a different etiology than the degeneration seen in people under the age of 65. Today some researchers question whether this differentiation serves any purpose other than indicating the age at which progressive dementia begins (Wells, 1978).

Postmortem examination of the brains of individuals who have had degenerative dementia shows many similarities. The brain has often decreased in size (atrophied) and weighs less than expected. The fissures are usually wider than normal, and the convolutions are narrowed. Depending upon the type of degenerative dementia, a variety of abnormalities may be found at the cellular level.

Presenile Dementia

Progressive degenerative disorders of the brain which begin before the age of 65 are relatively low in incidence. Two examples of these disorders are Huntington's chorea and Pick's disease.

Huntington's Chorea. Huntington's chorea strikes about 19 people per 100,000 (Heston, 1978). This rare disorder usually begins in the age range 30–40. The early signs include noticeable changes in personality. Common symptoms include depression, apathy, minor disorientation, and memory loss. As the disorder progresses, disorientation and memory loss become more severe, and involuntary, jerky motor movements of the arms, legs, neck, and facial muscles appear **(choreiform movements).** The disease progresses to a final vegetative state, and death occurs about 5–10 years after onset.

Huntington's chorea is inherited through a dominant genetic mechanism. The children of a parent who has Huntington's thus have a 50-percent chance of inheriting the disorder. Although we know that the disorder is inherited, we do not know what mechanism results in the deterioration of the brain tissue.

Recent studies have suggested several possible factors in the destruction of brain tissue in Huntington's chorea. Some studies have found a deficiency of the neurotransmitter GABA (gamma-amino-butyric acid) in some sections of the brains of victims of this disorder (e.g., Perry, Hansen, & Kloster, 1973). Other studies

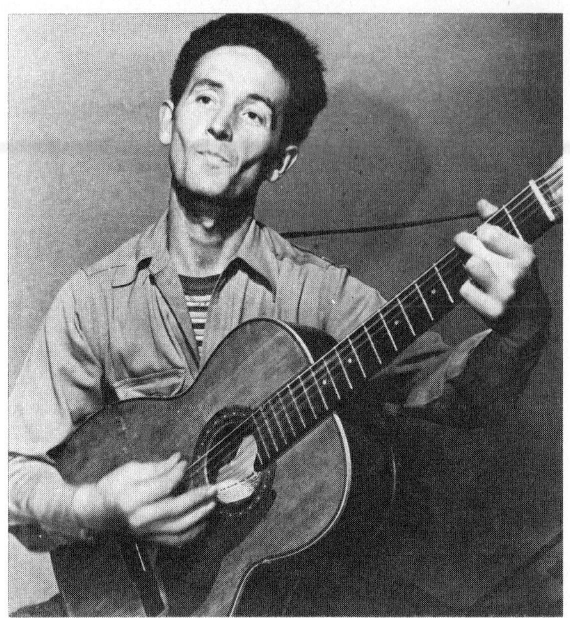

Woody Guthrie, a celebrated folksinger and song writer of the past, was a victim of Huntington's disease. His son, Arlo, also a professional singer, has a fifty-fifty chance of confronting the same fate as his father.

have found the presence of an abnormal protein in the brains of victims (e.g., Stahl & Swanson, 1974).

The presence of these abnormal proteins could explain the malfunction of neural tissue and even its destruction (Wells, 1978). However, the research is preliminary and needs further confirmation.

Pick's Disease. Unlike Huntington's chorea, spasmodic, involuntary muscle movements are rarely seen in Pick's disease. In Pick's disease, the motor and sensory areas of the brain are relatively unaffected, but the frontal and temporal lobe associative areas become severely atrophied. Women are twice as likely to develop this disorder as are men. Early signs of the dementia include lack of spontaneity, blunting of emotions, and loss of memory. The dementia progresses to severe memory loss, confusion, disorientation, and finally a weakened physical condition and death 4–6 years after onset. There is some evidence that Pick's disease may be transmitted by a dominant gene, like Huntington's chorea, but the evidence is not as strong (Heston, 1978; Poser, 1975).

Alzheimer's Disease and Senile Dementia

For many years, **Alzheimer's disease** was considered to be a presenile dementia distinguishable from the dementias seen in old age. However, recent studies have demonstrated that almost 80 percent of the individuals diagnosed as having senile dementia have a late-onset Alzheimer's disease (Liston, 1979; Strub, 1980). Individuals with presenile Alzheimer's disease and those with senile Alzheimer's disease have similar brain damage. Both groups have brain tissue that is characterized by the presence of two major types of degenerative changes: **senile plaques** and **neurofibrillary tangles.** Senile plaques are microscopic lesions in the nerve fiber. Neurofibrillary tangles consist of thickened, twisted, and distorted nerve fibers. If all patients with presenile Alzheimer's disease are counted with the 80 percent of senile elderly persons with this disorder, the importance of the disease becomes obvious: Between 880,000 and 1.2 million Americans have this disorder, making it the fourth or fifth most common cause of death (Katzman, 1976; Katzman & Karasu, 1975).

The symptoms of both early- and late-onset Alzheimer's disease (presenile Alzheimer's and senile Alzheimer's) are those of classic dementia. The early signs are forgetfulness or absentmindedness, problems in concentration, and irritability. Progressive worsening of these symptoms is usually accompanied by the individual's blaming others for one's own faults and problems. This projection of blame onto others often turns into a paranoid delusional system of beliefs about what others are doing. Personal habits such as hygiene deteriorate. Further development of the dementia is manifested by increasingly severe memory problems, confusion and disorientation, and obvious personality changes. Hallucinations may appear, and damage to the expressive and receptive communication centers of the brain may result in incomprehensible speech. The final outcome of the brain deterioration is stupor, coma, and death. From the time of onset, death may occur in as few as 4 years, or the progressive deterioration may last as long as 7–10 years. The following case illustrates the gradual onset and progressive deterioration in an individual diagnosed as having presenile Alzheimer's disease.

> Alice lived a normal life as a wife, homemaker, and mother until her late thirties. Her husband and two daughters described her as a friendly, warm, and quiet woman. At the age of 38, she seemed to become depressed, apathetic, and forgetful. A particularly disturbing behavior consisted of wandering away from home and entering nearby houses unannounced and uninvited. Her husband and teenaged daughters took her for evaluation to a local hospital after about a year of this behavior. At the hospital, she was diagnosed as having an anxiety neurosis and released.
>
> Alice's confusion and disorientation became worse during the next few months. Her housework and personal hygiene suffered, and she had to be constantly supervised. A readmission to the medical hospital and extensive tests revealed mild diffuse atrophy of the brain, and she was finally diagnosed as having presenile Alzheimer's disease.
>
> Her continued deterioration required that Alice be placed in a state mental hospital. The next four years were marked by increasing immediate and long-term memory deficits, confusion, disorientation, and emotional outbursts. Her judgment suffered, and she began to take others' possessions for her own, constantly paced or slept in a ward chair, and her rambling speech became incomprehensible. She could (or would) no longer dress herself or bathe.
>
> As two more years passed, Alice became incontinent and no longer fed herself. When fed by others, she would spit out the food. Lack of nourishment led to a physical decline, and she was fed through a tube. Alice's motor coordination became poor, her movements were slow, and her vocalization consisted of unintelligible crying noises.
>
> Alice was finally placed in a custodial nursing home. She cannot stand unsupported, is totally nonverbal, and has a vacant wide-eyed expression. Alice continues to be tubefed and her basic needs are cared for. Alice is now 49 years old; she has declined for 10 years.

When Alice dies, her family may allow the pathologist to perform an autopsy, which will examine her brain tissue. If large numbers of senile plaques and neurofibrillary tangles are found, the diagnosis of presenile Alzheimer's disease will be definitely confirmed. Postmortem examination is often the only sure procedure for diagnosing the type of dementia that an individual has suffered.

Everyone who reaches late middle age and old age develops senile plaques and neurofibrillary tangles, and loses brain cells (see Highlight 19.1). By the age of 65, about 70 percent of all individuals have these anatomic changes. However, normal (nondemented) subjects never have as many of these abnormalities as demented subjects (Tomlinson, 1977). Some experts wonder whether Alzheimer's disease is an accelerated form of aging(Strub, 1980). Another suggested cause is a slow-acting viral infection, to which some people may be more susceptible for genetic reasons (Cook & Austin, 1978). The exact etiology of presenile Alzheimer's and most senile dementia remains a mystery that will be solved only by further research.

EPILEPSY: A VERY SPECIAL GROUP OF BRAIN DISORDERS

The term **epilepsy** refers to a group of disorders which have a number of common features. The disorders are all characterized by recurring states of altered consciousness associated with sudden electrical discharges in some or most parts of the brain. These discharges have been described as an "electrical storm" or "short circuiting" in neural pathways. During the epileptic state, normal consciousness is interrupted; and in the most common type of epilepsy, there are extreme convulsive movements of the body. Depending upon the type of epilepsy, the state may last from less than a minute to several hours.

Major Types

Grand Mal. **Grand mal epilepsy** is the most common form of epilepsy. Its appearance is dramatic. In the course of normal activity, an individual with this disorder may suddenly lose consciousness. Typically, the individual

HIGHLIGHT 19.1
A POPULAR MISCONCEPTION: AGING, SENILE DEMENTIA, AND CEREBRAL ARTERIOSCLEROSIS

If you know many elderly people, you may have noticed that some have memory problems, absent-mindedness, and mild confusion of a less serious level than dementia. Others may present a clear picture of advancing senile dementia. Perhaps you have heard both groups of individuals described as suffering from "the effects of old age—you know, hardening of the arteries." "Hardening of the arteries" is a popular term for **cerebral arteriosclerosis.** In this condition, the arteries become inelastic, thickened, and in extreme cases, blocked. The subsequent reduced blood flow causes brain cells to die from lack of oxygenation and nutrition.

The belief that cerebral arteriosclerosis is the cause of most senility and senile dementia is a common misconception (Strub, 1980). Current expert opinion is that only a relatively few cases of senile dementia (8–10 percent) are due to this cause (Wells, 1978).

One cardiovascular disorder that does lead to a type of progressive dementia in the elderly consists of multiple minor or major strokes. A single major stroke may lead to a nonprogressive dementia if the brain damage is extensive. However, a series of strokes can lead to multi-infarct dementia. This disorder can be distinguished from other progressive dementias by its stepwise process. The cognitive damage is abrupt in onset, and then levels off or gets better. Another stroke or series of strokes leads to more damage and a reduction in functioning; function may improve, but is unlikely to reach its original level. Such deterioration is not slowly and smoothly progressive. The contrasting courses of the dementias are shown in the accompanying graphs.

When a stepwise process is observed, the dementia is likely to be due to cerebral strokes. Although such dementia is less common than other senile dementias, its accurate diagnosis is very important: Medical treatment of the cardiovascular problem may prevent further deterioration; and if the diagnosis of the process is early enough, dementia may be avoided entirely in some cases through effective medical treatment.

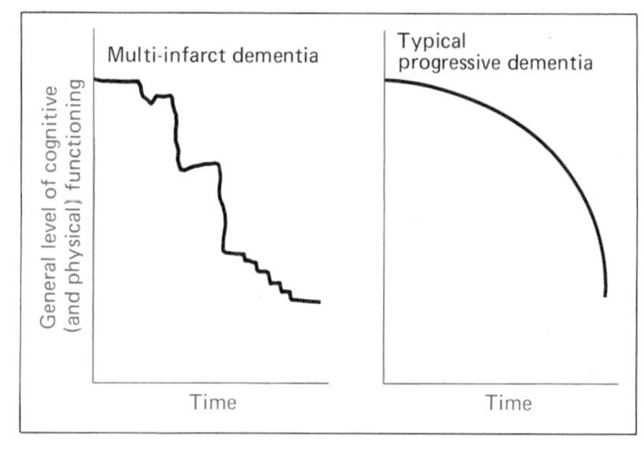

will become rigid, collapse to the floor if standing, and then experience violent jerking spasms of the voluntary musculature. Control over bowel and bladder may be lost, and breathing may become irregular. If the seizure is short, normal functioning may be regained very quickly. After longer seizures, an individual may fall into a very deep sleep for several hours before regaining full consciousness. At times, confusion, fatigue, and nausea may occur after the convulsion. These aftereffects may last a few minutes or hours; in unusual cases, they may last for several days. During a grand mal seizure, individuals may injure themselves while thrashing about, or may bite their tongues because of convulsive movements of the jaw muscles. Some epileptics experience an "aura" before the seizure, and can use it as a signal to prepare for the full attack. These auras are an early part of the seizure and consist of experiences such as headaches, dizziness, visual sensations (flashes of light or spots), humming or buzzing sounds, or peculiar odors or tastes.

Petit Mal. **Petit mal epilepsy** consists of a brief episode of a reduction in or loss of consciousness for a few seconds, sometimes up to half a minute. Major convulsions do not occur. The outward signs are usually a brief unresponsiveness, vacant look, sudden loss of posture or very mild brief jerking of the body. Petit mal epilepsy is more common in children than adults; because of its mildness, it may go undetected for long periods. In about half the cases, this disorder often disappears spontaneously when a child reaches puberty. However, the disorder may continue into adulthood, and some such individuals develop grand mal seizures in later life.

Psychomotor Epilepsy. The electrical disturbance in the brain which leads to psychomotor epilepsy is primarily localized in the left or right temporal lobes. Hence, it is sometimes referred to as **temporal lobe epilepsy.** In this disorder, the individual does not totally lose consciousness, but behaves as if in a trance. During the seizure, the person often engages in "automatic" behavior (i.e., behavior not under voluntary, conscious control). The seizure behavior may appear to be purposeful and organized, or it may be disoriented and confused. For example, the individual may dance, run, shout, and undress, or in a more disorganized manner might stare, mumble, drool, smack lips, and stumble into furniture. In some cases, there may be extreme fearfulness, temper outbursts, or belligerence, and the individual may seem to be hallucinating.

Causes

Although epileptic seizures are due to disorganized, relatively spontaneous firings of groups of neurons, the basic, causal mechanism for the disorganized action of the neurons is still unclear. One widely considered possibility is that these neurons are biochemically hypersensitive to stimulation (Pinkus & Tucker, 1978). They are more irritable than normal. In some cases, such hypersensitivity may be a result of a prior injury. Individuals who have experienced a physical trauma to the brain are more likely to develop a seizure disorder than those who have not experienced brain damage. This is such a common phenomenon that individuals who have suffered brain injury or undergone brain surgery are often placed on antiseizure medication as a routine precaution.

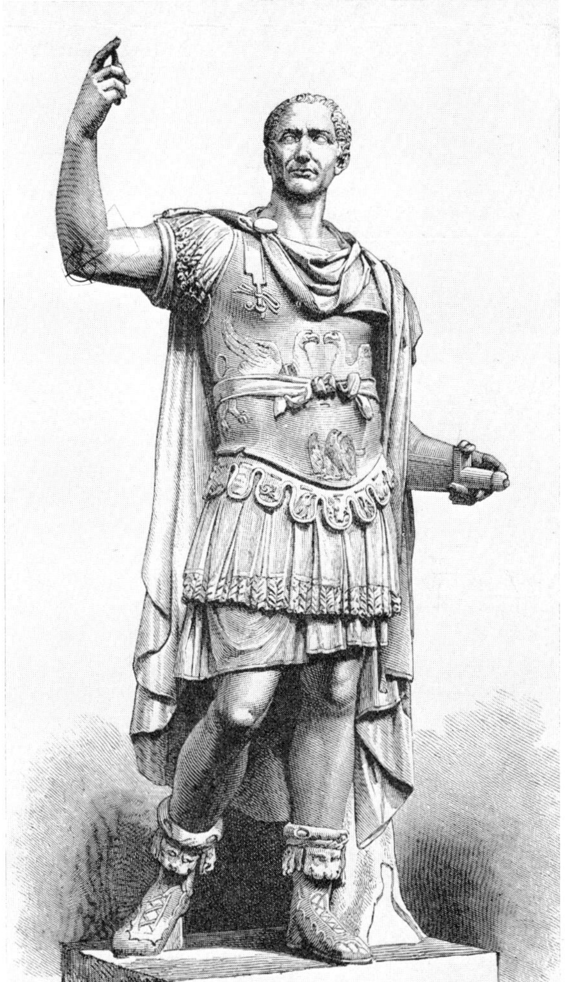

Julius Caesar is supposed to have suffered from epilepsy. Like most individuals with epilepsy, his disorder did not interfere with his living a productive life.

A large proportion of people with epilepsy have no signs of brain damage other than their seizure disorder or an abnormal EEG, or electroencephalogram (see Figure 19.2). Why do these individuals have hypersensitive neurons? Some studies have indicated that some forms of epilepsy, particularly the psychomotor type, may have a genetic component (Dejong & Sugar, 1972). Perhaps, in these cases, some biochemical defect is transmitted from parent to child. Yet in most cases of epilepsy of all types, no history of the disorder is found in the family prior to the involved individual, or in the affected individual's children. We still do not understand all the factors that can result in the development of neural hyperactivity and epilepsy.

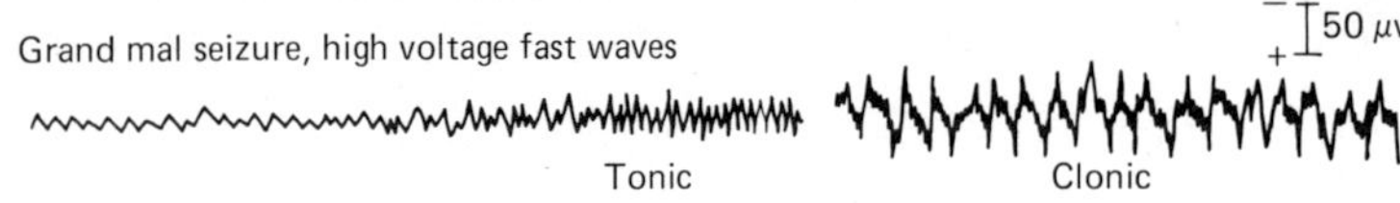

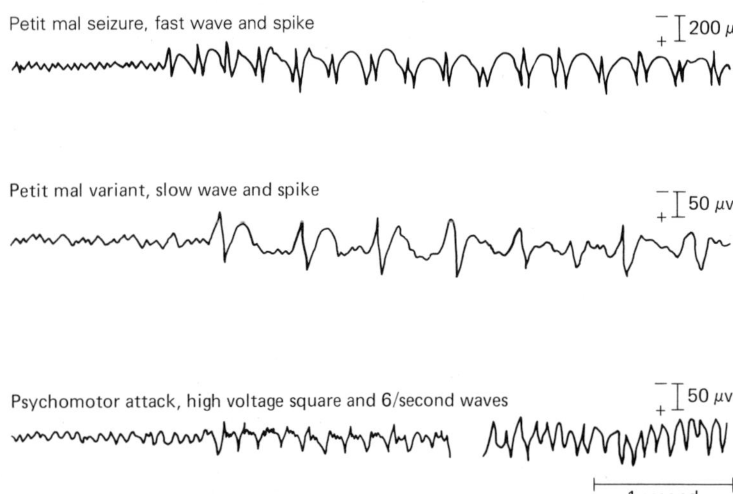

Figure 19.2.
The EEG (electroencephalogram) can be used to measure brain tissue electrical discharges characteristic of epileptic seizures. Specific types of discharges are usually associated with specific types of epilepsy, and may be present even when an immediate seizure is not occurring, aiding in diagnosis. However, only 1 in 10 people who has an abnormal brain-wave pattern actually has seizures. The EEG is not a foolproof diagnostic tool.
From Gibbs, Gibbs and Lennox (1939, p. 1112).

Managing Epilepsy

An individual with an epileptic disorder often must face a great deal of ignorance and prejudice among the general population, not to mention the embarrassment of "losing control" at inopportune times or in potentially dangerous settings (e.g., while driving a car). One false belief about epileptics is that they have an "epileptic personality," which contributes to their seizures. Supposedly, epileptics are overemotional, hostile, or suspicious. While some individuals with epilepsy have one or more of these characteristics, a more appropriate explanation may be that these elements are epileptic individuals' responses to others' reaction to their disorder, not an intrinsic aspect of the epilepsy.

About 80 percent of individuals with epilepsy can gain freedom from seizures by taking certain medications (Dilantin, Tridione, or Phenurone). Proper dosages of these medications can allow most epileptics to lead emotionally, cognitively, and behaviorally normal lives.

KEY TREATMENTS

The person who manifests an organic mental disorder often requires a variety of treatment approaches. Since the damage is organic, medical interventions may be required. However, many of the problems in organic mental disorder are due to psychological reactions to the loss of previous abilities, and are responsive to nonmedical interventions such as psychotherapy or behavior therapy and other environmental modifications. In this section, we will examine the contributions of both medicine and psychology to the treatment of these disorders.

Medical intervention

A major focus of medical intervention in organic mental disorder is on the identification of the underlying pathology. This is a critical activity, since rapid diagnosis may allow effective treatment of some conditions. In Table 19.1 some examples of organic mental disorder, typical underlying pathol-

Table 19.1
Organic mental disorder, underlying pathology, and common medical treatments

Organic mental disorder	*Example of underlying pathology*	*Medical treatment*
Delirium	Fever due to pneumonia	Antibiotics; sedative for moderate agitation
Amnestic syndrome	Thiamine deficiency and chronic alcohol use	Vitamin therapy
	Tumor	Surgery
Organic affective syndrome	Hypothyroidism	Thyroid medication
Organic personality syndrome	Benign frontal lobe tumor	Surgery
Dementia	Strokes due to high blood pressure	Treatment of high blood pressure
	Malignant tumor	Surgery, radiation, or chemotherapy

ogy, and common medical treatments are given. However, effective medical traetment of underlying pathology (such as a brain tumor) often does not "cure" the organic mental disorder. The underlying pathology may be treated and cured, but because of the extent of residual brain damage, the individual may continue to have a chronic brain syndrome. Medical treatment can have a range of effects:

1. The underlying pathology may be successfully treated, and the organic mental disorder may also remit. Delirium is a prime example of an organic brain syndrome that is very likely to clear up if the underlying pathology is treated. Other brain syndromes, such as those caused by some toxins or metabolic disturbances, may also respond well to medical treatment.
2. The underlying pathology may be successfully treated, but permanent damage to the brain may result in an ongoing organic mental disorder. Such an outcome may include successfully removed tumors, neurosyphilis, and multi-infarct dementia.
3. The underlying pathology may be so severe that medical treatment is ineffective, or the disorder may have no known treatment. The primary examples of this outcome are the degenerative disorders of presenile and senile dementia.

Chronic organic mental disorder is a major health care problem, especially among the elderly. Although the **degenerative dementias** cannot be reversed, many medical researchers are looking for treatments to reduce the impairment of senile dementia. Some researchers are studying the effects of a chemical called physostigmine on memory deficits in degenerative dementia. This drug appears to slightly increase memory performance in animals and normal humans. However, its effects are only temporary. The memory enhancement lasts only while the drug is being given intravenously, and decreases after about 15 minutes of continuous medication (Christie et al., 1981).

Unfortunately, physostigmine is not a useful treatment for memory disorder in degenerative dementia. Medical researchers will, however, continue to search for more effective, longer-lasting treatments for these disorders. Perhaps some aspects of dementia will be medically treatable in years to come (Wells, 1978).

Rehabilitation. Most body tissue regenerates when injured. If a finger is cut or scratched, new cells form during the healing process, and only a slight scar or no scar will remain. Brain cells, in contrast, do not regenerate. Once dead or destroyed, they are gone forever. However, when a part of the brain is damaged or destroyed, other parts of the brain may be able to take over some functions of the destroyed section. Some functions, once lost, can never be regained (e.g., loss of judgment because of frontal lobe damage does not appear to be relearnable).

The functions that appear most likely to be relearned include motor coordination, speech, and bowel and bladder control. A victim of a major stroke often has deficits in these areas, but the potential for long-term recovery of at least a portion of these abilities is good. The relearning is unlikely to be spontaneous. Brain-damaged persons require many months, even years, of structured practice in order to regain some of their predamage ability. The rehabilitation process can be frustrating and even physically painful, but if the training and practice do not occur, the functions may be lost permanently (C. B. Stevens, 1974).

Psychotherapy and behavior therapy

The verbal psychotherapies have been used to help organically damaged individuals. Emotional and motivational problems such as anger, depression, and despair may be alleviated through the process of sharing feelings and receiving understanding and support. The recognition that all physical disorders have a psychological component has led to a much wider availability of psychological treatment for individuals with chronic brain syndrome (and other chronic physical illnesses).

Behavioral therapy, like verbal psychotherapy, may assist the individual in making a better adjustment to the organic damage that has been suffered.

> At age 23, in 1964, Bob was involved in an auto accident that resulted in the destruction of one-fourth of his frontal lobes, damage to the motor cortex, and a two-month coma. Prior to the accident, he was employed as a factory worker and was engaged to be married. After his primary recovery, he received intensive physical therapy for approximately six months at a rehabilitation hospital. However, Bob's brain damage resulted in major deficits in speech, coordination, and ambulation. Since 1964 Bob has had numerous hospitalizations in state mental hospitals, usually with a diagnosis of organic brain syndrome without psychosis. Between hospitalizations, Bob has lived in various nursing homes. His admissions to the mental hospitals were precipitated by "combative" behavior. This combative behavior had been assumed to be due to his impulsivity and a "lack of control of rage" resulting from his organic damage.
>
> When seen, Bob was a patient on a medical unit because of his physical infirmity. He spent all his time in a wheelchair; his speech was difficult to understand; and his motor movements were relatively uncoordinated. The problem behavior was described as "extremely combative." His combativeness consisted of knocking down infirm patients and trying to punch staff. This behavior was subsequent to his various demands for constant attention not being met.
>
> A simple behavioral program was instituted with Bob. He was informed that knocking down other infirm patients and punching staff would result in the loss of privileges. He was also told that the absence of such behavior would result in his receiving a cigarette every 30 minutes, and one full day of no violence would be reinforced by a 30-minute meeting with a social worker (who happened to be a young attractive female). When the program began, Bob's average frequency of violence was between five and six incidents daily. Within five weeks, no incidents were occurring.
>
> After the aggresssion disappeared, a similar reinforcement program was begun to encourage Bob to take physical therapy, to practice rehabilitation exercises, and later to practice walking. In four months, Bob was able to walk while using crutches, something he had not done for several years. His heightened ability to control his temper, and his physical improvement, allowed him, at the age of 36, to leave the state hospital to live in a long-term community care facility, where he made a good adjustment.

For many years, Bob's physical disability and his combative rage were presumed to be due to irreversible organic brain damage. Some of his symptoms (such as his speech deficit and some motor uncoordination) were certainly due to such damage, and continued to be a problem. However, his combativeness and "inability" to walk responded to a behavioral treatment approach, suggesting that some of his behavior was due to reversible nonorganic factors.

Behavior therapy can also maximize the potential of individuals with degenerative disorders (Schaefer & Martin, 1969). When reinforcers are made contingent upon appropriate behavior, certain behaviors which are often presumed to be due to the deterioration of the brain can be changed. Bowel and bladder control may be reinstituted, hygiene improved, and some bizarre behaviors reduced. The implementation of a token economy can have broad effects on the functioning of wards of geriatric patients. Lest this give too optimistic an impression, we must remember that progressive brain deterioration will wipe out these gains in the long run. In addition, some organic deficits prevent effective learning. The individual with presenile or senile dementia who cannot store memories may never learn (remember) that keeping tidy results in reinforcement.

Even if not associated with specific reinforcers, some general environmental changes can help maximize the functioning of brain-damaged individuals. For example, individuals who have memory problems can be helped if calendars are available and others remind them what to do and where to be. Problems in speech comprehension may be alleviated if people talk slowly and clearly to the individual. Books with large print and large printed signs may help people read and find their way about. Patient and caring helpers can assist in reducing the psychological trauma of organic mental disorders. Too often, some modifiable aspects of brain-damaged individuals' behavior are attributed to the organic damage and left unchanged.

Summary

1. Disorders of thinking, feeling, and behaving which are mainly due to organic damage or dysfunction of brain tissue are known as organic mental disorders. These disorders are characterized by disturbances in: 1. orientation to time, place, or persons; 2. memory; 3. expressive or receptive communication; 4. sensory perception; 5. motor behavior; 6. intellectual functioning; and 7. emotion.

2. The pattern and extent of dysfunction depends on the location of the brain damage, the amount of damage, and the individual's vulnerability to the damage. This vulnerability is related to factors such as the individual's age at the time of damage and the person's general level of personality adjustment.

3. Organic mental disorder is manifested in syndromes, which are commonly occurring groupings of psychological or behavioral manifestations. The following syndromes are discussed in this chapter:

1. Delirium and dementia, two syndromes in which disturbances are seen in almost all functions.
2. Amnestic syndrome, in which the major disturbance involves loss of memory or loss of ability to store memory.
3. Organic hallucinosis, in which the individual hallucinates during a normal state of consciousness.
4. Organic affective syndrome, in which major disorders of mood (such as depression) occur.
5. Organic personality syndrome, in which the individual manifests a marked change in personality.
6. Intoxication or withdrawal, in which the individual manifests maladaptive behavior because of an intoxicated state, or a disturbed state due to the sudden cessation or reduced use of a chronically used intoxicating substance.

4. Organic mental disorder can be caused by any event or situation which leads to brain tissue damage or dysfunction.

5. Several disorders involving progressive deterioration of brain tissue exist. They are often called presenile or senile dementia, depending on whether the first signs appear before the age of 65 or after. Specific degenerative disorders have been identified on the basis of the various symptoms, courses, and types of tissue damage present.

6. A disorder of particular importance is Alzheimer's disease. This disease was once thought to be a presenile dementia, but the current opinion is that Alzheimer's disease and most senile dementias are the same disorder.

7. "Epilepsy" is the term applied to a disorder in which there are periodic alterations in the state of consciousness. The three most common forms of epilepsy are grand mal, petit mal, and psychomotor. Grand mal seizures involve major involuntary convulsive behavior, in addition to loss of awareness of surroundings. Petit mal epilepsy involves momentary lapses of consciousness. Psychomotor seizures involve a change in the level of consciousness, but no convulsions. Instead, the individual engages in "automatic" behavior, which may be organized but is more often confused and disorganized. Epilepsy may develop after known brain damage, but most epileptics do not have obvious structural damage to the brain. The only other sign of brain dysfunction they show are abnormal brain wave patterns on the electroencephalogram.

8. Organic mental disorder can often be treated if brain tissue has not been destroyed. However, if brain tissue is destroyed, there is no way to make new tissue replace the old. When some underlying organic disorder results in the dysfunction (rather than the destruction) of brain cells, treatment of the underlying disorder may reverse the organic disorder.

9. When irreversible brain damage occurs, organic mental disorder cannot be cured; but rehabilitation sometimes can maximize the individual's potential. Physical rehabilitation, for example, can help the individual to regain better motor coordination and speech skills. Psychotherapy and behavior therapy can motivate people to make successful use of the rehabilitation that is available to them. In addition, behavior therapy has been successful in keeping people functioning at a higher potential, rather than regressing to more disorganized levels of behavior. The success of behavior therapy with chronic, progressively deteriorating organic mental disorders is encouraging. However, no existing treatment approaches can reverse aspects of behavior which are due to the presence of destroyed or damaged brain tissue.

KEY TERMS

Cerebral metabolism. The process by which nutrients are used by brain cells to produce energy and waste products.

Degenerative disorder. A disorder that involves a progressive destruction of cellular structures in the brain, and a subsequent deterioration in cognitive functioning.

Endocrine dysfunction. A disorder in which the endocrine glands produce too much or too little of a hormone.

Neuropsychologist. A psychologist who specializes in the study and treatment of organic brain disorder.

Organic mental disorder. A mental disorder that is due to a known organic brain disorder.

Syndrome. A commonly occurring grouping of psychological or behavioral symptoms.

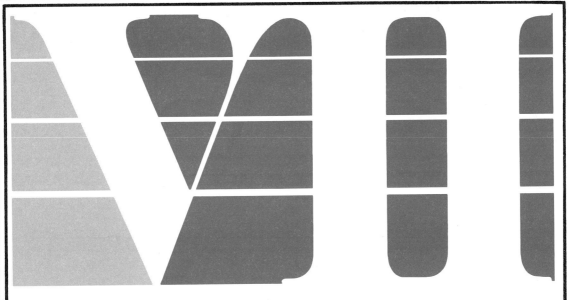

THERAPY AND TREATMENT IN THE SOCIAL CONTEXT

In Chapters 5–19, the application of a variety of treatment approaches to specific disorders has been presented. In Part VII two chapters are devoted to a general consideration of the application of treatment to abnormal behavior. These chapters focus primarily on a description and evaluation of different types of treatment approaches and on the delivery of treatment through organized social systems.

Chapter 20 covers three major types of treatments: biological approaches, insight-oriented psychotherapy, and behavioral therapy. Each treatment approach is briefly reviewed, and issues about its effectiveness are presented. Particular emphasis is given to the insight-oriented psychotherapies and behavioral therapies, and the ongoing concern with their effectiveness. An additional variable identified as important in these two treatment approaches is the characteristics of the therapist and Chapter 20 closes with this topic.

Abnormal behavior is a problem of social concern, and many organized systems provide care for people who have behavioral disorders. Chapter 21 describes these organized treatment delivery systems. The problems and potentials of psychiatric hospitalization, for example, have been and continue to be an area of controversy. The recent policy of deinstitutionalizating mental patients (their large-scale discharge to, and residence in, the general community) is presented, and the policy's benefits and problems are weighed. Chapter 21 describes the community mental health system, including new programs for the prevention of disordered behavior, which are alternatives to traditional residential treatment programs.

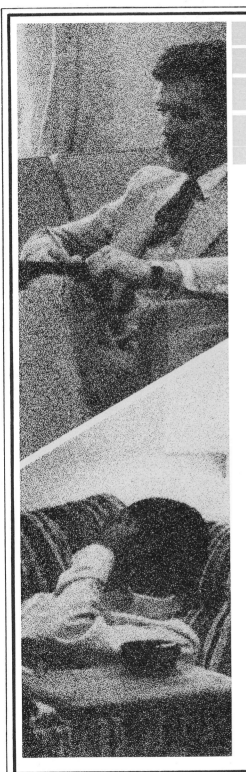

20

Therapeutic approaches and their effectiveness

- Biological therapies
- Insight-oriented psychotherapies
- Behavioral therapies
- What makes an effective therapist?
- A parting comment on the three therapies
- Summary
- Key Terms

The cognitive, emotional, and behavioral disorders that have been presented in this text disrupt the lives of millions of people. We know a great deal about these disorders, although many questions remain to be answered. Because these disorders result in so much suffering, many approaches have been developed to treat them. In Chapters 5–19, various treatments have been discussed for specific disorders (see Table 20.1). Now the major therapeutic approaches will be considered from a more general perspective, to enhance understanding of their similarities, differences, and effectiveness.

In this chapter, three general approaches to treatment will be examined. In each approach, different specific therapies will be covered. The major therapeutic approaches include **biological therapies, insight-oriented psychotherapies,** and **behavioral therapies.** The similarities and differences among these approaches on various dimensions are summarized in Table

Table 20.1
Treatments presented in previous chapters

Chapter and content[1]	*Type of treatment*		
	BIOLOGICAL	INSIGHTED-ORIENTED	BEHAVIORAL
5 Adjustment reaction/post traumatic stress		Problem-solving counseling, crisis intervention, hypnotism, psychodynamic therapy, group therapy	Stress inoculation training
6 Psychophysiological disorders	Disease-specific treatment	Psychodynamic therapy, hypnosis	Relaxation training, operant approaches, biofeedback
7 Anxiety disorder	Tranquilizer	Psychoanalysis, client-centered counseling	Biofeedback, systematic desensitization, exposure (flooding), response prevention, thought stopping; cognitive rehearsal
8 Somatoform and dissociative disorders		Psychodynamic therapy, hypnosis	Operant approaches
9 Psychosexual disorders	Sex reassignment surgery	Relationship counseling, sensate focusing, rape victim counseling	Systematic desensitization, operant approaches, aversion therapy, covert sensitization, orgasmic reconditioning
10 Substance abuse	Medical detoxification, methadone maintenance	Group psychotherapy, mutual help groups	Aversive conditioning, self-control training, self-monitoring
11 Personality disorders		Psychodynamic therapy	Cognitive-behavioral approaches

[1]Chapters 12 and 15 do not focus on treatment approaches.

20.2. This chapter will emphasize the insight-oriented therapies and behavioral therapies, since these two approaches are the most closely associated with the field of psychology.

BIOLOGICAL THERAPIES

Interviewer (I). What medications are you taking now?
Patient (P). Uh—when I'm down I take Elavil, otherwise I take Eskalith [lithium] to keep from getting manicky.
I. Does it work?
P. Fantastic! The Eskalith has changed my life. I don't get those crazy emotional highs anymore. My marriage is back together because my wife can tolerate me now, and I can hold a steady job.
I. What about your depressions?
P. Well, the Elavil doesn't help as much there. I still get depressed occasionally, but not like before, and I haven't had to have ECT for five years. I really didn't like to have that.

The previous chapters have demonstrated that many factors in addition to biological dysfunction contribute to disordered behavior. Yet biological therapies can have a profound impact on human behavior. Three types of biological treatment require consideration: the use of drugs (chemotherapy), electroconvulsive therapy (ECT), and psychosurgery.

Chemotherapy

The use of drugs to treat the symptoms of emotional disturbance is exceedingly common. In previous chapters the use of drugs in the treatment of anxiety, psychoses, depression, and mania has been described (see Table 20.1). Antianxiety agents such as Valium and Librium are among the most frequently prescribed medications in the United States. Some critics are

Chapter and content[1]	*Type of treatment*		
	BIOLOGICAL	INSIGHTED-ORIENTED	BEHAVIORAL
13 Schizophrenia	Major tranquilizers, electroconvulsive therapy	Psychoanalytic therapy, psychosocial therapy	Token economy, operant reinforcement, cognitive self-instruction
14 Paranoid psychoses	Chemotherapy	Psychodynamic therapy	Operant approach, attribution therapy
16 Affective disorders	Electroconvulsive therapy, chemotherapy	Psychodynamic therapy, A. T. Beck's cognitive therapy	Social skills reinforcement, operant reinforcement, helplessness reduction
17 Childhood disorders	Chemotherapy	Play therapy, psychoanalytic therapy, family therapy	Operant reinforcement, shaping, extinction, punishment
18 Mental retardation	Genetic counseling		General skills training, operant approaches
19 Organic mental disorder	Disease-specific treatment, chemotherapy, physical rehabilitation	Supportive psychotherapy	Operant approaches

Table 20.2
Summary of three approaches to treatment: biological, insight oriented, and behavioral

	Biological	*Insight oriented*		*Behavioral*
THEME	SOMATIC	DYNAMICAL SELF-UNDERSTANDING	EXPERIENTIAL SELF-UNDERSTANDING	BEHAVIOR
Prime concern	Biological dysfunction	Sexual repression	Alienation	Anxiety or specific observable behaviors
Concept of disorder or disturbance	Organic pathology: changes in structure or function of organic tissue or biological process.	Instinctual conflicts: early libidinal drives and wishes remain out of awareness (i.e., unconscious)	Existential despair: human loss of possibilities, fragmentation of self, lack of congruence with one's experiences	Learned behavior: excess or deficit behaviors environmentally reinforced or reinforced by cognitions
Concept of positive functioning	Absence of biochemical abnormality or structural abnormality	Resolution of underlying conflicts: victory of ego over id (i.e., ego strength)	Actualization of potential: self-growth, authenticity, and spontaneity	Behavior change: absence of specific problem behavior, reduction of anxiety, or learning of new behavior
Mode of change	Medication, physical treatment such as electroshock (ECT) or surgical intervention	Depth insight: understanding of the early past (i.e., intellectual-emotional knowledge)	Immediate experiencing: sensing or feeling in the immediate moment (i.e., spontaneous expression of experience)	Direct learning: behaving in the present (i.e., action or performance)
Time approach and focus	Nonhistorical, objective present	Historical: subjective past	Ahistorical: phenomenological moment	Nonhistorical: objective present
Type of treatment or intervention	Short-term or long-term; intense and/or maintenance	Long-term and intense; unstructured	Short-term and intense; unstructured	Short-term and structured
Therapist's task	Identify biological abnormality, choose and administer medical treatment	To comprehend unconscious mental content and its historical and hidden meanings	To interact in a mutually accepting atmosphere for arousal of self-expression (from somatic to spiritual)	To program, reward, inhibit, or shape specific behavioral responses to various external or internal stimuli
Primary tools and techniques	Medical intervention: diagnostic exam, physical tests, administration of medication or other medical treatment	Interpretation: free association, analysis of transference, resistance, slips, and dreams	Encounter: shared dialogue, experiments, or games; dramatization or playing out of feelings	Relearnings: systematic densitization, positive and negative reinforcements, shaping, conditioning, extinction
Approach	Medical: doctor-patient (i.e., expert-consumer) relationship	Medical: doctor-patient or parent-infant (i.e., authoritarian) therapeutic alliance	Existential: human peer–human peer or adult-adult (i.e., egalitarian) alliance	Educational: teacher-student or parent-child (i.e., authoritarian) learning alliance
Nature of relationship to outcome	Formal, but unnecessary for cure	Transferential and primary for cure: unreal relationship	Real and primary for change: real relationship	Usually exists, but is of secondary importance
Therapist's role and stance	Expert professional: objective, dispassionate, directive	Interpreter-reflector: indirect, dispassionate, or frustrating	Interactor-acceptor: mutually permissive or gratifying	Shaper-adviser: direct, problem solving, or practical

Adapted from Karasu (1977, p. 853)

concerned about overreliance on these chemical agents to deal with anxiety. Pills are an easy, convenient way of reducing anxiety, and people may prefer them over the difficult task of dealing with their emotional or behavioral problems. Antipsychotic drugs such as chlorpromazine (Thorazine) have been effective in the treatment of major psychoses, as we saw in Chapters 13, 14, and 16. Antidepressant medication such as Elavil has proven useful in the treatment of depression, and lithium carbonate (Eskalith) is often used to treat manic patients.

Although these drugs can be effective, they may have side effects. Use of the antianxiety agents can be addicting, and withdrawal symptoms can appear when the drugs are discontinued. Antipsychotic medication can lead to side effects that range from dryness of mouth to liver damage and tardive dyskinesia, a neuromuscular disorder. Drugs used in the treatment of depression may have unpleasant side effects such as blurred vision and confusion, and lithium use may lead to toxic effects as severe as death (see Chapters 13 and 16). The use of drugs to treat the symptoms of emotional disorder is not without its risks.

Many biologically oriented therapists feel that the effectiveness of the drugs balances the risks. There is no doubt that chemotherapy is more effective than the use of a **placebo** (an inert substance that the client believes is a real medication) (see Table 20.3). However, these drugs are not always effective. Antidepressants are ineffective for 15–30 percent of severely depressed people. Lithium does not work for 20 percent of the manic people with whom it is used. Even when taken continuously, antipsychotic medications do not prevent relapse in over 50 percent of treated individuals.

A major concern of nonbiologically oriented clinicians is that chemotherapy may reduce a patient's motivation to try other types of treatment. This may be a possibility for anxious or depressed individuals who find medication is effective in reducing their anxiety or lifting their depression. But in one of the few studies that examined this possibility, depressed people who received drug therapy continued to be motivated to identify and deal with the problems that led to their distress (Rounsaville, Klerman, & Weissman, 1981). Still, the use of drugs such as Valium and Librium is widespread, and most people who use these drugs to reduce anxiety do not go into other forms of treatment.

Table 20.3
Drug-placebo comparisons for frequently used substances

Drug (brand name in parentheses)	*Number of studies*	*Percent of studies in which drug was more effective than placebo*
Antianxiety agents		
Chlordiazepoxide (librium)	28	96
Diazepam (Valium)	18	89
Antidepressant agents		
Imipramine (Tofranil)	38	68
Amitriptyline (Elavil)	11	82
Antimania agent		
Lithium carbonate (Eskalith)	8	87
Antipsychotic agents		
Chlorpromazine (Thorazine)	66	83
Fluphenazine (Prolixin)	15	100

Based on Appelton and Davis (1973).

Electroconvulsive Therapy

The frequency of ECT has declined dramatically since the introduction of effective antipsychotic and antidepressive medication. During 1975–1976 ECT was used in 30 out of 36 New York hospitals; but it was used with only 1 percent of patients in public hospitals, 5 percent of patients in university hospitals, and 21 percent of patients in private, for-profit hospitals (Asnis, Fink, & Saferstein, 1978). Less than 4 percent of *all* new psychiatric hospital admissions received ECT.

Typically in ECT, the individual is given a muscle relaxant, electrodes are placed on one or both temples, and a .1–.5-second dose of 70–120 volts of electricity is administered. A course of treatment usually involves 5–10 separate ECT sessions over a two-week period. ECT appears most effective with severe depression. Some studies report that 60–90 percent of treated individuals improve dramatically (Fink, 1977; R. D. Weiner, 1979). ECT is less effective in the long run with schizophrenia (P. Taylor & Fleminger, 1980). The value of ECT with severe depressives is illustrated in the following short case:

> A 49-year-old woman was voluntarily hospitalized with her third severe depression in 7 years. Her depressive symptoms included severe early morning insomnia, anorexia [loss of appetite] and weight loss, and an inability to concentrate. The latter symptom was especially troublesome since the patient was a concert violinist who had become unable to perform because she could not concentrate on her music. Previous treatment with ECT at other institutions had offered rapid relief and a return of her ability to perform. The patient refused antidepressant medication, which had made her more agitated in the past, and requested ECT. She denied memory loss from her previous treatments. This patient responded to eight ECT sessions without memory loss or confusion and returned to an active teaching and performing career. (Salzman, 1977, p. 1006)

In this case, there were no adverse side effects. Many studies have demonstrated that memory impairment may occur on a short-term basis; and in rare instances, the lost memories will not return (Squire, Slater, & Miller, 1981). ECT is extremely controversial, in spite of its effectiveness with chronic, severe depression. Many problems are attributed to its use. Sipe (1979, p. 12) says, "ECT is a terrifying and often painful treatment which may violate a patient's civil rights. Side effects include amnesia, dizziness, and loss of appetite. ECT reduces a patient's dignity and its effectiveness is uncertain." Electroconvulsive therapy is a treatment that arouses angry opinions pro and con.

The mechanism by which ECT works is not clear, although some theorists suggest that ECT increases the availability of the neurotransmitters norepinephrine, dopamine, and serotonin in a part of the brain called the limbic system. Its usefulness has been amply demonstrated, while its risks demand caution in its application (see Chapters 13 and 16). ECT is definitely not on its way out, and some researchers are actively trying to reduce its risks by modifying characteristics of the electrical pulse used to induce the seizure. Some studies have found that modification of the electrical pulse may result in less confusion and memory impairment after treatment (Orpin, 1980).

Psychosurgery.

The psychosurgical procedures developed 45 years ago and used for 20 years are quite crude, compared to the procedures in use today (see Figure 20.1). In these early techniques, large areas of healthy brain tissue were destroyed in an attempt to drastically reduce behavior disorders. Psychosurgery is even more controversial than ECT. Many professionals react with strongly negative emotions to the idea of destroying brain tissue in order to change a person's behavior.

The early studies of psychosurgery demonstrated that while the target symptoms were often reduced, there were many serious side effects. Subjects often had serious memory deficits, were apathetic, and unable to care for themselves (Older, 1974). Although new techniques destroy only 5 percent as much tissue as the original approaches, the surgery remains drastic and irreversible, and most surgeons see it as a last resort. Psychosurgery is usually not done unless all other treatment approaches have been tried (e.g., after extensive trials of drugs, ECT, and psychotherapy) without relief of chronic symptoms.

> At 29, [Mrs. X] had the onset of the thought that she might contaminate her children with her vaginal secretions. Her obsession did not [respond] to intensive psychotherapy, including care by a psychoanalyst and ECT. Diagnosis was obsessive-compulsive neurosis with phobic manifestations. Psychosurgery was performed when she was 35 years old. Her follow up included the following: three years af-

Figure 20.1. Traditional lobotomy procedure. Thirty years ago, psychosurgical procedures destroyed large portions of brain tissue to obtain results. Today, more sophisticated procedures produce the same behavioral results with less damage to tissue.

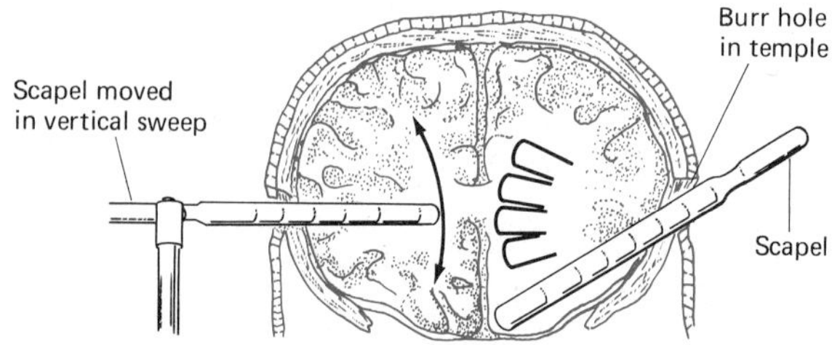

From W. Freeman and Watts (1950, Fig. 15).

ter the operation the patient had a child without any medical or psychiatric difficulty. Since her psychosurgery, she has seen a psychiatrist less than once a year. She was hospitalized at age 50 for ten days for depression. She currently admits to periodic mild anxiety feelings for which she takes an occasional tranquilizer. She has made an excellent adjustment living with her husband and family. (I. C. Bernstein, Callahan, & Jaranson, 1975, p. 1046)

It is difficult to objectively evaluate psychosurgery. Recent studies indicate that it effectively relieves symptoms in 50–75 percent of depressed, obsessional, or severely anxious individuals on whom it is performed (Kalinowsky, 1979; Shevitz, 1976). Psychosurgical results are usually poor with schizophrenic disorders. The idea of destroying brain tissue to change behavior is rejected by most clinicians on moral and ethical grounds. The effects of psychosurgery are permanent and irreversible, and even though new techniques may have fewer side effects, serious questions remain about the desirability of risking irreversible brain damage in order to change behavior.

Some Conclusions about Biological Therapies

1. The biological therapies are effective in the reduction of cognitive, emotional, and behavioral disorders.
2. They seem particularly useful in the most severe disorders such as psychoses.
3. The biological therapies pose substantial risk for the patient in terms of unpleasant or even dangerous or chronic side effects.
4. Contrary to popular belief, the biological therapies are not effective with every person and every disorder; a substantial number of people treated this way relapse, and in some the emotional disorder recurs even when treatment is continued.

INSIGHT-ORIENTED PSYCHOTHERAPIES

Interviewer (I). Why did you enter psychotherapy?
Patient (P). Things had been going badly for me. I was depressed and anxious most of the time, and I wasn't getting along with people I really cared about.
I. And how long has it been?
P. I've been seeing my therapist for almost four years.
I. How has it worked out?
P. Uh, there have been ups and downs. I'm not depressed anymore, and the anxiety that I feel is about like everyone else's. I guess the most important thing is that—uh—I feel I really understand why I was doing some of the things I was doing, and I'm handling my life better.
I. Four years is a long time. How long will you need to continue?
P. "Need" is a poor choice of words. I don't think I really need it anymore, but I still want it. I'm still learning things about myself, and improving my life. In terms of "need" or "pain" I could stop this week. (Laughs) Of course, my therapist might have a different idea about that! We haven't talked about termination yet.

Insight-oriented psychotherapy is a broad term for the treatment approaches traditionally thought of as verbal psychotherapy. These therapies are also often called **relationship therapies,** since many of them emphasize specific types of relationships between therapist and patient to facilitate the development of insight and behavior change. Over 100 different therapeutic approaches are in the category of insight-oriented psychotherapy (Parloff, 1975). Some have major theoretical differences from each other, while others are minor variations of similar themes. However, all these approaches consider the human relationship between therapist and subject, and the development of insight, as critical to therapy. In the process of an emotionally charged, confiding relationship, the client is helped to obtain new understanding about past or present attitudes, feelings, and behaviors. This new information, or insight, may be used to resolve problematic feelings in the context of the therapist-client relationship, and becomes the basis for trying out new behaviors that are more functional than the old.

The fact that insight-oriented therapies share some similarities should not disguise their differences. The underlying theoretical assumptions of many of these approaches may be very different. Thus, several types of insight therapies will be described.

Psychoanalysis

Psychoanalytic theory and therapy was once broadly accepted by psychologists. In 1960, 41 percent of clinical psychologists surveyed adhered to this theoretical orientation. Fifteen years later, another survey indicated that only 19 percent of clinical psychologists identified themselves with this approach (Garfield, 1981). However, many individuals in the helping professions of psychiatry, social work, and psychology still have a modified psychoanalytic or psychodynamic orientation.

Psychoanalytic therapy focuses on instinctual impulses, primarily sexual and agressive, which have been repressed into the unconscious, but which influence all behavior. Through a slow, intensive examination of historical life events, the client's repression of impulses is undone. The repressed material is brought into conscious awareness, where the ego can gain mastery over the id impulses. The client gains insight into the deep motivation of behavior and "works through" repressed feelings which surround the instinctual impulses that created turmoil during childhood. The tools that the psychoanalyst uses to achieve this goal are free association, transference, and interpretation.

In psychoanalysis, the patient traditionally reclines on a couch, with the analyst out of view. This particular seating arrangement is believed to facilitate free association.

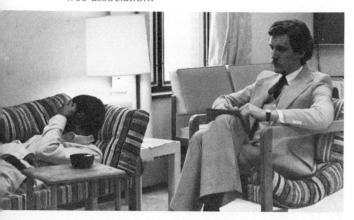

Free Association. Freud described free association as the royal road to the unconscious. In traditional analysis, the patient lies on a couch facing away from the analyst. This setting is thought to aid the patient to allow his or her thoughts to drift, and to speak whatever comes to mind. The uncensored speech of the patient provides the sensitive analyst with clues about the patient's deeper, repressed feelings and motivations. Greenson (1967) provides an example of free association and an analyst's sensitivity to, and interpretation of, the material.

> Mrs. K. . . . She begins the hour by saying she didn't feel like coming to the session. She has nothing on her mind, why don't I give her a hint as to what to talk about, her life is going along quite smoothly. . . . I was aware her tone had a quality of irritability and annoyance. So after some ten minutes of this, I intervene and say: "You seem annoyed." She answers: "I guess I am, but I don't know about what.". . .
>
> The patient is silent for a moment and then says suddenly: "Oh, I forgot to tell you my mother phoned me last night from New York." The patient then goes on to recount the phone conversation and her reactions to it in a steely, cold tone, in a stilted, jerky rhythm. . . [Later in the session Mrs. K. recounts a dream about swimming underwater in a scuba suit, while afraid that something nearby would blow up and injure her.]
>
> I say at this point: "You are afraid of what you are going to find under water, in your unconscious mind. You are scared, so you put on your rubber suit, so you won't feel things, so you won't get involved—in what?"
>
> The patient thinks a moment and says: "I'm tempted to run, to go back to how I was before analysis, being bored and empty. I'm tired of fighting and searching, I want to relax and take it easy. You're pushing me and I want you to do the work. . . ." [Pause.]
>
> I reply: "You're annoyed at me because I won't feed you; I won't be your good mommy." The patient literally shouts at me. "Don't say that word, I can't stand it. I hate it and you, too. Yes, I want you to help me but not just work for me; I want you to be warm and kind. All you do is work, work, work [pause] I guess you're right. I want you to take care of me like I take care of my baby. . . . (pp. 113–115)

With gentle prodding from the analyst, the associative process in this case, led to some very emotion-filled experiences for the patient. Why do you suppose the woman became so angry with the analyst at the end of the illustration? A psychoanalyst would describe this anger as a transference reaction.

Transference. A major factor in the psychoanalytic therapeutic approach is transference. As therapy progresses, the patient begins to behave irrationally towards the analyst, because of irrational emotional reactions. These reactions are due to the transference of emotions that the patient supposedly felt towards parents years before, onto the analyst. In Greenson's example, the patient's anger and hate towards the analyst is associated with his use of the word "mommy," and his refusal to "mother" her. The patient appears to be transferring her feelings about her parent onto the analyst. As transference reactions develop in analysis, they become powerful, emotionally charged situations which enable the analyst to offer interpretations of the patient's associations and emotional reactions. In Greenson's example, the analyst's interpretation results in the patient's recognition that she wants to be taken care of like a baby. The transference relationship may work in both directions. The analyst may develop a **countertransference** reaction with the patient. Countertransference means that the analyst transfers his or her irrational emotions onto the patient. Countertransference interferes with effective analysis. Analysts go through long years of their own analysis (often continuing all their working lives) in order to be able to avoid, or at least recognize and deal with, their own countertransference reactions.

Interpretation, Insight, and Working Through.

During the years of treatment of a patient, (most analysis takes three to five years) the analyst offers occasional interpretations of the free associative material, the transference reactions, and the patient's resistance to treatment. Effective interpretations (as in Greenson's case) must come at the right time, or the patient will resist them. Each interpretation should be at a level that will help the patient gain a little more self-understanding or insight. Insights are therapeutic if they are consistent, if they can be tested, and if they allow the person to interact with others in a more honest and meaningful manner (Karasu, 1977). Insight alone, however, may not be helpful. Insight must be associated with a corrective emotional process called **working through.** In this process, the patient gains effective self-understanding by repetitively reexperiencing repressed desires and emotions in a setting in which these can be reexamined, dealt with and placed at the service of the ego. When this occurs, the patient has a better chance at changing behavior.

The classical psychoanalytic approach has been modified by many analysts who followed Freud. They have become known as neo-Freudians (see Chapter 3). Freud's approach was rooted in a biological focus. Some neo-Freudians such as Karen Horney, Alfred Adler, and Harry Stack Sullivan emphasized interpersonal and social factors. Melanie Klein emphasized the adaptive functions of the ego. Carl Jung involved himself with the study of humans' evolutionary past and the idea of a collective unconscious transmitted across generations. Some modified the original psychoanalytic approach to make it less lengthy, the therapist more active, or to eliminate the traditional couch. In contrast to classical psychoanalysis, most psychoanalytically oriented psychotherapy today is short-term (two years or less). The therapist is more active, and the focus of the therapy is more on dealing with daily problems than on an extensive exploration of childhood memories through free association.

Existential and Humanistic Approaches

The psychoanalytic view that humans are virtually at the mercy of instinctual impulses and are unconscious of the deeper motivations of their behavior has been rejected by many therapists. The **humanistic** and **existential therapies** see human nature in a much more positive light. From these perspectives people are seen as active participants in their fate—striving, self-affirming, and self-actualizing creatures with nearly limitless capacity for growth. These types of therapy are closely associated with the philosophy of European existentialists such as Kierkegaard and Heidegger.

The humanistic and existential approaches are concerned with the process of "being" and "becoming": experiencing accurately what one is, what one can become, and "actualizing" one's potential. Pathology is seen as a result of being out of touch with what one is, a state of incongruence and blocked potential. Anxiety is a sign of incongruence or alienation from self and society. Therapeutic change occurs as a result of the *process* of *experiencing,* in which emotion and behavior are brought into awareness and are intensely felt. Change occurs within a meaningful relationship between therapist and client. This must be an emotionally arousing human relationship, in which each person tries to communicate honestly with the other, both verbally and nonverbally (Ford & Urban, 1965).

Existential therapist Len Bergantino (1981) describes what he calls an existential moment (or therapeutic experience) during the course of therapy:

> I remember going into a group as a co-therapist. The group has been meeting for about six months. One member of the group was in his late forties. He kept swinging his right arm, making a muscle, and letting everyone in the group know that he would punch anyone trying to get too close. Although this was only my second session in the group, there was something about this man that touched me deeply. I sensed this man's emotional starvation to be almost more severe than I could imagine. My instincts told me that he was bluffing about punching anyone. All I could feel was compassion for him. This compassion moved me to get off my chair when he was swinging his arm and, almost without realizing it, gently put my arm around his shoulder. At the same time I began to tell him that I could really sense his pain in being isolated and that even though he pretended to come across like a big mean ole bear, I could sense he was just a little pussy cat inside—and that I really liked him. He cried like a baby. That was the turning point in our relationship and in his relationships with other group members who were also touched by the moment. Both he and they were willing to make closer contact with each other. (p. 11)

By authentically expressing his feelings towards the client, Bergantino helped the man to get in touch with his inner feelings of emotional need and pain.

Humanistic and existential approaches have been described as a "third force" in psychology, since they reject the deteminism of both the psychoanalytic and behavioral approaches.

Client-Centered Therapy. Carl Rogers first introduced the client-centered approach under the term "nondirective therapy" in order to emphasize that the therapist does not dominate the therapeutic situation. The term "client" was used to encourage the view that the individual is not sick and is not a *patient* to be cured by some expert. In **client-centered therapy,** the role of the therapist is to provide a setting in which the client can engage in self-examination, achieve self-understanding, recognize the meaning of perceptions of the world, and one's place in it. At first, client-centered therapists focused on reflecting the client's feelings and clarifying the client's statements. These procedures were intended to communicate the therapist's understanding of the client's perceptions of life.

In time, client-centered therapy shifted from these techniques to an emphasis on the process of the therapist-client relationship, and thus on facilitative psychological attitudes held by the therapist. An effective therapist has *unconditional positive regard* for the client. This is an unqualified basic respect or valuing of the client as a person. Second, the therapist develops an *empathic understanding* of the client: an emotional and cognitive understanding of the client's *being* from the client's perspective, (walking in the other person's shoes, so to speak). The third attitude is *genuineness.* The therapist's verbal and nonverbal behavior must be consistent with her or his covert feelings, attitudes, and reactions.

The accepting, honest, human relationship offered by the client-centered therapist is a new experience for the client. The client has previously experienced relationships filled with *conditions* of *worth*: "I'll give you my love *if*. . . , you're a good boy as long as you. . ."; "Good girls don't think such thoughts. . . ." The genuine, caring relationship of the therapist promotes a natural process of growth, in which the client can contact his or her own inner being and bring the self-concept into congruence (a close fit) with behavior. For example, a client may discover that he or she can be angry with the therapist, who will not reject him or her. The client then no longer needs to seek approval from others, and can avoid conditions of worth (e.g., "If you get angry, people won't love you"), which lead to incongruent behavior.

The client-centered approach emphasizes therapy as a relationship between equals. The client and therapist form an alliance, rather than a teacher-student or doctor-patient relationship (in which one person supervises another). The therapist is not an emotionally distant expert who knows an esoteric technique, but is simply a person entering into a personal relationship with another person who can find out what is "best" for himself or herself, and grow in directions natural to the human organism.

Gestalt Therapy. Client-centered counseling's emphasis on the client's psychological present is shared by **gestalt therapy.** Both approaches avoid emphasizing the client's distant, childhood experiences. However, Gestalt therapy has a much greater emphasis on nonverbal aspects of therapy. It emphasizes activity over reflection, doing rather than talking, feeling rather than reasoning.

Gestalt therapy was developed primarily by the late Fritz Perls. It unites some aspects of psychoanalytic thinking (Perls's early training); the person-to-person relationship of Rogers; a concern for biological, visceral feelings; and Gestalt psychology. The concepts of Gestalt psychology which are relevant are those of figure and ground. Our current experiences are a *figure,* a foreground, which is perceived in the context of a *ground* (background), usually conceived of as feelings which are partly out of our awareness. The figure and ground together make the *Gestalt* (total experience). Therapy integrates the objective here-and-now experience with the undercurrents of emotion (our gut feelings).

Since Perls's death the most eminent Gestalt therapist is probably Walter Kempler (1973), who describes therapy as a highly emotional process:

> The task of therapy is to arouse . . . forgotten desires; to fire up abandoned conflict; and to keep all combatants at the front until everyone wins. (p. 70)

> When the conflict and struggle are insufficient to complete the process, another ingredient must be introduced. Fulfillment is replaced by grief. Then, the path from desire to calm is: desire-conflict-struggle-grief-calm. (p. 68)

> Crying, shouting, hating, screaming, and aching silently, are all parts of the necessary total work to be done. (p. 74) Such changes are not easily achieved. One must go through the rigors of hell each revealing inch of the way, experiencing the loss of treasured traits and valued virtues as though it were death itself. There are no volunteers. Everyone who goes is forced, either by an already existing unbearable pain inside himself, or by family, i.e., a significant other with whom he can not live and can not live without. And, as a rule, without a family to inspire the task, unbearable pain within is dealt with largely by denial, desensitization, and social achievement. (p. 78)

Denial and desensitization of feelings prevent an individual from fully experiencing his or her being. Social achievement is one strategy people can use to avoid honest emotion-filled relationships with others. It results in irrational concern about what others think of us; whether they approve of us. To come into contact with our being, we must get in touch with our gut-level feelings, some of which result from internalized representations of important others such as parents. One might, for example, have a deep feeling of inferiority and anger because of an internalized representation of a parent who treated one in a demeaning way during childhood. "Getting in touch" involves promoting an awareness of bodily sensations, posture, tension, movements, emotions, and one's internalized representations. When people get in touch with their emotions and internalized representations, and see why they behave as they do, they can change their behavior.

Gestalt therapy requires an active therapist. The therapist listens, interrupts, confronts, provokes, and directs in order to activate the client's emotions. Gestalt therapists emphasize getting the patient to focus on personal experiences and personalized statements. For example, the therapist may direct the patient to say

"I feel angry" rather than "It makes me angry." In sessions, the therapist may also encourage patients to exaggerate behaviors or emotions so that patients can get in touch with subtle undercurrents of feelings. The "empty chair" technique is often used to help people experience their internalized representations of others. The patient imagines that a significant person (e.g., his wife) is sitting in the chair; the patient tells the imaginary person his feelings towards her. Then the patient sits in the chair and role-plays the imagined person's response to what has been related. During the empty chair technique, very strong emotions often are experienced and expressed by the patient.

The process and techniques of Gestalt therapy are presumed to lead to an integration of feelings and behavior. The individual reaches a point where gut feelings can be recognized and accepted; and the shoulds, oughts, do's and don'ts internalized years before no longer determine the individual's behavior. The person can "be" with feeling, rather than "not be" with denial.

The Effectiveness of Insight-Oriented Psychotherapies

In the past several decades, hundreds of formal studies of the effectiveness of the verbal psychotherapies have been completed. These studies have examined either the improvement of patients receiving a particular psychotherapy, have compared several kinds of psychotherapy to each other, or have compared patient improvement in various kinds of psychotherapy to untreated control groups. The results from study to study have differed widely. Some have found that psychotherapy has no impact, others have found that certain psychotherapies are better than others, some have found that psychotherapy provides definite but limited improvement in patients. The lack of agreement in results is probably due to methodological flaws within most of these studies, and in differences in methodology between studies. Some of the problems in these studies include the following:

1. Limited scope. Many studies examined only one type of insight-oriented psychotherapy (e.g., only psychoanalysis or only client-centered counseling).
2. Limited subject samples. Some studies had only one type of patient (e.g., depressives or anxiety disorders). And subjects were often not representative of typical patients (many studies used college students who most clinicians would not have diagnosed as emotionally disturbed).
3. Inexperienced therapists. Many studies used psychology graduate students as the therapists.
4. Problems in definition. Definitions of improvement varied from study to study, or the definition was vague and hard to measure objectively.
5. Possible therapist's bias. Assessment of improvement was sometimes done by the involved therapist who had a stake in the outcome, and thus was likely to be biased.
6. Lack of a control group. Some studies had no control group to counter for spontaneous improvement.
7. Inadequate length of therapy. The researchers' resources sometimes limited the therapeutic interventions to a few weeks or months, an uncharacteristically short period for insight-oriented therapy.
8. Limited follow-up. Few studies compared treated subjects with control subjects on a periodic basis more than a few months after therapy was completed.

These types of flaws occur in studies which "prove" that insight-oriented therapy works, and in studies which "prove" that insight-oriented therapies are no better than spontaneous improvement (see Highlight 20.1). The contradictory results of these mostly flawed studies on the effectiveness of the insight-oriented therapies do not enable us to draw a firm conclusion about the therapeutic value of these approaches. However, the weight of the evidence seems to favor the tentative conclusion that the insight-oriented psychotherapies are more effective than no treatment.

M. L. Smith and Glass (1977) selected 375 outcome studies which compared the effects of at least one therapy treatment group to an untreated control group or to a group treated by a different type of therapy. Insight therapies and behavioral therapies were both represented in these studies. Smith and Glass used the data from the studies to calculate the size of the effects reported, and compared the effects to a wide range of variables including the type of therapy, length of therapy, experience

HIGHLIGHT 20.1
GETTING BETTER "SPONTANEOUSLY"

A wealth of studies have demonstrated that some emotionally disturbed individuals will get better "spontaneously," without treatment (e.g., Bergin & Lambert, 1978; Eysenck, 1969). In most untreated, **waiting list control** groups, **spontaneous remission** occurs in 30–45 percent of the subjects. A major concern in the evaluation of the biological, behavioral, and insight-oriented therapies is that these approaches be demonstrably superior to the spontaneous remission rate in "no-treatment," or waiting list control, groups. In our assessment of the relative superiority of treatment vs. no-treatment conditions, we have to remember that subjects in the no-treatment condition are not static while the study is going on. Many things happen that may have profound effects on their behavior and emotional adjustment. The fact that they have not received treatment in the experimental setting does not mean they will not find it somewhere else.

Spontaneous remission may be due to the individual entering into an informal "counseling" or "psychotherapeutic" relationship with a clergy member, friend, or teacher. It may be due to a religious "conversion," or to positive changes in school or work. These types of experiences may share many elements with formal insight-oriented psychotherapies or behavioral therapies. When someone becomes better adjusted through a spontaneous remission, it does not mean that the change had no cause. One important need in outcome research is to identify the events that lead to these "spontaneous" remissions. If we know what the causes are, and how they achieve their effect, we may be able to use them more formally to help people.

of the therapist, severity of the patient's disorder, and socioeconomic backgrounds of therapist and patient. When the effects were averaged, the typical person who had received therapy was found to be better off than 75 percent of the untreated controls. The average treated client experienced more fear and anxiety reduction than 83 percent of the controls. Almost the same percentage of treated clients experienced more improvement in self-esteem than did controls. Complicated statistical manipulations resulted in a conclusion that the behavioral and insight-oriented psychotherapies differed only negligibly in their relative effectiveness, with a slight advantage for behavioral approaches. The authors conclude that years of research demonstrate beneficial effects of the insight-oriented psychotherapies (M. L. Smith, Glass, & Miller, 1980).

We must keep in mind, however, that Smith and Glass (1977) combined data from studies that have been criticized as seriously flawed (Eysenck, 1978). In addition, the statistical analyses used by Smith and Glass have received a great deal of criticism (Gallo, 1978; Strahan, 1978). One critic has suggested that the conclusion which should be drawn from the data presented by Smith and Glass is that the effects of psychotherapy are not very powerful and that they do not justify the clients' expenditures of time and money (Rimland, 1979).

Glass and Smith (1978), in a reply to some of these criticisms, have pointed out that their findings in regard to the 375 studies closely parallel the findings of a study considered to be one of the best designed treatment outcome studies of psychotherapy. The study they mention is by R. B. Sloane and colleagues (1975). In this study, 90 nonpsychotic outpatients were randomly assigned to either a psychoanalytically oriented treatment condition, to a behavior therapy treatment, or to a low contact waiting list control group. The three groups were matched on a variety of factors such as sex and seriousness of symptoms. All were intelligent and well educated (good therapy candidates), but had "quite severe" anxiety symptoms or "personality disorders." The psychotherapists and the behavior therapists were highly experienced and well trained.

The subjects were followed up 4 and 12 months after treatment. Measures on standard psychological tests, self-ratings, ratings by friends and relatives, and ratings by an independent interviewer were compared to the same measures given prior to treatment. At the four-month follow-up, in both treatment groups (psychoanalytic and behavioral) 80 percent of the subjects were considered improved. However, 48 percent in the waiting list control group also were improved. At 12 months, the behavior therapy groups maintained a greater degree of improvement, but this finding was compromised by the fact that some subjects had received additional treatment. Sloane and colleagues concluded that both psychoanalytic psychotherapy and behavior therapy were effective, and no clear evidence showed that one was superior to the other (see Figure 20.2).

The subjects in the study were mailed a survey one year after the treatment began, which revealed a very interesting finding (R. B. Sloane et al., 1977). When asked what they felt was important out of 32 factors in the therapy, both the psychoanalytically treated and the behaviorally treated groups identified the same factors as most important: insight into their problems, the relationship with the therapist, the opportunity to ventilate feelings, and the development of confidence and trust in the therapist. The theoretical and technical focus of insight-oriented therapy and behavioral therapy were not rated as very important. The

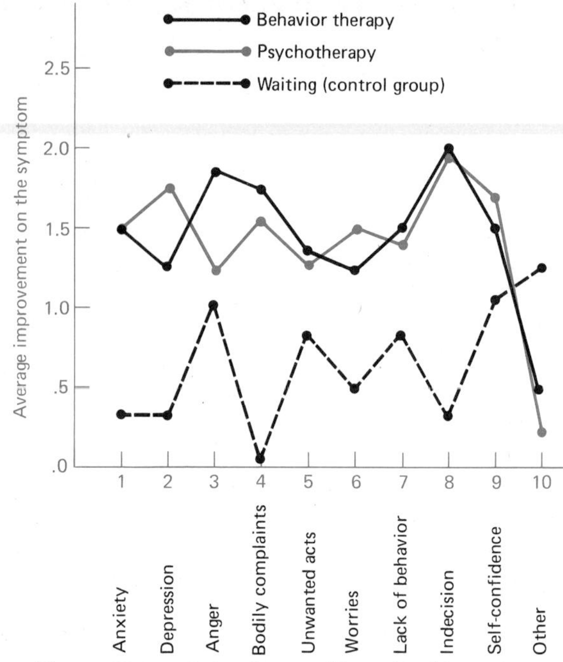

Figure 20.2. Behavior profiles of subjects in a psychotherapy outcome study at the end of treatment, showing amount of positive change. From R. B. Sloane et al. (1976, p. 333).

HIGHLIGHT 20.2
STRUCTURAL VARIATIONS IN PSYCHOTHERAPY

Group and Family Therapy

The classic type of psychotherapy is dyadic: one therapist works with one patient. But the therapy experience may involve more than one therapist working with more than one patient. Two common variations of this type are group therapy and family therapy.

In group therapy, one or more therapists meets with several unrelated patients in a group. Group therapy is done by therapists from virtually all theoretical backgrounds, but most would agree on the general advantages of the group setting. In group therapy, the patient quickly discovers that other people also have severe problems. Expression of one's problems brings reassurance from others that these problems are shared. By being able to share problems with others under the guidance of the therapist, the patient may experience an emotional release, or ventilation, and discover that emotional openness does not necessarily result in rejection. The group provides a microcosm in which the client can try out behaviors and receive feedback not only from the therapist but also from other group members. The peer pressure and peer support are powerful agents in behavior change. A major factor in group therapy is the possibility of vicarious learning or modeling. The patient can learn about emotional processes, problem solving, and behavior by observing others. Clients in groups often report that even though they have sat silently throughout several group sessions, they experienced the ebb and flow of the group and were learning about themselves and experiencing change.

Family therapy is a relatively recent development in psychotherapy, which has become much more popular since the 1960s. It is an outgrowth of the observation that family members have powerful influences on the behavior of the member who is in therapy. Many therapists have felt that the progress of patients has been undermined by family members during the periods between therapy sessions. Others observed that as the patient improved, another member in the patient's family became disturbed. D. Jackson (1965) introduced the term *family homeostasis* to refer to the behaviors of family members which serve to maintain a balance in family relationships.

Family therapists differ in their theoretical orientations, but most emphasize the importance of communication in families. The family is treated as a unit, with no members excluded from the session. The therapists (there are usually two, often one of each sex) act as models of communication. They emphasize direct communication with no hidden meanings or secret agenda. Verbal and behavioral incongruities are clarified and confronted. Insight-oriented or relationship therapists focus on emotional relationships in family interactions, while behavioral therapists focus on developing new reinforcement systems, and behavioral contracts between family members (see Chapter 17 for more on family therapy).

The Encounter Group Experience

Many of the principles and techniques of the insight-oriented or relationship therapies are utilized in encounter groups. Encounter groups are not formal psychotherapy, in fact, most encounter group leaders make a special effort to screen out from their groups people who need formal therapy. We might consider the encounter groups as "therapy for normals." The encounter group experience focuses on growth and self-actualization. These encounters are intense group relationships, which may involve marathon experiences (24 hours of constant contact). The groups use many procedures to attain the goals of self-awareness and open, honest relationships. Depending upon the group leader's orientation, participants in encounter groups may engage in physical exercises and touching (to enhance sensory awareness), verbal exchanges, meditation, and role playing. Some groups also use the controversial experience of nude encounters. Encounter groups have been hailed as the answer to modern alienation and isolation (C. R. Rogers, 1968) and criticized as a callous exploitation of therapeutic principles (Maliver, 1973). Many people have found encounters to be valuable personal experiences, but there are dangers. The intense relationships that develop in encounter groups can have both positive and negative effects. Negative effects can lead to deterioration in some individuals' functioning (probably in about 8–10 percent, according to many estimates; D. Hartley, Roback, & Abramowitz, 1976).

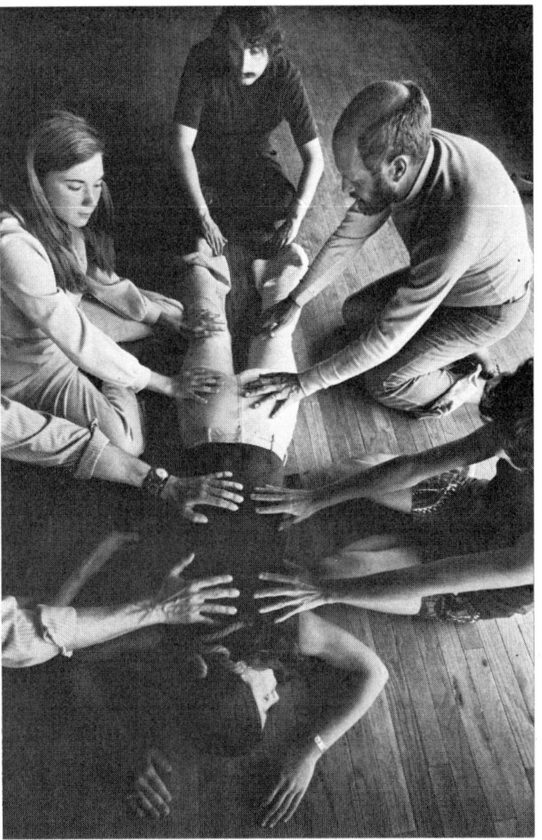

The encounter group experience involves many events that most of us do not have in our day-to-day lives.

Sloane et al. study has become a classic in the comparative evaluation of psychotherapy and behavior therapy. However, many people were reluctant to accept the conclusion of a single study. Now a recent study has substantially replicated the work of R. B. Sloane and colleagues. Cross, Sheehan, and Khan (1982) have reported on a study that is almost identical to the Sloane study in terms of methodology, subjects, control groups, and measurement techniques. In this recent study, psychodynamically oriented insight-therapy and social learning–oriented behavioral therapy were again found to be equally effective treatments. No significant differences were found in the two treatment groups at the end of three months of therapy or at a four-month and one-year follow-up. In addition, the relationship between client and therapist was again found to be very important to patients treated by both therapies.

Since both of the studies described above suggest that the quality or character of the relationship between patient and therapist is important in both insight-oriented therapy and behavioral therapy, one might ask if any warm, trusting relationship that focuses on the subject's problems would have worked as well as these formal therapies. This extremely important question will be returned to after the behavioral approaches are described.

A Consumer Perspective. Whether the insight-oriented therapies work can also be looked at from a consumer's perspective. People spend a great deal of time and large amounts of money on psychotherapy. Are they satisfied after it is finished? Many of them seem to be. Strupp, Fox, and Lessler (1969) sent surveys to 205 people who had been finished with psychoanalytic therapy for least one year. Returns were received from 131 people. Out of this group, 77 percent felt they had benefited either a fair amount (18 percent) or a great deal (59 percent). Eight percent thought they had benefited very little or not at all. The complaint or symptom that led these subjects to seek therapy had disappeared in 6 percent, was very greatly improved in 35 percent, considerably improved in 24 percent, and somewhat improved in 20 percent. In 9 percent it was not improved, and the symptom or complaint was worse in 2 percent. One client put it this way:

> I am a great deal more self-sufficient, so that my relationships are not based merely on need, but I can now be a part of a reciprocal situation. I can assume much more responsibility for my own actions and thus am better able to act rather than just react. My anger at my family has subsided, and I no longer feel that they are to blame for my unhappiness in any present sense. Most importantly, I am able to feel joy and pain, which even with the latter is good, because I'm living, and not just something parasitic. I can trust another person enough to care, and to risk the consequences of the caring. . . .
>
> Although problems still exist, I run no more. I find myself thinking back to my therapy sessions and trying to use what I learned there. I try to determine why certain situations cause problems for me and then determine what is the best way to handle them as they come. I now realize that nothing is really as "earth shattering" as it may seem at the time. . . . (Strupp et al., 1969, pp. 69–72)

Some Conclusions about Insight-Oriented Psychotherapies

1. The therapies seem to work better than no treatment.
2. They seem to work best with bright, articulate people.
3. Seriously disturbed people (e.g., psychotics) are less likely to benefit than are moderately disturbed people.
4. The specific theory and techniques of the treatment seem less important than the existence of a relationship between therapist and subject, although this does not mean that theory and technique have no importance.
5. Research currently cannot answer many important questions about the nature of effective insight-oriented therapy.

BEHAVIORAL THERAPIES

Interviewer (I). Ah, let's see . . . you have a phobia?

Patient (P). *Had* a phobia!

I. OK. Tell me something about it.

P. Well, I've had it since I was a kid, but it has gotten worse during the last four or five years. I couldn't stand to be in small spaces, and finally it was really interfering with my work, installing insulation. That's what finally got me to go see a psychologist.

I. And what did he do?

P. He was a she! She used something she called systematic desensitization. I would imagine things that made me real anxious and then used a procedure she taught me to relax [explains in more detail].

I. Did it work for you?

P. For sure! It took a while, I guess about a session a week for a little over three months . . . but today I don't get anxious at all, or feel closed in when I go in the same sort of places as before. Let's see, it's been three years now since the last time I saw her, but I still practice my relaxation exercise every once in a while.

Behavioral therapy has been defined in many different ways in the past 40 years (Farkas, 1980). Early definitions stressed the importance of learning theory and conditioning approaches in the reduction of anxiety. While these techniques continued to be used, operant behavioral approaches were developed, which focus on directly observable behavior and ignore the subjective experiences of the subject. More recently, many behavioral approaches have been developed which either use modeling (observational learning) or focus on the subject's cognitive processes as mediators of behavior.

The diversity of techniques and theories under the label of behavioral therapy have led one well-known behavior therapist to take a very general position on the definition of behavior therapy: Behavior therapists "place great value on meticulous observation, careful testing of hypotheses, and continual self-correction on the basis of empirically derived data" (Lazarus, 1977, p. 550). Most behavior therapists would not be satisfied with this broad statement. They would maintain that behavioral therapy is based on principles of learning with roots in experimental psychology; in contrast, the insight-oriented therapies are based on clinical and philosophical inference.

The most common behavioral therapies will now be described. These therapies are based on **counterconditioning,** operant learning principles, observational learning, and principles of cognitive behavior modification.

Counterconditioning and Extinction Procedures

Systematic Desensitization. Chapter 3 noted that Joseph Wolpe, a psychiatrist trained in South Africa, developed the technique of systematic desensitization. Wolpe (1958) proposed that the principle of **reciprocal inhibition,** which states that a behavior such as relaxation inhibits anxiety, could be applied to the treatment of anxiety-related disorders. The therapist and client first develop a hierarchy of anxiety-provoking stimuli. The therapist then trains the client in a relaxation procedure, which involves the alternate tensing and relaxing of muscle groups in a set pattern. Often this process is associated with relaxing mental imagery: lying on a sun-dappled beach, feeling warm summer breezes, hearing the gentle surf breaking on the sand. Several sessions may be devoted to this relaxation training, along with practice at home for 20–30 minutes a day. Once the patient has mastered the relaxation process, the desensitization begins.

During the process of systematic desensitization, the individual uses the relaxation procedure to become calm and is instructed to visualize the least anxiety-provoking item in the hierarchy. Often the patient experiences mild anxiety while imagining this, and the therapist guides him or her back through the relaxation procedure. The item is presented repeatedly, until the patient can maintain the relaxed, anxiety-free state while visualizing the previously anxiety-provoking stimuli. As each item is mastered, the patient moves up the hierarchy until even the most anxiety-provoking stimuli can be calmly visualized.

The use of imagery allows this procedure to deal with many anxiety-provoking stimuli that could not be re-created in the therapeutic setting. Some therapists move the therapy out of their office, and accompany the client into the actual anxiety-provoking situation. For example, a client with a phobia to elevators would be exposed to progressively more potentially anxiety-provoking situations involving elevators, while in the company of the therapist and while practicing the relaxation procedure. This would continue until the client could enter an elevator alone.

Flooding. Systematic desensitization starts with imagery low in anxiety-provoking content. **Flooding** (and variations called "implosive therapy" and "in vivo exposure") does just the reverse. It starts with the presentation of the most anxiety-provoking stimuli. The patient is "flooded" with the stimuli in a situation that is safe because of the therapist's presence. Flooding is based on the principle of extinction,

HIGHLIGHT 20.3
SYMPTOM SUBSTITUTION

As behavioral therapies became prominent, psychodynamically oriented therapists claimed that symptom substitution would occur in clients treated by behavior therapists. This criticism was based on the psychodynamic belief that maladaptive behavior is due to some underlying cause. If this cause were not dealt with, these therapists asserted, some new maladaptive behavior would appear to replace the one removed by the behavioral technique. The behavior therapists responded that since there is no underlying intrapsychic cause of misbehavior, symptom substitution should not occur.

So far, no studies have indicated that symptom substitution is a problem for clients treated with behavioral approaches. However, this does not mean that some clients treated with behavioral techniques do not develop other problems. An individual who is treated successfully for a phobia may, a year or two later, become depressed about other problems in his or her life. Such depression may be due to factors unrelated to the factors that led to the phobia, and thus cannot be considered to be symptom substitution.

which asserts that behavior will decrease in frequency if it is not reinforced. The anxiety response to a stimulus can be reinforced if people are allowed to remove themselves from the vicinity of the stimulus (leaving the area), or if they can avoid a stimulus by not thinking about it. Thus, the therapist who uses flooding keeps the patient thinking about, or in the presence of, the anxiety-provoking stimulus until the anxiety dissipates. The anxiety-provoking stimulus is not allowed to be reinforced through physical or mental avoidance. Repeated presentations of the stimulus and prevention of the avoidance response finally lead to a condition in which the presentation of the stimulus does not result in anxiety. Linden (1981) reviewed 39 studies of exposure-type treatments of phobic disorders and found that the lowest reported success rate was 58 percent, and many researchers reported reduction in symptoms in 75–100 percent of the people treated. Although some psychotherapists believed that new symptoms would be substituted for the eliminated behavior, this has apparently not occurred (see Highlight 20.3).

Aversive Counterconditioning. Systematic desensitization and flooding seek to eliminate an unpleasant previously conditioned state of anxiety that occurs in response to a particular stimulus. At times a behavior may occur which a client desires *not* to engage in. A therapist may try to create an unpleasant conditioned response that will result in the client avoiding the behavior. This **aversive counterconditioning** involves the repeated association of aversive experiences with a stimulus that was not previously avoided. The premise is that the stimulus newly associated with the aversive experience will acquire some of the aversive properties of the experience and be avoided. The aversive experience may be noxious smells, pain, or unpleasant reactions from the administration of drugs. In some cases, the individual may be required to imagine noxious experiences such as vomiting in association with the stimulus.

What kind of behaviors may be treated this way? Some of the behaviors dealt with in this manner are alcoholism, sexual fetishism, and pedophilia, or the sexual preference of adults for children (see Chapters 9 and 10). The behavior change in aversive counterconditioning is secondary to a change in response to a stimulus. The stimuli of alcohol, the fetish, or the child is associated with a noxious experience and is avoided, so that the problem behavior (drinking, fetishism, child molesting) does not have the opportunity to occur. Aversive counterconditioning is a somewhat controversial technique (as are all techniques that use "punishment" or noxious conditions). Many therapists (and laypeople) feel that the use of punitive or painful treatments is unethical or has the potential of being abused. Aversive counterconditioning has been particularly criticized when there is the slightest question whether the client was coerced into treatment by a social agency, parents, or the courts. The issue of involuntary treatment is a serious one, which will be discussed in Chapter 21.

Operant Behavior Therapy

Operant behavior therapy is the most behavioristic of the therapies. While not claiming that there are no mental events (since there obviously are), the operant behaviorist focuses exclusively on behavior that is observable and measurable.

Behaviors or responses (called *operants*) increase in frequency or decrease in frequency depending upon whether they are *reinforced*. When a behavior is reinforced in the presence of a particular stimulus (called a *discriminative stimulus*), the probability increases that the behavior will occur again when the stimulus recurs. If a response that occurs is only a poor approximation of a desired response, it may be *shaped*. **Shaping** means to reinforce responses successively, but the contingency for reinforcement becomes more stringent with each repetition. If undesirable responses occur, the absence of reinforcement will lead to *extinction* (i.e., the behavior will no longer occur after a number of trials with no reinforcement). The frequency of behaviors can be reduced through punishment in two ways. A behavior can be followed by an aversive stimulus such as an electric shock which will reduce the likelihood of the behavior recurring. A more common punishment approach is the use of *time-out from positive reinforcement* (either through fines, the removal of a toy, money, or something else of value; or the removal of the individual from a reinforcing situation).

Operant techniques are widely applied in treating major disorders, as we have seen in Chapters 13, 17, and 18, on schizophrenia, childhood disorders, and mental retardation, respectively. In addition, the techniques have contributed to the development of biofeedback techniques (see Highlight 20.4). The techniques

HIGHLIGHT 20.4
LEARNING PRINCIPLES AND BIOFEEDBACK

Biofeedback is the technique of using equipment (usually electronic) to reveal some internal physiological events, normal and abnormal, to individuals in the form of visual and auditory signals in order to teach them to manipulate these usually involuntary or unfelt events by manipulating the displayed signals (Basmajian, 1979). In the 1960s the study of human physiological measurement, operant conditioning, and classical conditioning merged to produce biofeedback therapy.

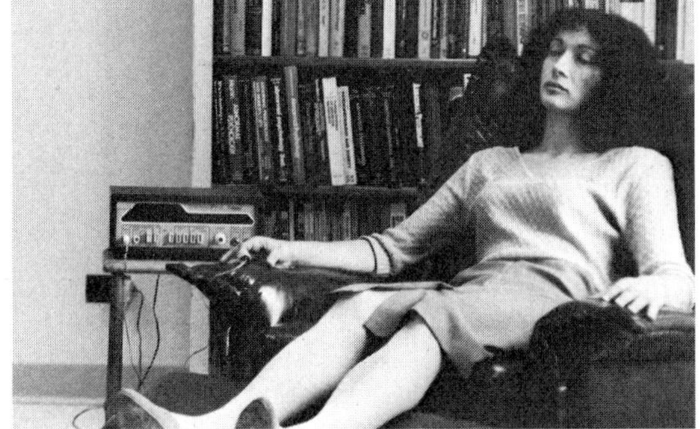

Many behaviorally-oriented psychologists use biofeedback equipment to facilitate the treatment of anxiety disorders. In the photo, the subject is connected to equipment which provides feedback regarding change in finger temperature. As finger temperature increases, it is a sign of relaxation.

The sensitive electronic equipment used in biofeedback provides the subject with a discriminative stimulus which would otherwise be unavailable. When a subject who expects to have the potential to change a physiological event hears or sees a signal indicating that the physiological change has occurred, we can infer that the signal also functions as a secondary reinforcer which strengthens the individual's response. The individual is reinforced for gaining control over internal processes. This inference has been questioned (D. Shapiro & Surwit, 1976). Biofeedback may work simply because it increases the availability of information, and allows the information to be processed more effectively (K. R. Gardner & Montgomery, 1977). The use and effectiveness of biofeedback are discussed in Chapters 6 and 7.

are broadly applicable to changing many forms of behavior. For example, how might we help a student who complains that she cannot study? One possibility would be to have the student come to our office each day to study for two hours. During the two hours we could reinforce her every 10 minutes, if she was studying when we observed her. As a reinforcer, we could give her $1 at every 10-minute interval that she was studying. A better procedure would be to check her *randomly* six times an hour (she might anticipate the more regular schedule and only study for the 1 minute before and after the regular 10-minute checks). If this was successful, we would use the principle of intermittent reinforcement and apply reinforcement on a variable basis. If she was studying when we checked, we would reinforce her sometimes and sometimes we would not. The learning that occurs under this type of reinforcement is much more resistant to extinction than that of other types.

The procedure described above has several disadvantages (besides costing the *therapist* $6 an hour). An important one is that the presence of the therapist is required. Another approach is to train an individual in self-control procedures. The troubled client is first taught the principles of operant learning. The client then establishes a baseline of the frequency of the behavior which is to be changed, and the circumstances during which it does and does not occur. The operant principles are then implemented under the guidance of the therapist. For example, a self-control program for increasing studying behavior follows:

1. Establish baseline of studying behavior and conditions under which it does or does not occur.
2. Change stimulus surroundings. Find a place to study free of interruptions and distraction.
3. Strengthen cues. Do no other activities at the study site. Do not sit there talking to friends, listening to the radio, and so on. Use the location for studying only.
4. Reinforcement. Study at the correct location for brief periods, then self-reinforce by doing something enjoyable.
5. Shaping. Increase study time a few minutes per day before stopping for reinforcement.
6. Intermittent reinforcement. When daily study time has increased substantially, reduce reinforcement to an intermittent basis.

Observational Learning

You have no doubt learned how to do something by watching someone else do it, and then modeling or imitating their behavior. This type of learning has been strongly emphasized by the social learning theorist Albert Bandura (1969). Let us look at **vicarious extinction** and **participant modeling,** two techniques which have been applied as therapies.

Vicarious Extinction. In **vicarious extinction,** a fear is reduced through the subject's obser-

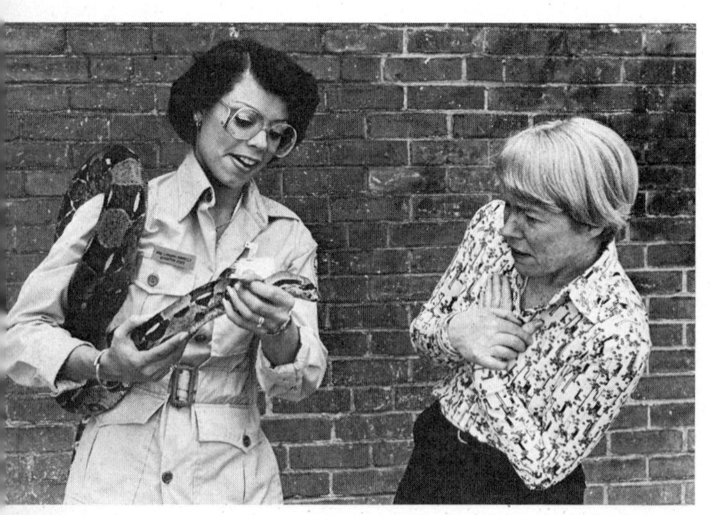

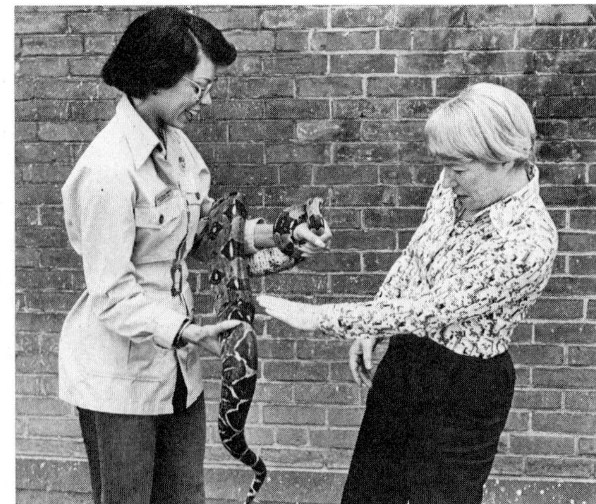

vation of other people interacting with the feared object with no aversive consequences. The procedure is often used with phobic children. Models, either on film or preferably in real life, interact with the phobic stimulus in a series of graduated steps in the presence of the phobic individual.

Participant Modeling. In **participant modeling,** the therapist models a series of behaviors for the subject, who then engages in the same series under the observation of the therapist. This technique can be used with many types of behaviors. For a phobia, the participant modeling procedure would work as follows: Suppose we are dealing with a fear of rats. While being observed by the client, the therapist would handle a rat in a series of graded conditions. The therapist would first touch the rat while wearing gloves, pick it up, hold it, put it down. Then the gloves would be removed and the rat picked up and held. At each step the rat would be handled more closely. After this demonstration, the client would go through the same series of incremental steps, until finally becoming able to handle the rat with no fear. Three to four hours of this type of training usually can extinguish most simple phobias. If the therapist is not comfortable with the phobic object, but tries to serve as a model anyway, the therapy appears to be unsuccessful. The client in that situation models the therapist's discomfort (Howard, 1975).

The Modification of Cognitions

The current interest in the role of cognitions in therapy is represented in two somewhat different approaches. The cognitive therapy of Aaron Beck and Albert Ellis's **rational-emotive therapy** both focus on cognitions, but do not emphasize the application of behavioral procedures such as observational learning, rehearsal, reinforcement, and desensitization. Beck and Ellis have been described as cognitive-*semantic* therapists because of their focus on primarily *verbal* therapy (Meichenbaum, 1977). **Cognitive-behavioral therapy** focuses on the importance of cognitions and the utility of techniques such as reinforcement, modeling, rehearsal, and desensitization in changing cognitions and behavior.

The cognitive therapy of Aaron Beck has been described extensively in Chapter 16 in the discussion of the treatment of depression. This section will focus on Albert Ellis's rational-emotive therapy as an example of a **cognitive-semantic therapy,** and on the cognitive-behavioral therapy of Donald Meichenbaum.

Participant modeling requires that the client face phobic fears through a series of steps which are first modeled by the therapist. However, the client ultimately must interact with the phobic stimulus, as depicted in these photos. (The therapist's overt reaction to the object of the client's phobia is a factor in the success of this therapy.)

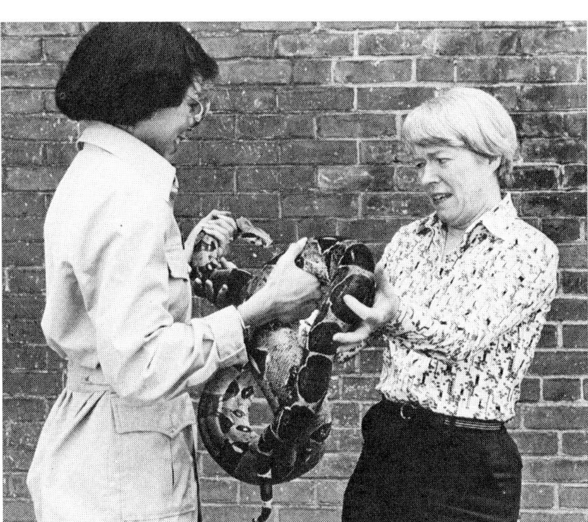

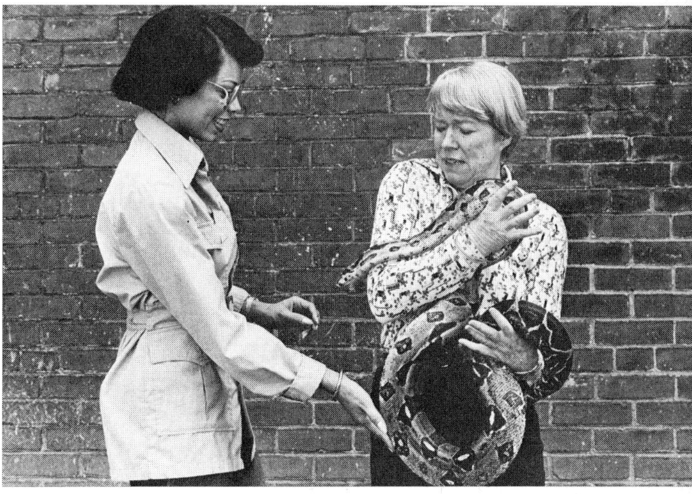

Rational-Emotive Therapy. Albert Ellis suggests that most, if not all, emotional suffering is due to the irrational ways that people perceive the world and to the irrational assumptions that they make. Examples of such assumptions are "Everyone or almost everyone must like me, and if they don't, it's horrible"; "I have to be a *big* success and if I'm not, I'm a failure." Ellis believes that people are preoccupied by "shoulds," "oughts," and "musts"; and people's self-worth is too often dependent on external events (being a success, being loved by others). The RET (rational-emotive therapy) therapist therefore tries to help clients change their irrational perceptions and assumptions and overcome the "shoulds" in their lives. The therapy process is characterized by a very directive relationship, in which the therapist first gets the client to talk about personal beliefs, then challenges them. The therapist may goad, provoke, and argue with the client; provide information; encourage new behavior; and assign homework. The therapist's goal is to help clients understand how they maintain irrational beliefs which create the emotional problems they are experiencing, and then to cultivate clients' ability to think more rationally.

Cognitive-Behavioral Therapy. Donald Meichenbaum and other cognitive-behavioral therapists try to increase the client's awareness of negative self-statements. However, these therapists focus on directly training their clients to use specific problem-solving and coping skills. The techniques of behavioral therapy such as observational learning, rehearsal, and reinforcement figure prominently in this approach. Meichenbaum (1977) suggests that three basic factors are involved in change: 1. the client's behaviors and the reactions they elicit in the environment; 2. the client's internal dialogue, or what the client says to himself before, accompanying, and following behavior; and 3. the client's cognitive structures (beliefs, feelings, and attitudes), which give rise to the specific internal dialogue.

In the first phase of cognitive-behavioral therapy, the therapist encourages the client to become a self-observer. The client must identify problem behaviors, thoughts, and reactions in need of change. In the second phase, the client is helped to create new cognitions, especially inner speech or self-talk, which are incompatible with the old self-defeating cognitions. In the third phase, the client is trained to produce new behaviors in the therapy session, and then in the everyday world. As the client's new behaviors are trained and practiced, the therapist reinforces them and the new inner speech. The extensive rehearsal of new behaviors distinguishes this approach from simple "positive thinking." Without extensive reinforced practice, thinking positively is unlikely to have a powerful effect on behavior. Some examples of positive self-talk which are used in the training of clients who need help in dealing with stressful experiences are provided in Table 20.4.

Effectiveness of Behavioral Therapies

The behavioral therapies have arisen from the scientific tradition, which emphasizes evaluation. They also have the advantage of focusing on goals which are more confidently measured than the goals of the insight-oriented therapies. The accurate measurement of change is easier in an observable behavior than in insights or emotions.

Studies of systematic desensitization have consistently demonstrated its effectiveness. A major study of desensitization (Paul, 1966) compared its effectiveness in the reduction of fear of public speaking with the effectiveness of insight-oriented psychotherapy. Desensitization and psychotherapy both were compared to a no-treatment control group and to an attention-placebo group. The attention-placebo group were people who were given a placebo tranquilizer and attention, but no other treatment. In this study, which used college students with a fear of public speaking, 100 percent of the desensitization group improved, while only 47 percent of the insight-oriented therapy and attention-placebo group and 17 percent of the no-treatment group, improved. Desensitization was obviously more effective than insight-oriented psychotherapy when limited to a short-term (five-hour) treatment. The results support Wolpe's (1958) early claims of improvement in 89 percent of the clinical cases with which he used this approach. Since the introduction of this technique, skilled behavior

Table 20.4
Examples of self-talk rehearsed by clients in Meichenbaum's stress-inoculation training

Preparing for a stressor
What is it you have to do?
You can develop a plan to deal with it.
Just think about what you can do about it. That's better than getting anxious.
No negative self-statements: Just think rationally.
Don't worry: Worry won't help anything.
Maybe what you think is anxiety is eagerness to confront the stressor.
Confronting and handling a stressor
Just "psych" yourself up, you can meet this challenge.
You can convince yourself to do it. You can reason your fear away.
One step at a time: You can handle the situation.
Don't think about fear; just think about what you have to do. Stay relevant.
This anxiety is what the doctor said you would feel. It's a reminder to use your coping exercises.
This tenseness can be an ally: a cue to cope.
Relax; you're in control. Take a slow deep breath.
Ah, good.
Coping with the feeling of being overwhelmed
When fear comes, just pause.
Keep the focus on the present; what is it you have to do?
Label your fear from 0–10 and watch it change.
You should expect your fear to rise.
Don't try to eliminate fear totally; just keep it manageable.
Reinforcing self-statements
It worked; you did it.
Wait until you tell your therapist about this.
It wasn't as bad as you expected.
You made more out of your fear than it was worth.
Your damn ideas—they're the problem. When you control them, you control your fear.
It's getting better each time you use the procedures.
You can be pleased with the progress you're making.
You did it!

Adapted from Meichenbaum (1977, p. 155).

therapists have consistently reported marked improvement in 80 percent of cases treated with systematic desensitization (Wolpe, 1981).

Flooding has been found in a number of studies to be equal in effectiveness to systematic desensitization in the treatment of phobias (Gelder et al., 1973). In addition, flooding, when combined with the prevention of the problem behavior, was effective in treating 86 percent of one group of individuals with obsessive-compulsive disorders (Foa & Goldstein, 1978). Such disorders are usually very resistive to treatment. In contrast to psychodynamically oriented treatment, which usually takes years to deal with such problems, the combined flooding/response prevention treatment consisted of 10–15 sessions over a two- to three-week period.

The operant approaches to treatment have been consistently effective in the treatment of some aspects of serious emotional disturbance (Ayllon & Azrin, 1968; Ayllon, Garber, & Allison, 1977; Paul & Lentz, 1977). Operant techniques have decreased or increased the frequency of a broad variety of behaviors in individuals who are schizophrenic, autistic, mentally retarded, or who have a variety of lesser disorders.

In Chapter 16 we saw that the cognitive-semantic approach of Aaron Beck has been successful in the treatment of mild and moderate depression. The cognitive-behavioral approaches have been effective in changing some behaviors in severe disorders such as schizophrenia (Meichenbaum & Cameron, 1973) and in disorders such as hyperactivity, social isolation, anxiety, and depression (Meichenbaum, 1977).

In evaluating the effectiveness of the insight-oriented psychotherapies, we reviewed the study by R. B. Sloane and colleagues (1975) which compared psychoanalytically oriented treatment, behavioral therapy, and a low contact, waiting list control group. In this study (one of the better outcome studies done to date) behavioral therapy resulted in an improvement in 80 percent of the subjects treated. Behavioral therapy was as effective as psychoanalytically oriented therapy and, at a 12 month follow-up, appeared to have more lasting effects. However, Sloane et al.'s demonstration that behavioral therapy was not dramatically more effective than psychoanalytically oriented therapy was a disappointment and a surprise for many behavior therapists. Some have had difficulty accepting this conclusion (see Eysenck, 1978; Wolpe, 1981). However, a more recent study by Cross et al. (1982) has added substantial support to this conclusion of Sloane's work.

If the behavioral therapies and the insight-oriented therapies are generally equally effective, perhaps the specific technique and theoretical foundation of the therapy are not the most important factors in therapeutic change. Some researchers have begun to examine therapist variables as important factors in the effectiveness of therapy.

Some Conclusions about Behavioral Therapies

1. The behavioral therapies have been demonstrated effective in changing behavior in both moderately and severely disturbed individuals.
2. Behavioral therapies have been reported to be particularly effective with disorders involving anxiety.
3. Behavioral therapies appear to be more quickly effective than insight-oriented psychotherapies, but insight-oriented therapists would say that the goals of behavior therapy are more limited.
4. Important questions remain about the degree to which the specific behavioral techniques are a critical factor, since some studies have suggested that the quality of the relationship between the behavioral therapist and the client is very important in successful treatment.

WHAT MAKES AN EFFECTIVE THERAPIST?

Insight-oriented psychotherapy and behavioral therapy are human enterprises. They share the characteristic of one person helping another, although each therapy's specific technology differs. Do the therapists who use these technologies differ on important dimensions? Is their behavior during a therapy session similar? In the outcome study of psychoanalytically oriented therapy and behavior therapy reported by R. B. Sloane and colleagues (1975), this question was addressed. The results were reported by Staples et al. (1975).

In Staples et al.'s study of therapist factors, three psychoanalytically oriented male psychotherapists and three male behavioral therapists each treated 10 patients. In each case, the fifth therapy session was audiotaped, and typewritten transcripts were made (60 tapes). The tapes and transcripts were rated by independent raters on therapist behaviors such as expression of self-congruence, empathy, unconditional positive regard, depth of interpersonal contact, degree of control, amount of speech and silence, information giving, question asking, and giving of support and approval. After four months, each therapist completed rating scales which indicated degree of attraction to the patient, including how much he liked the patient, how uncomfortable he felt with the patient, and how interesting he found the patient. After four months of treatment, each patient filled out two rating scales on the therapist. These scales indicated the patient's perception of the therapist's empathy, warmth, concreteness, self-congruence, degree of understanding, authoritarianism, amount of encouragement, and degree of critical hostility.

Staples and colleagues (1975) found differences in the way the therapy sessions were conducted, and in the patients' perceptions of their therapists. Behavioral therapists were more open about themselves, answered questions more freely, and became more personally involved with patients. Behavioral therapists were more directive, gave more advice, presented more information, and were more controlling of the content of the sessions than were psychotherapists. Psychotherapists were seen as less authoritarian and more encouraging of patients' independence. Therapists from both groups were perceived as warm and accepting of patients. Many of the differences in style between psychotherapists and behavioral therapists found in this study have also been found in other studies of therapist variables (Brunink & Schroeder, 1979; Greenwald et al., 1981). Behavioral therapists appear to be more active, directive, and advice-giving than psychotherapists.

A retrospective questionnaire answered by patients one to two years after the completion of therapy indicated that the most important factor in therapy in the patients' opinion was the encouragement, advice, and reassurance that they had received. They valued their therapists' understanding personality, and encouragement in facing their problems. A striking finding was that the patients saw the specific technical aspects of the therapy (e.g., dream analysis or conditioning) as less important than the general characteristics of the therapist. The differing theoretical background of the therapists, their different assumptions about the origin of human behavior, and their differing technical approach to therapy did not seem important to the patients; nor did these factors appear to make one therapy noticeably more effective than the other. Could the personal characteristics of therapists, which are unrelated to their theoretical orientation, be the most important factors in the successful treatment of patients?

Even before the 1975 study by Staples and colleagues, Truax and Carkhuff (1967) brought together a large amount of evidence which suggested that therapists who show high levels of genuineness, unconditional positive regard, and empathy—regardless of their theoretical orientation or particular therapy—had patients who improved to a greater extent than did the patients of therapists who did not have high levels of these characteristics. However, these characteristics (derived from client-centered therapy) only moderately correlated with positive therapy outcomes. Which other characteristics may also be important? Can certain personal characteristics yield effective therapy in the absence of formal, technical therapy skills? These important questions have been addressed in a well-designed study by Hans Strupp, one of the leading researchers in the area of psychotherapy.

Strupp and his associate Suzanne Hadley (1979) compared the effectiveness of an experienced group of either psychoanalytically oriented or experientially oriented psychotherapists with a group of untrained "therapists" and compared both groups to a low contact, waiting list control group. The untrained "therapists" were college professors with no special knowledge of psychology or experience in doing psychotherapy. They were selected because they had reputations of being interested in and accessible to their students; were known to be willing to listen to students' problems; and were described as warm, trustworthy people. College students were selected who were experiencing anxiety, depression, and a sense of isolation. These students were randomly assigned for therapy to either a trained psychotherapist, an untrained "therapist," or to the waiting list control group. At the end of the study, students in both therapy groups had improved more than the control group on most measures. However, there was no significant difference in the degree of improvement between students treated by the experienced psychotherapists and students treated by the psychologically untrained college professors.

Students from both treatment groups who improved the most had been treated by a therapist or professor who made active efforts to encourage the discussion of problems, dealt with here-and-now issues, and provided encouragement and information. Strupp and Hadley's study clearly demonstrates that factors outside formal therapeutic technique are important in psychotherapy. Does it demonstrate that formal theory, technique, and training are irrelevant to effective therapy? No, although it might suggest that an anxious, depressed, and lonely college student can benefit as much from being counseled by a warm, interested, and caring college professor as by an experienced psychotherapist.

Telch (1981) has warned that we cannot conclude that all therapy is equally appropriate for all types of disorders and all types of clients. We also cannot conclude that the therapist's personal variables (such as warmth, empathy, and amount of directiveness) are the *most* important factors in successful behavior change. The available reserach cannot support a firm conclusion in this direction. At the same time, the therapist's personal variables are extremely important and must be a focus of further research (Frank, 1979, 1981). In some types of therapies, the therapists's personality may be the most important factor; in other types of therapies, the therapist's qualities may be important but secondary to the technique.

We must also consider the relevance of the type of therapy and importance of the therapist's personal characteristics to the type of patient or client and the type of disorder being treated. Would a caring college professor be as effective as a trained psychotherapist in helping a suicidal student or a colleague with a paranoid psychosis? Would insight-oriented therapy be as effective as behavioral therapy in treating self-mutilative behavior? Would behavior therapy be as useful as insight-oriented therapy in dealing with a person with a multiple personality or with a disaster victim? What is the most useful and effective course of action for someone who is "moderately" depressed? Should this person see a psychiatrist and get a prescription for mood-elevating medication? Or should the individual seek out a psychoanalyst, a psychoanalytically oriented therapist, a Gestalt therapist, an operant behavior modifier, a cognitive-semantic therapist, a cognitive-behavioral therapist, or find a willing friend to talk to? Many questions such as these are currently being posed by outcome researchers in the field of psychotherapy.

A PARTING COMMENT ON THE THREE THERAPIES

The therapies discussed in this chapter—biological therapy, insight-oriented psychotherapy, and behavioral therapy—share a common purpose. All three have the goal of alleviating the human suffering that results from emotional, cognitive, and behavioral disorder. They differ widely in their basic conception of why these disorders occur, and in their approach to changing human behavior. In some not too distant future, there may be some significant integration and melding of all these approaches. Some theorists suggest that this is already occurring between insight-oriented psychotherapy and behavioral therapy (Krasner, 1978; Strupp 1979). In addition, many psychologists are becoming much more concerned with biological factors in human behavior. However, some differences among the therapies and their theories are considered irreconcilable by some experts (Messer & Winoker, 1980; Peele, 1981; Wolpe; 1981).

All of the therapies that have been discussed work. Some appear to work better with certain disorders, although such evidence is constantly being questioned and disputed by advocates of the approaches. The best studies available indicate that the therapies are equally effective on an overall basis. Overall, about 80 percent of the people treated improve, and 20 percent stay the same or get worse. About 30–40 percent of people who are not treated also improve. The overall effectiveness rates are no better for biological therapies than for relationship therapies—a fact that surprises many people.

Is therapy worth it? Of course, it is. If you had an emotional disorder and were told that without therapy you had 6 chances in 10 of staying miserable during the next year or two, but with therapy you had only 2 chances in 10 of the same fate, what would you do? I would very quickly find myself a compatible, experienced therapist and pay whatever I could afford for the treatment. Many people who cannot afford the cost of private treatment have the option of treatment services which are tax supported and publicly run. Treatment settings which offer these services are dealt with in Chapter 21.

Summary

1. The three major approaches in the treatment of abnormal behavior are the biological therapies, insight-oriented psychotherapies, and behavioral therapies. The biological therapies manipulate somatic processes. The insight-oriented psychotherapies focus on the therapeutic relationship between therapist and client, and the development of insight into the client's behavior. The behavioral therapies focus on the observable behavior of the client or on cognitions that mediate behavior.

2. Chemotherapy uses drugs to modify affect, thinking, and behavior. Psychoactive drugs have been consistently more effective than placebos, but are only effective with 70–80 percent of patients. A major concern about chemotherapy involves the unpleasant or dangerous side effects which can result from many of the medications. In addition, there is concern that chemotherapy reduces the patient's motivation to resolve the problems involved in the emotional disturbance.

3. Electroconvulsive therapy is used less frequently than in the past. Its mechanism of action is still unclear. Researchers continue to try to find ECT techniques that will minimize its side effects.

4. Psychosurgery is a controversial technique which continues to be used in a few centers around the country. New techniques have minimized its side effects, but this procedure is still used only with individuals with very severe pathology.

5. In psychoanalysis, therapists use the technique of free association to understand the unconscious dynamics of the client. The phenomenon of transference of feelings (which derive from previous life experiences) onto the therapist is a powerful therapeutic experience. Over time, the therapist interprets these feelings so that the patient can gain insight and work through them. If this approach is successful, the unconscious impulses and feelings can be placed in the service of the ego.

6. Humanistic or client-centered therapists see humans as naturally striving to grow in a positive direction, to self-actualize. Therapy is a process that maximizes this natural tendency. The client determines the content and direction of the process. The therapist concentrates on creating a therapeutic atmosphere in which the client can examine personal feelings and behavior. The therapist uses techniques such as reflection, clarification, and interpretation; more importantly, the therapist must communicate unconditional positive regard, empathy, and genuineness to the client.

7. Gestalt therapy, like client-centered counseling, focuses on current experience rather than the patient's past history. However, Gestalt therapy is more active and directive than client-centered counseling. The Gestalt therapist uses provocation, confrontation, and other directive techniques to arouse the client's emotions. One who is in the process of therapy integrates feeling and behavior, discovers one's "shoulds" and "oughts," and becomes free to be oneself.

8. Most studies on the outcome of psychotherapy are seriously flawed. Taken in total, they indicate that psychotherapy is more effective than no treatment, although it appears that even without treatment a significant number of people will get better.

9. One of the best controlled studies to date strongly suggests that psychotherapy and behavioral therapy are about equally effective. Insight-oriented or relationship therapy results in significant improvement in about 80 percent of the people treated who have problems with anxiety or depression, and who are intelligent, verbal, and motivated.

10. Behavior therapies are either based on a classical conditioning model, use procedures based on operant learning theory, and use observational learning (modeling) or use behavioral techniques which focus on cognitions as mediators of behavior.

11. In systematic desensitization, the patient is exposed to anxiety-provoking experiences in a series of graded steps from low anxiety to high. The exposure is associated with training in relaxation (a behavior incompatible with anxiety) at each step, so that the individual can finally be in the high-anxiety stimulus situation while remaining calm. Flooding begins with the most anxiety-provoking stimulus and maintains the person in it under the guidance of the therapist, until the anxiety dissipates or is extinguished. Both techniques have proven very useful in dealing with anxiety-related disorders such as phobias.

12. Aversive counterconditioning is a procedure in which a behavior is repeatedly associated with a noxious stimulus. It has been used to treat alcoholism, smoking, and socially unacceptable sexual behavior. This technique is controversial, particularly if the subject does not freely consent to the procedure.

13. Operant therapy applies principles of positive reinforcement, shaping, withdrawal of positive reinforcement, extinction, and punishment to behavior. Operant treatment focuses entirely on behavior and avoids dealing with mental concepts, since they are considered to be unmeasurable.

14. Observational learning principles are based on the recognition that people can learn by modeling the performance of others. Vicarious extinction can occur when we see people engage in activities which we fear, but which have no adverse effects on those we observe. Participant modeling is a procedure in which a therapist models a sequence of behaviors, then guides the client through the behaviors.

15. Cognitive-semantic therapy is an approach used by Aaron Beck and Albert Ellis. Ellis calls his approach rational-emotive therapy (RET). His therapy focuses on identifying the irrational assumptions that the patient holds.

16. Cognitive-behavioral therapists such as Donald Meichenbaum try to increase the client's awareness of cognitive self-talk, and its impact on behavior. The therapist teaches the client new positive self-statements, problem-solving skills, and coping strategies. The client rehearses new skills under the tutelage of the therapist, then tries them out in the everyday world.

17. The behavioral therapies, overall, are as effective as the insight-oriented psychotherapies, and may be more effective in dealing with such problems as phobias and anxiety reactions.

18. Operant approaches have proven very successful in the modification of specific behaviors in severe disorders.

19. The relatively equal effectiveness of the insight-oriented psychotherapies and the behavioral therapies has suggested to some researchers that the specific theories and techniques of therapies may be less important than the personal characteristics of the therapist. One well-designed study found that untrained therapists were as effective as those who were trained; effective therapists (trained and untrained) were willing to listen, were active, dealt with here-and-now issues, and provided a warm encouraging relationship.

20. We cannot conclude that technical expertise is not an important factor in the effectiveness of therapy. Further research is needed comparing the relative effectiveness of various types of therapies. Type of therapy needs to be evaluated in the context of the interaction between therapist characteristics, type of treatment, type of disorder, and degree of disorder.

KEY TERMS

Behavioral therapy. A treatment approach originally consisting of the use of principles of classical conditioning and operant conditioning. More recently it has expanded to include a wide range of techniques which emphasize changing behavior through the application of knowledge gained from experimental psychology.

Biological therapy. Therapy that manipulates biological conditions to change problem behavior.

Counterconditioning. The association of a new response with a previously conditioned stimulus.

Insight-oriented therapy. A treatment approach that focuses on the development of insight, or awareness and understanding, of one's own behavior in order to change behavior. Most insight therapies are verbal, and use the development of an emotional relationship between patient and therapist to enhance insight and create change. These therapies are sometimes called relationship therapies.

Placebo. An inert substance (like sugar), or "therapy" which if it effects a change in behavior, does so because the person *expects* it to, rather than because of any intrinsic therapeutic effect of the substance or "therapy." Placebos are often used in treatment outcome studies. The active treatment is compared to the effect of the placebo to determine the importance of the patients expectation that treatment will improve their condition.

Spontaneous remission. A reduction in symptoms which is not due to formal therapies. The person appears to "just get better," but the remission probably is due to some positive change in the person's life.

Waiting list control. A control group in studies of the effects of treatment. The person is assigned to a waiting list during the course of the study and receives no treatment until after the completion of the study. This type of control group allows the experimenter to measure the effects of the passage of time during the course of the study.

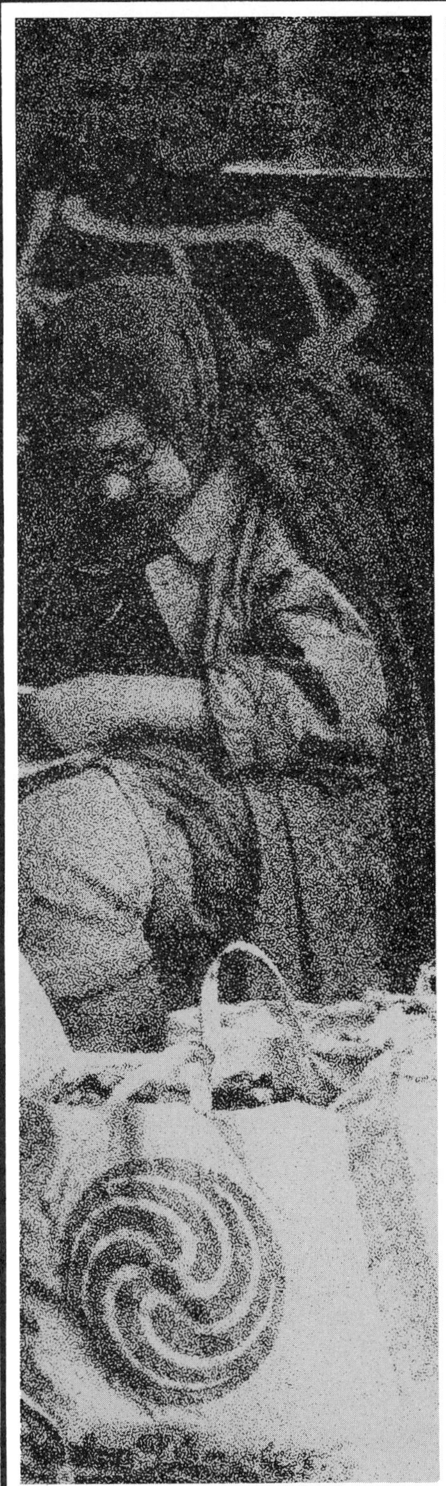

21

Treatment within the social context

- The hospital as a treatment setting
- Before and after the hospital: community mental health
- Social control and behavior change
- Alternatives to traditional solutions
- The problem of dealing with abnormal behavior
- Summary
- Key terms

> "Jan Vorelissen, of Amesland, Complayning to ye Court that his son Erik is bereft of his naturall Senses and is turned quyt madd and yt, he being a poore man is not able to maintaine him; Ordered: yt three or four persons bee hired to build a little block-house at Amesland for to put in the said madman."
>
> To meet the cost of building the block-house and the maintenance of Erik, a small tax was levied on the community. (Deutsch, 1937, p. 42)

The treatment of abnormal behavior occurs within a social context. For many people, an emotional disorder is primarily a personal problem. These people seek treatment out of their own volition (although perhaps at the suggestion or insistance of a friend or relative). If the individual can afford it, the treatment is likely to occur in a private practice setting. The person locates and is treated by a therapist on a fee-for-service basis. A person who cannot afford to pay for such services may obtain them from organizations that are supported by charitable donations or public tax money.

Some individuals' behavior causes personal problems for them and serious problems for the people around them. These individuals are often identified as *requiring* some formal social intervention, whether they want it or not. In Colonial Pennsylvania, in 1676, Erik Vorelissen was confined to a block-house at the commu-

Table 21.1
Some comparisons between private and public treatment facilities for the mentally ill

	Private		*Public*
	General hospital psychiatric unit	Mental hospital	County, state and federal mental hospitals
Patients and sources of funding	The poor, funded by tax money; middle class, funded by insurance; upper class, privately funded.	Middle class, funded by insurance for 30–90 days; upper class, self-funded for as long as necessary.	Mostly poor, without resources; middle class who have used up insurance; some previously upper class who have exhausted other options.
Causes of admission	Acute severe emotional or behavioral disturbance.	Acute severe emotional or behavioral disturbance. People who need and can afford long-term care.	Some acute emotional or behavioral disturbance, many who have had previous hospitalizations in private sector and have run out of money. Severe behavioral disorders that present danger to self or others. People who have not significantly benefited from treatment during other admissions.
Legal classification of patients	Mostly voluntary; some are treated for short time on emergency, compulsory basis.	Mostly voluntary; a few are treated for moderate to long periods involuntarily under court order.	Some voluntary. Others remain "voluntary" under grudging recognition that the courts would commit them for involuntary treatment if they refused. Many are involuntary, treated against their wishes under court order.
Type of treatment	Usually medication and/or ECT. Some crisis counseling.	Medication and ECT. Milieu therapy. Psychodynamically oriented psychotherapy.	Medication. ECT much less likely. Range from custodial care to intensive psychotherapy and behavior therapy.

nity's expense, because of his problem behavior, and because his family was poor and unable to care for him. Erik's behavior was a problem for himself, his family, and his community. Organized treatment of abnormal behavior today reflects a continuing concern for social control of deviant behavior and for the welfare of the individual. At times it is very difficult to tell where one concern leaves off and the other begins.

In this chapter, the major components of today's organized mental health care system are presented. The necessity for these services and their problems will be considered. Some current issues about the right to change people's behavior will be presented, some alternatives to traditional services will be described, and the possibility of effective prevention of abnormal behavior will be considered.

THE HOSPITAL AS A TREATMENT SETTING

For at least 700 years, Western socieites have had special settings to which people with problem behaviors could be sent for some sort of care. The association of hospitals with medical treatment is a much more recent phenomenon. The word "hospital" in fact, is derived from the word "hospice," which referred to a shelter or lodging for travelers, children, or the poor. It has much the same meaning as "asylum" (a place of protection and safety), another word used to refer to some institutions that provided care for the emotionally disturbed. Hospices, asylums, and mental hospitals began as social institutions which offered two services to the community: social control of some individuals

	Private		*Public*
	General hospital psychiatric unit	Mental hospital	County, state and federal mental hospitals
Length of treatment or residence	A few days to a few weeks.	Some a few days to a few weeks. Many about 90 days (until insurance runs out). Some with good financial resources may be treated for 1 to several years.	Some a few days to a few weeks. Most admissions are for 2 to 3 months. A significant pool of very disturbed, residual residents may spend years in residence.
Environment	Small number of patients; large number of staff. Very similar to regular medical hospital unit.	Small number of patients; very well staffed with well-paid, highly trained experts. Often a country estate/lodge atmosphere.	Large numbers of patients. comparatively poor staffing, fewer highly trained professionals, especially in state-operated facilities. Physical plant usually older, less well maintained.
Costs	Similar to medical hospital unit. \$150–\$200 per day. Cost per 8-day to 2-week treatment length about \$1,500–\$3,000. Paid by insurance, by family, or occasionally by government.	Basic room and board usually \$200–\$300 per day. Some much higher. Therapy costs extra. Total monthly cost \$6,000 and up. Typical \$20,000 cost for insurance-covered 3-month stay.	Varies from state to state—\$80 per day is not atypical—some states much lower, a few higher. Monthly expense to state per patient can be \$2,000–\$3,000. Patients with resources must reimburse state for a portion (e.g., in Illinois, a patient with personal funds can be billed a maximum of about 1,000 per month.)

whose behavior caused problems in the community, and the provision of a humane environment in which these people could live. For the past 200 years, treatment has also been an important function of hospitals. The modern mental hospital must balance all three goals: 1. the provision of social controls, 2. the maintenance of a humane environment, and 3. the treatment of behavior disorders.

Several types of settings provide residential treatment for people who manifest abnormal behavior. Publicly funded, government-operated mental hospitals are perhaps the most publicized. In addition, private mental hospitals provide both short-term and long-term treatment to individuals who can afford the extremely costly treatment. In recent years, a tremendous number of general community hospitals also have opened psychiatric units that offer short-term treatment to emotionally or behaviorally disturbed individuals. Table 21.1 summarizes some differences in these three types of facilities.

Going to the Mental Hospital

People are admitted to mental hospitals (or the psychiatric units of medical hospitals) under a variety of circumstances. These people usually have a serious and long-standing emotional or behavioral problem that has recently become more of a problem for them; or they have a serious disturbance that has rapidly "appeared" (acute onset) and become worse.

Some people evaluate themselves and decide that they need hospitalization. More often, someone else (perhaps a relative) is alarmed at the person's emotional pain or behavioral disturbance and convinces the person to seek admission to the mental hospital. Some individuals may be in private or clinic treatment with a psychiatrist or psychotherapist, who sees that the person's problem behavior is getting worse (despite therapy) and who convinces the patient that admission to a hospital is necessary.

Most patients in mental hospitals go there voluntarily. However, many voluntary patients stay only because they are aware that if they tried to leave, the staff (usually with good clinical reasons; see Highlight 21.1) would try to have them committed. Many seriously disturbed people resist admission to residential treatment settings. Involved friends, relatives, and therapists cannot convince such persons that hospitalization is needed. Other disturbed individuals may engage in bizarre behaviors that draw the attention of the police, who may decide that these persons should go to a mental hospital, rather than be jailed for a minor offense. In these situations, if individuals manifest evidence that they present a danger to others or to themselves because of their mental disturbance, they may be committed to a hospital against their wishes through a legal process that includes many checks and balances.

Private Residential Treatment

The General (Medical) Hospital Psychiatric Unit. In the past two decades, a general movement towards more community care for mental illness has resulted in dramatic growth in the number of general hospital psychiatric units. In 1963 there were 465 psychiatric inpatient units in general hospitals; by 1979 there were 1045 (American Hospital Association, 1980). This type of program offers short-term intensive care for about 30 percent of moderately and severely disturbed individuals who are psychiatric inpatients (Keill, 1981). General hospital psychiatric units are heavily staffed and offer treatment composed of chemotherapy, family counseling, and crisis intervention. These programs focus on a reintegration of the individual's functioning at a level prior to the onset of the acute disorder for which treatment was sought. In many instances, this goal can be achieved (at least the major symptoms diminish) in 7–14 days. The individual is then usually referred for outpatient services with a private practitioner or with the staff of a community mental health center. Programs of this type usually refuse admission to patients who are not voluntary (a major exception is California, where most programs accept involuntary patients) and who may require longer treatment (Leeman, 1980). The severity of involuntary patients' disorders and the programmatic changes that these individuals require are believed to be beyond the treatment capacity of most such programs (Leeman & Berger, 1980).

When disturbed individuals are turned away from psychiatric units because they will not voluntarily accept treatment, or because their

HIGHLIGHT 21.1
LEGAL STATUS OF ADMISSIONS TO MENTAL HOSPITALS

State governments have established different types of admissions to protect certain rights of people who admit themselves or are admitted by others to residential treatment settings. The specific details of admission status vary from state to state, but generally encompass the following three categories.

1. Voluntary admission. The individuals admit themselves for treatment on their own decision. They have the right to leave at any time. The facility does not have the right to detain them unless the best judgment of the professional staff is that these patients are so disturbed that they might harm themselves (e.g., commit suicide) or someone else. In this case, the facility can hold the individuals for a short time (e.g., 48 hours) against their wills in a status called an emergency admission.
2. Emergency admission. Individuals can be admitted without their consent (or can be prevented from ending a voluntary admission) if clinical judgment (or obvious behavior) indicates that they are dangerous to themselves (suicidal) or to others. Individuals may also be kept against their will if they would endanger themselves through extreme neglect. For example, some patients are so disturbed or out of contact that they might walk in front of a speeding car. A mental health professional (in some states only a psychiatrist, in others also a clinical psychologist) must file a petition in a court of law, usually within 48 hours after such an emergency admission in order to keep a person on an involuntary status. Otherwise, the individual must be release.
3. Involuntary hospitalization. Individuals may be admitted involuntarily for longer than the emergency status period if they continue to present a danger to themselves or others because of their mental condition. This type of admission must be formally done by a court of law. Usually two psychiatrists or a psychiatrist and a psychologist must fill out a legal document (called a petition) documenting the dangerousness of the patient, and submit it to a judge in open court. The patient has the right to legal representation (the court provides a public defender if the individual cannot afford private counsel), the right to call witnesses, and the right to a jury trial or hearing. The final decision for or against **involuntary treatment** of the individual is made by the jury and/or judge, not by the mental health professionals.

disorder is not likely to remit within a few weeks, the usual alternative is their admission to a state-operated mental hospital. However, some individuals who would not benefit from the short-term treatment of the general hospital psychiatric unit may be treated in a private mental hospital if they have the necessary financial resources.

The Private Mental Hospital. There are approximately 180 private mental hospitals in the United States; they provide 3–5 percent of the inpatient psychiatric care given in this country (Taube & Redick, 1977). About two-thirds are operated as profit-making organizations, and one-third are operated by nonprofit groups such as churches or foundations (Witkin, 1977). Private mental hospitals are usually small, well staffed, and provide intensive treatment to individuals who need and can afford moderately long hospital stays. Almost 95 percent of the patients in private mental hospitals are discharged in less than four months (Gibson, 1978). The other 5 percent may spend up to a year or more in treatment if they have enough funds available. The treatments offered cover a wide range, including intensive individual psychotherapy, chemotherapy, group psychotherapy, family therapy, and ECT. Most (70 percent) of the patients receive three or more types of formal therapy and are also involved in many other daily activities such as sporting events, dances, art, and school. Private mental hospitals have two to three times as many treatment staff as the typical public mental hospital.

Although those who are admitted to private mental hospitals may be very disturbed, they are usually voluntary patients. Depressed individuals comprise over 40 percent of admissions. Of the rest, about 10 percent are alcoholics; 6 percent have adjustment reactions; 5

percent manifest personality disorders; 16 percent have drug problems, organic brain disorders, or neuroses such as obsessive compulsive disorder; and approximately 20 percent are diagnosed as schizophrenic (R. W. Gibson, 1978). In contrast, over 50 percent of admissions to many public mental hospitals are diagnosed as schizophrenic.

Issues Regarding the Private Sector. The treatment services offered by psychiatric units in general hospitals and by private mental hospitals are important aspects of organized mental health care. The short-term intensive care in psychiatric units appears to be important in reducing many individuals' need for long-term hospitalization. Private mental hospitals provide humane intensive care for a small population who can personally afford the cost, or who have extensive health insurance coverage. However, both types of facilities do not accept the cases that many professionals consider the most difficult. People with serious chronic behavioral disorder who may present a danger to themselves or to others, individuals who will not voluntarily accept treatment, and the poor must be treated elsewhere. These individuals and others (including patients treated in the private sector who do not improve) may ultimately be admitted to a public mental hospital.

Public Residential Treatment

There are over 300 county, state, and federal mental hospitals and residential facilities for the mentally retarded. The large majority are state operated. On any day, almost 150,000 people are residents in public mental hospitals, and almost 140,000 are in residential facilities for the retarded (Braddock, 1981). Public mental hospitals provide services for almost one-half of all people who require inpatient care for emotional or behavioral disorder. Publicly funded residential facilities provide services to a wide range of people. Most have severe emotional and behavioral disorders (see Table 21.2). Public facilities have the task of dealing with individuals who have not been accepted by other facilities, who have been treated by other facilities with little success, or who cannot afford other alternatives. Considering the difficulty of the task, one might expect public facilities to be provided with many resources in the form of well-trained staff who are competitively paid, access to the best equipment and supplies, and a modern well-maintained physical plant. Unfortunately, that is rarely the case. Public mental hospitals have seldom been a priority funding item in the eyes of county, state, and federal officials.

Table 21.2
Major categories of admissions to Illinois state mental hospitals in September 1981

Catagories	*Percent of admissions*
Organic brain syndrome	3
Nonpsychotic disorders (e.g., alcoholism, dysthymic disorder, anxiety disorder, personality disorder)	33
Psychotic disorders (schizophrenia, schizophreniform disorder, schizoaffective disorder, major affective disorder, paranoid disorders)	64

Based on *Monthly Statistics* (1981).

From their beginnings, public mental hospitals have been accused (usually rightfully so) of being little more than warehouses providing **custodial care.** In the past, little treatment occurred, and patients were sometimes abused and were often kept locked up long after their major symptoms had faded. These facilities were described as **total institutions** (Goffman, 1961), where residents developed a pattern of adjustment that included dependency and a sense of helplessness—elements which were then seen as part of their illness (Gruenberg, 1969). So many problems developed in such facilities that some experts argued that they should all be closed and some alternative treatment setting developed (Albee, 1968).

Public mental hospitals reached a peak census of 559,000 patients in 1955. Following the introduction of psychotropic medications in the late 1950s, many psychosocial treatment techniques began to be used in these facilities. Because of these changes, patients were more rapidly discharged into the community, and the average stay of newly admitted patients decreased. A process known as **deinstitutionalization** had begun. By 1980 the inpatient census of public mental hospitals had decreased from the 1955 peak by almost 75 percent. The decline in population and length of stay was associated with at least two factors. One was the community mental health movement, with its new focus on the provision of treatment services in community mental health centers and in short-term community inpatient units. A second was the increased restrictiveness of laws regarding involuntary admissions to mental hospitals. The laws made such admission more difficult unless patients were dangerous or suicidal. During the reduction in patient census, a few public mental hospitals closed. Most have remained in operation. They are smaller than before, and are somewhat better staffed today, but still are poor in resources.

A Public Mental Hospital. Treatment today in public mental hospitals is not very different from that in private hospitals, with the significant exception of resources. There is less of everything. One would find almost universal usage of chemotherapy. Fewer patients would be receiving individual psychotherapy and other psychosocial treatments than in private facilities. Staffing in the public mental hospital is usually a major problem. There are less staff members and a lower proportion of well-trained professionals. The therapy that public mental health patients receive is likely to be less intensive or less frequent, and more likely to be done by staff who are not professionals.

Some hospitals have programs called **therapeutic communities.** In this approach, developed by psychiatrist Maxwell Jones (1953), patients become actively involved in running the treatment program. Staff attempt to interact with patients as equals, rather than as authoritarian experts who "know best." As many issues as possible are decided by patient committees, including important decisions such as who will receive passes to leave the grounds and, in some programs, who is ready for discharge. Allowing the patients to make such decisions is believed to strengthen their self-esteem and ability to accept responsibility. An environment (milieu) is developed which is thought to be generally therapeutic. Such programs are sometimes called **milieu therapy.** Milieu programs or therapeutic communities are difficult to run, especially when patients are severely impaired. Although the effectiveness of milieu therapy has not been clearly demonstrated, its humanizing value in large institutions cannot be denied.

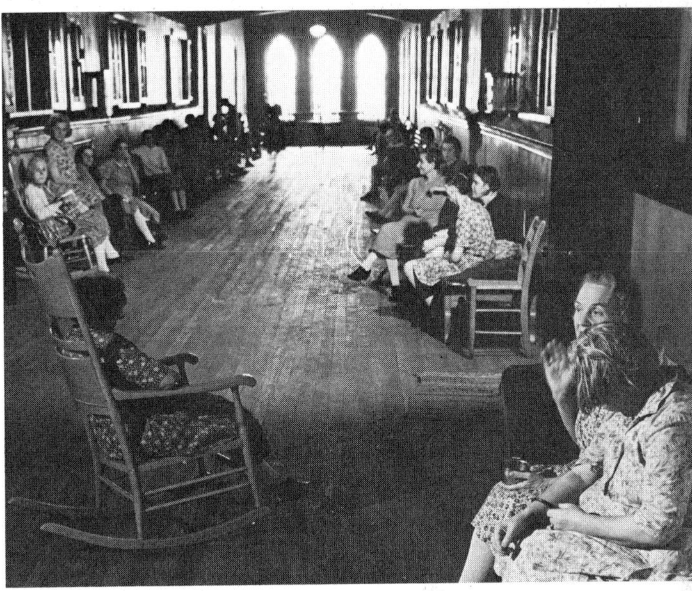

In the 1930s and 1940s, public mental hospitals became extremely overcrowded.

In Chapter 13, the application of operant learning principles in the treatment of schizophrenia was discussed. Many public mental hospitals have programs which use these principles in a **token economy;** in this system, desired behaviors and unacceptable behaviors are clearly specified. Patients can obtain tokens (conditional reinforcers) for engaging in desired or appropriate behaviors. These tokens can be redeemed for such reinforcers as snacks and privileges. Tokens can be taken away (or withheld) when inappropriate behavior occurs, and can be used to incrementally shape behavior. Controlled evaluations of token economies have demonstrated their usefulness in modifying the behaviors of groups of individuals (Atthowe & Krasner, 1968; Patterson, 1976). The effective token economy, however, requires constant monitoring, and supervision of staff (Carsrud, Carsrud, & Dodd, 1980; Patterson, 1976). A common problem in such programs is that the token system becomes a routine that staff assume will run automatically.

Token economies can be effective in changing behavior within the hospital unit. Yet many have questioned how much generalization of such learning will occur when the patient is discharged into a setting where token reinforcement is not available. A limited token economy may effectively change specific behaviors of patients in mental hospitals, yet may not impact significantly on the overall functioning of the individual (Biklen, 1976). Gordon Paul and Robert Lentz (1977) developed an intensive social learning program that seemed to have broad effects on patients' inhospital and postdischarge functioning. Their work has become a modern classic, and similar programs have been implemented in a number of public mental hospitals.

The social learning approach implemented by Paul and Lentz was compared with a milieu program (therapeutic community) and a hospital unit that provided chemotherapy and little else but unstructured ward routines. The social learning program was based on a token economy that rewarded patients for engaging in specific appropriate behaviors. However, the program also rewarded patients for engaging in social interaction, communication, vocational and homemaking training, and many other skills needed for life in the community. Like the milieu program, the social learning program emphasized "normalization" of the ward environment. Patients and staff called each other by first names, staff wore street clothes rather than uniforms, and patients were called "residents." The three different programs were evaluated on many measures over a 54-month period.

Figure 21.1 illustrates the differences in overall functioning of subjects on the three units at each 6-month evaluation. The social learning program was markedly more effective after only 6 months, and continued to improve until the 12-month point. A decrease in effectiveness in the social learning program which occurred later was primarily due to the difficulty in dealing with assaultive behavior, a problem finally handled by using a **time-out technique** (withdrawal of positive reinforcement). Even during that period, however, the social learning program was more effective than milieu therapy or routine ward treatment. The effects of the social learning program appear to have generalized after discharge. More residents were discharged from the social learning program than from the milieu program or the routine treatment ward, and one-third more of those discharged from the social learning program stayed out of the hospital for at least 3 months. The success of this approach with chronic mental patients (in the 1977 Paul and Lentz study, the average length of hospitalization had been 14 years), is impressive. Today, many public mental hospitals have mounted similar programs for their seriously impaired residents.

Problems for the Public Mental Hospital.

Many positive changes in public mental hospitals have occurred since the early 1960s. When current conditions are compared to conditions prevalent 20 years ago, the changes are obvious. The modern public mental hospital is smaller, better staffed, has more well-trained professionals, and more active treatment programs than the public mental hospital of 20 years ago. In a typical state hospital, admission rates have increased by 300 percent in 20 years. The average length of stay of a patient has decreased from 20 years to seven months, and most patients stay less than two months (Redlich & Kellert, 1978). However, the readmission rates of discharged patients have increased dramatically. About 60 percent of admissions are people who have been hospitalized before. Patients are treated and discharged, but most have to be readmitted after spending some time in the community. The changes have not resolved all of the problems present in public mental hospitals.

Talbot (1980) has identified types of problems which prevent the public mental hospital from developing the kind of services necessary to provide adequate treatment. Two problems seem particularly important:

1. The public mental hospital must provide services for the treatment failures of all the other systems. These patients manifest very severe behavioral and emotional disorders, and are the most difficult to treat. About 35 percent of the patients admitted to public mental hospitals have been hospitalized against their will.

2. Public mental hospitals are low in resources. State and federal legislators (and the citizens who elect them) do not give public mental hospitals high priority in the budget. Effective treatment programs are expensive, perhaps far more expensive than the public is willing to pay.

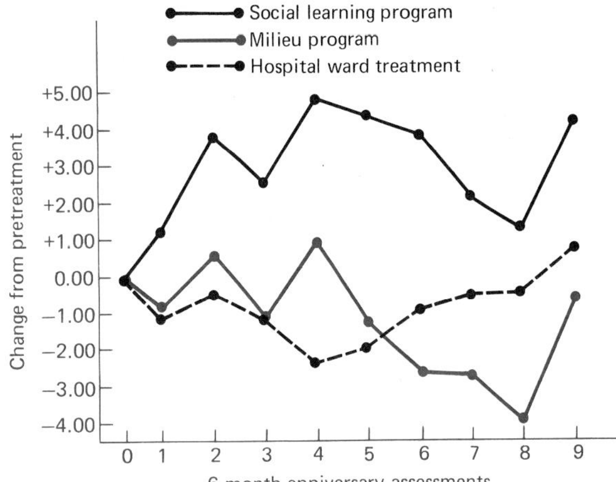

Figure 21.1. Change in overall resident functioning in social learning program, milieu program, and routine treatment ward.
For each program, $n = 28$.
Adapted from Paul and Lentz (1977, p. 374).

BEFORE AND AFTER THE HOSPITAL: COMMUNITY MENTAL HEALTH

In the mid 1950s, a great deal of dissatisfaction arose over the availability of treatment for emotional and behavioral disorders (see Highlight 21.2). Few services were available with the exception of private practitioners and inpatient mental hospitals. In 1963, recognition of the need for additional services led to the development of a system of care based in the community, rather than in long-term residential facilities.

The new system consisted of comprehensive community mental health centers, which were supported by tax dollars. This new approach was expected to make the public mental hospital obsolete, so that the state tax money used to support the mental hospital would ultimately replace the federal money used to fund the new centers. The centers were to provide community-based services in at least five areas: 1. inpatient services, 2. outpatient services, 3. emergency services, 4. pre- and posthospital care, and 5. education and mental health consultation. It was planned that 2000 such centers would be opened. However, by 1980, only enough funds for about 600 centers had been made available, and funding for many more appeared doubtful. The underlying philosophy of this movement towards community services for the mentally ill was that almost all, if not all, people with emotional or behavioral disor-

HIGHLIGHT 21.2
SHOULD PUBLIC MENTAL HOSPITALS BE CLOSED?

George Albee (1968) has proposed that public mental hospitals be taken apart "stone by stone and then, like the city of Carthage, plowed three feet under and sowed with salt." His emphatic statement reflects the belief of many mental health professionals and laypersons that the public mental hospital has so many historical problems that it can never provide a valuable treatment function.

There is little doubt that the public mental hospital setting can be dehumanizing and impersonal, and that generally less treatment is offered than in the best of the private sector. Furthermore, many people who would have been treated in public mental hospitals in the past can be treated in community settings. Still, tens of thousands of people manifest behaviors that will not be tolerated in community treatment facilities. Our society requires that these people be treated somewhere, and the public mental hospital is the only place available for such treatment. Certainly, public mental hospitals cannot and should not be closed until alternative settings that *can* effectively deal with this group of people have been developed. At the same time, people should not be admitted to public mental hospitals unless it is certain that they cannot be treated in a less restrictive setting.

ders could be treated on a short-term basis and did not require extensive hospitalization.

More treatment occurs on an outpatient basis today than 25 years ago. In 1955, 23 percent of all therapy was done on an outpatient basis (Bassuk & Gerson, 1978). In 1980 almost 70 percent occurred on an outpatient basis (Redlich & Kellert, 1978). The treatment provided within the community mental health center consists primarily of short-term supportive psychotherapy and chemotherapy based on the techniques discussed in Chapter 20. In addition, there is a major focus on crisis intervention (resolving problems before they become established as long-term disorders) and prevention of major emotional disorders. Ideally, an individual with serious problems would be able to obtain needed services before having to go to a public mental hospital, and thus the hospitalization would be prevented. Individuals discharged from inpatient treatment would be able to obtain ongoing treatment after discharge to reduce the likelihood of readmission. The people who are at high risk for hospitalization would be maintained at a more functional level in the community.

The community mental health movement has not been entirely successful. In recent years, for example, admissions to public mental hospitals have increased, not decreased. A major criticism of community mental health centers has been that they have focused their resources on providing care for moderately disturbed middle-class people who are interested in verbal psychotherapy (Chu & Trotter, 1974). Some very innovative programs have been established for high risk populations, but most of the chronically disabled people discharged from mental hospitals in the process of deinstitutionalization do not appear to be served by many community mental health centers.

Figure 21.2. Reduction in patient census of county, state, and federal mental hospitals during the deinstitutionalization era of community mental health.

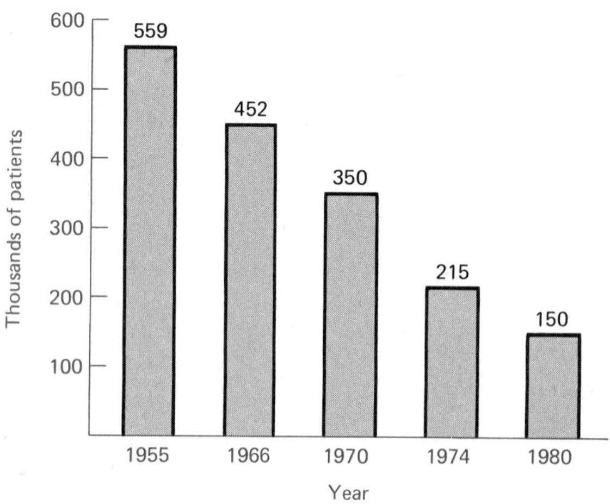

Problems in Deinstitutionalization

Where did all the people who were in mental hospitals in 1955 go? Where are the people who have developed chronic schizophrenia and other long-term disorders since 1955? Most of them are not regularly seen at community mental health centers. The reduction in patient populations of mental hospitals since 1955 (see Figure 21.2) cannot be taken as a sign that these types of individuals no longer exist.

In the two decades that mental hospital populations have been shrinking, there has been a corresponding increase in the number of privately owned, for-profit facilities called nursing homes or sheltered care facilities. These facilities originally provided a place for the chronically physically ill and elderly to live and receive minimal nursing care. Today almost one-third of the residents in these facilities are under the age of 65 and are diagnosed as mentally ill or mentally retarded (Bassuk & Gerson, 1978).

Although some of these private facilities are very good and provide active treatment programs, most appear to be very much like the custodial wards of the old mental hospitals. The staff are not experienced or trained to work with emotional and behavioral disorders, there are even fewer staff than in public mental hospitals, and the primary (often only) treatment is chemotherapy (M. Jones, 1975). Talbot (1979) has described this situation as a national disgrace. Have we simply exchanged the problem of the public mental hospital for the problem of the community nursing home? It appears so. In spite of the expansion in service delivery through the community mental health movement, many ex-mental patients live lives of quiet desperation and isolation in the deteriorating neighborhoods of major cities (Edelson, 1976).

SOCIAL CONTROL AND BEHAVIOR CHANGE

Many of the behaviors discussed in this text are not defined as personal problems by the person who manifests them. Society defines the behavior as problematic, and creates a system for dealing with people who manifest it. From this perspective, organized mental health services often act as agents of social control. As more has been learned about human behavior, more behaviors have been defined as requiring therapeutic intervention because they are seen as being due to biological malfunction or psychological disturbance. Whether persons want to change is often not the issue. We require that people change "for their own good." In the following two examples, people were hospitalized for treatment against their will. Neither person wanted to be treated, but release from the hospital depended on their cooperation and acceptance of medication and counseling.

> An elderly woman barricades herself in her apartment, and stops answering the door and the telephone. A neighbor becomes concerned after hearing strange wailing sounds coming from the apartment in the middle of the night, and calls the police. The police break into the apartment and find the old woman sitting in a corner. She babbles incomprehensibly in response to their questions. They take her to a local mental hospital for admission. At the hospital, she protests that no one has the right to put her in "this place."
>
> A man goes to a local mental health clinic and tells his social worker that the voice of his dead uncle is making him do things. He shows the social worker a butcher knife that he is carrying for protection from "evil" people, and asks the social worker if she is evil. The social worker suggests that he needs to see the doctor about his medication; he refuses; the police are called; and he is taken to the state mental hospital for admission.

If an individual is emotionally or behaviorally disturbed and desires treatment, few questions are raised about the therapist's right to try to change the person's behavior. However, when individuals behave in such a way that others (e.g., relatives, mental health professionals, or a court of law) require that they be treated involuntarily, against their will, the social control aspects of treatment raise many questions. There have been numerous abuses of involuntary confinement for the ostensible purpose of treatment (see Highlight 21.3). Concern about the abridgement of the rights of the mentally ill has become a major issue in mental health care in recent years.

The Rights of the Mentally Ill

The rights of the mentally ill are now in a process of clarification and expansion. Some mental health professionals would say that the pendulum has swung too far: Because of changes in mental health legislation, some people who should be treated are not being treated. These professionals believe that mental patients have gained the "right to rot" (Appelbaum & Gutheil, 1980).

How disturbed must people be before others have the right to force them into a treatment setting? For commitment, most state laws require that people's behavior present a serious danger to others or themselves (because of mental illness), or that people be so disturbed that they cannot care for themselves. These criteria may seem clear, but mental health professionals often have difficulty making accurate judgments on these issues.

What are the signs of dangerousness? Verbal threats? Argumentative behavior? Does actual physical violence have to occur? These issues have not been clarified by courts of law, so mental health professionals use their "best clinical judgment." When made, errors usually predict potentially dangerous behavior in people who are not actually dangerous to themselves or others. Mental health professionals want to avoid the risk of unfortunate events such as the following:

> Passersby and station personnel observe that a young woman has been spending several days at Union Station in Washington, D.C. Her behavior appears strange to others. She is finally befriended by a newspaper reporter who becomes aware that her perception of her situa-

HIGHLIGHT 21.3
KENNETH DONALDSON: TREATMENT OR IMPRISONMENT?

Kenneth Donaldson was involuntarily hospitalized on January 3, 1957. His father had petitioned the court of Pinellas County, Florida, for Kenneth's admission and the presiding judge ordered that Kenneth be hospitalized. Donaldson was diagnosed as manifesting paranoid schizophrenia, and the judge believed that he could be dangerous, based on the testimony of a psychiatrist. The judge told Kenneth that he would be sent to the hospital for a "few weeks" to "take some of this new medication" (Brooks, 1974). Kenneth Donaldson was not released until 1971, after he had instituted a law suit to force the state of Florida to let him out. Because of his religion (Christian Science), Donaldson refused to accept either medication or ECT during his almost 15 years of hospitalization. No other therapy was offered to him. But at no time in the 15 years was there a record of Donaldson ever engaging in a physically dangerous act towards others or himself. Donaldson's complaints and allegations of being locked up unjustly were brushed off by staff as being paranoid delusional symptoms.

Kenneth Donaldson sued the doctors responsible for his treatment for $38,500. The case was appealed by the doctors to the Supreme Court, which ruled in 1975 that individuals who are involuntarily confined in a mental hospital have the right to treatment that will provide a realistic opportunity of a cured or improved mental condition. Donaldson later settled with the physicians for a sum of $20,000.

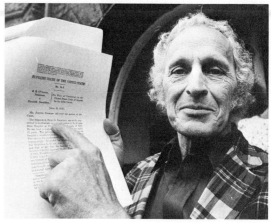

Kenneth Donaldson, 1975.

tion is profoundly unrealistic and that she is, in fact, delusional. He persuades her to accompany him to St. Elizabeth's Hospital, where she is examined by a psychiatrist who recommends admission. She refuses hospitalization and the psychiatrist allows her to leave. [The psychiatrist has no legal right to keep her against her will if she is not dangerous to herself or others.] She returns to Union Station. A few days later she is found dead, murdered, on one of the surrounding streets (Chodoff, 1976, p. 496).

In spite of the problems related to involuntary treatment, no one seriously suggests that it should not be used. However, because it is such a serious interference in personal liberty, the legal rights of patients are being emphasized—especially their right to receive treatment and their right to refuse treatment.

The Right to Treatment. No individual should be involuntarily confined because of a cognitive, emotional, or behavioral disorder unless treatment appropriate to the disorder is provided. The presence of mental illness does not justify confinement against an individual's will if treatment is not provided. In the past, people could be locked away in custodial hospitals which had no treatment services. Today, if society requires that an individual be involuntarily hospitalized, it has the obligation to offer treatment services.

The Right to Refuse Treatment. It might seem that an individual should have the right to refuse any sort of unwanted treatment. After all, you do not *have* to have surgery if a doctor tells you that you need it, do you? We do have the right to be physically sick, don't we? In fact, there are times when we do not have the right to refuse treatment. If we have a highly contagious disease that presents a public health hazard, we can be legally forced to have treatment. In a similar vein, people have the right to refuse treatment for mental disorder. However, if their mental disorder presents a serious danger to themselves or to others, the treatment can be given against their will. Again the issue of dangerousness becomes a critical factor in determining what can legally be done; and the mental health professional has the difficult task of deciding if the individual is, in fact, dangerous.

Many of the criticisms of human rights violations in involuntary treatment center on the prediction of dangerousness. The bulk of the evidence indicates that mental health professionals are not especially accurate in predicting which chronic patients will be dangerous at some distant time (Shah, 1977, Steadman & Cocozza, 1974). When such predictions are made, the mental health professional identifies a high number of **false positives:** people identified as dangerous who never engage in dangerous acts. John Monahan (1978), however, suggests that short-term predictions in emergency situations may be more accurate. Virtually no research has been done on the accuracy of short-term prediction of dangerousness in extremely disturbed individuals, although the prediction of dangerousness in this situation is extremely relevant for mental health treatment.

The rights of mental patients are now much clearer than they have been in the past. This does not mean that their rights are not being violated; there is still a gulf between the laws and reality (Meisel, 1975). Mental health professionals, attorneys, and judges must still struggle with questions about the conditions that legally justify limiting an individual's freedom in order to change disordered behavior.

Criminal Acts, the Law, and Mental Health

An accepted concept in our system of justice is that before an individual can be judged guilty of a criminal act he or she must be responsible for the behavior. In addition, in order to be tried in a court of law, the individual must be competent to understand the legal proceedings. Mental health professionals have become involved in both these issues.

Competency to Stand Trial. The individual's guilt or innocence cannot be resolved until she or he is found competent to stand trial. At any time in public mental hospitals, there are about 15,000 individuals who are charged with crimes, but who are considered to be incompetent to stand trial (Pendleton, 1980). A sample case follows:

> A young man is arrested because he fits the description of a rapist who attacked a 13-year-old girl in full view of several witnesses. At a court hearing, a psychiatrist and psychologist testify that the young man is a disturbed schizophrenic who thinks that the officers of the court are demons, and who "knows" that his attorney is the devil's disciple. In view of this testimony, the court concludes that the young man is not competent to stand trial. He is committed to a mental hospital until the time that he becomes competent to stand trial.

To be competent, one's mental illness must not interfere with the ability to cooperate in one's defense. The person must understand the charges and the consequences of a guilty verdict; the person also must understand the purpose of the trial and the roles of the various members of the court. The person does not have to be "cured" or "normal." About 90 percent of the individuals not originally found competent become competent to stand trial after treatment (Pendleton, 1980).

The Insanity Defense. In some cases, an individual is ultimately found competent to stand trial, but then found **not guilty by reason of insanity** (NGRI). An example follows:

> She seemed little different from any other mother at the nursery school—at least not until she and her children had not appeared for two weeks and she was found sitting in her apartment, with the children dead, hanging from coat hooks in the closet. The world was an evil place, you see . . . and the children had to be saved from it. She had killed them because God had commanded her to send them to him. Even now she could hear the roaring voice of the "evil ones" who were frustrated because she had cheated them of her children.

Because testimony was presented that this young woman was so mentally disordered at the time of the killings that she was not responsible for her behavior, she was not convicted of the crime or sent to prison. Instead she was committed to a mental hospital for treatment. Thirty-six months later she was discharged as recovered; she now lives in a midwestern city.

The successful use of **insanity** as a defense is rare. Less than 1 percent of defendants in murder trials use this defense. It is however, controversial, and cases in which it is used often get major publicity. "Insanity" is a legal term, not a scientific one. Our legal system has traditionally provided the possibility of a defect of reasoning due to mental disorder to be used as a defense in criminal cases. Until recent years, individuals who were found not guilty by reason of insanity generally wound up imprisoned in mental hospitals for longer periods than they would have spent in prison if they had been convicted. Currently, the increased emphasis on patient rights has resulted in rulings in many jurisdictions which require that such people be released if their mental disorder no longer presents an immediate threat to others (Herbert, 1979).

The release of such individuals from mental hospitals within a "short" time (usually several years) of their trial has resulted in a great deal of adverse public reaction. Although such individuals were found not to have been responsible for their acts, the public apparently does not want them to be free. In response to this feeling, some state legislatures (e.g., Michigan and Illinois) have enacted laws that allow a finding of **guilty but mentally ill** (GMI). Under this finding individuals can be treated, but when treatment has been completed, they are kept in prison to serve the remaining portion of judicial sentence, with the same possibility of parole or release as any other prison inmates convicted of the same offense.

The treatment of individuals who have been found incompetent to stand trial, not guilty by reason of insanity, or guilty but mentally ill, is complicated by their legal status. As with other involuntary patients, the therapist may have to treat someone who does not believe he or she should be treated. When individuals accept that they have committed the act, they may become extremely depressed. It is especially difficult for people to deal with their feelings about killing a family member. When these issues can be worked through, the therapist and patient may be left facing an outcome which may be more negative than time spent in a mental hospital. The individual who is now competent to stand trial may have to go to court, where she or he expects to be found guilty. If already tried, the individual may know that recovery means a transfer to prison. Either of these possibilities may work against effective treatment. In addition, the therapist is likely to have personal concerns about the patient's stability. One must be very sure of one's clinical judgment to recommend the discharge of an individual who is known to have committed an act such as murder.

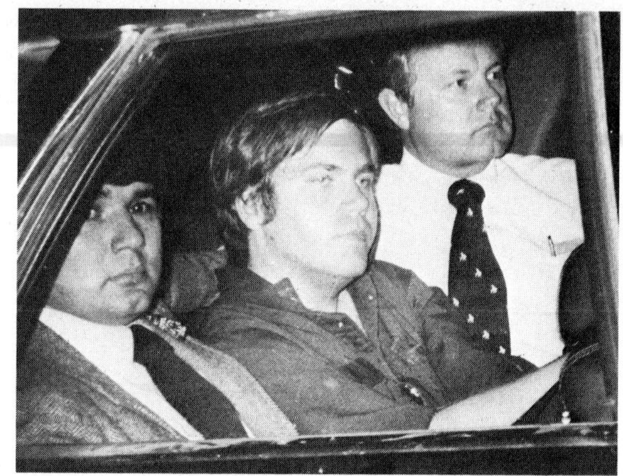

On June 21, 1982, John W. Hinckley, Jr., charged with shooting President Ronald Reagan and three other men, was found not guilty by reason of insanity. Four of the defense psychiatric experts claimed that Hinckley suffered from severe mental illnesses, including process schizophrenia. Prosecution psychiatrists, however, said Hinckley was suffering only minor personality disorders and minor depression. The jury verdict prompted angry demands in Congress for sharply limiting the law which permits the insanity plea. The photo shows Hinckley (center) flanked by Federal agents, being driven from U.S. District Court on March 30, 1981.

The loose confederation of agencies and systems that make up mental health services in the United States has many problems. The problems seem to impact most severely on public mental hospitals. The other mental health service systems have the option (and usually exercise it) of funneling the most difficult chronic, high risk patients to the public mental hospital, especially when such persons resist treatment. The problem is compounded by the courts, who commit the patients both civilly and in criminal cases, demand that treatment be given, and act as a guardian of the rights of all patients. Do we expect too much of these facilities, considering the amount of resources our government provides? In the long run, society's expectations of the public mental hospital may have to change. As more and more alternatives to hospitalization are developed in the community, perhaps public mental hospitals will deal only with legally involuntary patients. The emphasis on safeguarding the rights of the involuntary mental patient may lead to an insistence on funding adequate resources for this group of people. In the long run, the public mental hospital may come to provide a limited but adequate service as one part of the mental health treatment system.

ALTERNATIVES TO TRADITIONAL SOLUTIONS

Public and private mental hospitals, psychiatric units in general hospitals, private therapists in the community, and many comprehensive community mental health centers all offer relatively traditional treatment services. The awareness of professionals and laypeople that these systems are only partial solutions to the problem of abnormal behavior has led to the development of many alternatives. Three examples of the many types of alternatives are lodge programs for chronic ex-patients, self-help groups, and programs for the prevention of abnormal behavior.

Alternative Living for the Ex-Mental Patient

In the mid-1960s psychologist George Fairweather created an alternative living situation for ex-mental patients (Fairweather et al., 1969). It became known as a community "lodge" program. Chronic male patients in a federal mental hospital were trained in homemaking, vocational, and social interaction skills. A cohesive sense of group identity was established with these men. The goal was for the men to become a small, self-supporting society, almost a family. This was followed by the rental of a whole motel and the development of a small business (lawn care) which these men could operate as a group. The men were discharged from the hospital and moved to the motel. The living situation and business were coordinated by the men, under the supervision of a professional mental health worker. As the men became self-supporting over a period of several years, the supervision and guidance of the professional was withdrawn and the men were left on their own. Not all the men were able to maintain themselves outside the hospital, but many were.

This communal living experiment demonstrated that most chronically disabled mental patients can live outside a hospital setting, work, and manage their own behavior. They can even manage the complexities of a group living situation and run their own business. The success of the program has led to the development of many similar lodge-type programs around the country which provide a nonhospital, nonnursing home, environment for ex-mental patients.

New Support Systems

Self-help groups have become an important avenue of assistance for individuals with behavioral and emotional problems. It has been estimated that over 500,000 such groups are

This patient of a state mental hospital is employed in a furniture repair shop. He lives in a half-way house on the hospital grounds.

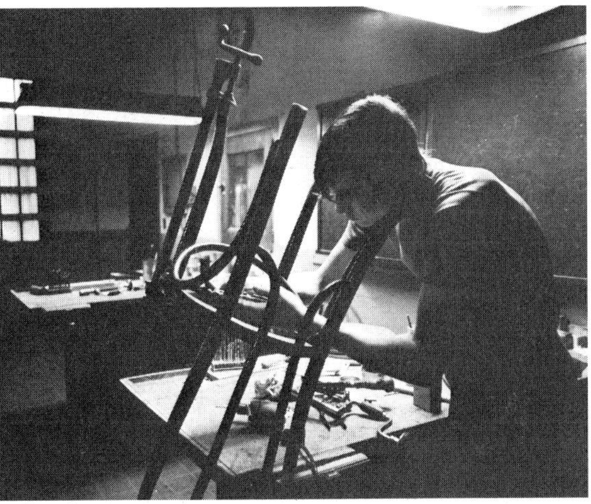

currently in operation in the United States (Riessman, 1979). The classic example of a self-help organization is Alcoholics Anonymous (AA). In self-help groups individuals with problems gather together in a relatively permanent relationship to provide each other with mutual support and assistance in dealing with any one or a number of life's problems. Many of these groups are openly antagonistic or hostile to the traditional solutions offered by professionals. Gartner and Riessman (1977), two important proponents of mutual help or self-help groups have acknowledged the dangers associated with an overreliance on self-help groups to solve human problems. The self-help approach for example, may result in "victim blaming." A person who does not improve may be told by peers that she or he simply has not tried hard enough. In addition, a mutual help group may foster unnecessary dependence, rather than growth and individuality.

Prevention As An Alternative Approach

Once abnormal behavior has become established, effective treatment is not an easy task. It would be better if we could prevent the occurrence of abnormal behavior or mental disorder in the first place (Bloom, 1981). Prevention can be grouped into three levels: primary, secondary, and tertiary. Most of the treatment approaches discussed in this text fall into the secondary and tertiary categories. **Tertiary prevention** focuses on reducing the rate of residual defects from mental disorder, after treatment has been completed. **Secondary prevention** involves early identification of the development of a problem in behavior, and the implementation of approaches that will prevent the development of a full-blown disorder. **Primary prevention** is the process of identifying and eradicating the causes of disorders in order to lower their incidence of occurrence.

Examples of primary prevention include the following:

1. Genetic counseling to reduce the incidence of some types of mental retardation.
2. Educational programs on the dangers of various types of substance abuse.
3. Programs in training positive parenting skills.
4. Cognitive stimulation programs for children at risk for cultural-familial retardation.
5. Work-safety education programs for workers who deal with toxic chemicals that can lead to organic brain syndrome.
6. Senior citizen programs for the elderly to prevent social isolation.

Examples of secondary prevention include the following:

1. Early identification of childhood problems (phobias, school refusal, withdrawal) and implementation of treatment.
2. Early identification of mental retardation and implementation of social and educational training.
3. Early identification of major emotional disorder in adults and treatment (such as early treatment of the first signs of depression).
4. Crisis intervention for individuals who are faced with stressful experiences such as job loss, family deaths, illness, major disasters.
5. Hospitalization and effective treatment of major mental disorders.

Examples of tertiary prevention include the following:

1. Vocational training for recovered ex-mental patients.
2. Self-help groups for individuals who have recovered from emotional or behavioral disorders (for example, weight reduction maintenance groups; Alcoholics Anonymous).
3. Sheltered workshops for the mentally retarded.
4. Community lodge programs for ex-mental patients.

The Impact of Alternative Solutions

It is extremely difficult to assess the overall effects of alternative solutions and preventive approaches to the problem of abnormal behavior (Lamb & Zusman, 1981). Individual programs have been demonstrated effective in reaching their goal. For example, the community lodge program developed by George Fairweather reduced the likelihood that its members would be rehospitalized. An excellent example of an effective primary prevention program is the routine screening of infants for PKU (phenylketonuria), one cause of mental retardation. In Chapter 18 we saw that the detection of this abnormality allows a dietary treatment that can keep mental retardation from developing in children who have this problem.

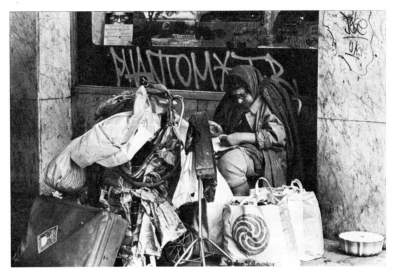

The discharge of large numbers of ex-mental patients into large urban areas has resulted in the existence of many homeless street people, who are unable to properly provide for themselves. Alternative living situations are desperately needed.

Often, the broad-scale mandated implementation of alternative approaches to deal with or treat abnormal behavior has unexpected results. In the 1960s and 1970s, comprehensive community mental health centers were considered to be a bold new approach—an alternative to the mental health services system then current. It was presumed that community treatment services would make state mental hospitals obsolete, and introduce a new era in treating human problems. These expectations were unfulfilled. In fact, as a result of the community mental health movement, admissions to public mental hospitals have increased. Deinstitutionalization has resulted in large numbers of ex-mental patients living in custodial nursing homes and "sheltered" homes or worse, wandering the streets. They went out of the custodial wards in mental hospitals and *into* custodial wards in the community. On the positive side, community mental health centers have brought services to large numbers of people who were not served or were underserved before the centers opened, and these centers have prevented the institutionalization of many people.

Alternative solutions to dealing with abnormal behavior seem to be effective in reaching limited goals. They may have a broad impact on changing the mental health services system. However, their impact has yet to be adequately evaluated (Braun et al., 1981).

THE PROBLEM OF DEALING WITH ABNORMAL BEHAVIOR

Abnormal behavior can be a concern for virtually everyone. A glance through a major daily newspaper reveals how frequent such behavior is. More personally, each of us may have concerns about our own functioning; or we may have a close friend, relative, or acquaintance who seems to have a problem similar to some described in this book. Many people have asked why these problems cannot be treated or solved more quickly, more effectively, and with fewer negative consequences.

Research and Services

In spite of all that we know (and we know a great deal), we have much more to learn about human behavior. The science of human behavior is young, and the right questions often have not been asked. Frequently, when the right questions have been asked, they have not been asked in a way that a useful answer can be found. The painstaking accumulation of knowledge continues, and many professionals consider the current times to be among the most exciting in the study of human behavior. We seem to be beginning to ask at least some of the right questions in the right way.

Many of the disorders that people experience have fairly effective treatments. However, these treatments often cannot be effectively delivered to those who need them. The numbers of trained personnel and good facilities are limited. The primary problem in this delivery is money. The best services are available only to those who can pay. Taxpayers (you and I) seem to be unwilling to foot the bill for much more than already exists in the way of public services. Some pessimists believe that no amount of money, no matter how huge, would be enough to provide services for all those who have cognitive, emotional, and behavioral problems.

Values and Judgments

The things that we do about certain behaviors depend on the values and attitudes of the society that we live in. We make judgments based on values and attitudes about what "should" be done. To use an extreme example, what should we do about "criminal" behavior? Is the armed robber or murderer "sick," is the behavior learned, or is the perpetrator "bad"? Should the criminal be treated, reeducated, or punished? What should we do when some people manifest bizarre behaviors which are simply unappealing? Should we force them to change against their will? Should the "community" be forced to become more accepting of these behaviors? The scientific study of human behavior can answer some of our questions about the reasons why people behave the way they do, and about how we can change behavior with the best chance of success. Whether we will make a major effort to use this knowledge on a broad scale to grapple with the important problems of our citizens depends on many other factors.

SUMMARY

1. Organized treatment of abnormal behavior reflects a concern for providing social control of deviant behavior and a concern for the welfare of the individual.

2. Voluntary admission to a public or private mental hospital may occur either when an individual evaluates himself as needing inpatient treatment, or when other people such as family, friends, or the court persuade the individual to admit himself. If necessary, admission may occur involuntarily by order of a court.

3. Psychiatric units in general medical hospitals have multiplied in the past 20 years. These facilities provide short-term intensive treatment, and can accept emergency admissions around the clock.

4. Most patients can recover substantially in the general psychiatric unit in one to two weeks, and return to the community for outpatient care.

5. The general hospital psychiatric unit usually does not treat patients whose disturbance is likely to require lengthy treatment or patients who must be treated involuntarily.

6. The private mental hospital provides services to about 3–5 percent of the people who require inpatient care. These facilities are usually small, well staffed, and have intensive programs. Treatment in such hospitals is extremely expensive. Private mental hospitals usually will not accept patients who are resistant to treatment.

7. There are approximately 150,000 inpatients in public mental hospitals. Public mental hospitals are required to accept disturbed individuals who cannot afford treatment elsewhere, those whose disorder requires lengthy treatment, and those who must be treated against their will.

8. Public mental hospitals have had the difficult task of providing services without necessary resources. They have often been accused of being custodial warehouses. Conditions have improved dramatically in these facilities since the deinstitutionalization of chronic patients, but these institutions are still resource poor.

9. Many hospitals have developed therapeutic communities or milieu therapy; these programs allow patients to have more control over their lives. A major emphasis in many hospitals is the application of behavioral therapy programs called token economys. Some hospitals have instituted social learning programs which use token economys, but also focus on the teaching and development of skills important for survival in the community after discharge. These programs have been effective with many patients.

10. Comprehensive community mental health centers were developed as one aspect of the community mental health movement. These facilities provide varied services, including: 1. inpatient services (usually in conjunction with a general hospital psychiatric unit), 2. outpatient services, 3. emergency services, 4. pre- and posthospital care, and 5. education and mental health consultation.

11. The community mental health center was intended to make public mental hospitals obsolete. The centers have not achieved this goal; and they have been criticized for focusing on services to moderately disturbed middle-class people, rather than to the type of person who is likely to be admitted to a public mental hospital. In spite of this criticism, many innovative programs have been implemented.

12. Deinstitutionalized mental patients have often been discharged into community settings that many professionals consider to be no better than a custodial ward in a mental hospital.

13. Problems in the provision of treatment in mental hospitals have led to the current emphasis on the rights of mental patients. People can be involuntarily hospitalized if they present a danger to themselves or to others. The definition and prediction of dangerousness is a difficult task for mental health professionals. The level of accuracy of these judgments has been constantly criticized.

14. Two types of patients who have an involvement with the criminal courts must be treated by public mental hospitals. People are admitted to mental hospitals who are incompetent to stand trial because of mental illness. If and when they achieve competency, they will be tried for their alleged criminal behavior. A second group consists of those who have been found either not guilty by reason of insanity (NGRI) or guilty but mentally ill (GMI). These individuals are hospitalized after their trial. If treatment is successful, people found NGRI will be discharged into the community, and those found GMI will serve any remaining portion of their sentence before being released from custody.

15. Concerns over the problems of traditional solutions to abnormal behavior have led to the development of alternative programs. New programs such as community lodges for ex-mental patients, and support systems such as self-help groups hold some promise for providing services to disturbed individuals.

16. The difficulty in treating abnormal behavior has stimulated a search for ways to prevent the development of abnormal behavior. Three levels of prevention are commonly identified. Primary prevention identifies and eradicates the basic causes of abnormal behavior. Secondary prevention involves early identification and treatment of the disorder. Tertiary prevention consists of reducing the residual defects which may be present after a disorder has been treated.

17. Dealing with the problem of abnormal behavior is a difficult and complicated task. Although we know a great deal about human behavior, our knowledge is limited. The delivery of services to those who need them is compromised by major deficits in our resources of staff and facilities. Many questions remain about what we should or should not do about certain human behaviors; such questions arise out of our values and attitudes.

KEY TERMS

Custodial care. The provision of care and custody rather than treatment. The emphasis is on isolating the person from the community, providing food and lodging, but not on active treatment.

Deinstitutionalization. The movement of the focus of treatment and care from large residential institutions to community based organizations.

Insanity. A legal term which means that a person is not responsible for his or her behavior if that behavior is due to mental illness.

Involuntary treatment. Treatment administered against the individual's will; usually by court order.

Milieu therapy. A treatment approach that attempts to make the total environment therapeutic.

Total institution. An institutional setting in which most aspects of the person's life are controlled by others. Examples include military service, prisons, and mental hospitals.

GLOSSARY

Abnormal Deviating from the norm.

Abnormal psychology A subfield of psychology that focuses on behavior that is distressing to a person or society or which is otherwise identified as abnormal. Psychologists who specialize in this area are usually called clinical psychologists.

Abstinence Not engaging in a behavior. Usually used in the context of avoiding an intoxicating drug.

Acute hallucinosis A state of drug intoxication characterized by hallucinations.

Acute schizophrenia Schizophrenia characterized most typically by sudden onset and severe symptoms.

Adaptive behavior Behavior that allows or helps a person adjust to new situations or increased demands.

Addictive personality A particular personality type that is more likely to lead to addiction.

Adjustment disorder Disordered behavior or symptoms that are a result of major life changes or stressors. Reduction in stress typically leads to decrease in symptoms.

Adrenaline A hormone secreted by the adrenal medulla during strong emotions. Also called epinephrine.

Affect Emotion or feeling.

Affective disorders Disturbances in mood that are associated with changes in behaving and thinking.

Agoraphobia Fear of open places that may become so severe that a person cannot leave his or her house.

Alcoholic personality See addictive personality.

Alcoholics Anonymous A self-help group that is organized and operated by alcoholics with the goal of maintaining sobriety.

Alcoholism The excessive consumption of alcohol to the extent that it seriously interferes with personal, social, or occupational functioning; or the physiological dependence on alcohol.

Alzheimer's disease A progressive dementia characterized by specific neurological degeneration.

Amnestic syndrome Loss of memory due to organic damage to brain tissue.

Amniocentesis Sampling of fluid that surrounds the fetus so that fetal cells can be tested for chromosomal defects.

Amphetamine A drug that produces a stimulating effect.

Amphetamine psychosis A psychotic disorder characterized by hallucinations and persecutory delusions that can result from chronic use of amphetamines.

Anaclitic depression Major depression that sometimes occurs when an infant is separated from its mother for long periods of time.

Anal stage According to psychoanalytic theory, the period when the anus becomes the center for gratification. Pleasure derives from the expulsion or retention of feces.

Analgesic A substance or event that leads to insensitivity to pain.

Anhedonia The inability to experience pleasure or joy.

Animal magnetism A force similar to magnetism believed to be present in animals and humans by followers of Anton Mesmer.

Anticipatory anxiety Anxiety experienced in anticipation of some event.

Antipsychotic drugs Drugs that reduce the symptoms of psychosis.

Antisocial personality disorder A disorder that is marked primarily by antisocial behavior without shame or remorse

Anxiety Feelings of fear and apprehension often associated with signs of autonomic nervous system arousal.

Anxiety disorder Disorder in which anxiety is the dominant symptom.

Aphasia Loss or inability to communicate in language symbols through speech or writing due to organic brain disorder.

Apraxia Inability to engage in a familiar sequence of behaviors due to organic brain damage.

Arousal dysfunction Psychosexual disorder in which the individual experiences lessened or no sexual arousal.

Asylums Institutions that offered asylum or sanctuary to disadvantaged people, particularly the mentally disturbed.

Attribution theory Theory that people attribute their behavior to specific aspects of themselves or their environment and that the attributes people think exist can then influence subsequent behavior.

Aura Subjective sensations like odors, sounds, or visual experiences that precede migraine headaches or epileptic seizures.

Autism Thinking and behaving is dominated by inner processes with little relationship to reality.

Autonomic nervous system The part of the nervous system that regulates involuntary processes like glandular secretion, visceral muscle contraction, heart rhythm, and rate.

Aversive counterconditioning Also called aversive conditioning. The pairing of a noxious or unpleasant stimulus with a behavior in order to decrease the frequency of that behavior.

Aversive stimulation Application of a noxious, unpleasant stimulus.

Aversive treatment See aversive counterconditioning.

Avoidance learning The process in which an organism learns to avoid an unpleasant experience by making a different response.

Avoidant personality disorder A personality disorder characterized by extreme sensitivity to rejection and avoidance of relationships, even though the person wants to have relationships with others.

Barbiturate A class of drugs that have a sedative effect and which can lead to psychological and physical dependence.

Baseline observation A procedure in which the base rate of a behavior is observed and recorded.

Behavior disorder A disorder manifested in behavior.

Behavioral interview A clinical interview in which the focus is on identifying specific problem behaviors and the reinforcement contingencies that led to or maintain the behavior.

Behavioral medicine An area of specialization that

focuses on the effects of behavior on physical health and illness and on treatment approaches that have a behavioral orientation.

Behavioral assessment An assessment approach that emphasizes the observation of behavior as opposed to the assessment of intrapsychic events.

Behavioral therapies Treatment approaches that are based on principles of learning.

Biofeedback The use of instrumentation to provide information to a person on biological processes that are not usually available to the person's awareness.

Biological therapies Treatment that consists of biological interventions like the administration of medication.

Bipolar affective disorder A disorder in which a person has at least one disturbance of mood that consists of mania and one that consists of depression.

Bisexual A preference for sexual partners of both sexes.

Blood alcohol content The level of alcohol in the blood that is measured as a percent of the total volume of blood.

Blunted affect A noticeably reduced emotional range.

Borderline personality disorder A personality disorder characterized by intense, variable relationships with others, and labile emotions.

Cardiovascular system A major organ system composed of the heart, arteries, veins, and capillaries.

Case study An approach to studying human behavior that focuses on intensive studies of individuals.

Castration Removal of the male's testes, which results in lowered levels of male sexual hormones.

Castration anxiety In the psychoanalytic framework, castration anxiety refers to the fears a boy has about being castrated by his father because the boy has sexual feelings toward his mother.

Catatonic excitement An agitated state seen in some catatonic schizophrenics.

Catatonic immobility A condition in which a person with catatonic schizophrenia becomes unresponsive and physically immobile.

Catatonic schizophrenia A type of schizophrenia characterized by immobility or excitement and at times strange mannerisms or repetitious stereotyped behavior.

Cathartic method A technique that encourages the extensive ventilation of buried feelings, leading to a sense of release.

Cerebral arteriosclerosis A disorder in which fatty deposits adhere to the walls of the vascular system and reduce blood flow.

Cerebral metabolism The process in which brain cells "burn fuel" (use nutrients) to produce energy.

Choreiform movements Involuntary movements, most noticeably writhing movements of the limbs, due to organic brain disorder.

Chromosomes Structures in the cells that carry genetic information. There are 23 pairs of chromosomes in human cells.

Clang association A symptom consisting of mental associations that result in speech having a nonsensical rhyming quality.

Classical conditioning The process in which a stimulus (later called a conditioned stimulus) is paired repeatedly with an unconditioned response. The conditioned stimulus eventually elicits a conditioned response (previously the unconditioned response).

Client-centered therapy A type of humanistic therapy, developed by Carl Rogers, that emphasizes an accepting atmosphere on the part of the therapist and lets clients make their own decisions.

Clinical interview An interview that has the goal of obtaining relevant historical and current life information in order to identify a client's problems and plan treatment.

Close binding mother A mother who becomes overly involved with a child, and creates a greater than normal dependence in the child.

Cocaine A major stimulant drug that induces a sense of euphoria or well-being.

Cocaine psychosis A psychotic state of hallucinations, delusions, and agitation that may result from cocaine intoxication.

Cognitions Mental events including thoughts, attitudes, beliefs, and expectations.

Cognitive behavior modification A treatment approach that emphasizes changing cognitions and using behavioral techniques to modify behavior.

Cognitive behavioral therapy See cognitive behavior modification.

Cognitive learning Learning that involves cognitions in determining behavior.

Cognitive rehearsal A technique in which a person rehearses behavior mentally.

Cognitive-semantic therapy A treatment approach that attempts to change cognitions primarily through verbal therapy, although some practice of behavior may be involved.

Cognitive theory See cognitive learning.

Collective unconscious Carl Jung's concept of a racial unconscious transmitted from generation to generation that all people share.

Compulsions Behavior that an individual feels compelled to perform in spite of its irrationality.

Compulsive personality disorder A personality disorder characterized by long-standing compulsiveness in behavior and emotional aloofness.

Concussion Temporary disruption of consciousness due to a blow to the head. No permanent physical damage occurs to the brain.

Condition of worth A term of Carl Rogers that describes a condition placed on a person by a significant person like a parent. The condition determines the person's sense of worth, for example, "I'll value you *if* you never get angry."

Conditioned Repeated pairing of a stimulus with a response so that the stimulus comes to elicit the response with high probability.

Conditioned response A response that is elicited by a conditioned stimulus.

Conditioned stimulus An initially neutral stimulus that becomes capable of eliciting a conditioned response after repeated pairing with an unconditioned stimulus.

Conditioning See classical conditioning and operant learning.

Conscience The aspect of the superego that determines whether behaviors are experienced as proper.

Consensual validation The confirmation of experiences, beliefs, or attitudes through the discovery that other people share them.

Control group A group of subjects in an experiment that are not subject to the variable being introduced. The control group is the standard against which the experimental group is compared.

Contusion A bruise in the brain tissue.

Conversion disorder A disorder involving physical symptoms that have no physical cause. The name derives from one theory that psychological problems are *converted* into physical manifestations.

Coronary artery disease Disease of the arteries often called "hardening of the arteries."

Correlational chart A graphic representation of correlated measurements.

Correlation coefficient A statistical measurement of the degree to which two variables are related. Correlations range between +1.00 and −1.00.

Counterconditioning A process in which a conditioned response is replaced with an incompatible response through a new conditioning process.

Countertransference The transference of irrational feelings by the *therapist on to* the patient. Countertransference is believed by psychoanalytically oriented therapists to interfere with effective therapy.

Covert sensitization The association of unpleasant mental images with undesirable behavior in order to reduce the frequency of that behavior.

Crazy A popular colloquialism for psychotic or otherwise disturbed behavior.

Crisis A period of psychological disequilibrium that occurs in the face of severe stress.

Crisis decompensation Deterioration of functioning during a time of crisis.

Crisis intervention counseling Counseling that has the goal of intervening in crisis behavior in order to prevent the development of lasting problems.

Cross-dress To wear the clothing of a member of the opposite sex.

Cultural-familial retardation Pertaining to genetic and social or cultural factors that may result in mental retardation.

Cultural relativism The position that normality or abnormality of behavior is relative to the culture in which the person has developed.

Custodial care Provision for physical needs without active treatment.

Cyclothymic disorder A disorder of mood in which mood alternates between highs and lows but which is not severe enough to be considered a *full* bipolar affective disorder.

Defense mechanisms Behaviors used to avoid anxiety-provoking experiences. The term derives from psychoanalytic theory positing that the person is not aware of the reason for the behavior.

Degenerative dementia Deterioration in cognitive functioning due to organic brain deterioration that continues to progress.

Deinstitutionalization The process of discharging long-term patients from mental hospitals into the community for less restrictive treatment.

Delirium A state of fluctuating confusion and disorientation due to probable metabolic disturbance in brain function.

Delirium tremens A state of delirium and psychotic behavior resulting from chronic alcoholism that may appear when the person stops drinking.

Delusion A fixed false belief not shared by others.

Delusion of jealousy A false belief that a spouse or love is unfaithful that persists in spite of evidence to the contrary.

Dementia Deterioration in intellectual functioning and behavior due to organic disturbance of the brain.

Dementia praecox An early term for what is now called schizophrenia.

Demonic possession Possession of the soul by a demon who can then control a person's behavior.

Dependence In the context of drug use, the term refers to a physiological need for the drug in order to avoid withdrawal symptoms.

Dependent personality disorder A personality disorder in which extremely dependent behavior is a long-term characteristic of a person.

Dependent variable A variable that is measured after manipulation of an independent variable to determine if any change has occurred.

Depersonalization disorder A disorder in which a person experiences a sense of unreality.

Depression A disorder characterized by sadness, guilt, apathy, and dejection.

Depressogenic schemata Aaron Beck's term for patterns of thinking that may lead to depressive feelings.

Derailment A symptom of thought disorder seen in schizophrenia in which the individual is unable or unwilling to maintain a logical stream of thought. Their train of thought "derails."

Detoxification The process of reducing the toxic or intoxicating levels of a drug in a person's body.

Developmental period The period of life during which most psychological and physical development occurs. It is usually presumed to end around the age of 18 to 21. However, many current theorists think that psychological development continues throughout life.

Deviant Deviating from the norm.

Diagnosis The process of arriving at an identification of a disorder that a person has, or the disorder itself.

Diagnostic nomenclature A system for naming disorders.

Diathesis A predisposition toward a disorder.

Dilate To increase in size.

Discriminative stimulus A stimulus that acts as a signal that a certain behavior will lead to a particular consequence such as reinforcement.

Displacement The shifting of emotions from one object, person, or situation to another. Usually the second object, person, or situation is less threatening than the first.

Dissociation A state in which a person continues to act but the behavior is not available to normal awareness.

Dissociative disorders See dissociation.

Dopamine A neurotransmitter that is present in the brain and which may be in excess in schizophrenia.

Double-bind A type of relationship characterized by conflicting messages. The relationship is confusing but important and the person cannot escape it.

Double-blind study A type of study in which the subjects *and* the experimenter are blind to (do not know) which subjects are receiving the actual treatment and which are getting a placebo.

Down's syndrome A type of mental retardation due to the presence of an extra chromosome.

Drift phenomenon An explanation of the higher incidence of schizophrenia in lower socioeconomic classes proposing that some schizophrenics drift into lower classes because they cannot adjust to the expectations of middle- and upper-class existence.

Dyspareunia A sexual disorder characterized by pain during sexual activity.

Dysthymic disorder Mild to moderate depression.

Echolalia A symptom consisting of the repetitive echoing of what another person says rather than responding with rational speech.

Echopraxia The mechanical repetition of the behavior of another person when that behavior occurs.

Ego According to psychoanalytic theory, that part of the personality that mediates among id impulses, the superego, and reality.

Ego alien Foreign to the person's view of himself or herself.

Ego defenses See defense mechanisms.

Ego dystonic homosexuality Homosexuality that is upsetting to the person who exhibits it.

Ego ideal Types of behavior that are characteristic of what the person sees as the higher values in life.

Ego syntonic Acceptable or fitting in with the person's conception of himself or herself.

Egocentricity Self-centeredness.

Ejaculatory dysfunction A disorder of sexual functioning in which the male most typically ejaculates prematurely, but in some cases it consists of an inability to ejaculate.

Electra conflict A conflict in girls between sexual desire for their fathers and the threat of punishment for those forbidden feelings.

Electroconvulsive therapy A treatment in which electrical current is passed between electrodes placed on the temple. The current causes random firing of brain neurons.

Electrodermal response A change in skin resistance to the passage of electrical current that occurs when there is autonomic nervous system arousal.

Electroshock treatment See electroconvulsive therapy.

Emotional disorder A general term for many disorders that consist of disturbances of emotion or behavior.

Emotional numbness The lack of emotional feeling sometimes seen in persons who have experienced a disastrous event.

Empathy A deep sense of understanding of another person's experiences.

Endocrine system A system of glands that produces hormones.

Endogenous depression A depression in which no precipitating environmental causes can be found.

Endorphin A biochemical substance produced by the body that has some effects similar to an opiate.

Enkephalin Type of biochemical substance that includes endorphins.

Enuresis Prolonged bladder incontinence past the usual age at which bladder control is developed.

Epidemiological research The study of the distribution, incidence, and associated variables of illness.

Epilepsy A disorder that consists of convulsions and loss of consciousness, alterations in consciousness, or automatic behavior.

Erectile dysfunction A sexual disorder of males in which penile erection is absent or only partial during sexual activity.

Essential hypertension Chronic high blood pressure in the absence of known physical disorder.

Exhibitionism In the context of a sexual disorder, the exposing of one's genitals in unacceptable circumstances.

Existential therapy Therapy that focuses on peoples' alienation from others and on developing the ability to be authentic in one's relationships.

Exogenous depression A depression that was apparently precipitated by external stresses or losses.

Exorcism A ritual that has the goal of casting a devil or demon out of a presumably possessed individual.

Expectancy The expectations held toward a person.

Experimental group The group of subjects that are

given the experimental manipulation in an experiment.

Extinction Repeated presentation of a stimulus without reinforcement of a subsequent response. Without reinforcement the response decreases in frequency and finally does not occur. It becomes extinguished.

False positive The positive prediction that an event will occur that turns out to be false.

Family therapy Therapy that involves virtually all members of a family in the therapy process.

Fetal alcohol syndrome A syndrome of birth defects due to chronic abuse of alcohol by the mother during pregnancy.

Fetish Use of a nonliving object or an unusual part of the human body to enhance sexual gratification.

Fever treatments A treatment for general paresis in the 1920s, 1930s, and 1940s, which consisted of inducing a high fever in patients. Use of the treatment generalized to other major disorders.

Fight or flight response Reaction of the autonomic nervous system to stressful circumstances that includes changes in blood flow, heart rate, muscle tension, and other functions.

Flashback The sudden imaginal recurrence of a past experience.

Flooding A treatment technique that consists of keeping the patient in the presence of an anxiety-provoking stimulus until the anxiety decreases.

Free association A technique of psychoanalysis in which the patient is encouraged to say whatever comes to mind without censoring it.

Ganglia Bundles of nerve terminals.

Gastric acids Acids that assist in the digestion of food in the gastrointestinal tract.

Gender identity disorder A disorder of subjective sexual identity.

General adaptation syndrome A syndrome identified by Hans Selye that occurs when people are under stress and which leads to lessened resistance to physical disease.

General paresis A disorder due to invasion of the brain by syphilis organisms. It is also called neurosyphilis.

Generalized anxiety disorder The chronic experience of anxiety that is not associated with a particular situation or object.

Genes Carriers of genetic information that are in the chromosomes.

Genetic counseling Counseling of individuals who may or do carry genes that may produce birth defects in their children.

Genital stage A psychosexual stage according to Freud during which mature sexuality develops after puberty.

Genotype The inherited potential to develop certain characteristics.

Gestalt therapy A therapy developed by Fritz Perls that emphasizes here and now experiences.

Grand mal epilepsy Epilepsy that consists of a convulsive seizure and loss of consciousness.

Grandiose thinking Believing that one has special importance beyond the reality of the situation.

Guilty but mentally ill A legal finding in a court trial that the person is guilty of the crime but should receive special treatment because he or she was mentally ill at the time of the act.

H-Y antigen Hormonal substance that is important in the development of physical sexual characteristics.

Habituation The decrease in intensity or frequency of a response due to the repeated presentation of the eliciting stimulus.

Hallucinations The experience of perceptions or sensations from an external source when no actual source exists.

Hallucinogen A drug that induces major changes in sensation and perception.

Hara-kiri A ritualized form of suicide in Japanese culture used when the individual has "lost face."

Hebephrenia A subtype of schizophrenia characterized by severe personality disorganization, inappropriate behavior, and affect of silliness. In DSM-III it is called disorganized schizophrenia.

Hemodialysis Removal of toxins or waste products from the blood by artificial means, usually by passing the blood through fine filters in a dialysis machine.

Heterogeneity The condition of many differences among concepts, objects, and so on that have been lumped together in one group. Heterogeneity within groups is undesirable in classification systems.

High risk population A group of subjects who for some reason can be identified as being at greater risk than the random population for a disease or disorder.

High risk studies The study of high risk populations.

Histrionic personality disorder A personality disorder characterized by self-centered, dramatic emotional reactions and behavior, as well as dependency.

Homeostatic The condition of being in balance or equilibrium. A homeostatic mechanism strives to maintain homeostasis.

Homogeneity The condition of having similarity between members of a class.

Homosexuality Sexual preference for members of the same sex.

Hormone A biochemical substance secreted by hormone glands that have wide-ranging effects on the physiological functioning of the body.

Humanistic approach An approach emphasizing that people should be viewed as unique individuals, each of whom is valuable in his or her own right and who can determine his or her own fate.

Humanistic psychology See humanistic approach.

Humors Substances once presumed to be important in determining health, sickness, and behavior. Classic humors were blood, phlegm, black bile, and yellow bile.

Hyperactivity A disorder characterized by high levels of activity, restlessness, and poor attention span and concentration.

Hyperkinetic syndrome See hyperactivity.

Hypervigilance An unusual sensitivity to the actions of others and their possible relationship to oneself.

Hypnotic induction The process of facilitating the presence of a hypnotic state in a subject.

Hypnotism The use of hypnosis, a trancelike state induced through suggestion in the subject.

Hypochondriasis A disorder or trait that results in an individual being overly preoccupied with the physical functions of the body and fearful of developing or having a physical disease.

Hypothalamus A part of the brain implicated in the autonomic nervous system response, in possible eating disorders, and in emotion.

Hypothesis A statement that is tested in research.

Hysteria A label applied to behavior that is stereotypic of the dependent female or applied to disorders that involve bodily symptoms or altered states of consciousness.

Hysterical personality See histrionic personality disorder.

Iconic storage Short-term storage of mental representations of perceptions.

Id According to psychoanalytic theory, part of the personality that consists of instinctual impulses that demand immediate gratification.

Ideas of reference The belief or "feeling" that events have special meaning about oneself.

Identification The process of taking in or incorporating into the personality characteristics of an important person. In psychoanalytic theory it is seen as an important defense mechanism.

Idiot savant A retarded individual, usually at the moderate level, who possesses an unusual skill or ability.

Inappropriate affect The expression of emotions that are not appropriate for a situation.

Independent variable The variable that is manipulated in an experiment.

Infantile autism A severe disorder that begins early in childhood (often before the age of 3) that consists of extreme social unresponsiveness and strange behavior.

Illusion A misinterpretation of actual stimuli.

Immunology The study of the functions of the immune system of the body that fights disease.

Impotence The inability of the male to attain an erection sufficient to complete the sexual act.

Incest Sexual behavior between close blood relatives.

Incest taboo Cultural prohibitions against incest.

Insidious Slow, subtle development of unpleasant or bad consequences.

Insight-oriented psychotherapies Psychotherapy that emphasizes the development of self-understanding, usually in the context of an intense relationship with a therapist.

Instrumental learning Learning to make a response or emit a behavior that has an effect on the environment that is reinforcing.

Insulin shock A convulsive therapy that consists of the administration of insulin until the person enters a coma.

Intellectualization The isolation and walling off of emotions by focusing on *thinking about* things rather than by allowing oneself to emotionally experience them.

Intelligence quotient A numerical estimate of relative intellectual ability. It is usually based on a normal probability distribution with the number 100 used as the midpoint of the distribution of scores.

Intelligence test A test, usually standardized, that measures samples of the abilities that are presumed to reflect intelligence.

Intermittent schedule of reinforcement Schedule of reinforcement in which not every correct response is reinforced.

Internist A physician who specializes in internal medicine.

Intracranial pressure The pressure of the cerebral fluid within the cranial cavity.

Intrapsychic Mental events that are not directly observable, including wishes, beliefs, thoughts, and according to psychoanalytic theory, unconscious events.

Introjected objects A psychoanalytic term that refers to objects (people) whose characteristics have been taken into the personality of a person.

Intrusive thoughts Thoughts that seem to intrude upon one's thinking. The person experiences these intrusive thoughts as persistent and usually unpleasant.

Involuntary treatment Treatment against a person's will.

LSD Lysergic acid diethylamide, an hallucinogen.

La belle indifference A blasé lack of concern seen in many people with conversion disorder.

Labile Rapidly changing or variable.

Latency The period of childhood that Freud believed consisted of a lack of sexual interest.

Law of effect A behavior law formulated by E. L. Thorndyke that states in essence that behavior is determined by its effect on the environment.

Lead encephalitis An inflammation of brain tissue due to the toxic effects of ingestion of lead.

Learned helplessness A reaction of helplessness that is learned through experiencing inescapable aversive events about which the individual believes he or she can do nothing.

Learning theory A general term for types of theories that propose ways in which behavior is learned according to principles established in psychological laboratory experimentation.

Libido A psychoanalytic term that refers to a reservoir of psychic energy.

Life instincts In psychoanalytic theory, those instincts that motivate pleasure-seeking and sexual behavior.

Limbic system Part of the lower brain associated with some emotional and motivational functions.

Lithium carbonate A trace element used to treat mania.

Liver cirrhosis A condition in which damage to liver tissue occurs.

Lobotomy The surgical removal or cutting of areas of the brain in order to treat disordered behavior.

Looseness of association See derailment.

Magical thinking A type of thinking characterized by belief in superstition and other irrational beliefs.

Maladaptive Characterized by a relative inability to adapt to changing life circumstances, or behavior that results in detrimental consequences.

Malingering Intentional faking of abnormal behavior or physical illness.

Mania A disorder characterized by elation, euphoria, grandiosity, and at times irritability and hostility.

Manic-depressive psychosis See bipolar affective disorder.

Manie sans délire Early term for antisocial personality (insanity without confusion).

Marihuana The leaves of the *Cannabis Sativa* plant that contains a psychoactive substance.

Masochism Obtaining sexual gratification or enhancement of pleasure by having pain inflicted upon oneself.

Medical disease model The view that abnormal behavior is like a physical disease.

Melancholia A term for severe depression with psychotic symptoms.

Mental illness A term for disturbed emotions or behavior implying that it is a sickness like any other physical problem.

Mental retardation An intellectual level that is at most an IQ of 70 or below, beginning during the developmental period, and which is associated with deficits in social adaptation.

Mescaline A hallucinogen present in a cactus.

Methadone maintenance A treatment for heroin addiction in which the addict is given methadone, which prevents physical withdrawal but in moderate doses does not produce psychological effects.

Metrazol shock A convulsive therapy induced by the administration of a camphor derivative called metrazol.

Milieu therapy A treatment approach in which people are given responsibility for many aspects of decision making and staff relate more as equals than as experts.

Modeling Learning through observing the example of other people. Similar to imitative learning but broader in implication.

Monozygotic twins Twins who develop from the union of a single egg and sperm.

Mood congruent Consistent with a mood.

Moral anxiety Anxiety over violating moral standards learned from parents.

Moral treatment Term used to describe treatment in asylums in the nineteenth century when inmates were treated with greater humanism and dignity then before.

Multi-axial diagnostic system A diagnostic system in which several factors are classified on different axes.

Multiple personality A dissociative disorder in which a person develops two or more distinct personalities that alternate in control of behavior.

Mutism The unwillingness or inability to speak.

Narcissistic personality disorder A personality disorder characterized by self-centeredness, self-importance, and minimal care for others.

Narcotic A drug that induces a drowsy, floating feeling and can reduce the perception of pain. Taken for its pleasurable feelings, a narcotic can lead to psychological and physical dependence.

Neo-Freudian A term used to label psychoanalytically oriented theorists who modified Freud's theories.

Neurofibrillary tangles A characteristic sign of some types of degenerative dementia. Under microscopic examination, tangled fibers appear in the nerve cells.

Neurologist A physician who specializes in the treatment of organic disorders of the nervous system.

Neuron An individual nerve cell.

Neuropsychologist A psychologist who has specialized in brain-behavior relationships.

Neurosis A term often used generally to categorize nonpsychotic disorders that primarily involve excessive anxiety, fear, or depression. Because the term is associated with psychoanalytic theory, its use is becoming less widespread by theorists of other persuasions and is no longer used in DSM-III.

Neurosyphilis Syphilis affecting the central nervous system. See general paresis.

Neurotic anxiety In the psychoanalytic view, anxiety that is irrational or due to unconscious conflict.

Neurotic needs Needs that result from unresolved unconscious conflicts.

Neurotransmitter A biochemical substance that acts as a transmitter across a synaptic cleft from one neuron to another.

Nihilistic delusion A fixed belief that the world no

longer exists or that things in it such as people are dead or unreal.

Norepinephrine A hormone that acts as a biochemical neural transmitter.

Normal Not deviating from the norm. Behavior that is not disturbed.

Normal probability curve A bell-shaped distribution usually found when a large sample of people are measured on many characteristics.

Norms A standard based on the commonness of a behavior.

Not guilty by reason of insanity A legal finding in a trial that absolves a person of legal guilt for the commission of an act if the person, due to the presence of mental illness, was determined to be unable to conform his or her behavior to the law.

Objective personality test A test of personality in which the items and responses are standardized through the administration of the test to large numbers of people and which do not require subjective interpretation by the examiner.

Observational learning Learning that occurs through the observation of a model that engages in the behavior to be learned.

Obsessions Thoughts and impulses that are recognized as irrational but which the person cannot discard.

Obsessive-compulsive disorder A disorder consisting either of obsessions or compulsive behaviors or both.

Oedipus conflict Relating to the Oedipal period or conflict that involves sexual impulses toward the parent of the same sex.

Operant behavior therapy Therapy based on the principles of operant learning.

Operant learning Learning that occurs because a response (operant) is reinforced by a change in the environment.

Opiate A type of drug that reduces pain and can lead to euphoria, for example, morphine and heroin.

Opioids See opiate.

Oral stage From birth to about one year old. The period that Freud believed was characterized by "sexual" gratification through stimulation of the mouth.

Organic mental disorder Abnormal behavior associated with organic brain dysfunction.

Organic viewpoint The view that abnormal behavior has a primarily organic cause.

Organic wisdom A concept of Carl Rogers that the organism (person) has an innate awareness of what is good for it.

Organism A living being.

Orgasmic dysfunction A disorder in which there is an inability to achieve a satisfactory orgasm.

Orgasmic reconditioning A conditioning procedure that uses masturbation to condition sexual arousal to acceptable sexual objects and to reduce sexual arousal to less acceptable objects.

Orthomolecular psychiatry A viewpoint in psychiatry that abnormal behavior is due primarily to deficits in vitamins and trace elements in the body. The view is controversial.

Over-the-counter drugs Drugs that can be legally purchased over the counter without a physician's prescription, for example, aspirin.

PCP Phencyclidine (street name, angel dust). An animal tranquilizer which produces disorientation, confusion, and stupor in humans.

Panic disorder An anxiety disorder in which the person is subject to unpredictable attacks of severe anxiety.

Paranoia A disorder characterized by well-organized delusions (fixed, false beliefs), occasionally with hallucinations.

Paranoid Characterized by suspiciousness and beliefs of persecution by others.

Paranoid disorders A group of disorders that includes paranoid state, paranoia, and shared paranoid disorder.

Paranoid personality disorder A personality disorder consisting of chronic suspiciousness and aloofness.

Paranoid pseudocommunity The actually unrelated group of people that the paranoid individual perceives as joined in a conspiracy against him or her.

Paranoid schizophrenia A subtype of schizophrenia characterized by paranoid beliefs of a simple and disorganized type associated with the personality disorganization of schizophrenia.

Paranoid state Paranoia that has a relatively sudden onset, often associated with major life changes or stress.

Paraphilias Sexual behavior that involves preference for nonhuman objects, the need for pain or humiliation, or nonconsenting relationships.

Parasympathetic nervous system Division of the autonomic nervous system that is primarily associated with maintaining bodily systems in a homeostatic balance that conserves energy.

Parataxic distortion A term coined by H. S. Sullivan to identify reactions that are primarily based on fantasy rather than on reality.

Participant modeling A treatment approach in which the subject first views then participates in the behaviors of a model.

Passive-aggressive personality disorder A disorder that consists of chronic passive stubbornness or subtle obstruction of demands placed on an individual.

Pedophilia erotica A term now in disuse, used to label sexual preference for children.

Pellagra A disorder caused by a vitamin deficiency that, aside from its physical symptoms, can result in psychosis.

Penis envy In Freudian theory, the female child is believed to envy the male's penis (father's) and if this is not resolved she becomes competitive with males in adult life. The concept is currently disputed.

Pepsinogen An enzyme important in digestion of food.

Personality disorder A disorder consisting of enduring personality traits that result in maladaptive behavior.

Personality inventory A psychological test that inventories personality by the presentation of many items that are usually answered simply yes, no, or don't know.

Personality trait A long-term characteristic of a person's personality functioning.

Pervasive developmental disorder A disorder beginning in childhood in which severe behavioral problems occur in all areas of functioning.

Petit mal epilepsy A seizure disorder in which there is no convulsion but there is momentary loss of awareness.

Phallic stage A psychoanalytic psychosexual stage of development during which the Oedipal conflict is important.

Phenomenal field The totality of an individual's experience at any one moment.

Phenothiazine A class of drugs used in treating schizophrenia, also called ataraxic drugs, antipsychotic drugs, or major tranquilizers.

Phenotype The actual physical and behavioral characteristics of an individual that are the result of an interaction of genetic endowment and environmental experience.

Phenylketonuria (PKU) A recessively transmitted disorder of protein metabolism that uncorrected can lead to mental retardation.

Phobia An irrational fear associated with a particular object or situation.

Phobic disorder See phobia.

Physiological predisposition A physical defect that leaves a person vulnerable to a disorder.

Placebo Any ineffective treatment (inert pill or other therapy) that is used to control for a subject's expectation that he or she will get better because of the treatment. If the subject does improve, it is due to the placebo effect or expectation held by the subject.

Play therapy A treatment approach for children that uses play as a vehicle for the therapy.

Pleasure principle In psychoanalytic theory, the principle that id impulses seek immediate gratification.

Post traumatic stress disorder An adjustment reaction following a major stressor such as a natural disaster or combat.

Postnatal The period following birth.

Predisposition A factor that makes it more likely that an individual will develop a disorder under certain conditions, such as stress.

Preliminary crystalization In the development of paranoid beliefs, the point at which the person mistakenly realizes that others are to blame for his or her troubles.

Premorbid Prior to the development of an illness.

Premorbid competence The level of coping skills or adjustment prior to the onset or appearance of symptoms of a disorder.

Prenatal Prior to birth.

Preparedness theory The theory that individuals are prepared through either innate factors or psychological variables to respond with greater autonomic reactions to some stimuli rather than to others.

Presenile dementia Degenerative dementia that begins prior to the age of 65.

Primary antisocial personality Antisocial behavior that is associated with lack of remorse, shame, and guilt.

Primary prevention Activities that focus on the prevention of problems that can ultimately lead to the development of disordered behavior.

Primary process thinking Irrational thinking or images that are characteristic of the id impulses.

Proband In a genetic study, the individual who is used as the comparison or index case to which other individuals (often the person's twin) are compared.

Process schizophrenic A schizophrenic disorder that develops gradually over a period of years, characterized by poor premorbid competence.

Projection The attribution of an impulse, belief, or feeling onto another person when in fact the person projecting it has the impulse, belief, or feeling but does not recognize it. Considered a defense mechanism by psychoanalytic theorists.

Projective tests A personality evaluation technique in which it is presumed that people project important aspects of themselves onto ambiguous stimuli.

Prototype classification A classification approach that does not require absolute heterogeneity or homogeneity. Overlap between categories is acceptable on some variables.

Pseudoneurological Having the appearance of a

neurological problem but actually nonorganic in origin.

Pseudopregnancy False pregnancy in which actual pregnancy symptoms appear.

Psilocybin A hallucinogen derived from a mushroom.

Psychedelic Having an effect on the mind. Usually used in the context of hallucinogenic drugs.

Psychic determinism The position that all behavior is ultimately determined by unconscious events in the mind and that there is no free will.

Psychoanalysis A theoretical and therapeutic approach developed by Sigmund Freud.

Psychogenic amnesia Amnesia due to psychological rather than to organic factors.

Psychogenic fugue A state of altered consciousness in which the individual leaves his or her familiar surroundings, assumes a new identity, and does not have conscious awareness of the old life and identity.

Psychogenic pain disorder A disorder in which a person has pain with no organic cause, or organically caused pain is experienced as much more severe than the organic damage would warrant.

Psychomotor retardation The slowing of physical and psychological processes.

Psychopathology The manifestation of emotional or behavioral disorder.

Psychopathy A term sometimes used to refer to antisocial personality disorder.

Psychophysiological disorders Disorders in which there is actual physical tissue change or damage associated with psychological factors or stress.

Psychosexual disorder A disorder that involves sexual dysfunction due to psychological factors rather than to organic factors.

Psychosexual dysfunction See psychosexual disorder.

Psychosexual stages In Freudian theory, psychosexual development occurs through the resolution of five stages: oral, anal, phallic, latency, and genital.

Psychosis A general term for severe disorders that involve more or less personality disorganization, hallucinations, and delusions.

Psychosocial support system The network of people who care about a person and who can offer emotional and social support to the person during times of stress.

Psychosomatic A somewhat out-of-date term for psychophysiological disorders.

Psychotic Manifesting a psychosis.

Psychotic depression Severe depression associated with loss of contact with reality, hallucinations, and delusions.

Psychotropic drugs Drugs that affect the mind.

Random sample The selection of a sample of individuals or other objects of study from a larger population strictly on the basis of chance.

Rape Forcible sexual intercourse with a nonconsenting person.

Rating scale A set of items that allows an individual to rate himself or herself or others along a continuum for one or more variables.

Rational-emotive therapy A treatment approach developed by Albert Ellis that emphasizes both emotional and cognitive change by using primarily verbal techniques.

Rationalization A defense mechanism in which a person gives a good reason for behavior rather than the real reason.

Reaction formation A psychoanalytic defense mechanism in which a person reacts to unconscious wishes by behaving in an opposite manner in order to guard against the expression of the desires of the unconscious.

Reactive schizophrenia One categorization of schizophrenia that is applied when the onset of the disorder is sudden and associated with some life stress.

Reality anxiety Anxiety that is due to actual dangers such as being threatened by an armed robber or a dog known to be vicious.

Reality testing Behavior that tests the reality of one's perceptions by gaining obvious or subtle feedback.

Reciprocal inhibition A principle used in systematic desensitization positing that anxiety is inhibited by antagonistic responses like relaxation.

Regression In psychoanalytic theory, a defense against anxiety that consisted of reverting to less mature types of behaviors that were previously satisfying.

Reinforcement A consequence (contingency) following a response that increases the likelihood that the response will occur in the future in similar situations.

Relaxation therapy A therapy that emphasizes the learning of a procedure for relaxation that can be used to decrease or prevent anxiety.

Relaxation training See relaxation therapy.

Reliability The degree to which a measurement yields the same result when repeatedly applied to the same data.

Reliable See reliability.

Repression The act of pushing unacceptable or painful experiences, desires, or impulses into the unconscious or out of conscious awareness.

Reversal design An experimental design in which behavior is measured, conditions are changed, behavior is remeasured, and then the conditions are *reversed* back to the original conditions and behavior is measured once again.

Rh factor A measurement of the presence or absence of certain antibodies in the blood of a woman. If the Rh antibodies are present, a fetus may have problems in obtaining sufficient oxygen in its blood.

Role enactment The degree to which a person behaves in expected ways when performing social roles such as "mother" or "policeman" or "doctor."

Role expectations The expectations that members of a culture hold for social roles such as policeman, husband, or child.

Ruminative thinking Mental rehashing of past or future behavior, problems, and so on.

Sadomasochist An individual who obtains sexual gratification through both the infliction and receipt of pain.

Schizoid Characterized by withdrawal, seclusiveness, oversensitivity, and eccentricity.

Schizoid personality disorder A personality disorder characterized by schizoid behavior.

Schizophrenia A severe disorder that consists of personality disorganization, withdrawal, blunted or flat affect, disordered thought process, and hallucinations and delusions.

Schizophrenic disorder See schizophrenia.

Schizophrenic spectrum disorders Disorders seen in relatives of schizophrenics at a greater frequency than the general population. Includes schizotypal and schizoid personality disorders, among others.

Schizophreniform disorder A disorder similar to schizophrenia that has a relatively sudden onset and is of short rather than chronic duration.

Schizophrenogenic Leading to the development of schizophrenia.

Schizotypal personality disorder A personality disorder consisting of egocentricity, seclusiveness, and eccentric thought and behavior.

School phobia Irrational fear of school attendance.

Secondary antisocial personality An individual characterized by antisocial behavior that is due to other disorders such as depression.

Secondary prevention Early identification and treatment of disorders before they can become chronic.

Secondary process thinking Reality-oriented thinking processes characteristic of the ego.

Sedative A drug that can induce a relaxed state and sleep.

Self-actualization motive The fulfilling of one's full potential.

Self-concept An individual's sense of identity.

Self-help group A group of individuals who band together for mutual assistance and support in dealing with a problem.

Self-instructional training A cognitive behavioral approach for teaching an individual to modify his or her cognitions and behavior.

Self-mutilation The purposeful injury of one's own body.

Senile dementia Progressive degenerative dementia that first becomes apparent after the age of 65.

Senile plaques Microscopic sign of senile dementia that consists of deposits of foreign substances in nerve cells.

Sensate focus A type of training that emphasizes deriving pleasure from touching and being touched by a partner, at first with no pressure to culminate in sexual intercourse.

Separation anxiety Anxiety experienced when separated from someone a person is dependent on.

Serotonin A neurotransmitter.

Serum cholesterol The level of cholesterol in the blood.

Sex reassignment surgery Surgery that changes the sexual genitalia of males to females and vice versa. A treatment for gender identity disorder.

Sexual sadism Sexual enhancement from the infliction of pain.

Sexual surrogate The controversial use of a paid individual to train a person in sexual techniques through practice of sexual intercourse.

Shaping Training of behavior in which successively closer approximations of the target behavior are reinforced until the desired behavior has been "shaped."

Shared paranoid disorder A paranoid disorder in which the delusional system is shared by two or more persons.

Simple phobia Irrational fear of a specific object such as a spider or snake.

Social learning theory Learning theory whose major proponent is Albert Bandura. The theory accepts concepts of classical and operant conditioning but also emphasizes modeling and cognitive learning.

Social phobia Irrational fear of social situations such as public speaking.

Societal-reaction theory A theory that abnormal behavior is a reaction to the expectations of complex social systems.

Sociopathy Another term for antisocial personality disorder.

Somatic Pertaining to the body.

Somatic delusion A fixed, false belief whose content revolves around bodily complaints.

Somatization disorders Disorders that involve concerns about physical functioning and misinterpretation of physical sensations.

Somatoform disorders Disorders of psychological origin that take the form of physical symptoms when there is no organic change.

Somnambulism Sleepwalking as a dissociative experience in adults.

Spectator role Taking a distant, evaluative role while engaging in sexual intercourse, which complicates anxiety over sexual functioning.

Spontaneous remission Recovery from a disorder with little or no treatment.

St. Vitus dance A form of mass madness in medieval times.

Startle response Sudden involuntary behavioral reaction to unexpected stimuli.

State anxiety Anxiety primarily due to the current conditions the person is experiencing rather than to long-term personality variables.

Stereotypic behavior Frequent repetition of behavior in a mechanistic fashion.

Stress The perception that events are disruptive and threatening.

Stress inoculation training A cognitive behavioral technique that teaches people to change their cognitions in order to deal with stress in more effective ways.

Sublimation Defense mechanism through which id impulses are directed into socially valued pursuits such as art and the composition of music.

Substance use disorders Disorders involving the abuse of substances that have effects on the psychological functioning of the individual.

Sudden death Death that occurs unexpectedly under conditions of intense emotion.

Superego In psychoanalytic theory, that part of the personality that is made up of the conscience and the ideal values incorporated from the parents.

Supportive psychotherapy Psychotherapy that has the goal of providing support while an individual resolves problems or weathers a crisis. It is usually of short term.

Survival guilt A sense of guilt experienced by survivors of a disaster when their behavior has not met their own expectations. The guilt often involves wondering why the person has survived while others have died.

Survivor shame See survivor guilt.

Survivor syndrome See survivor guilt

Sympathetic nervous system The division of the autonomic nervous system that activates many bodily systems under conditions of stress. The activation of these systems is called the fight or flight response.

Syndrome A group of symptoms that occur together in a disorder.

Syphilis A parasite infection transmitted through sexual contact. A venereal disease.

Systematic desensitization A behavioral technique in which relaxation is used to densensitize a person to stimuli that elicit anxiety.

Tactile insensitivity A lack of sensitivity to touch.

Tarantism A term used in southern Europe referring to mass madness during the medieval era.

Tardive dyskinesia A neurological disorder that is a side effect of antipsychotic medication. It is characterized by involuntary muscle tremors and movements, especially in the face and tongue.

Temperament Characteristic emotional tone, level of tension, and behavior that is apparent from birth.

Temporal lobe Portion of the brain located roughly in the area of the temple.

Temporal lobe epilepsy Epilepsy in which the locus of the disturbance first occurs in the temporal lobe. It is sometimes characterized by impulsive or apparently automatic behavior during the seizure.

Tertiary prevention Treatment aimed at reducing the long-term effects of chronic mental disorder.

Thanatos In psychoanalytic theory, thanatos is the death instinct.

Theory Systematically organized body of knowledge, assumption, and principles that is used to analyze, predict, or explain a set of phenomena.

Therapeutic community See milieu therapy.

Thought stopping A technique for stopping unwanted thoughts.

Time-out technique A technique utilizing the withdrawal of the opportunity for obtaining positive reinforcement in order to decrease the frequency of occurrence of undesirable behavior.

Token economy An organized system of reinforcement using tokens such as plastic chips or play money that can be redeemed for commodities, privileges, or access to activities.

Tolerance The development of a condition in which increasing dosages of a drug are required to obtain equivalent effects.

Total institution An institution that has control over most aspects of an individual's life. Examples include the army, prisons, and mental hospitals.

Trait anxiety Anxiety that is apparently due to long-term aspects of the individual's personality.

Tranquilizing medication Medication that reduces the subjective sense of anxiety.

Transference In psychoanalytic therapy, the transference of irrational feelings by the patient onto the therapist.

Transsexualism A disorder in which an individual experiences himself or herself as being a member of the sex opposite to his or her anatomical sexual endowment.

Transvestites Individuals who cross-dress in order to enhance sexual gratification.

Trephining An ancient treatment in which a hole was bored or chipped in a person's skull, probably to release a demon believed to be possessing the person.

Type A behavior A characteristic style of behavior that consists of driven overcommitment to activities like work and an inability to relax.

Uncomplicated bereavement The normal emotional mourning process that occurs when a loved one has died.

Unconditioned response A response elicited by a stimulus.

Unconditioned stimulus A stimulus that elicits a response.

Unconscious conflicts Conflict between unconscious impulses and the threat of punishment that would occur if the impulses were expressed. The person is not aware of the conflict.

Unconscious processes Psychological processes of which the subject is not aware.

Undifferentiated schizophrenia A subtype of schizophrenia that is characterized by a mixture of symptoms seen in the other schizophrenic subtypes.

Undoing A defense mechanism consisting of behaviors that are intended to atone for past misdeeds, real or imagined.

Unipolar depression Depression that is not associated with episodes of mania.

Vagal nerve Nerve that is important in the activity of the heart muscle.

Vaginismus A disorder consisting of an involuntary contraction of the muscles in the lower third of the vagina that results in difficult or painful intercourse or makes penetration impossible.

Valid See validity.

Validity The degree to which a measuring device actually measures what it is supposed to measure.

Vasodilation Enlargement of the diameter of blood vessels that increases blood flow.

Vicarious extinction The extinction of a behavior that occurs when one observes the behavior being extinguished in another person (a model).

Visceral organs The organs in the abdominal cavity (stomach, intestines, liver, kidneys, etc.).

Voluntary musculature The striated muscles over which people have voluntary control.

Voodoo death Death that results from a voodoo curse when the subject of the curse believes in voodoo and expects to die.

Voyeurism The enhancement of sexual gratification through secret viewing of another person disrobing or of persons engaging in sexual activity.

Vulnerability hypothesis A model of major disorders proposed by Joseph Zubin. Individuals have predispositions that leave them more or less vulnerable to the development of a psychological disorder.

Waiting list control group In treatment evaluation studies, a group placed on a waiting list to which the treatment group can be compared. Any change in the waiting list control group subjects is usually attributed to the passage of time.

Waxy flexibility A symptom of catatonia in which the person can be molded into positions as if made of wax and will stay in the position for long periods.

Wernicke's area A part of the brain important in verbal comprehension.

Withdrawal The pulling back from social interaction into an existence of isolation from others.

Working through Confronting and reliving painful experiences until more adaptive ways of behaving and relating are developed.

Zeitgiest The spirit of a particular time in history.

BIBLIOGRAPHY

A.A.M.D. *Manual on terminology and classification in mental retardation.* Special Publication No. 2. Washington, D.C.: American Association on Mental Deficiency, 1977 revision.

Abel, E. L. Fetal alcohol syndrome: Behavioral teratology. *Psychological Bulletin,* 1980, *87*(1), 29–50.

Abel, G. G. Physiological evaluation of the sexual offender. *Tenth Annual Conference on Law, Psychiatry and Mental Health,* Chicago, 1979.

Abel, G. G., Barlow, D. H., Blanchard, E. B., & Guild, D. The components of rapists' sexual arousal. *Archives of General Psychiatry,* 1977, *34*(7), 895–903.

Abel, G. G., & Blanchard, E. B. The role of fantasy in the treatment of sexual deviation. *Archives of General Psychiatry,* 1974, *30*(4), 467–475.

Abel, G. G., Blanchard, E. B., & Becker, J. V. An integrated treatment program for rapists. In R. T. Rada (Ed.) *Clinical aspects of the rapist.* New York: Grune & Stratton, 1978.

Abood, L. G. Some chemical concepts of mental health and disease. In *The effect of pharmacologic agents on the nervous system,* vol. 37. Proceedings of the Association for Research in Nervous and Mental Disease. Baltimore: Williams & Wilkins, 1959.

Abrams, R., & Taylor, M. A. Unipolar mania: A preliminary report. *Archives of General Psychiatry,* 1974, *30*(4), 441–443.

Abramson, L. Y., Seligman, M. E. P., & Teasdale, J. D. Learned helplessness in humans: Critique and reformulation. *Journal of Abnormal Psychology,* 1978, *87*(1), 49–74.

Achté, K. A., Lonnquist, J., Pilreola, D., & Niskanen, P. Course and prognosis of schizophrenic psychosis in Helsinki. *Psychiatric Journal of the University of Ottawa,* 1979, *4*(4), 344–348.

Ackerman, P. T., Dykman, R. A., & Peters, J. E. Teenage status of hyperactive and non-hyperactive learning disabled boys. *American Journal of Orthopsychiatry,* 1977, *47(4),* 577–596.

Ackley, D. C. A brief overview of child abuse. *Social Casework,* 1977, *58*(1), 21–24.

Acosta, F. X., Yamamoto, J., & Wilcox, S. A. Application of electromyographic biofeedback to the relaxation training of schizophrenic, neurotic, and tension headache patients. *Journal of Consulting and Clinical Psychology,* 1978, *46*(2), 383–384.

Adams, J. E., & Lindemann, E. Coping with long term disability, In G. V. Coelho, D. A. Hamburg, and J. E. Adams (Eds.) *Coping and adaptation.* New York: Basic Books, 1974.

Adams, M. S., & Neel, J. V. Children of incest. *Pediatrics,* 1967, *40,* 55–62.

Adams, P. L. *Obsessive children.* New York: Brunner/Mazel, 1973.

Adler, G. The psychotherapy of schizophrenia: Semrad's contributions to current psychoanalytic concepts. *Schizophrenia Bulletin,* 1979, *5*(1), 130–137.

Agras, W. S., Sylvester, D., & Oliveau, D. C. The epidemiology of common fears and phobias. *Comprehensive Psychiatry,* 1969, *10,* 151–156.

Agras, W. S., Taylor, C. B., Kraemer, H. C., Allen, R. A., & Schneider, J. A. Relaxation training: Twenty-four-hour blood pressure reductions. *Archives of General Psychiatry,* 1980, *37*(8), 859–863.

Ainsworth, M. D. S., Blehar, M. C., Waters, E., & Wall, S. *Patterns of attachment: A psychological study of the strange situation.* Hillsdale, N.J.: Erlbaum, 1978.

Akhter, S., Wig, N. N., Varma, V. K., Pershad, D., & Verma, S. K. A phenomenological analysis of symptoms in obsessive-compulsive neurosis. *British Journal of Psychiatry,* 1975, *127*(2), 342–348.

Akil, H., Watson, S., Sullivan, S., & Barchas, J. D. Enkephalin-like material in normal human cerebrospinal fluid: Measurement and levels. *Life Sciences,* 1978, *23*(1), 121–126.

Akiskal, H. S., Djenderedjian, A. H., Rosenthal, R. H., & Khavi, M. K. Cyclothymic disorder: Validating criteria for inclusion in the bipolar affective group. *American Journal of Psychiatry,* 1977, *134*(11), 1227–1233.

Akiskal, H. S., & McKinney, W. T. Overview of recent research on depression. *Archives of General Psychiatry,* 1975, *32*(2), 285–304.

Albee, G. W. Myths, models and manpower. *Mental Hygiene,* 1968, *52,* 2–10.

Albert, N. Evidence of depression in an early adolescent school population. *Unpublished manuscript.* Villanova, Penn., 1973.

Alexander, F. *Psychosomatic medicine.* New York: Norton, 1950.

Alexander, F. G., & Selesnick, S. T. *The history of psychiatry.* New York: Harper & Row, 1968.

Allerton, W. S. Psychiatric casualties in Vietnam. *Roch Medical Image and Commentary*, 1970, *12*(8), 27.

Allport, G. W. *Pattern and growth in personality.* New York: Holt, Rinehart and Winston, 1961.

Allport, G. W. An autobiography. In G. W. Allport (Ed.) *The person in psychology: Selected essays.* Boston: Beacon Press, 1968.

American Hospital Association. *Hospital statistics.* Chicago, 1980.

Andrasik, F., & Holroyd, K. A. A test of specific and nonspecific effects in the biofeedback treatment of tension headache. *Journal of Consulting and Clinical Psychology*, 1980, *48*(5), 575–586.

Angrist, B., & Gershon, S. The phenomenology of experimentally induced amphetamine psychosis: Preliminary observations. *Biological Psychiatry*, 1970, *2*, 97–107.

Angrist, B., Lee, H. K., & Gershon, S. The antagonism of amphetamine induced symptomatology by a neuroleptic. *American Journal of Psychiatry*, 1974, *131*(7), 817–819.

Anonymous. First person account: After the funny farm. *Schizophrenia Bulletin*, 1980, *6*(3), 544–546.

(Anonymous), J., Chambers, W. M., & Janzan, W. B. The eclectic and multiple therapy of a shoe fetishist. *American Journal of Psychotherapy*, 1976, *30*(2), 317–326.

Appel, P. W., & Kaestner, E. Interpersonal and emotional problem solving among narcotic drug abusers. *Journal of Consulting and Clinical Psychology*, 1979, *47*(6), 1125–1127.

Appelbaum, P. S., & Gutheil, T. G. The Boston state hospital case: "Involuntary mind control," the constitution, and the "right to rot." *American Journal of Psychiatry*, 1980, *137*(6), 720–723.

Appelbaum, S. A. To define and decipher the borderline syndrome. *Psychotherapy: Theory, research and practice*, 1979, *16*(4), 364–370.

Appenzeller, O. Getting a sorehead from banging it on the wall. *Headache*, 1973, *13*, 131–132.

Appleton, W. S., & Davis, J. M. *Practical clinical psychopharmacology.* New York: Medcom, 1973.

Arieti, S. *Interpretation of schizophrenia.* New York: Brunner, 1966.

Arieti, S. Psychotherapy of severe depression. *American Journal of Psychiatry*, 1977, *134*(8), 864–868.

Arieti, S. Psychotherapy of schizophrenia: New and revised procedures. *American Journal of Psychotherapy*, 1980, *34*(4), 464–476.

Asarnow, R. F., & Mac Crinnon, D. J. Residual performance deficit in clinically remitted schizophrenics: A marker of schizophrenia. *Journal of Abnormal Psychology*, 1978, *87*(6), 597–608.

Asarnow, R. F., Steffy, R. A., & Mac Crimmon, D. J. An attentional assessment of foster children at risk for schizophrenia. *Journal of Abnormal Psychology*, 1977, *86*(2), 267–275.

Asnis, G. M., Fink, M., & Saferstein, S. ECT in metropolitan New York hospitals: A survey of practice, 1975–1976. *American Journal of Psychiatry*, 1978, *135*(4), 479–482.

Asp, D. R. Effects of alcoholics' expectation of a drink. *Journal of Studies on Alcohol*, 1977, *38*(9), 1790–1795.

Astor, M. H. An introduction to biofeedback. *American Journal of Orthopsychiatry*, 1977, *42*(4), 615–625.

Atthowe, J. M., & Krasner, L. Preliminary report on the application of contingent reinforcement procedures (token economy) on a "chronic" psychiatric ward. *Journal of Abnormal Psychology*, 1968, *78*(1), 37–43.

Avery, D., & Winoker, G. The efficacy of electroconvulsive therapy and anti-depressants in depression. *Biological Psychiatry*, 1977, *12*, 507–523.

Avery, D., & Winoker, G. Suicide, attempted suicide, and relapse rates in depression. *Archives of General Psychiatry*, 1978, *35*(6), 749–753.

Ayllon, T., & Azrin, N. H. The measurement and reinforcement of behavior of psychotics. *Journal of the Experimental Analysis of Behavior*, 1965, *8*, 357–383.

Ayllon, T., & Azrin, N. H. *The token economy: A motivational system for therapy and rehabilitation.* New York: Appleton-Century-Crofts, 1968.

Ayllon, T., Garber, S. W., & Allison, M. G. Behavioral treatment of childhood neurosis. *Psychiatry*, 1977, *40*, 315–322.

Ayllon, T., Haughton, E., & Hughes, H. B. Interpretation of symptoms: Fact or fiction? *Behavior, Research, and Therapy*, 1965, *3*(1), 1–8.

Ayllon, T., & Micheal, J. The psychiatric nurse as a behavioral engineer. *Journal of the Experimental Analysis of Behavior*, 1959, *2*, 323–334.

Ayllon, T., Smith, D., & Rogers, M., Behavioral management of school phobia. *Journal of Behavioral Therapy and Experimental Psychiatry*, 1970, *1*, 125–138.

Azrin, N. H., Gottlieb, L., Hughart, L., Wesolowski, M. D., & Rahn, T. Eliminating self-injurious behavior by educative procedures. *Behavior Research, and Therapy*, 1975, *3*, 101–111.

Azrin, N. H., & Thienes, P. M. Rapid elimination of enuresis by intensive learning without a conditioning apparatus. *Behavior Therapy*, 1978, *9*, 342–354.

Baechler, J. *Suicides.* New York: Basic Books, 1979.

Bakal, D. A. Headache: A biopsychological perspective. *Psychological Bulletin*, 1975, *82*, 367–382.

Bale, R. N., Van Stone, W. W., Kuldau, J. M., Engelsing, T. M. J., Elashoff, R. M., & Zarcone,

V. P. Therapeutic communities vs. methadone maintenance—A prospective controlled study of narcotic addiction treatment: Design and one year follow-up. *Archives of General Psychiatry,* 1980, *37*(2), 179–193.

Ban, T. A. *Recent advances in the biology of schizophrenia.* Springfield, Ill.: Thomas, 1973.

Ban, T. A., & Lehmann, H. E. Nicotinic acid in the treatment of schizophrenia. *Canadian Psychiatric Association Journal,* 1970, *15,* 499–500.

Bandura, A. A social learning interpretation of psychological dysfunction. In P. London and D. Rosenhan (Eds.) *Foundations of abnormal psychology.* New York: Holt, Rinehart and Winston, 1968.

Bandura, A. *Principles of behavior modifications.* New York: Holt, Rinehart and Winston, 1969.

Bandura, A. *Social learning theory.* Morristown, N.J.: General Learning Press, 1971.

Bandura, A. *Social learning theory.* Englewood Cliffs, N.J.: Prentice-Hall, 1977.

Bandura, A. The self-system in reciprocal determinism. *American Psychologist,* 1978, *33,* 344–358.

Bandura, A. Self-efficacy mechanisms in human agency. *American Psychologist,* 1982, *37*(2), 122–147.

Bandura, A. Ross, D., & Ross, S. A. Imitations of film-mediated aggressive models. *Journal of Abnormal Psychology,* 1963, *66*(1), 3–11.

Barber, T. X. *Hypnosis: A scientific approach.* New York: Van Nostrand Reinhold, 1969.

Barber, T. X. *LSD, marihuana, yoga, and hypnosis.* Chicago: Aldine, 1970.

Barkley, R. A. A review of stimulant drug research with hyperactive children. *Journal of Child Psychology and Psychiatry,* 1977, *18,* 137–165.

Barlow, D. H. Increasing heterosexual responsiveness in the treatment of sexual deviation: A review of the clinical and experimental evidence. *Behavior Therapy,* 1973, *4,* 655–671.

Barlow, D. H., Abel, G. G., & Blanchard, E. B. Gender identity change in transsexuals. *Archives of General Psychiatry,* 1979, *36*(9), 1001–1007.

Barlow, D. H., Leitenberg, H., & Agras, W. S. Experimental control of sexual deviation through manipulation of the noxious scene in covert sensitization. *Journal of Abnormal Psychology,* 1969, *74*(7), 596–601.

Barlow, D. H., Reynolds, E. J., Agras, S. Gender identity change in a transsexual. *Archives of General Psychiatry,* 1973, *28*(4), 569–578.

Barlow, D. H., & Wolfe, B. E. Behavioral approaches to anxiety disorders: A report on the NIMH-Suny, Albany research conference. *Journal of Consulting and Clinical Psychology,* 1981, *49*(3), 448–454.

Barnes, F. A psychiatric unit serving an international community. *Hospital & Community Psychiatry,* 1980, *31*(11), 756–758.

Baroff, G. S. *Mental retardation: Nature, cause, and management.* Washington, D.C.: Hemisphere Press, 1974.

Baroja, J. C. *The world of witches.* London: Weidenfeld and Nicolson, 1964.

Baron, R. A., & Byrne, D. *Social psychology: Understanding human interaction* (2nd ed.). Boston: Allyn & Bacon, 1977.

Bartop, R. W., Luckhurst, E., Kiloh, I. G., & Penny, R. Depressed lymphocyte function after bereavement. *The Lancet,* April 16, 1977, pp. 834–836.

Basmajian, J. V. (Ed) *Biofeedback—Principles and practice for clinicians.* Baltimore: Williams & Wilkins, 1979.

Basmajian, J. V. Introduction: Principles and background. In J. V. Basmajian (Ed) *Biofeedback—Principles and practice for clinicians.* Baltimore: Williams & Wilkins, 1979.

Bassuk, E. L., & Gerson, S. Deinstitutionalization and mental health services. *Scientific American,* 1978, *238*(2), 46–54.

Bateson, G., Jackson, D. D., Haley, J., & Weakland, J. Toward a theory of schizophrenia. *Behavioral Science,* 1956, *1,* 241–264.

Bayh, B. Interview. Barbiturate abuse held U.S. epidemic. *Los Angeles Times,* December 5, 1972, p. 9.

Bebbington, P. E. The efficacy of alcoholics anonymous: The elusiveness of hard data. *British Journal of Psychiatry,* 1976, *128,* 572–580.

Beck, A. T. *Depression: Clinical, experimental and theoretical aspects.* New York: Harper & Row, 1967.

Beck, A. T. The development of depression: A cognitive model. In R. J. Friedman and M. M. Katz (Eds.) *The psychology of depressions: Contemporary theory and research.* Washington, D.C.: Winston, 1974.

Beck, A. T. *Cognitive therapy and the emotional disorders.* New York: International Universities Press, 1976.

Beck, A. T., Laude, R., & Bohnert, M. Ideational components of anxiety neurosis. *Archives of General Psychiatry,* 1974, *31*(3), 319–325.

Beck, A. T., & Rush, A. J. A cognitive model of anxiety formation and anxiety resolution. In I. G. Sarason and C. D. Spielberger (Eds.) *Stress and anxiety,* vol. 2, New York: Wiley, 1975.

Beck, A. T., Rush, A. J., Shaw, B. F., & Emery, G. *Cognitive therapy of depression.* New York: Guilford Press, 1980.

Beck, A. T., Ward, C. H., Mendelson, M., Mock, J. E., & Erbaugh, J. K. Reliability of psychiatric diagnosis: II. A study of consistency of clinical judgments and ratings. *American Journal of Psychiatry,* 1962, *119*(2), 351–357.

Beck, J. C., Golden, S., & Arnold, F. An empirical investigation of psychotherapy with schizophrenic patients. *Schizophrenia Bulletin,* 1981, *7*(2), 241–247.

Becker, E. *The denial of death.* New York: Free Press, 1974.

Beech, H. R., & Perigault, J. Toward a theory of obsessional disorder. In H. R. Beech (Ed.) *Obsessional states.* London: Methuen, 1974.

Begelman, D. A. Misnaming, metaphors, the medical model and some muddles. *Psychiatry,* 1971, *34*(1), 38–58.

Beit-Hallahni, B. Psychological theories and correctional practice: A historical note. *Correctional and Social Psychiatry and the Journal of Behavior Technology, Methods and Therapy,* 1976, *22*(1), 38–39.

Bell, A. P., & Weinberg, M. S. *Homosexualities: A study of diversity among men and women.* New York: Simon & Schuster, 1978.

Bell, E., Jr. The basis of effective military psychiatry. *Diseases of the Nervous System,* 1958, *19*(7), 283–288.

Bellak, L. *The porcupine dilemma.* New York: Citadel Press, 1970.

Bemporad, J. R., Dunton, H. D., & Spady, F. W. The treatment of a child foot fetishist. *American Journal of Psychotherapy,* 1976, *3*(2), 303–316.

Benda, C. E., Squires, N. D., Ogonik, M. J., & Wise, R. Personality factors in mild mental retardation: 1. Family background and sociocultural patterns. *American Journal of Mental Deficiency,* 1963, *68*(1), 11–17.

Bender, L. The family patterns of 100 schizophrenic children observed at Bellevue, 1935–1952. *Journal of Autism and Childhood Schizophrenia,* 1974, *4,* 279–292.

Benedict, R. Anthropology and the abnormal. *Journal of Genetic Psychology,* 1934a, *10,* 59.

Benedict, R. *Patterns of culture.* Boston: Houghton Mifflin, 1934b.

Benson, H. *The relaxation response.* New York: Morrow, 1975.

Bentler, P. M., & Prince, C. Personality characteristics of male transvestites: III. *Journal of Abnormal Psychology,* 1969, *74*(2), 140–143.

Bergantino, L. *Psychotherapy, insight, and style: The existential moment.* Boston: Allyn & Bacon, 1981.

Berger, D. M. The survivor syndrome: A problem of nosology and treatment. *American Journal of Psychotherapy,* 1977, *31*(2), 238–251.

Berger, K., & Zarit, S. Late life paranoid states: Assessment and treatment. *American Journal of Orthopsychiatry,* 1978, *48*(3), 528–537.

Bergin, A. E., & Lambert, M. J. The evaluation of therapeutic outcomes. In S. L. Garfield and A. E. Bergin (Eds.) *Handbook of psychotherapy and behavior change.* New York: Wiley, 1978.

Bernstein, G. A. Physician management of incest situations. *Medical Aspects of Human Sexuality,* 1979, *13*(11), 66–87.

Bernstein, I. C., Callahan, W. A., & Jaranson, J. M. Lobotomy in private practice. *Archives of General Psychiatry,* 1975, *32*(8), 1041–1047.

Bertelson, A., Harvald, A., & Hauge, M. A Danish twin study of manic-depressive disorders. *British Journal of Psychiatry,* 1977, *130,* 330–351.

Berzins, J. I., Rors, W. F., English, G. E., & Haley, J. V. Subgroups among opiate addicts: A typological investigation. *Journal of Abnormal Psychology,* 1974, *83*(1), 65–73.

Bettelheim, B. Individual and mass behavior in extreme situations. *Journal of Abnormal and Social Psychology,* 1943, *38*(4), 417–452.

Bettelheim, B. *The informed heart.* New York: Free Press, 1960.

Bettelheim, B. *The empty fortress.* New York: Free Press, 1967.

Bettelheim, B. *A home for the heart.* New York: Knopf, 1973.

Betz, B. J. Curtain on schizophrenia: A twenty-five-year clinical follow up. *American Journal of Psychotherapy,* 1980, *34*(2), 252–260.

Bieber, I. A discussion of homosexuality: The ethical challenge. *Journal of Consulting and Clinical Psychology,* 1976, *44*(2), 163–167.

Bieber, I. Commentary: The new "Kinsey Institute" study of homosexuality. *Medical Aspects of Human Sexuality,* 1978, *12*(9), 43–45.

Bieber, I., & Bieber, T. Heterosexuals who are preoccupied with homosexual thoughts. *Medical Aspects of Human Sexuality,* 1975, *9*(4), 152–168.

Bieber, I., Dain, H. J., Dince, P. R., Drellich, M. G., Grand, H. C., Gundlach, R. H., Kremer, M. W., Rifkin, A. H., Wilbur, C. B., & Bieber, T. B. *Homosexuality: A psychoanalytic study.* New York: Basic Books, 1962.

Bigelow, G., & Griffiths, R. An intensive teaching unit for severely and profoundly retarded women. In T. Thompson and J. Grabowski (Eds.) *Behavior modification of the mentally retarded* (2nd ed.). New York: Oxford University Press, 1977.

Biklen, D. P. Behavior modification in a state mental hospital: A participant-observer's critique. *American Journal of Orthopsychiatry,* 1976, *46*(1), 53–61.

Bild, K. & Adams, H. E. Modification of migraine headaches by cephalic blood volume, pulse, and EMG biofeedback. *Journal of Consulting and Clinical Psychology,* 1980, *48*(1), 51–57.

Birch, H. G., Richardson, S. A., Baird, D., Harobin, G., & Illsley, R. *Mental subnormality in the commu-*

nity: A clinical and epidemiological study. Baltimore: Williams & Wilkins, 1970.

Blanchard, E. B., & Young, L. D. Clinical applications of biofeedback training: A review. *Archives of General Psychiatry,* 1974, *30*(5), 573–589.

Blaney, P. H. Contemporary theories of depression: Critique and comparison. *Journal of Abnormal Psychology,* 1977, *86*(3), 203–223.

Bleuler, E. *Dementia Praecox or the group of schizophrenias.* New York: International Universities Press, 1950.

Bleuler, M. The offspring of schizophrenics. *Schizophrenia Bulletin,* Spring 1974, no. 8, pp. 93–107.

Bleuler, M. On schizophrenic psychosis. *American Journal of Psychiatry,* 1979, *136*(11), 1403–1409.

Bliss, E. L. Multiple personalities: A report of 14 cases with implications for schizophrenia and hysteria. *Archives of General Psychiatry,* 1980, *37*(12), 1388–1397.

Block, H. S. Army clinical psychiatry in the combat zone, 1967–1968. *American Journal of Psychiatry,* 1969, *126*(3), 289–298.

Bloom, B. L. The logic and urgency of prevention. *Hospital & Community Psychiatry,* 1981, *32*(12), 839–842.

Blum, J. D. On changes in psychiatric diagnosis over time. *American Psychologist,* 1978, *33*(11), 1017–1031.

Boas, F. *Mind of primitive man.* New York: Macmillan, 1919.

Bogdan, R., & Taylor, S. The judged, not the judges: An insider's view of mental retardation. *American Psychologist,* 1976, *31*(1), 47–52.

Bolter, J. F., & Hannon, R. Cerebral damage associated with alcoholism: A reexamination. *The Psychological Record,* 1980, *30*(1), 165–179.

Bond, I. K., & Hutchinson, H. C. Application of reciprocal inhibition therapy to exhibitionism. In L. P. Ullmann and L. Krasner (Eds.) *Case studies in behavior modification.* New York: Holt, Rinehart and Winston, 1965.

Borus, J. F. Incidence of maladjustment in Vietnam returnees. *Archives of General Psychiatry,* 1974, *30*(4), 554–557.

Bowers, K. S. Situationism in psychology: An analysis and a critique. *Psychological Review,* 1973, *80,* 307–336.

Bowers, K. S., & Kelly, P. Stress, disease and hypnosis. *Journal of Abnormal Psychology,* 1979, *88*(5), 490–505.

Bowlby, J. Separation anxiety. *International Journal of Psychoanalysis,* 1960, *41*(1), 1–25.

Bowlby, J. *Attachment and loss, vol. 2: Separation.* New York: Basic Books, 1973.

Braddock, D. Deinstitutionalization of the retarded: Trends in public policy. *Hospital & Community Psychiatry,* 1981, *32*(9), 607–615.

Braden, W., Stillman, R. C., & Wyatt, R. J. Effects of marijuana on contingent negative variations and reaction times. *Archives of General Psychiatry,* 1974, *31*(4), 537–541.

Braukmann, C. J., Fixsen, D. L., Phillips, E. L., & Wolf, M. M. Behavioral approaches to treatment in the crime and delinquency field. *Criminology,* 1975, *13,* 299–331.

Braun, P., Kochansky, G., Shapiro, R., Greenberg, S., Gudeman, J. E., & Shore, M. F. Overview: Deinstitutionalization of psychiatric patients, a critical review of outcome studies. *American Journal of Psychiatry,* 1981, *138*(6), 736–749.

Brecher, E. M. So why do heroin addicts drop dead? *New York Times Magazine* November 19, 1972, pp. 108–116.

Breggin, R. "The second wave." *Mental Hygiene,* 1973, *57*(1), 11–13.

Briddell, D. W., & Wilson, G. T. The effects of alcohol and expectancy set on male sexual arousal. *Journal of Abnormal Psychology,* 1976, *85*(2), 225–234.

Brill, N. Q. Gross stress reaction II: Traumatic war neurosis. In A. M. Freedman and H. I. Kaplan (Eds.) *Comprehensive textbook of psychiatry.* Baltimore: Williams & Wilkins, 1967.

British glossary of psychiatric terminology. British General register office, London, 1968.

Brodie, H. K. H., Gartrell, N., Doering, C., & Rhue, T. Plasma testosterone levels in hexterosexual and homosexual men. *American Journal of Psychiatry,* 1974, *131*(1), 82–83.

Bronfenbrenner, U. Is early intervention effective? In S. Ryan. (Ed.) *A report on longitudinal evaluations of preschool programs,* vol. 2. Washington, D.C.: Office of Child Development, 1974.

Brooks, A. D. *Law, psychiatry and the mental health system.* Boston: Little, Brown, 1974.

Brown, S. A., Goldman, M. S., Inn, A., & Anderson, L. R. Expectations of reinforcement from alcohol: Their domain and relation to drinking patterns. *Journal of Consulting and Clinical Psychology,* 1980, *48*(4), 419–426.

Brownmiller, S. *Against our will: Men, women and rape.* New York: Simon & Schuster, 1975.

Bruch, H. *The golden cage: The enigma of anorexia nervosa.* Cambridge, Mass.: Harvard University Press, 1978.

Brunink, S. A., & Schroeder, H. E. Verbal therapeutic behavior of expert psychoanalytically oriented, gestalt, and behavior therapists. *Journal of Consulting and Clinical Psychology,* 1979, *47,* 567–574.

Bryant, G., & Cirel, P. An exemplary project: A community response to rape. *National Law Enforce-*

ment Assistance Administration. Washington, D.C., 1977.

Buck, F. A test of heightened external responsiveness in an alcoholic population. *Journal of Abnormal Psychology,* 1979, *88*(4), 361–368.

Buckalew, L. W. Alcohol: A description and comparison of recent scientific vs. public knowledge. *Journal of Clinical Psychology,* 1979, *35*(2), 459–463.

Bucher, B., & Lovaas, O. I. Use of aversive stimulation in behavior modification. In M. R. Jones (Ed.) *Miami symposium on the prediction of behavior, 1967.* Miami: University of Miami Press, 1968.

Budzynski, T. H. Biofeedback strategies in headache treatment. In J. V. Basmajian (Ed.) *Biofeedback principles and practice for clinicians.* Baltimore: Williams & Wilkins, 1979.

Bunge, R. G. Variations in male genitals which make coitus difficult. *Medical Aspects of Human Sexuality,* 1970, *4*(11), 120–132.

Bunney, W. E., Jr., Murphy, D. L., Goodwin, F. K., & Borge, G. F. The "switch process" in manic depressive illness: A systematic study of sequential behavioral changes. *Archives of General Psychiatry,* 1972, *27*(3), 295–302.

Burgess, A. W. Family reaction to homicide. *American Journal of Orthopsychiatry,* 1975, *45*(3), 391–398.

Burgess, A. W., & Holmstrom, L. L. Coping behavior of the rape victim. *American Journal of Psychiatry,* 1976, *133*(4), 413–418.

Burros, W. M. The growing burden of impotence. *Family Health,* 1974, *6*(5), 18–21.

Busse, E. W., & Pfeiffer, E. Functional psychiatric disorders in old age. In E. W. Busse and E. Pfeiffer (Eds.) *Behavior and adaptation in late life* (2nd ed.). Boston: Little, Brown, 1977.

Byassee, J. E. Essential hypertension. In R. B. Williams, Jr. and W. D. Gentry (Eds.) *Behavioral approaches to medical treatment.* Cambridge, Mass.: Ballinger, 1977.

Cadoret, R. J. Evidence for genetic inheritance of primary affective disorder in adoptees. *American Journal of Psychiatry,* 1978, *135*(4), 463–464.

Cadoret, R. J. Psychopathology in adopted away offspring of biologic parents with antisocial behavior. *Archives of General Psychiatry,* 1978, *35*(2), 176–184.

Cadoret, R. J., & Cain, C. Sex differences in prediction of antisocial behavior in adoptees. *Archives of General Psychiatry,* 1980, *37*(10), 1171–1175.

Cadoret, R. J., Cain, C., & Groves, W. M. Development of alcoholism in adoptees raised apart from alcoholic biologic relatives. *Archives of General Psychiatry,* 1980, *37*(5), 561–563.

Cahalan, D. Subcultural differences in drinking behavior in U.S. national surveys and selected European studies. In P. E. Nathan and G. A. Marlott (Eds.) *Alcoholism: New directions in behavioral research and treatment.* New York: Plenum Press, 1978.

Callahan, F. J., & Leitenberg, H. Aversion therapy for sexual deviation: Contingent shock and covert sensitization. *Journal of Abnormal Psychology,* 1973, *81*(1), 60–73.

Cameron, N. *The psychology of behavior disorder.* Boston: Houghton Mifflin, 1947.

Cameron, N. Paranoid reactions. In A. Freedman and H. Kaplan (Eds.) *Comprehensive textbook of psychiatry.* Baltimore: Williams & Wilkins, 1967.

Cameron, N., & Magaret, A. *Behavior pathology.* Boston: Houghton Mifflin, 1957.

Cancro, R. Genetic evidence for the existence of subgroups of the schizophrenic syndrome. *Schizophrenia Bulletin,* 1979, *5*(3), 454–459.

Canning, J., & Canning, C. *The gift of mother.* Boston: Developmental Evaluation, Childrens Hospital Medical Center, 1975.

Cannon, W. Voodoo death. *Psychosomatic Medicine,* 1957, *19,* 182–190.

Cantor, N., Smith, E. E., French, R., & Mezzich, J. Psychiatric diagnosis as prototype categorization. *Journal of Abnormal Psychology,* 1980, *89*(2), 181–193.

Cantwell, D. P. Psychiatric illness in the family of hyperactive children. *Archives of General Psychiatry,* 1972, *27,* 414–417.

Cantwell, D. P., Baker, L., & Rutter, M. Family factors. In M. Rutter and E. Schopler (Eds.) *Autism: A reappraisal of concepts and treatment.* New York: Plenum Press, 1978.

Caplan, G. *Principles of preventative psychiatry.* New York: Basic Books, 1964.

Caramazza, A., & Berndt, R. S. Semantic and syntactic processes in aphasia: Review of the literature. *Psychological Bulletin,* 1978, *85,* 898–918.

Carlin, A. S., Bakker, C. B., Halpern, L., & Post, R. D. Social facilitation of marijuana intoxication: Impact of social set and pharmacological activity. *Journal of Abnormal Psychology,* 1975, *80*(2), 132–140.

Carlson, A. Antipsychotic drugs, neurotransmitters, and schizophrenia. *American Journal of Psychiatry,* 1978, *135*(2), 164–173.

Carlson, G., & Goodwin, F. K. The stages of mania: A longitudinal analysis of the manic episode. *Archives of General Psychiatry,* 1973, *28*(2), 221–228.

Carpenter, W. T., Strauss, J. S., & Bartko, J. J. The diagnosis and understanding of schizophrenia. Part I. Use of signs and symptoms for the identification of schizophrenic patients. *Schizophrenic Bulletin,* winter 1974, no. 11, p. 47.

Carpenter, W. T., Strauss, J. S., & Mulch, S. Are there pathognomic symptoms of schizophrenia? *Archives of General Psychiatry,* 1973, *29*(3), 443–449.

Carr, A. T. Compulsive neurosis: Two psychophysiological studies. *Bulletin of the British Psychological Society*, 1971, *24*(3), 256–257.

Carr, A. T. Compulsive neurosis: A review of the literature. *Psychological Bulletin*, 1974, *81*, 311–319.

Carsrud, A. L., Carsrud, K. B., & Dodd, B. G. Randomly monitored staff utilization of behavior modification techniques: Long term effects on clients. *Journal of Consulting and Clinical Psychology*, 1980, *48*(6), 704–710.

Cassel, J. The contribution of the social environment to host resistance. *American Journal of Epidemiology*, 1976, *104*(1), 107–123.

Cedercreutz, C. Hypnotic treatment of 100 cases of migraine. In F. H. Frankel and H. S. Zamansky (Eds.) *Hypnosis at its bicentennial*. New York: Plenum Press, 1978.

Chamberlin, B. C. The psychological aftermath of disaster. *Journal of Clinical Psychiatry*, 1980, *41*(7), 238–244.

Chambers, C. D., Griffey, M. S. Use of legal substance within the general population: The sex and age variables. *Addictive Diseases*, 1975, *2*(1), 7–19.

Chapman, L. J. Recent advances in the study of schizophrenic cognition. *Schizophrenia Bulletin*, 1979, *5*(4), 568–580.

Chapman, L. J., & Chapman, J. P. Illusory correlations as an obstacle to the use of valid psychodiagnostic signs. *Journal of Abnormal Psychology*, 1969, *74*(2), 271–287.

Chapman, L. J., & Chapman, J. P. *Disordered thoughts in schizophrenia*. Englewood Cliffs, N.J.: Prentice-Hall, 1973.

Chein, L., Gerard, D., Lee, K., & Rosenfeld, E. *The road to H*. New York: Basic Books, 1964.

Chesno, F. A., & Kilmann, D. R. Effects of stimulation intensity on sociopathic learning. *Journal of Abnormal Psychology*, 1975, *84*(1), 144–151.

Chess, S. The plasticity of human development. *American Academy of Child Psychiatry*, 1978, *17*(1), 80–91.

Chess, S., & Thomas, H. Differences in outcome with early intervention in children with behavior disorders. In M. Roff, L. N. Robins, and M. Pollack (Eds.) *Life history research in psychopathology*. Minneapolis: University of Minnesota Press, 1972.

Chodoff, P. The German concentration camp as a psychological stress. *Archives of General Psychiatry*, 1970, *22*(1), 78–87.

Chodoff, P. The diagnosis of hysteria: An overview. *American Journal of Psychiatry*, 1974, *131*(7), 1073–1078.

Chodoff, P. The case for involuntary hospitalization of the mentally ill. *American Journal of Psychiatry*, 1976, *133*(5), 496–501.

Christie, J. E., Shering, A., Ferguson, J., & Glen, A. I. M. Physostigmine and arecoline: Effects of intravenous infusions. *British Journal of Psychiatry*, 1981, *138*(1), 46–50.

Chu, F. D., & Trotter, S. *The madness establishment: Ralph Nader's study group report on the National Institute of Mental Health*. New York: Grossman Press, 1974.

Claridge, G. Psychosomatic relations in physical disease. In H. J. Eysenck (Ed.) *Handbook of abnormal psychology*. London: Pitman, 1973.

Cleckley, H. M. *The caricature of love*. New York: Ronald Press, 1957.

Cleckley, H. M. *The mask of sanity* (5th ed.). St. Louis: Mosby, 1976.

Cloninger, C. R., Reich, T., & Guze, S. B. Genetic-environmental interaction and antisocial behavior. In R. D. Hare and D. Schalling (Eds.) *Psychopathic behavior*. New York: Wiley, 1978.

Cobb, S. Social support as a moderator of life stress. *Psychosomatic Medicine*, 1976, *38*(3), 300–314.

Cobb, S., & Rose, R. M. Hypertension, peptic ulcer, and diabetes in air traffic controllers. *Journal of the American Medical Association*, 1973, *224*(4), 489–492.

Coelho, G. V., & Adams, J. E. Introduction. In G. V. Coelho, D. A. Hamburg, and J. E. Adams (Eds.) *Coping and adaptation*. New York: Basic Books, 1974.

Cohen, D. B. On the etiology of neurosis. *Journal of Abnormal Psychology*, 1974, *83*(5), 473–479.

Cohen, M. L., Garofolo, R., Boucher, R., & Seghorn, T. The psychology of rapists. In S. A. Pasternack (Ed.) *Violence and victims*. New York: Spectrum, 1975.

Cohen, M. L., Seghorn, T., & Calmas, W. Sociometric study of the sex offender. *Journal of Abnormal Psychology*, 1969, *74*(2), 249–255.

Cohen, M. M., Marinello, M. J., & Bock, N. Chromosomal damage in leukocytes induced by Lysergic acid. *Science*, 1967, *155*, 1417–1419.

Cohen, S. The hallucinogens. In W. G. Clark and J. del Giudice (Eds.) *Principles of psychopharmacology*. New York: Academic Press, 1970.

Cohen, S. Cocaine. *Journal of the American Medical Association*, 1975, *236*(1), 74–75.

Cohen, S. Angel dust. *Journal of the American Medical Association*, 1977, *238*(6), 515–516.

Cohn, N. *The pursuit of the millenium*. New York: Oxford University Press, 1970.

Colby, K. M. *Artificial paranoia: A computer simulation of paranoid process*. New York: Pergamon Press, 1975.

Colby, K. M. Clinical implications of a simulation model of paranoid process. *Archives of General Psychiatry*, 1976, *33*, 854–857.

Colby, K. M. Appraisal of four psychological theories of paranoid phenomena. *Journal of Abnormal Psychology*, 1977, *86*(1), 54–59.

Collison, D. A. Which asthmatic patients should be treated by hypnotherapy. *Medical Journal of Australia,* 1975, *1,* 776–781.

Connolly, J. A. Intelligence levels of Down's syndrome children. *American Journal of Mental Deficiency,* 1978, *83*(2), 193–196.

Cook, R. H., & Austin, J. H. Precautions in familial transmissible dementia: Including Alzheimer's disease. *Archives of Neurology,* 1978, *35*(11), 697–698.

Cooper, J. E., Kendell, R. E., Gurland, B. J., Sharpe, L., Copeland, J. R. M., & Simon, R. *Psychiatric diagnosis in New York and London.* London: Oxford University Press, 1972.

Corsellis, J. A. N. The neuropathology of dementia. *Age and Aging* (Supplement), 1977, *6,* 20.

Cory, C. T. Newsline: The long lived urged to work. *Psychology Today,* September 1980, *14*(4), 21.

Costello, L. G. A critical review of Seligman's laboratory experiments on learned helplessness and depression in humans. *Journal of Abnormal Psychology,* 1978, *87*(1), 21–31.

Coyne, J. C. Depression and the response of others. *Journal of Abnormal Psychology,* 1976, *85*(2), 186–193.

Craft, M. D. *Ten studies into psychopathic personality.* Bristol, England: Wright, 1965.

Crissey, M. S. Mental retardation: Past, present and future. *American Psychologist,* 1975, *30*(8), 800–808.

Cromwell, R. L., De Amicis, L., Hayes, T., & Briggs, D. Reaction time cross-over. A vulnerability index: Mean reaction time, a symptom severity index. *Psychopharmacology Bulletin,* 1979, *15*(1), 24–25.

Cross, D. G., Sheehan, P. W., & Khan, J. A. Short and long term follow-up of clients receiving insight oriented therapy and behavior therapy. *Journal of Consulting and Clinical Psychology,* 1982, *50*(1), 103–112.

Culliton, B. J. Pot facing stringent scientific examination. *Science News,* 1970, *97*(4), 102–105.

The curse of hyperactivity. *Newsweek Magazine,* June 23, 1980, pp. 59–62.

Dahlstrom, W. G. MMPI handbook, vol. II: A sneak preview. *Ninth Annual MMPI Symposium,* Los Angeles, Calif., 1974.

Dain, N. *Concepts of insanity in the United States, 1789–1865.* New Brunswick: Rutgers University Press, 1964.

Davison, G. Differential relaxation and cognitive restructuring in therapy with a "paranoid schizophrenic" or "paranoid state." *Proceedings of the 74th Annual Convention of the American Psychological Association, 1966.*

Davison, G. Homosexuality: The ethical challenge. *Journal of Consulting and Clinical Psychology,* 1976, *44*(2), 151–162.

Davison, G. Not can but ought: The treatment of homosexuality. *Journal of Consulting and Clinical Psychology,* 1978, *46*(2), 170–172.

de Araujo, G., Van Arsdel, P. P., Jr., Holmes, T. H., & Dudley, D. L. Life changes, coping ability and chronic intrinsic asthma. *Journal of Psychosomatic Research,* 1973, *17,* 359–363.

De Betz, B. Brief guide to office counseling: Gender disorders. *Medical Aspects of Human Sexuality,* 1975, *9*(4), 87–88.

De Leon, G., & Sacks, S. Conditioning functional enuresis: A four year follow-up. *Journal of Consulting and Clinical Psychology,* 1972, *39,* 299–300.

de Piano, F. A., & Salzberg, H. C. Clinical applications of hypnosis to three psychosomatic disorders. *Psychological Bulletin,* 1979, *86*(6), 1223–1235.

Debray, Q. A genetic study of chronic delusions. *Neuropsychobiology,* 1975, *1,* 313–321.

Dejong, R. N., & Sugar, O. *The yearbook of neurology and surgery.* Chicago: Yearbook Medical, 1972.

Dekker, E., & Groen, J. Reproducible psychogenic attacks of asthma. *Journal of Psychosomatic Research,* 1956, *1,* 58–67.

Dekker, E., Pelser, H. E., & Groen, J. Conditioning as a cause of asthmatic attacks. *Journal of Psychosomatic Research,* 1957, *2,* 97–108.

Delong, G. R. A neuropsychological interpretation of infantile autism. In M. Rutter and E. Schopler (Eds.) *Autism: A reappraisal of concepts and treatment.* New York: Plenum Press, 1978.

Depue, R. A., & Monroe, S. M. Learned helplessness in the perspective of the depressive disorders: Conceptual and definitional issues. *Journal of Abnormal Psychology,* 1978, *87*(1), 3–20.

Derogatis, L. R., & Meyer, J. K. The invested partner in sexual disorders: A profile. *American Journal of Psychiatry,* 1979, *136*(12), 1545–1549.

Deutsch, A. *The mentally ill in America: A history of their care and treatment from colonial times.* New York: Doubleday, Doran, 1937.

Diagnostic and statistical manual of mental disorders (2nd ed.). Washington, D.C.: American Psychiatric Association, 1968.

Diaz-Buxo, J. A., Candle, J. A., Chandler, J. T., Farmer, C. D., & Holbrook, W. D. Dialysis of schizophrenic patients: A double-blind study. *American Journal of Psychiatry,* 1980, *137*(10), 1220–1222.

Dimsdale, J. E. The coping behavior of Nazi concentration camp survivors. *American Journal of Psychiatry,* 1974, *131*(7), 792–797.

Dimsdale, J. E. Emotional causes of sudden death. *American Journal of Psychiatry,* 1977, *134*(12), 1361–1366.

Dinaburg, D., Glick, I. D., & Feigenbaum, E. Marital therapy of women alcoholics. *Journal of Studies on Alcohol,* 1977, *38*(7), 1247–1258.

Doane, J. A. Family interaction and communication deviance in disturbed and normal families: A review of research. *Family Process,* 1978, *17,* 357–376.

Dohrenwend, B. S. Life events as stressors: A methodological inquiry. *Journal of Health and Social Behavior,* 1973, *14,* 167–175.

Dohrenwend, B. P., & Dohrenwend, B. S. Social and cultural influences on psychopathology. In M. R. Rosenzweig and L. W. Porter (Eds.) *Annual review of psychology.* Palo Alto, Calif.: Annual Reviews, 1974.

Dole, V. P., Nyswander, M., & Warner, A. Successful treatment of 750 criminal addicts. *Journal of the American Medical Association,* 1968, *206,* 2709–2711.

Doll, E. A. *Measurement of social competence: A manual for the Vineland social maturity scale.* Circle Pines, Minn.: American Guidance Service, 1953.

Dor-Shav, N. K. On the long range effects of concentration camps internment on Nazi victims: 25 years later. *Journal of Consulting and Clinical Psychology,* 1978, *46*(1), 1–11.

Doughty, P. L., Carter, W. E., Coggins, W. J., & Page, J. B. Marijuana—Here to stay? *APA Monitor,* 1976, *7*(1), 5; 10.

Drillien, C. M. The incidence of mental and physical handicaps in school age children of very low birth weight: II. *Pediatrics,* 1967, *39,* 238–247.

DSM-I *Diagnostic and statistical manual of mental disorders.* Washington, D.C.: American Psychiatric Association, 1952.

DSM-II *Diagnostic and statistical manual of mental disorders (2nd ed.).* Washington, D.C.: American Psychiatric Association, 1968.

DSM-III. *Diagnostic and statistical manual of mental disorders (3rd ed.).* Washington, D.C.: American Psychiatric Association, 1980.

Dunbar, F. *Psychosomatic diagnosis.* New York: Harper & Row, 1943.

Dunham, H. W. *Community and schizophrenia.* Detroit: Wayne State University Press, 1965.

Dunner, D. L., Stallone, F., & Fieve, R. R. Lithium carbonate and affective disorders V: A double blind study of prophylaxis of depression in bipolar illness. *Archives of General Psychiatry,* 1976, *33*(1), 117–120.

Dye, O. A., Saxon, S. A., & Milby, J. R. Long term neuropsychological deficits after traumatic head injury with comatosis. *Journal of Clinical Psychology,* 1981, *37*(3), 472–477.

Earls, F. Prevalence of behavior problems in 3-year-old children. *Archives of General Psychiatry,* 1980, *37*(10), 1153–1157.

ECT Task Force. *Report 14.* American Psychiatric Association, Washington, D.C., 1978.

Edelson, M. Alternative living arrangements. In H. R. Lamb and Associates (Eds.) *Community survival for long term patients.* San Francisco: Jossey-Bass, 1976.

Edwards, G. The meaning and treatment of alcohol dependence. *British Journal of Psychiatry,* Special Publication, 1975, no. 9, pp. 239–251.

Eggers, C. Course and prognosis of childhood schizophrenia. *Journal of Autism and Childhood Schizophrenia,* 1978, *8*(1), 21–36.

Eilbracht, A., & Thompson, T. Behavioral intervention in a sheltered work activity setting for retarded adults. In T. Thompson and J. Grabowski (Eds.) *Behavior modification of the mentally retarded. (2nd ed.)* New York: Oxford University Press, 1977.

Eisenberg, L. School phobia: A study in the communication of anxiety. *American Journal of Psychiatry,* 1958, *114,* 712–718.

Elgin Daily Courier News. *Psychiatrists say dissident general sane.* May 17, 1979, p. 7.

Ellenberg, L., Rosenbaum, G., Goldman, M. S., & Whitman, R. D. Recoverability of psychological functioning following alcohol abuse: Lateralization effects. *Journal of Consulting and Clinical Psychology,* 1980, *48*(4), 503–510.

Ellington, R. J. Incidence of EEG abnormality among patients with mental disorders of apparently nonorganic origin: A critical review. *American Journal of Psychiatry,* 1954, *11*(2), 263–275.

Ellis, A. H. *Reason and emotion in psychotherapy.* New York: Stuart Press, 1962.

Ellis, A. H. Rational-emotive therapy. In R. J. Corsini (Ed.) *Current psychotherapies.* Itasca, Ill.: Peacock, 1973.

Ellsworth, R. B. *The MACC behavioral adjustment scale: Revised 1971 manual.* Los Angeles: Western Psychological Corp., 1971.

Elmore, A. M. A comparison of the psychophysiological and clinical response to biofeedback for temporal pulse amplitude reduction and biofeedback for increases in hand temperature in the treatment of migraine. Unpublished doctoral dissertation, State University of New York at Stony Brook, 1979.

Engel, B. T. Behavioral applications in the treatment of patients with cardiovascular disorders. In J. V. Basmajian (Ed.) *Biofeedback-principles and practice for clinicians.* Baltimore: Williams & Wilkins, 1979.

Engel, E. One hundred years of cytogenetic studies in health and disease. *American Journal of Mental Deficiency,* 1977, *82*(2), 109–116.

Engel, G. Sudden and rapid death during psychological stress. *Annals of Internal Medicine,* 1971, *74,* 721–728.

Engs, R. Drinking patterns and drinking problems of college students. *Journal of Studies on Alcohol,* 1977, *38*(11), 2144–2156.

Epstein, A. W. Fetishism. In R. Slovenko (Ed.) *Sexual behavior and the law.* Springfield, Ill.: Thomas, 1965.

Epstein, C. J., & Golbus, M. S. Prenatal diagnosis of genetic diseases. *American Scientist,* 1977, *65,* 703–711.

Erikson, E. H. *Childhood and society* (2nd ed.). New York: Norton, 1964.

Evans, R. B. Childhood parental relationships of homosexual men. *Journal of Consulting and Clinical Psychology,* 1969, *33*(1), 129–135.

Exner, J. E. *The Rorschach: A comprehensive system.* New York: Wiley, 1974.

Exner, J. E. *The Rorschach: A comprehensive system, vol. 2: Current research and advanced interpretation.* New York: Wiley, 1978.

Eysenck, H. J. *Handbook of abnormal psychology.* New York: Basic Books, 1961.

Eysenck, H. J. *The effects of psychotherapy.* New York: Science House, 1969.

Eysenck, H. J. The learning theory model of neurosis: A new approach. *Behavioral Research and Therapy,* 1976, *14,* 251–267.

Eysenck, H. J. Comment: An exercise in mega-silliness. *American Psychologist,* 1978, *33*(5), 517.

Eysenck, H. J., & Eysenck, S. B. G. *Personality structure and measurement.* London: Routledge & Kegan Paul, 1968.

Fagan, T. J., & Lira, F. T. The primary and secondary sociopathic personality: Differences in frequency and severity of antisocial behaviors. *Journal of Abnormal Psychology,* 1980, *89*(3), 493–496.

Fairweather, G. W., Sanders, D. H., Cressler, D. L., & Maynard, H. *Community life for the mentally ill: An alternative to institutional care.* Chicago: Aldine, 1969.

Farber, I. E., Harlow, H. F., & West, L. J. Brainwashing, conditioning, and DDD (debility, dependency, and dread). *Sociometry,* 1956, *19,* 271–285.

Farberow, N. L. Mental health response in major disasters. *The Psychotherapy Bulletin,* fall 1977, *10*(4), 10–19.

Faris, R. E. L., & Dunham, H. W. *Mental disorders in urban areas: An Ecological study of schizophrenia and other psychosis.* Chicago: University of Chicago Press, 1939.

Farkas, G. M. An ontological analysis of behavior therapy. *American Psychologist,* 1980, *35*(4), 364–374.

Farmer, P. M., Peck, A., & Terry, R. D. Correlations among numbers of neuritic plaques, neurofibrillary tangles, and the severity of senile dementia. *Journal of Neuropathological and Experimental Neurology,* 1976, *35,* 367.

Feeney, D. M. The marijuana window: A theory of cannabis use. *Behavioral Biology,* 1976, *18,* 455–471.

Feighner, J. P. Nosology: A voice for a systematic data-oriented approach. *American Journal of Psychiatry,* 1979, *136*(9), 1173–1174.

Feingold, B. F. Hyperkinesis and learning disabilities linked to artificial food flavors and colors. *American Journal of Nursing,* 1975, *75,* 797–803.

Feldman, M. P. *Criminal behavior: A psychological analysis.* London: Wiley, 1977.

Fenz, W. Strategies for coping with stress. In I. G. Sarason and C. D. Spielberger (Eds.) *Stress and anxiety,* vol. 2. New York: Wiley, 1975.

Ferber, A., Mendelsohn, M., & Napier, A. *The book of family therapy.* New York: Science House, 1972.

Ferster, C. B. Positive reinforcement and behavioral deficits of autistic children. *Child Development,* 1961, *32,* 437–456.

Fields, S. Folk healing for the wounded spirit. *Innovations,* 1976, *3*(1), 2–24.

Fieve, R. R. Lithium for manic disorders: Challenge to electroshock therapy? *New York State Journal of Medicine,* 1971, *71*(18), 2219–2222.

Fieve, R. R., Dunner, D. L., Kumbarachi, T., & Stallone, F. Lithium carbonate in affective disorders IV. A double blind study of prophylaxis in unipolar recurrent depression. *Archives of General Psychiatry,* 1975, *32*(12), 1541–1544.

Fieve, R. R., Rosenthal, D., & Brill, H. (Eds.) *Genetic research in psychiatry.* Baltimore: Johns Hopkins University Press, 1975.

Figley, C. R. Psychosocial adjustment among Vietnam veterans: An overview of the research. In C. R. Figley (Ed.) *Stress disorders among Vietnam veterans: Theory, research and treatment.* New York: Brunner/Mazel, 1978.

Fillmore, K. M. Drinking and problem drinking in early adulthood and middle age: An exploratory 20 year follow up study. *Quarterly Journal of Studies in Alcoholism,* 1974, *35,* 819–840.

Filskov, S., & Goldstein, S. G. Diagnostic validity of the Halstead-Reitan neuropsychological battery. *Journal of Consulting and Clinical Psychology,* 1974, *42*(3), 382–388.

Fink, M. Myths of "shock therapy." *American Journal of Psychiatry,* 1977, *134*(9), 991–996.

Fink, M. A history of convulsive therapy. *The Psychiatric Journal of the University of Ottawa,* 1979, *4*(1), 105–110.

Fisch, M., Goldfarb, A., & Shahinian, S. Chronic brain syndrome in the community aged. *Archives of General Psychiatry,* 1968, *18,* 739–745.

Fischer, M. Genetic and environmental factors in schizophrenia. *Acta Psychiatrica Scandinavica,* Supplement 238, 1973.

Fleiss, J. L., Gurland, B. J., & Goldberg, K. Independence of depersonalization-derealization. *Journal of Consulting and Clinical Psychology,* 1975, *43*(1), 110–111.

Flynn, J. P. Recent findings related to wife abuse. *Social Casework*, 1977, *58*(1), 13–20.

Foa, E. G., Steketee, G., & Milby, J. B. Differential effects of exposure and response prevention in obsessive-compulsive washers. *Journal of Consulting and Clinical Psychology*, 1980, *48*(1), 71–79.

Foa, E. G., & Goldstein, A. Continuous exposure and complete response prevention in the treatment of obsessive-compulsive neurosis. *Behavior Therapy*, 1978, *9*, 821–829.

Fogelson, D. L., Marder, S. R., & Van Putten, T. Dialysis of schizophrenia: Review of clinical trials and implications for further research. *American Journal of Psychiatry*, 1980, *137*(5), 605–606.

Folstein, S., & Rutter, M. Infantile autism: A genetic study of 21 twin pairs. *Journal of Child Psychology and Psychiatry*, 1977, *18*, 297–321.

Fontana, A. F., Hughes, L. A., Marcus, J. L., & Dowds, B. N. Subjective evaluations of life events. *Journal of Consulting and Clinical Psychology*, 1979, *47*(5), 906–911.

Ford, D., & Urban, H. *Systems of psychotherapy: A comparative study.* New York: Wiley, 1965.

Fordyce, W. E. *Use of the MMPI in the assessment of clinical pain.* Nutley, N.J.: Roch Laboratories Monograph, 1979.

Frances, A. The DSM-III personality disorders section: A commentary. *American Journal of Psychiatry*, 1980, *137*(9), 1050–1054.

Frances, R. J., Timm, S., & Bucky, S. Studies of familial and non-familial alcoholism: I. Demographic studies. *Archives of General Psychiatry*, 1980, *37*(5), 564–566.

Frank, J. D. The present status of outcome studies. *Journal of Consulting and Clinical Psychology*, 1979, *47*(2), 310–316.

Frank, J. D. Reply to Telch. *Journal of Consulting and Clinical Psychology*, 1981, *49*(3), 476–477.

Frederick, C. Current trends in suicidal behavior in the United States. *American Journal of Psychotherapy*, 1978, *37*(2), 172–200.

Freedman, B., & Chapman, L. J. Early subjective experience in schizophrenic episodes. *Journal of Abnormal Psychology*, 1973, *82*(1), 46–54.

Freedman, D. Ethnic differences in babies. *Human Nature*, January 1979, pp. 36–43.

Freeman, W., & Watts, J. W. *Psychosurgery in the treatment of mental disorders and intractable pain.* (2nd ed.). Springfield, Ill.: Thomas, 1950.

Freud, S. *The basic writings of Sigmund Freud.* Transl. A. A. Brill. New York: Modern Library, 1938.

Freudenberger, H. J. The dynamics and treatment of the young drug abuser in an Hispanic therapeutic community. *Journal of Psychedelic Drugs*, 1975, *7*(3), 273–280.

Freund, G. Chronic central nervous system toxicity of alcohol. *Annual Review of Pharmacology*, 1973, *13*(2), 217–227.

Friar, L. R., & Beatty, J. Migraine: Management by trained control of vasoconstriction. *Journal of Consulting and Clinical Psychology*, 1976, *44*(1), 46–53.

Frick, O. L. Immediate hypersensitivity. In H. H. Fundenberg, D. P. Stites, J. L. Caldwell, and J. V. Wells (Eds.) *Basic and clinical immunology.* Los Altos, Calif.: Lange, 1976.

Friday, N. *My secret garden.* New York: Trident Press, 1973, pp. 88–92.

Friedman, M., & Rosenman, R. H. *Type A behavior and your heart.* New York: Knopf, 1974.

Friedman, P., & Linn, L. Some psychiatric notes on the Andrea Doria disaster. *American Journal of Psychiatry*, 1957, *114*(4), 426–432.

Fromm-Reichmann, F. *Psychotherapy with schizophrenics.* New York: International Universities Press, 1952.

Fuller, G. D. Current status of biofeedback in clinical practice. *American Psychologist*, 1978, *33*(1), 39–48.

Galanter, M., Stillman, R., Wyatt, R. J., Vaughan, T. B., Weingartner, H., & Nurnberg, F. L. Marihuana and social behavior: A controlled study. *Archives of General Psychiatry*, 1974, *30*(4), 518–519.

Gallo, P. S. Comment: Metaanalysis—A mixed metaphor? *American Psychologist*, 1978, *33*(5), 515–517.

Garber, H., & Heber, F. R. The Milwaukee project: Indications of the effectiveness of early intervention in preventing mental retardation. In P. Mitler (Ed.) *Research and practice in mental retardation*, vol. 1. Baltimore: University Park Press, 1977, pp. 119–127.

Gardner, K. R., & Montgomery, P. S. *Clinical biofeedback: A procedural manual.* Baltimore: Williams & Wilkins, 1977.

Gardner, L. I., & Neu, R. L. Evidence linking an extra Y chromosome to sociopathic behavior. *Archives of General Psychiatry*, 1972, *26*(3), 220–222.

Garfield, S. L. Psychotherapy: A 40 year appraisal. *American Psychologist*, 1981, *36*(2), 174–183.

Garmezy, N. Process and reactive schizophrenia: Some conceptions and issues. *Schizophrenia Bulletin*, fall 1970, no. 2, pp. 30–74.

Gartner, A., & Riessman, F. *Self-help in the human services.* San Francisco: Jossey-Bass, 1977.

Geer, J. H., Davison, G. C., & Gatchel, R. I. Reduction of stress in humans through non-veridical perceived control of aversive stimulation. *Journal of Personality and Social Psychology*, 1970, *16*, 731–738.

Gelder, M. G., Bancroft, J. H., Gath, D. H., Johnston, D. W., Matthews, A. M., & Shaw, P. M. Specific and nonspecific factors in behavioral therapy. *British Journal of Psychiatry*, 1973, *123*, 445–462.

Gelles, R. J. *The violent home.* Beverly Hills, Calif.: Sage, 1972.

Gendreau, P., & Gendreau, L. P. A theoretical note on personality characteristics of heroin addicts. *Journal of Abnormal Psychology,* 1973, *82*(1), 139–140.

Gerard, D. L., & Houston, L. G. Family setting and the social ecology of schizophrenia. *Psychiatric Quarterly,* 1953, *27*(1), 97–101.

Gergen, K. J. Social psychology as history. *Journal of Personality and Social Psychology,* 1973, *26,* 309–320.

Getz, W., Wiessen, A. E., Sue, S., & Ayers, A. *Fundamentals of crisis counseling.* New York: Lexington Books, 1974.

Giaretto, H. Humanistic treatment of father-daughter incest. In R. E. Helfer and C. H. Kempe (Eds.) *Child abuse and neglect: The family and the community.* Cambridge, Mass.: Ballinger, 1978.

Gibbs, F. A., Gibbs, E. L., & Lennox, W. G. Influence of the blood sugar level on the wave and spike formation in petit mal epilepsy. *Archives of Neurology and Psychiatry,* 1939, *41*(6), 1111–1116.

Gibson, R. W. Private psychiatric hospitals: Excellence is their watchword. *American Journal of Psychiatry,* 1978, *135,* Supplement, 17–21.

Gift, T. E., Strauss, J. S., Kokes, R. F., Harder, D. W., & Ritzer, B. A. Schizophrenia: Affect and outcome. *American Journal of Psychiatry,* 1980, *137*(5), 580–585.

Ginsberg, G. L., Frosch, W. A., & Shapiro, T. The new impotence. *Archives of General Psychiatry,* 1972, *26*(3), 218–219.

Glass, A. J. Principles of combat psychiatry. *Military Medicine,* July 1955, *117,* 27–33.

Glass, D. C. *Behavior patterns, stress, and coronary disease.* Hillsdale, N.J.: Erlbaum, 1977.

Glass, D. C., Contrada, R., & Snow, B. Stress, Type A behavior and coronary disease. *Weekly Psychology Update, Biomedia,* 1980, *1*(1), 1–7.

Glass, G. V., & Smith, M. L. Comment: Reply to Eysenck. *American Psychologist,* 1978, *34*(4), 517–519.

Glenn, J. F. Microphallneurosis. *Medical Aspects of Human Sexuality,* 1972, *6*(9), 190–200.

Goffman, E. *Asylums: Essays on the social situation of mental patients and other inmates.* Garden City, N.Y.: Doubleday-Anchor, 1961.

Gold, M. W. Stimulus factors in skill training of retarded adolescents on a complex assembly task. *American Journal of Mental Deficiency,* 1972, *76,* 517–526.

Gold, M. W. Research on the vocational habilitation of the retarded: The present, the future. In N. R. Ellis (Ed.) *International review of research in mental retardation.* New York: Academic Press, 1973.

Golden, K. M. Voodoo in Africa and the United States. *American Journal of Psychiatry,* 1977, *134*(12), 1425–1427.

Goldfried, M. R., & Davison, G. C. *Clinical behavior therapy.* New York: Holt, Rinehart and Winston, 1976.

Goldfried, M. R., & Kent, R. N. Traditional versus behavioral personality assessment: A comparison of methodological and theoretical assumptions. *Psychological Bulletin,* 1972, *77,* 409–420.

Goldstein, A. G. Hallucinatory experience: A personal account. *Journal of Abnormal Psychology,* 1976, *85*(4), 423–429.

Golin, S., Terrell, F., Weitz, J., & Drost, P. The illusion of control among depressed patients. *Journal of Abnormal Psychology,* 1979, *88*(4), 454–457.

Goodwin, D. W. Alcoholism and heredity: A review and hypothesis. *Archives of General Psychiatry,* 1979, *36*(1), 57–61.

Goodwin, D. W., Powell, B., Hill, S. Y., Lieberman, W., & Viamontes, J. Effect of alcohol on dissociated learning in alcoholics. *Journal of Nervous and Mental Disease,* 1974, *158*(2), 198; 201.

Goodwin, F. K., & Athanasios, P. Z. Lithium in the treatment of mania. *Archives of General Psychiatry,* 1979, *36*(7), 840–844.

Goodwin, J. The etiology of combat related post-traumatic stress disorders. In T. Williams (Ed.) *Post traumatic stress disorders of the Vietnam veteran.* Cincinnati, Ohio: Disabled American Veterans, 1980.

Gottesman, I., & Shields, J. *Schizophrenia and genetics: A twin vantage point.* New York: Academic Press, 1972.

Gove, W. R., & Tudor, J. F. Adult sex roles and mental illness. *American Journal of Sociology,* 1973, *78,* 812–835.

Grace, W. J., & Graham, D. T. Relationships of specific attitudes and emotions to certain bodily diseases. *Psychosomatic Medicine,* 1952, *14,* 243–251.

Graham, D. L., & Cross, W. C. Values and attitudes of high school drug users. *Journal of Drug Education,* 1975, *5*(1), 97–107.

Graham, D. T. Health, disease and the mind body problem: Linguistic parallelism. *Psychosomatic Medicine,* 1967, *29*(1), 52–71.

Graham, D. T. Psychosomatic medicine. In N. S. Greenfield and R. A. Sternback (Eds.) *Handbook of psychophysiology.* New York: Holt, Rinehart and Winston, 1972.

Graham, D. T., Stern, J. A., & Winoker, G. Experimental investigation of the specificity of attitude hypothesis in psychosomatic disease. *Psychosomatic Medicine,* 1958, *20,* 446–457.

Graham, F. V., Ernhart, C. B., Craft, M., & Berman, P. W. Brain injury in the preschool child: Some developmental considerations. *Psychological Monographs,* 1963, *77,* 573–574.

Graham, J. R. The Minnesota multiphasic personality inventory. In B. B. Wolman (Ed.) *Clinical diagnosis of mental disorders: A handbook.* New York: Plenum Press, 1978.

Graham, J. R., & Wolff, H. G. Mechanism of migraine headache and action of ergotamine tartrate. *Archives of Neurology and Psychiatry,* 1938, *39,* 737–763.

Gralnick, A. Management of character disorders in a hospital setting. *American Journal of Psychotherapy,* 1979, *33*(1), 54–66.

Gray, J. *The psychology of fear and stress.* New York: McGraw-Hill, 1971.

Green, M. H., & Dupont, R. L. Heroin addiction trends. *American Journal of Psychiatry,* 1974, *13*(5), 545–550.

Green, R. Viewpoints: What are your feelings toward sex change surgery? *Medical Aspects of Human Sexuality,* 1971, *5*(6), 126–129.

Green, R. *Sexual identity conflict in children and adults.* New York: Basic Books, 1974.

Green, R., Newman, L. E., & Stoller, R. J. Treatment of boyhood transsexualism. *Archives of General Psychiatry,* 1972, *26*(3), 213–217.

Green, S. Study of parental loss in neurotics and sociopaths. *Archives of General Psychiatry,* 1964, *11*(2), 177–180.

Greenberg, I. Clinical correlates of fourteen-and-six-cycles-per-second positive EEG spiking and family pathology. *Journal of Abnormal Psychology,* 1970, *76*(3), 403–412.

Greenberg, J. How accurate is psychiatry? *Science News,* 1977, *112,* 28–29.

Greenson, R. R. *The technique and practice of psychoanalysis,* vol. 1. New York: International Universities Press, 1967.

Greenwald, D. P., Kornblith, S. J., Hersen, M., Bellack, A. S., & Himmelhock, J. M. Differences between social skills therapists and psychotherapists in treating depression. *Journal of Consulting and Clinical Psychology,* 1981, *49*(5), 757–759.

Greer, W., & Cobbs, P. *Black rage.* New York: Bantam Press, 1968.

Greilsheimer, H., & Groves, J. E. Male genital self-mutilation. *Archives of General Psychiatry,* 1979, *36*(4), 441–446.

Griffith, J. D., Cavanaugh, J., Held, J., & Oates, J. A. Dextroamphetamine, evaluation of psychotomimetic properties in man. *Archives of General Psychiatry,* 1972, *26*(1), 97–100.

Griffith, J. J., Mednick, S. A., Schulsinger, F., & Diderichsen, B. Verbal associative disturbance in children at high risk for schizophrenia. *Journal of Abnormal Psychology,* 1980, *89*(2), 125–131.

Grinspoon, L. *Marihuana reconsidered.* Cambridge, Mass.: Harvard University Press, 1971.

Groth, N., & Burgess, A. W. Male rape: Offenders and victims. *American Journal of Psychiatry,* 1980, *137*(7), 806–810.

Groth, N., Burgess, A. W., & Holmstrom, L. L. Rape: Power anger and sexuality. *American Journal of Psychiatry,* 1977, *134*(11), 1239–1243.

Gruenberg, E. M. The social breakdown syndrome—Some origins. *American Journal of Psychiatry,* 1967, *123*(6), 726–730.

Gruenberg, E. M. From practice to theory: Community mental health services and the nature of psychoses. *The Lancet,* April 5, 1969, pp. 721–724.

Grunebaum, H., & Perlman, M. S. Paranoia and naivete. *Archives of General Psychiatry,* 1973, *28*(1), 30–32.

Grusec, J., Mischel, W. Models' characteristics as determinants of social learning. *Journal of Personality and Social Psychology,* 1966, *4,* 211–215.

Guerra, F. *The pre-Colombian mind.* New York: Seminar Press, 1971.

Guilford, J. P. *Fundamental statistics in psychology and education* (3rd ed.). New York: McGraw-Hill, 1956.

Guze, S. B., Goodwin, D., & Crane, J. Criminality and psychiatric disorders. *Archives of General Psychiatry,* 1969, *20*(4), 583–591.

Gynther, M. D., & Gynther, R. A. Personality inventories. In I. B. Weiner (Ed.) *Clinical methods in psychology.* New York: Wiley, 1976.

Haier, R. J., Rosenthal, D., & Wender, P. H. MMPI assessment of psychopathology in the adopted away offspring of schizophrenics. *Archives of General Psychiatry,* 1978, *35*(2), 171–175

Hall, R. C. W., & Malone, P. T. Psychiatric effects of prolonged Asian captivity: A two year follow up. *American Journal of Psychiatry,* 1976, *133*(7), 786–790.

Halleck, S. L. Another response to "homosexuality: The ethical challenge." *Journal of Consulting and Clinical Psychology,* 1976, *44*(2), 167–170.

Hamburger, R. N. Allergy and the immune system. *American Scientist,* 1976, *64,* 157–164.

Hamilton, J. W. Voyeurism: Some clinical and theoretical considerations. *American Journal of Psychotherapy,* 1972, *26*(2), 277–287.

Hanson, D. R., Gottesman, I. I., & Hester, L. L. Some possible childhood indicators of adult schizophrenia inferred from children of schizophrenics. *British Journal of Psychiatry,* 1976, *129*(1), 142–154.

Harbin, H. T., & Madden, D. J. Battered parents: A new syndrome. *American Journal of Psychiatry,* 1979, *136*(10), 1288–1291.

Hare, R. D. *Psychopathy: Theory and research.* New York: Wiley, 1970.

Hare, R. D. Anxiety, stress, and psychopathology. In I. G. Sarason and C. D. Spielberger (Eds.) *Stress and anxiety,* vol. 2. New York: Wiley, 1975.

Hare, R. D. Psychophysiological studies of psychopathy. In D. C. Forles (Ed.) *Clinical applications of psychophysiology.* New York: Columbia University Press, 1978.

Harford, T. C., Dorman, N., & Feinhandler, S. J. Alcohol consumption in bars: Validation of self-reports against observed behavior. *Drinking and Drug Practicum Surveyor,* 1976, no. 11, pp. 13–15.

Harlow, H. F., & Harlow, M. K. Effects of various mother infant relationships on Rhesus monkey behaviors. In B. M. Foss (Ed.) *Determinants of infant behavior IV.* London: Methuen, 1969.

Harper, R. *Psychoanalysis and psychotherapy: 36 systems.* Englewood Cliffs, N.J.: Prentice-Hall, 1960.

Harris, B. Whatever happened to little Albert? *American Psychologist,* 1979, *34*(1), 151–160.

Harrow, M., Grinker, R. R., Holzman, P. S., & Kayton, L. Anhedonia and schizophrenia. *American Journal of Psychiatry,* 1977, *134*(7), 794–797.

Hartley, D., Roback, H. B., & Abramowitz, S. I. Deterioration effects in encounter groups. *American Psychologist,* 1976, *31*(3), 247–255.

Hastings, D. W. Viewpoints: What are your feelings toward sex change surgery? *Medical Aspects of Human Sexuality,* 1971, *5*(6), 135–136.

Hathaway, S. R. Where have we gone wrong? The mystery of the missing progress. In J. N. Butcher (Ed.) *Objective personality assessment: Changing perspective.* New York: Academic Press, 1972.

Hathaway, S. R., & McKinley, J. C. *Multiphasic personality inventory.* New York: The Psychological Corp., 1943.

Haynes, S. N., Griffin, P., Mooney, G., & Parise, M. Electromyographic biofeedback and relaxation instruction in the treatment of muscle contraction headache. *Behavior Therapy,* 1975, *6,* 672–678.

Heath, R. G., Martens, S., Leach, B. E., Cohen, M., & Feigley, L. A. Behavioral changes in nonpsychotic volunteers following administration of taraxein, a substance obtained from serum of schizophrenic patients. *American Journal of Psychiatry,* 1958, *114*(8), 917–920.

Heaton, R. K., & Victor, R. G. Personality characteristics associated with psychedelic flashbacks in natural and experimental settings. *Journal of Abnormal Psychology,* 1976, *85*(1), 83–90.

Heber, R. *Epidemiology of mental retardation.* Springfield, Ill.: Thomas, 1970.

Heber, R., & Garber, H. Prevention of cultural-familial retardation. In A. Jeger and R. Slotnick (Eds.) *Community health: A behavioral-ecological perspective.* New York: Plenum Press, 1980.

Heilbrun, A. B. Psychopathy and violent crime. *Journal of Consulting and Clinical Psychology,* 1979, *47*(3), 509–516.

Heilbrun, A. B., & Heilbrun, K. S. Content analysis of delusions in reactive and process schizophrenics. *Journal of Abnormal Psychology,* 1977, *86*(6), 597–608.

Heilbrun, K. S. Silverman's subliminal psychodynamic activation: A failure to replicate. *Journal of Abnormal Psychology,* 1980, *89*(4), 560–566.

Helzer, J. E., & Winoker, G. A family interview study of male manic depressives. *Archives of General Psychiatry,* 1974, *31*(1), 73–77.

Henderson, D. K., & Gillespie, R. D. *Textbook of psychiatry* (10th ed.). London: Oxford University Press, 1969.

Herbert, W. States ponder notion of criminal insanity. *APA Monitor,* April 1979, pp. 8–9.

Hersen, M. The behavioral treatment of school phobia: Current techniques. *The Journal of Nervous and Mental Disease,* 1971, *153*(2), 99–106.

Hersen, M., & Bellack, A. S. *Behavioral assessment: A practical handbook.* New York: Pergamon Press, 1976.

Hersen, M., Gullich, E. L., Matherne, P. M., & Harbert, T. L. Instructions and reinforcement in the modification of a conversion disorder. *Psychological Reports,* 1972, *31*(6), 719–722.

Heston, L. L. Psychiatric disorders in foster home reared children of schizophrenic mothers. *British Journal of Psychiatry,* 1966, *112,* 819–825.

Heston, L. L. The clinical genetics of Pick's disease. *Acta Psychiatrica Scandinavica,* 1978, *57,* 202–206.

Hilberman, E. Rape: The ultimate violation of self. *American Journal of Psychiatry,* 1976, *133*(4), 436–437.

Hilgard, E. R. *Hypnotic susceptibility.* New York: Harcourt Brace Jovanovich, 1965.

Hilgard, E. R. Pain as puzzle for psychology and physiology. *American Psychologist,* 1969, *24*(1), 103–113.

Hilgard, E. R., MacDonald, H., Morgan, A. H., & Johnson, L. S. The reality of hypnotic analgesia: A comparison of highly hypnotizables with simulators. *Journal of Abnormal Psychology,* 1978, *87*(2), 239–246.

Hirshfield, M. *Sexual anomalies and perversions.* New York: Emerson Books, 1948.

Hiscock, M., Kinsbourne, M., Caplan, B., & Swanson, J. M. Auditory attention in hyperactive children: Effects of stimulant medication on dichotic listening performance. *Journal of Abnormal Psychology,* 1979, *88*(1), 27–32.

Hodges, W. F. The psychophysiology of anxiety. In M. Zuckerman and C. D. Spielberger (Eds.) *Emotions and anxiety: New concepts, methods and applications.* Hillsdale, N.J.: Erlbaum, 1976.

Hoenig, J. Etiological research in transsexualism. *The Psychiatric Journal of the University of Ottawa,* 1981, *6*(2), 184–189.

Hoffer, A. The effect of nicotinic acid on the frequency and duration of rehospitalization of schizophrenic patients: A controlled comparison study. *International Journal of Neuropsychiatry,* 1966, no. 2, 234–240.

Hoffer, A., Osmond, H., Callbeck, M. J., & Kahan, I. Treatment of schizophrenia with nicotinic acid and nicotinamide. *Journal of Clinical Experimental Psychopathology,* 1957, *18*(11), 131–158.

Hoffman, E., & Reeves, R. An idiot savant with unusual mechanical ability. *American Journal of Psychiatry,* 1979, *136*(5), 713–714.

Hofling, C. K. *Textbook of psychiatry for medical practice,* (3rd ed.). Philadelphia: Lippincott, 1975.

Hofmann, A. Psychotomimetic drugs: Chemical and pharmacological aspects. *Acta Physiological et Pharmacoligica Neerlandia,* 1959, *8,* 240–258.

Hollister, L. E. Clinical evaluation of naltrexone treatment of opiate-dependent individuals. *Archives of General Psychiatry,* 1978, *35*(3), 335–340.

Holmes, T. H., & Rahe, R. H. The social readjustment rating scale. *Journal of Psychosomatic Research,* 1967, *11,* 213–218.

Hopkins, W. P., & Fine, H. J. The end of Jim Morrison: A schizoid suicide—A phenomenological study in object relations. *Psychotherapy: Theory, Research and Practice,* 1977, *4*(4), 423–427.

Hoppe, K. D. Chronic reactive aggression in survivors of severe persecution. *Comprehensive Psychiatry,* 1971, *12*(3), 230–237.

Horn, A. S., & Snyder, S. H. Chloropromazine and dopamine: Conformational similarities that correlate with the antischizophrenic activity of phenothiazine drugs. *Proceedings of the National Academy of Sciences,* 1971, *68,* 2325–2328.

Horn, J. M., Loehlin, J. C., & Willerman, L. Intellectual resemblance among adoptive and biological relatives: The Texas adoption project. *Behavior Genetics,* 1979, *9,* 177–207.

Horton, P. Normality—toward a meaningful construct. *Comprehensive Psychiatry,* 1971, *12*(1), 1–21.

Horvey, S. C. Hypnotics and sedatives. In L. S. Goodman and A. Gilman (Eds.) *The pharmacological basis of therapeutics* (5th ed.). New York: Macmillan, 1975.

Houlihan, J. P. Heterogeneity among schizophrenic patients: Selective review of recent findings (1970–1975). *Schizophrenia Bulletin,* 1977, *3*(2), 246–258.

Howard, G. *Participant modeling in the treatment of rat phobias.* Unpublished doctoral dissertation. Southern Illinois University, 1975.

Howland, J. S. The use of hypnosis in the treatment of a case of multiple personality. *Journal of Nervous and Mental Disease,* 1975, *161*(2), 138–142.

Huesmann, L. R. (Ed.) Special issue: Learned helplessness as a model of depression. *Journal of Abnormal Psychology,* 1978, *87*(1), 1.

Hugdahl, K., Fredrikson, M., & Ohman, A. Preparedness and arousability as determinants of electrodermal conditioning. *Behavior Research and Therapy,* 1977, *15,* 345–353.

Hugdahl, K., & Karker, A. C. Biologic vs. experiential factors in phobic conditioning. *Behavior Research and Therapy,* 1981, *19*(2), 109–115.

Hughes, J. Isolation of an endogenous compound from the brain with properties similar to morphine. *Brain Research,* 1975, *88,* 295–308.

Hunt, D. D., & Hampson, J. L. Follow up of 17 biologic male transsexuals after sex reassignment surgery. *American Journal of Psychiatry,* 1980, *137*(4), 432–438.

Hunt, M. *Sexual behavior in the seventies.* Chicago: Playboy Press, 1974.

Hunter, E. J. The Vietnam POW veteran: Immediate and long term effects. In C. R. Figley (Ed.) *Stress disorders among Vietnam veterans.* New York: Brunner/Mazel, 1978.

Hutchings, B., & Mednick, S. A. Registered criminality in the adoptive and biological parents of registered male adoptees. In S. A. Mednick, F. Schulsinger, and J. Bell (Eds.) *Genetics, environment and psychopathology.* New York: Elsevier-North Holland, 1974.

Ince, L. P. Behavior modification of sexual disorders. *American Journal of Psychotherapy,* 1973, *27*(3), 446–451.

Inhelder, B. *The diagnosis of reasoning in the mentally retarded* (2nd ed.). New York: Chandler, 1968.

Inouye, E. Similarity and dissimilarity of schizophrenia in twins. *Proceedings of the Third International Congress of Psychiatry, 1961,* vol. 1. Montreal: University of Toronto Press, 1963, pp. 524–530.

Jackson, D. The study of the family. *Family Process,* 1965, *4*(1), 1–19.

Jacobson, A., Kales, J. D., & Kales, A. Clinical and electrophysiological correlates of sleep disorders in children. In A. Kales (Ed.) *Sleep: Physiology and pathology.* Philadelphia: Lippincott, 1969.

Jacobson, A. M., Manschreck, T. C., & Silverberg, E. Behavioral treatment for Raynaud's disease: A comparative study with long term follow up. *American Journal of Psychiatry,* 1979, *136*(6), 844–846.

Jahoda, M. *Current concepts of positive mental health.* New York: Basic Books, 1959.

James, K. L. Incest: The teenager's perspective. *Psychotherapy: Theory, Research and Practice,* 1977, *14*(2), 146–155.

Janisse, M. P. The relationship between pupil size and anxiety: A review. In I. G. Sarason and C. D. Spielberger (Eds.) *Stress and anxiety,* vol. 3. New York: Wiley, 1976.

Janzen, C. Families in the treatment of alcoholism. *Journal of Studies on Alcohol,* 1977, *38*(1), 114–130.

Jarvik, L. F., Klodin, V., & Matsuyama, S. S. Human

aggression and the extra Y chromosome: Fact or fantasy? *American Psychologist*, 1973, *28*(8), 674–682.

Jarvik, M. E. The behavioral effects of psychotogens. In R. C. DeBold and R. C. Leaf (Eds.) *LSD, man and society*. Middletown: Connecticut Wesleyan Press, 1968.

Jarvis, V. Countertransference in the management of school phobia. *Psychoanalytic Quarterly*, 1964, *33*, 411–419.

Jeans, R. F., I. An independently validated case of multiple personality. *Journal of Abnormal Psychology*, 1976, *85*(3), 249–255.

Jeffee, S. *Narcotics—An American plan*. New York: Erikson, 1966.

Johnson, W. G., Ross, J. M., & Mastria, M. A. Delusional behavior: An attributional analysis of development and modification. *Journal of Abnormal Psychology*, 1977, *86*(4), 421–426.

Jones, E. The cocaine episode. In L. Trilling and S. Marcus (Eds.) *The life and works of Sigmund Freud*. New York: Basic Books, 1953.

Jones, K. L., & Smith, D. W. Recognition of the fetal alcohol syndrome in early infancy. *The Lancet*, 1973, *2*, 994–1001.

Jones, M. *The therapeutic community*. New York: Basic Books, 1953.

Jones, M. Community care for chronic mental patients: The need for a reassessment. *Hospital & Community Psychiatry*, 1975, *26*(2), 94–98.

Jones, M. C. Personality correlates and antecedents of drinking patterns in adult males. *Journal of Consulting and Clinical Psychology*, 1968, *32*(1), 2–12.

Jones, M. C. Personality antecedents and correlates of drinking patterns in women. *Journal of Consulting and Clinical Psychology*, 1971, *36*(1), 61–70.

Jones, M. C. Albert Peter and J. B. Watson. *American Psychologist*, 1974, *29*(8), 581–583.

Judd, L. L., & Grant, I. Brain dysfunction in chronic sedative users. *Journal of Psychedelic Drugs*, 1975, *7*(2), 143–149.

Kafrissen, S. R., Heffron, E. G., & Zusman, J. Mental health problems in environmental disasters. In H. L. P. Resnik and H. L. Ruben (Eds.) *Emergency psychiatric care: The management of mental health crisis*. Bowie, Md.: Charles Press, 1975.

Kales, J. D., Kales, A., Soldatos, C. R., Chamberlin, K., & Martin, E. D. Sleepwalking and night terrors related to febrile illness. *American Journal of Psychiatry*, 1979, *136*(9), 1007–1014.

Kalinowsky, L. B. Psychosurgery: The past twenty years. *Psychiatric Journal of the University of Ottawa*, 1979, *4*(1), 111–113.

Kallmann, F. J. *Heredity in health and mental disorder*. New York: Norton, 1953.

Kanner, L. Autistic disturbances of affective content. *Nervous Child*, 1943, *2*, 217–250.

Kanner, L. Follow-up study of eleven autistic children originally reported in 1943. *Journal of Autism and Childhood Schizophrenia*, 1971, *1*(2), 119–145.

Kanner, L., Rodriguez, A., & Alexander, B. How far can autistic children go in matters of social adjustment? *Journal of Autism and Childhood Schizophrenia*, 1972, *2*(1), 9–33.

Kantor, R. E., Wallner, J. M., & Winder, L. L. Process and reactive schizophrenia. *Journal of Consulting Psychology*, 1953, *17*(1), 157–162.

Kaplan, H. S. *The new sex therapy*. New York: Brunner/Mazel, 1974.

Kaplan, H. S. *The illustrated manual of sex therapy*. New York: Quadrangle/New York Times Book, 1975.

Kaplan, H. S. Interview: "Quack" sex therapy. *Medical Aspects of Human Sexuality*, 1977, *4*(2), 32–47.

Kaplan, H. S. Interview: Inhibited sexual desire. *Medical Aspects of Human Sexuality*, 1979, *13*(11), 26–47.

Kaplan, N. M. *Your blood pressure: The most deadly high: A physician's guide to controlling your hypertension*. New York: Medcom, 1974.

Karasu, T. B. Psychotherapies: An overview. *American Journal of Psychiatry*, 1977, *134*(8), 851–863.

Karasu, T. B. Psychotherapy of the psychosomatic patient. *American Journal of Psychotherapy*, 1979, *33*(3), 354–364.

Kasl, S. V., & Cobb, S. Blood pressure changes in men undergoing job loss: A preliminary report. *Psychosomatic Medicine*, 1970, *6*(1), 95–106.

Katkin, E. S. Electrodermal lability: A psychophysiological analysis of individual differences in response to stress. In I. G. Sarason and C. D. Spielberger (Eds.) *Stress and anxiety*, vol. 2. New York: Wiley, 1975.

Katzman, R. The prevalence and malignancy of Alzheimer's disease. *Archives of Neurology*, 1976, *33*(2), 217–218.

Katzman, R., & Karasu, T. B. Differential diagnosis of dementia. In W. S. Fields (Ed.) *Neurological and sensory disorders in the elderly*. New York: Stratton Intercontinental Medical Book, 1975.

Kaufman, E. The abuse of multiple drugs: I. Definition, classification and extent of problem. *American Journal of Drugs and Alcohol Abuse*, 1976, *3*(2), 279–292.

Kazdin, A. E. The failure of some patients to respond to token programs. *Journal of Behavior Therapy and Experimental Psychiatry*, 1973, *4*(1), 7–14.

Kazdin, A. E., & Wilcoxon, L. A. Systematic desensitization and nonspecific treatment effects: A methodological evaluation. *Psychological Bulletin*, 1976, *83*, 729–758.

Keane, T. M., & Lisman, S. A. Alcohol and social anxiety in males: Behavioral, cognitive, and physiological effects. *Journal of Abnormal Psychology,* 1980, *89*(2), 213–223.

Keill, S. L. The general hospital as the core of the mental health services system. *Hospital & Community Psychiatry,* 1981, *32*(1), 776–778.

Keith, S. J., Gunderson, J. G., Reifman, A., Buchsbaum, S., & Mosher, L. R. Special report: Schizophrenia 1976. *Schizophrenia Bulletin,* 1976, *2*(4), 509–564.

Kellner, R. Psychotherapy in psychosomatic disorders: A survey of controlled studies. *Archives of General Psychiatry,* 1975, *32*(8), 1021–1028.

Kempler, W. *Principles of Gestalt family therapy.* Oslo, Norway: A. S. Joh. Nordahls Trykken, 1973.

Kendall, R. E. *The role of diagnosis in psychiatry.* Oxford: Blackwell Scientific, 1975.

Kendler, K. S., Gruenberg, A. M., & Straus, J. S. An independent analysis of the Copenhagen sample of the Danish adoption study of schizophrenia: II. The relationship between schizotypal personality disorder and schizophrenia. *Archives of General Psychiatry,* 1981a, *38*(8), 982–984.

Kendler, K. S., Gruenberg, A. M., & Straus, J. S. An independent analysis of the Copenhagen sample of the Danish adoption study of schizophrenia: III. The relationship between paranoid psychosis (delusional disorder) and the schizophrenia spectrum disorders. *Archives of General Psychiatry,* 1981b, *38*(8), 985–987.

Kendler, K. S., & Hays, P. Paranoid psychosis (delusional disorder) and schizophrenia: A family history study. *Archives of General Psychiatry,* 1981, *38*(4), 547–551.

Kennedy, W. A. School phobia: Rapid treatment of fifty cases. *Journal of Abnormal and Social Psychology,* 1965, *70,* 285–289.

Kephart, W. M. Sex and the divorced man. *Medical Aspects of Human Sexuality,* 1972, *6*(9), 173.

Kessler, P., & Neale, J. M. Hippocampal damage and schizophrenia: A critique of Mednick's theory. *Journal of Abnormal Psychology,* 1974, *83*(2), 91–96.

Kessler, S. The genetics of schizophrenia: A review. *Schizophrenia Bulletin,* 1980, *6*(3), 404–416.

Kety, S. S. Progress toward an understanding of the biological substrates of schizophrenia. In R. Fieve, D. Rosenthal, and H. Brill (Eds.) *Genetic research in psychiatry.* Baltimore: Johns Hopkins University Press, 1975.

Kety, S. S., Rosenthal, D., Wender, P. H., & Schulsinger, F. Studies based on a total sample of adopted individuals and their relatives: Why they were necessary, what they demonstrated and failed to demonstrate. *Schizophrenia Bulletin,* 1976, *2,* 413–428.

Khavari, K. A., Mabry, E., & Humes, M. Personality correlates of hallucinogen use. *Journal of Abnormal Psychology,* 1977, *86*(2), 172–178.

Kiev, A. Transcultural psychiatry: Research problems and perspectives. In S. C. Plog, and R. B. Edgerton (Eds.) *Changing perspectives in mental illness.* New York: Holt, Rinehart and Winston, 1969.

Kinsey, A. C., Pomeroy, W. B., & Martin, C. E. *Sexual behavior in the human male.* Philadelphia: Saunders, 1948.

Kinsey, A. C., Pomeroy, W. B., Martin, C. E., & Gebhard, P. H. *Sexual behavior in the human female.* Philadelphia: Saunders, 1953.

Kinsman, R. A., Spector, S. L., Shucard, D. W., & Luparello, T. J. Observations on patterns of subjective symptomatology of acute asthma. *Psychosomatic Medicine,* 1974, *36*(2), 129–143.

Kittrie, N. N. *The right to be different: Deviance and enforced therapy.* Baltimore: Johns Hopkins University Press, 1971.

Klebanoff, L. D. A comparison of parental attitudes of mothers of schizophrenics, brain injured and normal children. *American Journal of Orthopsychiatry,* 1959, *24,* 445–454.

Kleeman, S. T. Psychiatric contributions in the treatment of asthma. *Annals of Allergy,* 1967, *25,* 611–619.

Klein, D. Psychosocial treatment of schizophrenia or psychosocial help for people with schizophrenia? *Schizophrenia Bulletin,* 1980, *6*(1), 122–130.

Kluver, H. *Mescal and mechanisms of hallucinations.* Chicago: University of Chicago Press, 1966.

Knight, R. A., Roff, J. D., Barrnett, J., & Moss, J. L. Concurrent and predictive validity of thought disorder and affectivity: A 22-year follow-up of acute schizophrenics. *Journal of Abnormal Psychology,* 1979, *88*(1), 1–12.

Kojak, G., & Canby, J. P. Personality and behavior patterns of heroin-dependent American service men in Thailand. *American Journal of Psychiatry,* 1975, *132*(3), 246–250.

Kolb, L. C. *Noyes modern clinical psychiatry* (7th ed.). Philadelphia: Saunders, 1968.

Kopel, S., & Arkowitz, H. The role of attribution and self-perception in behavior change: Implications for behavior therapy. *Genetic Psychology Monographs,* 1975, *92*(2), 175–212.

Korchin, S. *Modern clinical psychology: Principles of intervention in the clinic and community.* New York: Basic Books, 1976.

Kormos, H. R. The nature of combat stress. In C. R. Figley (Ed.) *Stress disorders among Vietnam veterans.* New York: Brunner/Mazel, 1978.

Kornetsky, C. *Pharmacology: Drugs affecting behavior.* New York: Wiley, 1976.

Kornetsky, C., & Orzack, M. H. Physiological and

behavioral correlates of attention dysfunction in schizophrenic patients. *Journal of Psychiatric Research,* 1978, *14,* 69–79.

Kovacs, M. The efficacy of cognitive and behavior therapies for depression. *American Journal of Psychiatry,* 1980; *137*(12), 1495–1504.

Kovacs, M. & Beck, A. T. Maladaptive cognitive structures in depression. *American Journal of Psychiatry,* 1978, *135*(5), 525–533.

Kovacs, M., Rush, A. J., Beck, A. T., & Hollon, S. Depressed outpatients treated with cognitive therapy or pharmacotherapy. *Archives of General Psychiatry,* 1981, *38*(1), 33–39.

Kozol, H. L. Myths about the sex offender. *Medical Aspects of Human Sexuality,* 1971, *5*(6), 51–62.

Kraines, S. H. *The therapy of the neuroses and psychoses.* Philadelphia: Lea & Febiger, 1957.

Kramer, J. C., Fishman, V. S., & Littlefield, D. C. Amphetamine abuse: Pattern and effects of high dose taken intravenously. *Journal of American Medical Association,* 1967, *201*(1), 305–309.

Krasner, L. The future and the past in the behaviorism-humanism dialogue. *American Psychologist,* 1978, *33*(9), 799–804.

Krauthamer, C. The personality of alcoholic middle-class women: A comparative study with MMPI. *Journal of Clinical Psychology,* 1979, *35*(2), 442–448.

Kringlen, E. *Heredity and environment in the functional psychoses.* London: Heinemann, 1967.

Kristt, O. A., & Engel, B. T. Learned control of blood pressure in patients with high blood pressure. *Circulation,* 1975, *51,* 370–378.

Kroll, J. A reappraisal of psychiatry in the middle ages. *Archives of General Psychiatry,* 1973, *29*(3), 276–283.

Krueger, D. W. Symptom passing in a transvestite father and three sons. *American Journal of Psychiatry,* 1978, *135*(6), 739–742.

Krueger, D. W. The differential diagnosis of proverb interpretation. In W. E. Fann, I. K. Karacan, A. Pokorny, and R. L. Williams (Eds.) *Phenomenology and treatment of schizophrenia.* New York: Spectrum, 1978.

Kübler-Ross, E. *On death and dying.* New York: Macmillan, 1969.

Kunnes, R. Double-dealing in dope. *Human Behavior,* 1973, *2*(10), 22–27.

Kuriansky, J. B., Deming, W. E., & Gurland, B. J. On trends in the diagnosis of schizophrenia. *American Journal of Psychiatry,* 1974, *131*(3), 402–428.

Kushner, F. H. All of us bear the scars. *U.S. News and World Report,* April 16, 1973, *74*(16), p. 41.

Kutash, I. L., Kutash, S. B., Schlesinger, L. B., & Associates. *Violence.* San Francisco: Jossey-Bass, 1978.

Lacey, J. I. Somatic response patterning and stress: Some revisions of activation theory. In M. H. Appley and R. Trumball (Eds.) *Psychological stress.* New York: McGraw-Hill, 1967.

Lackman, S. J. *Psychosomatic disorders: A behavioristic interpretation.* New York: Wiley, 1972.

Lader, M., & Mathews, H. Physiological changes during spontaneous panic attacks. *Journal of Psychosomatic Research,* 1970, *14*(4), 377–382.

Laing, R. D., & Esterson, A. *Sanity, madness, and the family.* New York: Basic Books, 1971.

Lamb, H. R., & Zusman, J. A. New look at primary prevention. *Hospital & Community Psychiatry,* 1981, *32*(12), 843–848.

Lambert, M. M., Sandoval, J., & Sassone, D. Prevalence of hyperactivity in elementary school children as a function of social system defenses. *American Journal of Orthopsychiatry,* 1978, *48,* 446–463.

Langer, E. J., & Abelson, R. P. A patient by any other name . . .: Clinic group difference in labeling bias. *Journal of Consulting and Clinical Psychology,* 1974, *42*(1), 4–9.

Larkin, A. R. The form and content of schizophrenic hallucinations. *American Journal of Psychiatry,* 1979, *136*(7), 940–943.

LaRusso, L. Sensitivity of paranoid patients to nonverbal cues. *Journal of Abnormal Psychology,* 1978, *87*(5), 463–471.

Laughlin, H. P. *The neurosis in clinical practice.* Philadelphia: Saunders, 1956.

Lazarus, A. H. Has behavior therapy outlined its usefulness? *American Psychologist,* 1977, *33*(7), 550–554.

Lazarus, R. S. Psychological stress and coping in adaptation and illness. *International Journal of Psychiatry in Medicine,* 1974, *5*(2), 321–333.

Leeman, C. P. Involuntary admissions to general hospitals: Progress or threat? *Hospital & Community Psychiatry,* 1980, *31*(5), 315–318.

Leeman, C. P., & Berger, H. S. The Massachusetts psychiatric society's position paper on involuntary psychiatric admissions to general hospitals. *Hospital & Community Psychiatry,* 1980, *31*(5), 318–324.

Lehrer, P. M. Physiological effects of relaxation in a double-blind analog of desensitization. *Behavior Therapy,* 1972, *3*(2), 193–208.

Leitenberg, H. Behavioral approaches to treatment of neurosis. In H. Leitenberg (Ed.) *Handbook of behavior modification and behavior therapy.* Englewood Cliffs, N.J.: Prentice-Hall, 1976.

LeJeune, R., & Alex, N. On being mugged: The event and its aftermath. *Urban Life and Culture,* 1973, pp. 259–287.

Lemberg, R. W. Multi-sensory hallucinatory experiences: A diary account. *American Journal of Psychotherapy*, 1978, *32*(3), 457–468.

Lemert, E. M. *Human deviance, social problems, and social control.* Englewood Cliffs, N.J.: Prentice-Hall, 1967.

Leon, C. A. "El Duende" and other incubi: Suggestive interactions between culture, the devil, and the brain. *Archives of General Psychiatry*, 1975, *32*(2), 155–162.

Leon, G. R., Gillum, B., Gillum, R., & Gouze, M. Personality stability and change over a 30-year period—Middle age to old age. *Journal of Consulting and Clinical Psychology*, 1979, *47*(3), 517–524.

Leopold, R. L., & Dillon, H. Psychoanatomy of a disaster: A long term study of post-traumatic neurosis in survivors of a marine explosion. *American Journal of Psychiatry*, 1963, *119*(10), 913–921.

Lerro, F. A., Hurnyak, M. M., & Patterson, C. Successful use of thermal biofeedback in severe adult asthma. *American Journal of Psychiatry*, 1980, *137*(6), 735–736.

Lester, D. The myth of suicide prevention. *Comprehensive Psychiatry*, 1972, *13*(6), 555–560.

Levenson, R. W., Sher, K. J., Grossman, L. M., Newman, J., & Newlin, D. B. Alcohol and stress response dampening: Pharmacological effects, expectancy, and tension reduction. *Journal of Abnormal Psychology*, 1980, *89*(4), 528–538.

Levine, D. S., & Willver, S. G. *The cost of mental illness.* 1974. Mental Health Statistical Note No. 125, National Institute of Mental Health. Washington, D.C., 1976.

Levitz, L. S., & Ullman, L. P. Manipulations of indications of disturbed thinking in normal subjects. *Journal of Consulting and Clinical Psychology*, 1969, *33*(7), 633–641.

Levy, L., & Rowitz, L. *The ecology of mental disorder.* New York: Behavioral Publications, 1973.

Levy, L., & Rowitz, L. Mapping out schizophrenia. *Human Behavior*, 1974, *3*(5), 602–611.

Lewin, B. I. *The psychoanalysis of elation.* New York: Norton, 1950.

Lewinsohn, P. M. A behavioral approach to depression. In R. J. Friedman and M. M. Katz (Eds.) *The psychology of depression: Contemporary theory and research.* Washington, D.C.: Winston, 1974.

Lewinsohn, P. M. The behavioral study and treatment of depression. In M. Hersen, R. M. Eisler, and P. M. Miller (Eds.) *Progress in behavior modification.* New York: Academic Press, 1975.

Lewinsohn, P. M., Mischel, W., Chaplin, W., & Barton, R. Social competence and depression: The role of illusory self-perceptions. *Journal of Abnormal Psychology*, 1980, *89*(2), 203–212.

Lezak, M. D. *Neuropsychological assessment.* New York: Oxford University Press, 1976.

Liberman, D. A. Behaviorism and the mind: A (limited) call for a return to introspection. *American Psychologist*, 1979, *34*(4), 319–333.

Liberman, R. P. Behavior therapy for schizophrenia. In L. J. West and D. E. Flinn (Eds.) *Treatment of schizophrenia: Progress and prospects.* New York: Grune & Stratton, 1976.

Lidz, T., Flech, S., & Cornelison, A. *Schizophrenia and the family.* New York: International Universities Press, 1965.

Liem, J. H. Effects of verbal communications of parents and children: A comparison of normal and schizophrenic families. *Journal of Consulting and Clinical Psychology*, 1974, *42*(3), 438–450.

Liem, J. H. Family studies of schizophrenia: An update and commentary. *Schizophrenia Bulletin*, 1980, *6*(3), 429–455.

Lifton, R. *Death in life: The survivors of Hiroshima.* London: Weidenfeld and Nicholson, 1969.

Lifton, R. J. The "gook syndrome" and "numbed warfare." *Saturday Review*, December 1972, *55*(47), 66–72.

Lifton, R. J., & Olson, E. The human meaning of total disaster. *Psychiatry*, 1976, *39*(1), 1–18.

Lindemann, E. Symptomatology and management of acute grief. *American Journal of Psychiatry*, 1944, *101*(9), 141–148.

Linden, W. Exposure treatments for focal phobias: A review. *Archives of General Psychiatry*, 1981, *38*(7), 769–775.

Lin-fu, J. S. Undue absorption of lead among children: A new look at an old problem. *New England Journal of Medicine*, 1972, *286*, 702–710.

Lipowski, Z. J. Organic brain syndromes: Overview and classification. In D. F. Benson and D. Blumer (Eds.) *Psychiatric aspects of neurological disease.* New York: Grune & Stratton, 1975.

Lipowski, Z. J. A new look at organic brain syndromes. *American Journal of Psychiatry*, 1980, *137*(6), 674–678.

Lipscomb, T. R., & Nathan, P. E. Blood alcohol level discrimination: The effects of family history of alcoholism, drinking pattern and tolerance. *Archives of General Psychiatry*, 1980, *37*(5), 571–576.

Lipscomb, T. R., Nathan, P. E., Wilson, G. T., & Abrams, D. B. Effects of tolerance on the anxiety-reducing function of alcohol. *Archives of General Psychiatry*, 1980, *37*(5), 577–582.

Liston, E. H. The clinical phenomenology of presenile dementia: A critical review of the literature. *Journal of Nervous and Mental Disease*, 1979, *167*, 329–336.

Litman, R. E. Suicide as acting out. In E. S. Shneidman, N. L. Farberow, and R. E. Litman (Eds.) *The psychology of suicide.* New York: Science House, 1970.

Little, L. M., & Curran, J. P. Covert sensitization: A clinical procedure in need of some examination. *Psychological Bulletin,* 1978, *85,* 513–531.

Lloyd, C. Life events and depressive disorder reviewed: I. Events as predisposing factors. *Archives of General Psychiatry,* 1980a, *37*(5), 529–535.

Lloyd, C. Life events and depressive disorder reviewed: II. Events as precipitating factors. *Archives of General Psychiatry,* 1980b, *37*(5), 541–548.

Lobitz, W. C., & Lobitz, G. K. Clinical assessment in the treatment of sexual dysfunction. In J. LoPiccolo and L. LoPiccolo (Eds.) *Handbook of sex therapy.* New York: Plenum Press, 1978.

Loh, H. H., Brase, D. A., & Associates. Beta-endorphin in vitro inhibition of striatal dopamine release. *Nature,* 1976, *264,* 567–568.

LoPiccolo, J. Direct treatment of sexual dysfunction. In J. LoPiccolo and L. LoPiccolo (Eds.) *Handbook of sex therapy.* New York: Plenum Press, 1978.

Lotter, V. Factors related to outcome in autistic children. *Journal of Autism and Childhood Schizophrenia,* 1974, *4,* 263–277.

Lotter, V. Follow-up studies. In M. Rutter and E. Schopler (Eds.) *Autism: A reappraisal of concepts and treatment.* New York: Plenum Press, 1978.

Lovaas, O. I., Berberich, J., Perloff, B., & Schaeffer, B. Acquisition of imitative speech by schizophrenic children. *Science,* 1966, *151,* 705–707.

Lovaas, O. I., Koegel, R. L., & Schreibman, L. Stimulus overselectivity autism: A review of research. *Psychological Bulletin,* 1979, *86,* 1236–1254.

Lovaas, O. I., Schreibman, L., & Koegel, R. L. A behavior modification approach to the treatment of autistic children. *Journal of Autism and Childhood Schizophrenia,* 1974, *4,* 111–129.

Lown, B., Desilva, R. A., Reich, P., & Murawski, B. J. Psychophysiologic factors in sudden cardiac death. *American Journal of Psychiatry,* 1980, *137*(11), 1325–1335.

Ludwig, A. M. Altered states of consciousness. *Archives of General Psychiatry,* 1966, *15*(9), 225–234.

Ludwig, A. M., Wikler, A., & Stark, L. H. The first drink: Psychobiological aspects of craving. *Archives of General Psychiatry,* 1974, *30*(4), 539–547.

Ludwig, L. D. Elation-depression and skill as determinants of desire for excitement. *Journal of Personality,* 1975, *43*(1), 1–22.

Luparello, T. J., McFadden, E. R., Lyons, H. A., & Bleecker, E. R. Psychologic factors and bronchial asthma. *New York State Journal of Medicine,* 1971, *71,* 2161–2165.

Luria, A. R. *The working brain: An introduction to neuropsychology.* New York: Basic Books, 1973.

Luria, Z., & Osgood, C. F. IV. Postscript to "the three faces of Evelyn." *Journal of Abnormal Psychology,* 1976, *85*(3), 276–286.

Lyght, C. E. (Ed.) *The Merck manual of diagnosis and therapy* (11th ed.). Rahway, N.J.: Merck, Sharpe and Dohme Research Laboratory, 1966.

Lykken, D. T. A study of anxiety in the sociopathic personality. *Journal of Abnormal and Social Psychology,* 1957, *55*(1), 6–10.

Macdonald, J. M. False accusations of rape. *Medical Aspects of Human Sexuality,* 1973, *7*(5), 170.

Macdonald, J. M. *Indecent exposure.* Springfield, Ill.: Thomas, 1973.

Madden, J., Levenstein, P., & Levenstein, S. Longitudinal I.Q. outcomes of the mother-child home program. *Child Development,* 1976, *47,* 1015–1025.

Maher, B. A. *Principles of psychopathology.* New York: McGraw-Hill, 1966.

Maher, B. A. Delusional thinking and cognitive disorders. In H. London and R. E. Nisbett (Eds.) *Thought and feeling.* Chicago: Aldine, 1974.

Mahoney, M. J. *Cognition and behavior modification.* Cambridge, Mass.: Ballinger, 1974.

Maisch, H. *Incest.* New York: Stein & Day, 1972.

Maisto, S. A., Lauerman, R., & Adesso, V. S. A comparison of two experimental studies of the role of cognitive factors in alcoholics' drinking. *Journal of Studies on Alcohol,* 1977, *38*(1), 145–149.

Maliver, B. L. *The encounter game.* New York: Stein & Day, 1973.

Maloney, M. P., & Ward, M. P. *Psychological assessment: A conceptual approach.* New York: Oxford University Press, 1976.

Maloof, B. A. Alcohol stress and coping: An examination of the differential impact of alcohol on the ability of alcoholics and nonalcoholics to cope with a stressful situation. Doctoral Dissertation. Brandeis University (University microfilms no. 75-16040), 1975.

Malpass, R. S. Theory and method in cross-cultural psychology. *American Psychologist,* 1977, *32*(12), 1069–1079.

Mann, D. Marijuana alert II: More of the grim story. *Reader's Digest,* November 1980, pp. 65–71.

Manschreck, T. C., & Petri, M. The paranoid syndrome. *The Lancet,* July 29, 1978, pp. 251–253.

Margulies, R. Z., Viessler, R. C., & Kanded, D. B. A longitudinal study of onset of drinking among high school students. *Journal of Studies on Alcohol,* 1977, *38*(5), 897–912.

Marks, I. Behavioral psychotherapy of adult neurotics. In S. L. Garfield and A. E. Bergin (Eds.) *Handbook of psychotherapy and behavior change: An empirical analysis.* New York: Wiley, 1978.

Marks, I., & Gelder, M. Transvestitism and fetishism: A clinical and psychological change during faradic aversion. *British Journal of Psychiatry*, 1967, *113*, 711–729.

Marks, I. M., & Lader, M. Anxiety states (anxiety neurosis): A review. *Journal of Nervous and Mental Diseases*, 1973, *156*(1), 3–18.

Marmor, J., Gould, R. E., Friedman, R. L., & Clark, T. E. Viewpoints: What distinguishes "healthy" from "sick" sexual behavior? *Medical Aspects of Human Sexuality*, 1977, *11*(10), 67–77.

Marshall, W. L. A combined treatment approach to the reduction of multiple fetish related behaviors. *Journal of Consulting and Clinical Psychology*, 1974, *24*(4), 613–616.

Martin, M. H. Muscle-contraction headache. *Psychosomatic*, 1972, *13*(1), 16–19.

Maslow, A. H. *Motivation and personality*. (2nd ed.). New York: Harper & Row, 1970.

Maslow, A. H., & Mittleman, B. *Principles of abnormal psychology*. New York: Harper & Row, 1951.

Masserman, J. H. *Principles of dynamic psychiatry* (2nd ed.). Philadelphia: Saunders, 1961.

Massie, H. N. Blind ratings of mother-infant interactions in home movies of prepsychotic and normal infants. *American Journal of Psychiatry*, 1978, *135*, 1371–1374.

Masters, W. H., & Johnson, V. E. *Human sexual response*. Boston: Little, Brown, 1966.

Masters, W. H., & Johnson, V. E. *Human sexual inadequacy*. Boston: Little, Brown, 1970.

Masters, W. H., & Johnson, V. E. *The pleasure bond: A new look at sexuality and commitment*. Boston: Little, Brown, 1975.

Masters, W. H., & Johnson, V. E. *Homosexuality in perspective*. Boston: Little, Brown, 1979.

Masuda, M., Lin, K. M., & Tazuma, L. Adaptation problems of Vietnamese refugees: II. Life changes and perception of life events. *Archives of General Psychiatry*, 1980, *37*(4), 447–450.

Matarazzo, J. D. The interview: Its reliability and validity in psychiatric diagnosis. In B. Wolman (Ed.) *Clinical diagnosis of mental disorder: A handbook*. New York: Plenum Press, 1978.

Matefy, R. E. Operant conditioning procedure to modify schizophrenic behavior: A case report. *Psychotherapy: Theory, Research, and Practice*, 1972, *9*(3), 226–230.

Matefy, R. E., Hayes, C., & Hirsch, J. Psychedelic drug flashbacks: Attentional deficits? *Journal of Abnormal Psychology*, 1979, *88*(2), 212–215.

Matelzky, B. M. Assisted covert sensitization in the treatment of exhibitionism. *Journal of Consulting and Clinical Psychology*, 1974, *42*(1), 34–40.

Mattusek, P. Late symptomatology among former concentration camp inmates. In S. Arieti (Ed.) *The world biennial of psychiatry and psychotherapy*. New York: Basic Books, 1971.

Maugh, T. H. II. Marihuana: The grass may no longer be greener. *Science*, 1974a, *185*, 683–685.

Maugh, T. H. II. Marihuana (II): Does it damage the brain? *Science*, 1974b, *185*, 775–776.

May, J. T., & Sprague, H. A. Chronic stress as a predictor of family health action and health stress. In I. G. Sarason and C. D. Spielberger (Eds.) *Stress and anxiety*, vol. 3. New York: Wiley, 1976.

May, R. Existential psychology. In T. Millon (Ed.) *Theories of psychopathology and personality*. Philadelphia: Saunders, 1973.

McCabe, M., Fowler, R., Caldoret, R., & Winoker, G. Symptom differences in schizophrenia with good and poor prognosis. *American Journal of Psychiatry*, 1972, *128*(10), 1239–1243.

McCall, R. J. *The varieties of abnormality: A phenomenological analysis*. Springfield, Ill.: Thomas, 1975.

McCary, J. L. *Human sexuality* (2nd ed.). New York: Van Nostrand, 1973.

McClelland, D. C. Sources of hypertension in the drive for power. Presented at the Kittay Scientific Foundation Symposium, *Psychopathology and human adaptation*. New York, 1975.

McClelland, D. C. Inhibited power motivation and high blood pressure in men. *Journal of Abnormal Psychology*, 1979, *88*(2), 182–190.

McCord, W., Porta, J., & McCord, J. The family genesis of psychosis. *Psychiatry*, 1962, *25*(1), 60–71.

McCulloch, M. J., & Feldman, M. P. Aversion therapy in the management of 43 homosexuals. *British Medical Journal*, 1967, *2*, 594–630.

McDaniel, J. G. Misery loves company. *Journal of the Medical Association of Georgia*, 1976, *65*(1), 97–98.

McDavid, J. W., & Harari, H. *Social psychology: Individuals, groups, societies*. New York: Harper & Row, 1968.

McLemore, C. W., & Benjamin, L. S. Whatever happened to interpersonal diagnosis? A psychosocial alternative to DSM-III. *American Psychologist*, 1979, *34*(1), 17–34.

McNeil, E. B. *The quiet furies: Man and disorder*. Englewood Cliffs, N.J.: Prentice-Hall, 1967.

McReynolds, W. T. Letters to the editor: Psychologists' reactions to DSM-III. *American Journal of Psychiatry*, 1980, *137*(11), 1468.

Mechanic, D. (Coordinator) Report of the task panel on the nature and scope of the problems. *Presidents Commission on Mental Health*, vol. 2. Washington, D.C.: U.S. Government Printing Office, 1978, pp. 1–138.

Mednick, S. A. A learning theory approach to research in schizophrenia. *Psychological Bulletin*, 1958, *55*, 316–327.

Mednick, S. A., & Schulsinger, F. Some premorbid characteristics related to breakdown in children with schizophrenic mothers. In D. Rosenthal and

S. S. Kety (Eds.) *The transmission of schizophrenia.* Oxford: Pergamon Press, 1968.

Mednick, S. A., & Schulsinger, F. A. Learning theory of schizophrenia: Thirteen years later. In M. Hammes, K. Salzinger, and S. Sutton (Eds.) *Psychopathology: Contributions from the social, behavioral and biological sciences.* New York: Wiley, 1973.

Mednick, S. A., Schulsinger, H. E., & Schulsinger, F. Schizophrenia in children of schizophrenic mothers. In A. Davids (Ed.) *Child personality and psychopathology: Current topics,* vol. 2. New York: Wiley, 1975.

Meehl, P. E. Schizotaxia, schizotypy, schizophrenia. *American Psychologist,* 1962, *17*(8), 827–838.

Mehr, J. *Human services: Concepts and intervention strategies.* Boston: Allyn & Bacon, 1980.

Meichenbaum, D. A self-instructional approach to stress management: A proposal for stress inoculation training. In C. D. Spielberger and I. G. Sarason (Eds.) *Stress and anxiety,* vol. 1. New York: Halsted Press, 1975.

Meichenbaum, D. *Cognitive-behavior modification: An integrated approach.* New York: Plenum Press, 1977.

Meichenbaum, D., & Cameron, R. Training schizophrenics to talk to themselves: A means of developing attentional controls. *Behavior Therapy,* 1973, *4,* 515–534.

Meichenbaum, D., Turk, D., & Burstein, S. The nature of coping with stress. In I. G. Sarason and C. D. Spielberger (Eds.) *Stress and anxiety,* vol. 2. New York: Wiley, 1975.

Meisel, A. Rights of the mentally ill: The gulf between theory and reality. *Hospital & Community Psychiatry,* 1975, *26*(6), 349–353.

Meiselman, K. C. Inducing "schizophrenic" association in normal subjects. *Journal of Abnormal Psychology,* 1978, *87*(3), 291–293.

Meissner, W. W. *The paranoid process.* New York: Jason Aronson, 1978.

Mendels, J. *Concepts of depression.* New York: Wiley, 1970.

Mendels, J., Stennett, J. L., Burns, D., & Frazer, A. Amine precursors and depression. *Archives of General Psychiatry,* 1975, *32*(1), 22–30.

Mendelson, M. Intrapersonal psychodynamics of depression. In F. F. Flack and S. C. Draghi (Eds.) *The nature and treatment of depression.* New York: Wiley, 1975.

Mental retardation activities of the U.S. Department of Health, Education, and Welfare. Washington, D.C.: U.S. Government Printing Office, 1963.

Merbaum, M., & Hefez, A. Some personality characteristics of soldiers exposed to extreme war stress. *Journal of Consulting and Clinical Psychology,* 1976, *44*(1), 1–6.

Mercer, J. The myth of 3% prevalence. In G. Tarjan, K. R. Eyman, and C. E. Meyers (Eds.) *Sociobehavioral studies in mental retardation.* Washington, D.C.: American Association on Mental Deficiency, 1973.

Messer, S. B., & Winoker, M. Some limits to the integration of psychoanalytic and behavior therapy. *American Psychologist,* 1980, *35*(9), 818–829.

Meyer, V., & Chesser, E. S. *Behavior therapy in clinical psychiatry.* Baltimore: Penguin Press, 1970.

Meyer-Bahlburg, H. F. L. Sex hormones and female homosexuality: A critical examination. *Archives of Sexual Behavior,* 1979, *8*(1), 101–118.

Meyers, A., Mercatoris, M., & Sciota, A. Use of covert self-instruction for the elimination of psychotic speech. *Journal of Consulting and Clinical Psychology,* 1976, *44,* 480–483.

Mezzich, A. C., & Mezzich, J. E. Diagnostic reliability of childhood and adolescence behavior disorders. *American Psychological Association, 87th Annual Convention,* New York, 1979.

Michaelson, G. Short term effects of behavior therapy and hospital treatment of chronic alcoholics. *Behavior Research and Therapy,* 1976, *14*(1), 69–72.

Miele, F. Cultural bias in the WISC. *Intelligence,* 1979, no. 3, 149–164.

Milgram, N. A. Cognition and language in mental retardation: Directions and implications. In D. K. Routh (Ed.) *The experimental psychology of mental retardation.* Chicago: Aldine, 1973.

Miller, E. *Clinical neuropsychology.* Hammondsworth, England: Penguin Books, 1972.

Miller, J. Helping the suicidal client: Some aspects of assessment and treatment. *Psychotherapy: Theory, Research and Practice,* 1980, *17*(1), 94–100.

Miller, W. R. Behavioral treatment of problem drinkers: A comparative outcome study of three controlled drinking therapies. *Journal of Consulting and Clinical Psychology,* 1978, *46*(1), 74–86.

Miller, W. R., & Joyce, M. A. Prediction of abstinence, controlled drinking, and heavy drinking outcomes following behavioral self-control training. *Journal of Consulting and Clinical Psychology,* 1979, *47*(4), 773–775.

Millon, T. *Disorders of personality DSM-III: Axis II.* New York: Wiley, 1981.

Mirsky, I. A. Physiologic, psychologic, and social determinants in the etiology of duodenal ulcer. *American Journal of Digestive Diseases,* 1958, *3*(3), 285–314.

Mischel, W. Towards a cognitive social learning reconceptualization of personality. *Psychological Review,* 1973, *80,* 252–283.

Mischel, W. *Introduction to personality* (2nd ed.). New York: Holt, Rinehart and Winston, 1976.

Monahan, J. Prediction research and the emergency commitment of dangerous mentally ill persons: A reconsideration. *American Journal of Psychiatry,* 1978, *135*(2), 198–201.

Money, J. Sexual dimorphism and homosexual gender identity. *Psychological Bulletin,* 1970, *74,* 425–440.

Money, J. Viewpoints: What are your feelings towards sex change surgery? *Medical Aspects of Human Sexuality,* 1971, *5*(6), 135.

Monthly statistics. Illinois Department of Mental Health and Developmental Disabilities, Springfield, Ill.: September 1981.

Montigny, C. D., & Aghajanian, G. K. Tricyclic antidepressants: Long term treatment increases responsivity of rat forebrain neurons to serotonin. *Science,* 1978, *202,* 1303–1305.

Morishima, A. Artistic talent at I.Q. 47: His spirit raises the ante for retardates. *Psychology Today,* June 1975, pp. 72–73.

Morishima, A., & Brown, L. F. An idiot savant case report: A retrospective view. *Mental Retardation,* 1976, *13,* 46–47.

Morishima, A., & Brown, L. F. A case report on the artistic talent of an autistic idiot savant. *Mental Retardation,* 1977, *15,* 33–36.

Morse, R. Post operative delirium: A syndrome of multiple causation. *Psychosomatics,* 1970, *11,* 164–168.

Morse, W. The education of socially maladjusted and emotionally disturbed children. In W. Cruickshank and G. Johnson (Eds.) *Education of exceptional children and youth* (2nd ed.). Englewood Cliffs, N.J.: Prentice-Hall, 1967.

Mosher, D. L., & O'Grady, K. E. Homosexual threat, negative attitudes towards masturbation, sex guilt, and males' sexual and affective reactions to explicit sexual films. *Journal of Consulting and Clinical Psychology,* 1979, *47*(5), 860–873.

Mosher, L. R., & Keith, S. J. Research on the psychosocial treatment of schizophrenia: A summary report. *American Journal of Psychiatry,* 1979, *136*(5), 623–631.

Moss, A., & Wyner, B. Tachycardia in house officers presenting cases at grand rounds. *Annals of Internal Medicine,* 1970, *72,* 255–256.

Mowrer, O. H. On the dual nature of learning—A reintegration of "conditioning" and "problem solving." *Harvard Educational Review,* 1947, *17,* 102–148.

Mowrer, O. H., & Mowrer, W. Enuresis: A method for its study and treatment. *American Journal of Orthopsychiatry,* 1938, *8,* 436–447.

Mucha, T. F., & Reinhardt, R. F. Conversion reactions in student aviators. *American Journal of Psychiatry,* 1970, *127*(3), 493–497.

Mules, J. E., Hague, W. H., & Dudley, D. L. Life change: Its perception and alcohol addiction. *Journal of Studies on Alcohol,* 1977, *38*(3), 487–493.

Mulford, H. A. Stages in the alcoholic process: Towards a cumulative nonsequential index. *Journal of Studies on Alcohol,* 1977, *38*(3), 563–583.

Mulvihill, J. J., & Yeager, A. M. Fetal alcohol syndrome. *Teratology,* 1976, *13,* 345–348.

Munzinger, H. The adopted childs I.Q.: A critical review. *Psychological Bulletin,* 1975, *82,* 623–659.

Murphy, H. B. M. Cultural factors in the genesis of schizophrenia. In D. Rosenthal and S. S. Kety (Eds.) *The transmission of schizophrenia.* New York: Pergamon Press, 1968.

Murphy, H. B. M., Witthower, E. D., Fried, J., & Ellenberger, H. A cross-cultural survey of schizophrenic symptomatology. *International Journal of Social Psychology,* 1963, *9*(2), 237–249.

Murray, H. A. (Ed.) *Explorations in personality.* New York: Oxford University Press, 1938.

Mussen, P. H., Conger, J. J., & Kagen, J. *Child development and personality* (4th ed.). New York: Harper & Row, 1974.

Naditch, M. P., & Fenwick, S. LSD flashbacks and ego functioning. *Journal of Abnormal Psychology,* 1977, *86*(4), 352–359.

Nahas, G. G. Marihuana. *Journal of the American Medical Association,* 1975, *233*(1), 79–80.

Naroll, R. Cultural determinants and the concept of the sick society. In S. C. Plog and R. B. Edgerton (Eds.) *Changing perspectives in mental illness.* New York: Holt, Rinehart and Winston, 1969.

National Institute of Mental Health. *Research in the service of mental health.* DHEW Publication no. (ADM 75-236). Washington, D.C.: Superintendent of Documents, 1975.

Neale, J. M. Perceptual span in schizophrenia. *Journal of Abnormal Psychology,* 1971, *77*(2), 196–204.

Negrete, J. C. Aspects psychologiques dans l'etiologie de l'alcoolisme. (Psychological aspects in the etiology of alcoholism). *Toxicomanies,* 1973, *6,* 149–155.

Neisworth, J. T., & Moore, F. Operant treatment of asthmatic responding with the parent as therapist. *Behavior Therapy,* 1972, *3*(1), 95–99.

Nelson, H. High blood pressure found in third of adults in survey. *Los Angeles Times,* March 27, 1973, p. 3.

Nelson, J. C., & Charney, D. S. The symptoms of major depressive illness. *American Journal of Psychiatry,* 1981, *138*(1), 1–13.

Nemetz, G. H., Craig, K. D., & Reich, G. Treatment of female sexual dysfunction through symbolic modeling. *Journal of Consulting and Clinical Psychology,* 1978, *46*(1), 62–73.

Neugebauer, R. Medieval and early modern theories

of mental illness. *Archives of General Psychiatry,* 1979, *36,* 477–483.

Newman, L. E., & Stoller, R. J. Nontranssexual men who seek sex reassignment. *American Journal of Psychiatry,* 1974, *131*(4), 437–441.

News from the World of Medicine. Could you be scared to death? *Reader's Digest,* June 1980, *116*(698), 183.

NIAA. *National Institute on Alcohol Abuse and Alcoholism.* Report. Washington, D.C.: U.S. Government Printing Office, 1978.

NIDA. *Marihuana and health.* National Institute on Drug Abuse. Rockville, Md., 1977.

NIDA. *Drug abuse statistics in 1977.* Washington, D.C., 1978.

Norman, W. T. Psychometric considerations for a revision of the MMPI. In J. N. Butcher (Ed.) *Objective personality assessment: Changing perspectives.* New York: Academic Press, 1972.

Notman, M. T., & Nadelson, C. C. The rape victim: Psychodynamic considerations. *American Journal of Psychiatry,* 1976, *133*(4), 408–412.

Obe, G., & Herha, J. Chromosomal damage in chronic alcohol users. *Humangenetik,* 1975, *29*(1), 191–200.

O'Connor, J. A comprehensive approach to the treatment of ulcerative colitis. In O. W. Hill (Ed.) *Modern trends in psychosomatic medicine,* vol. 2. New York: Appleton-Century-Crofts, 1970.

Offit, A. K. *The sexual self.* Philadelphia: Lippincott, 1977.

Öhman, A., Erixon, G., & Löfberg, I. Phobias and preparedness: Phobic versus neutral pictures as conditioned stimuli for human autonomic responses. *Journal of Abnormal Psychology,* 1975, *84*(1), 41–45.

Older, J. Psychosurgery: Ethical issues and a proposal for control. *American Journal of Orthopsychiatry,* 1974, *44*(5), 661–674.

Orpin, J. A. Electroconvulsive therapy: New techniques. *Psychiatric Journal of the University of Ottawa,* 1980, *5*(3), 162–165.

Osgood, C. E., Luria, Z., Jeans, R. F., & Smith, S. W. The three faces of Evelyn: A case report. *Journal of Abnormal Psychology,* 1976, *85*(3), 247–286.

Parad, H., & Resnik, H. L. P. The practice of crisis intervention in emergency care. In H. L. P. Resnik and H. L. Ruben (Eds.) *Emergency psychiatric care.* Bowie, Md.: Charles Press, 1975.

Parker, E. S., & Noble, E. P. Alcohol consumption and cognitive functioning in social drinkers. *Journal of Studies on Alcoholism,* 1977, *38*(7), 1224–1232.

Parloff, M. *Twenty-five years of research in psychotherapy.* New York: Albert Einstein College of Medicine, Department of Psychiatry, October 17, 1975.

Patel, C. H., & North, W. R. Randomized controlled trial of yoga and biofeedback in management of hypertension. *The Lancet,* 1975, *2*(2), 93–95.

Patterson, R. L. *Maintaining effective token economies.* Springfield, Ill.: Thomas, 1976.

Paul, G. L. *Insight vs. desensitization in psychotherapy.* Stanford, Calif.: Stanford University Press, 1966.

Paul, G. L., & Lentz, R. J. *Psychosocial treatment of chronic mental patients: Milieu vs. social learning programs.* Cambridge, Mass.: Harvard University Press, 1977.

Pauly, I. B. Viewpoints: What are your feelings toward sex change surgery? *Medical Aspects of Human Sexuality,* 1971, *5*(6), 129–130.

Pauly, I. B. Female transsexuals. *Archives of Sexual Behavior,* 1974, *3,* 487–526.

Paykel, E. S., Myers, J. K., Lindenthal, J. J., & Tanner, J. Suicide feelings in the general population: A prevalence study. *British Journal of Psychiatry,* 1974, *124,* 460–469.

Pearse, B. A., Walters, E. D., Sargent, J. D., & Meers, M. Intensive biofeedback for treatment of migraine headache. Presented at the Sixth Annual Biofeedback Research Society Meeting. Monterey, Calif., February 1975.

Peele, S. Reductionism in the psychology of the eighties: Can biochemistry eliminate addiction, mental illness, and pain? *American Psychologist,* 1981, *36*(8), 807–818.

Pendleton, L. Treatment of persons found incompetent to stand trial. *American Journal of Psychiatry,* 1980, *137*(9), 1048–1100.

Perrucci, R. *Circle of madness.* Englewood Cliffs, N.J.: Prentice-Hall, 1974.

Perry, T. L., Hansen, S., & Kloster, M. Huntington's chorea: Deficiency of Y-aminobutyric acid in the brain. *New England Journal of Medicine,* 1973, *228,* 337–342.

Pert, C. B., & Snyder, S. H. Opiate receptor: Demonstration in nervous tissue. *Science,* March 9, 1973, *179,* 1011–1014.

Peters, J. E., & Stern, R. M. Specificity of attitude hypothesis in psychosomatic medicine: A reexamination. *Journal of Psychosomatic Research,* 1971, *15,* 129–135.

Peters, M. Aversive conditioning and alcoholism: A nineteenth century case report. *Canadian Psychological Review,* 1976, *17*(1), 61.

Petrich, J., & Holmes, T. H. Life change and onset of illness. *Medical Clinics of North America,* 1977, *61,* 825–836.

Philips, I. Childhood depression: Interpersonal interaction and depressive phenomena. *American Journal of Psychiatry,* 1979, *136*(8), no. 8, 511–515.

Philipps, R. J. An experimental investigation of suggestion and relaxation in asthmatics. Unpublished doctoral dissertation. Kingston, Ont.: Queens University, 1970.

Piaget, J. *The construction of reality in the child.* New York: Basic Books, 1954.

Piaget, J. Piaget's theory. In P. H. Mussen (Ed.) *Carmichael's manual of child psychology* (3rd ed.). New York: Wiley, 1970.

Piggott, L. R. Overview of selected basic research in autism. *Journal of Autism and Developmental Disorders,* 1979, *9,* 199–218.

Pihl, R. O., & Sigal, H. Motivation levels and the marihuana high. *Journal of Abnormal Psychology,* 1978, *87*(2), 280–285.

Pines, M. Mental health meeting on brain research sparks optimism. *A.P.A. Monitor,* 1981, *12*(2), 6.

Pinkus, J. H., & Tucker, G. J. *Behavioral neurology* (2nd ed.). New York: Oxford University Press, 1978.

Piotrowski, Z. A. Unsuspected and pertinent microfacts in personology. *American Psychologist,* 1982, *37*(2), 190–196.

Pittel, S. M., & Hofer, R. The transition to amphetamine abuse. In D. E. Smith and D. R. Wesson (Eds.) *Uppers and downers.* Englewood Cliffs, N.J.: Prentice-Hall, 1973.

Poeck, K. Modern trends in neuropsychology. In A. Benton (Ed.) *Contributions to clinical neuropsychology.* Chicago: Aldine, 1968.

Pokorny, A. D., Thornby, J., Kaplan, H. B., & Ball, D. Prediction of chronicity in psychiatric patients. *Archives of General Psychiatry,* 1976, *33*(8), 932–937.

Polansky, N. A., Borgman, R. D., & DeSaix, C. *Roots of futility.* San Francisco: Jossey-Bass, 1972.

Porsolt, R. D., LePichon, M., & Jalfre, M. Depression: A new animal model sensitive to antidepressant treatments. *Nature,* 1977, *266,* 730–732.

Poser, C. M. The presenile dementias. *Journal of the American Medical Association,* 1975, *233*(1), 81–84.

Post, R. M. Cocaine psychosis: A continuum model. *American Journal of Psychiatry,* 1975, *132*(3), 225–231.

Post, R. M., Fink, E., Carpenter, W. T., & Goodwin, F. K. Cerebrospinal fluid amine metabolites in acute schizophrenia. *Archives of General Psychiatry,* 1975, *32,* 1063–1069.

Potash, H., & Brunell, L. Multiple conjoint psychotherapy with folie á deux. *Psychotherapy: Theory, Research and Practice,* 1974, *11*(3), 270–276.

Powell, D. H. A pilot study of occasional heroin users. *Archives of General Psychiatry,* 1973, *28*(4), 586–594.

Prange, A. J. The use of drugs in depression: Its theoretical and practical basis. *Psychiatric Annals,* 1973, *32*(2), 56–75.

Price, K. P. The application of behavior therapy to the treatment of psychosomatic disorders: Retrospect and prospect. *Psychotherapy: Theory, Research and Practice,* 1974, *11*(2), 138–155.

Price, R. H. Psychological deficit vs. impression management in schizophrenic word association performance. *Journal of Abnormal Psychology,* 1972, *79*(1), 132–137.

Prigatano, G. P., & Johnson, H. J. Autonomic nervous system changes associated with a spider phobic reaction. *Journal of Abnormal Psychology,* 1974, *83*(2), 174.

Purcell, K., Brady, K., Chai, H., Muser, J., Moek, L., Gordon, N., & Means, J. The effect on asthma in children on experimental separation from the family. *Psychosomatic Medicine,* 1969, *31,* 144–164.

Quay, H. Psychopathic personality as pathological stimulation seeking. *American Journal of Psychiatry,* 1965, *122*(2), 180–183.

Rabkin, J. G. Criminal behavior of discharged mental patients: A critical appraisal of the research. *Psychological Bulletin,* 1979, *86,* 1–27.

Rachman, S. Sexual fetishism: An experimental analogue. *Psychological Record,* 1966, *16,* 293–296.

Rachman, S. Obsessional ruminations. *Behavior, Research and Therapy,* 1977, *9,* 229–235.

Rachman, S., & Hodgson, R. J. *Obsessions and compulsions.* Englewood Cliffs, N.J.: Prentice-Hall, 1980.

Rachman, S. J. *Fear and anxiety.* San Francisco, Calif.: Freeman, 1978.

Rada, R. T. (Ed.) *Clinical aspects of the rapist.* New York: Grune & Stratton, 1978.

Rahe, R. Life changes and subsequent illness reports. In E. K. Gunderson and R. H. Rahe (Eds.) *Life stress and illness.* Springfield, Ill.: Thomas, 1974.

Rahe, R., Mahan, J. L., & Arthur, R. J. Prediction of near-future health change from subjects preceding life changes. *Journal of Psychosomatic Research,* 1970, *14,* 401–406.

Rahe, R., & Romo, M. Recent life changes and the onset of myocardial infarction and sudden death in Helsinki. In E. K. Gunderson and R. Rahe (Eds.) *Life stress and illness.* Springfield, Ill.: Thomas, 1974.

Rainer, J. D. Heredity and character disorders. *American Journal of Psychotherapy,* 1979, *33*(1), 6–16.

Rattan, R. B., & Chapman, L. J. Associative intrusions in schizophrenic verbal behavior. *Journal of Abnormal Psychology,* 1973, *82*(1), 169–173.

Redlich, F., & Kellert, S. R. Trends in American mental health. *American Journal of Psychiatry,* 1978, *135*(1), 22–28.

Reed, E. W., & Reed, S. C. *Mental retardation: A family study.* Philadelphia: Saunders, 1965.

Rees, L. The importance of psychological, allergic, and infective factors in childhood asthma. *Journal of Psychosomatic Research,* 1964, *7,* 253–262.

Refsum, S. Genetic aspects of migraine. In P. J. Vinken and G. W. Bruyn (Eds.) *Handbook of clinical neurology,* vol. 5. New York: Wiley, 1968.

Regier, D. A., Goldberg, I. O., & Taube, C. A. The defacto U.S. mental health services systems: A public health perspective. *Archives of General Psychiatry,* 1978, *35,* 685–693.

Rehm, L. P., & Kornblith, S. J. Behavior therapy for depression: A review of recent developments. In M. Hersen, R. M. Eisler, and P. M. Miller (Eds.) *Progress in behavior modification,* vol. 7. New York: Academic Press, 1979.

Reicher, J. W. Psychoanalytically oriented treatment of offenders diagnosed as developmental psychopaths: The mesdagklinick experience. *International Journal of Law and Psychiatry,* 1979, *2,* 87–98.

Reid, W. H. The sadness of the psychopath. *American Journal of Psychotherapy,* 1978, *32*(4), 496–509.

Reilly, S. S., & Muzekari, L. H. Responses of normal and disturbed adults and children to mixed messages. *Journal of Abnormal Psychology,* 1979, *88*(2), 203–208.

Reiser, M. F. Changing theoretical concepts in psychosomatic medicine. In S. Arieti (Ed.) *American handbook of psychiatry,* vol. 4. New York: Basic Books, 1975.

Reitan, R. M., & Davison, L. A. (Eds.) *Clinical neuropsychology.* Washington, D.C.: Winston, 1974.

Repp, A. Communication: Observations of a day at Bicetre. *Journal of Applied Behavioral Analysis,* 1977, *10*(3), 548.

Research in the service of mental health. National Institute of Mental Health. DHEW Publication no. (ADM 75-236). Washington, D.C.: Superintendent of Documents, 1975.

Richter, C. On the phenomenon of sudden death in animals and man. *Psychosomatic Medicine,* 1957, *19,* 190–198.

Riess, D. The family and schizophrenia. *American Journal of Psychiatry,* 1976, *133*(2), 181–185.

Riessman, F. Self-help. In S. Alley, J. Blanton, and R. E. Feldman (Eds.) *Paraprofessionals in mental health.* New York: Human Services Press, 1979.

Rimland, B. *Infantile autism.* New York: Appleton-Century-Crofts, 1964.

Rimland, B. Comment: Death knell for psychotherapy? *American Psychologist,* 1979, *34*(2), 192.

Rinkel, M. Psychedelic drugs. *American Journal of Psychiatry,* 1966, *122,* 1415–1416.

Roberts, A. H. *Brain damage in boxers.* London: Pitman, 1969.

Robinowitz, R., Woodward, W. A., & Penk, W. E. MMPI comparison of black heroin users volunteering or not volunteering for treatment. *Journal of Consulting and Clinical Psychology,* 1980, *48*(4), 540–542.

Robins, L. N. *Deviant children grown up.* Baltimore: Williams & Wilkins, 1966.

Robinson, N. M., & Robinson, H. B. *The mentally retarded child* (2nd ed.). New York: McGraw-Hill, 1976.

Rogers, C. R. *Counseling and psychotherapy.* Boston: Houghton Mifflin, 1942.

Rogers, C. R. *Client-centered therapy: Its current practice, implications, and theory.* Boston: Houghton Mifflin, 1951.

Rogers, C. R. A theory of therapy, personality and interpersonal relationships, as developed in the client-centered framework. In S. Koch (Ed.) *Psychology: A study of a science,* vol. 3. New York: McGraw-Hill, 1959.

Rogers, C. R. *On becoming a person: A therapist's view of psychotherapy.* Boston: Houghton Mifflin, 1961.

Rogers, C. R. Interpersonal relationships: Year 2000. *Journal of Applied Behavioral Sciences,* 1968, *4,* 265–280.

Rosen, E., Fox, R. E., & Gregory, I. *Abnormal psychology* (2nd ed.). Philadelphia: Saunders, 1972.

Rosenkrans, M. A. Imitation in children as a function of perceived similarity to a social model and vicarious reinforcement. *Journal of Personality and Social Psychology,* 1967, *7,* 307–315.

Rosenman, R. H., Friedman, M., Strauss, R. et al. A predictive study of coronary heart disease: The western collaborative group study. *Journal of the American Medical Association,* 1964, *189*(1), 15–22.

Rosenthal, D. *Genetic theory and abnormal behavior.* New York: McGraw-Hill, 1970.

Rosenthal, D. A program of research on heredity in schizophrenia. *Behavioral Science,* 1971, *16,* 191–201.

Rosenthal, D., Wender, P. H., Kety, S. S., Schulsinger, F., Welner, J., & Rieder, R. Parent-child relationships and psychopathological disorder in the child. *Archives of General Psychiatry,* 1975, *37,* 466–476.

Rosenthal, R. Covert communication in the psychological experiment. *Psychological Bulletin,* 1967, *67,* 356–367.

Rosenthal, R. H., & Allen, T. W. The examination of attention, arousal, and learning dysfunction of hyperkinetic children. *Psychological Bulletin,* 1978, *85,* 689–715.

Rosenthal, R. H., Rosenthal, C. F. Types of frigidity. *Medical Aspects of Human Sexuality,* 1975, *9*(5), 116–125.

Ross, A. O. *Psychological disorders of children.* New York: McGraw-Hill, 1980.

Rotter, J. B., & Hochreich, D. J. *Personality.* Glenview, Ill.: Scott, Foresman, 1975.

Rounsaville, B. J., Klerman, G. L., & Weissman, M. M. Do psychotherapy and pharmacotherapy for depression conflict? Empirical evidence from a clinical trial. *Archives of General Psychiatry,* 1981, *38*(1), 24–29.

Rubel, A. J. The epidemiology of a folk illness: Susto in Hispanic America. *Ethnology,* 1964, *2,* 286–293.

Rubin, V., & Comitas, L. *Ganja in Jamaica: A medical anthropological study of chronic marijuana use.* The Hague: Mouton, 1975.

Rudin, E. *Zur verebieng und neurentstehung der dementia praecox.* Berlin: Springer, 1916.

Rule, G. B., & Nesdale, A. R. Environmental stressors, emotional arousal and aggression. In I. G. Sarason and C. D. Speilberger (Eds.) *Stress and anxiety,* vol. 3. New York: Wiley, 1976.

Russ, K. L., Hammer, R. L., & Adderton, M. Clinical follow-up. Treatment and outcome of functional headache patients treated with biofeedback. Presented at the Eighth Annual Meeting of the Biofeedback Society of America. Orlando, Fla., March 1977.

Rutter, M. The development of infantile autism. *Psychological Medicine,* 1974, *4,* 147–163.

Rutter, M. *Helping troubled children.* New York: Plenum Press, 1975.

Ryckman, R. M. *Theories of personality.* New York: Van Nostrand, 1978.

Saccuzzo, D. P. Input capability and speed of processing in mental retardation: A reply to Stanovich and Purcell. *Journal of Abnormal Psychology,* 1981, *90*(2), 172–174.

Saccuzzo, D. P., Kerr, M., Marcus, H., & Brown, R. Input capability and speed of processing in mental retardation. *Journal of Abnormal Psychology,* 1979, *88*(4), 341–345.

Sackheim, H. A., Nordlic, J. W., & Gur, R. C. A model of hysterical and hypnotic blindness: Cognition, motivation, and awareness. *Journal of Abnormal Psychology,* 1979, *88*(1), 474–489.

Safer, D. A familial factor in minimal brain dysfunction. *Behavior Genetics,* 1973, *3,* 175–186.

Sagarin, E. Viewpoints: What are your feelings toward sex change surgery? *Medical Aspects of Human Sexuality,* 1971, *5*(6), 130–135.

Salzman, C. ECT and ethical psychiatry. *American Journal of Psychiatry,* 1977, *134*(9), 1006–1009.

Salzman, C. The use of ECT in the treatment of schizophrenia. *American Journal of Psychiatry,* 1980, *137*(9), 1032–1041.

Salzman, L. F., & Klein, R. H. Habituation and conditioning of electrodermal responses in high risk children. *Schizophrenia Bulletin,* 1978, *4,* 210–222.

Sarbin, T. R. The scientific status of the mental illness metaphor. In S. C. Plog and R. B. Edgerton (Eds.) *Changing perspectives in mental illness.* New York: Holt, Rinehart and Winston, 1969.

Sartorius, N., Shapiro, R., & Jablensky, A. The international pilot study of schizophrenia. *Schizophrenia Bulletin,* winter 1974, no. 11, 21–34.

Satterfield, J. H., Cantwell, D. P., Saul, R. E., & Yusin, A. Intelligence, academic achievement, and EEG abnormalities in hyperactive children. *American Journal of Psychiatry,* 1974, *13*(4), 391–395.

Scarf, M. Images that heal: A doubtful idea whose time has come. *Psychology Today,* September 1980, *14*(4), 45–46.

Scarr, S. Genetics and the development of intelligence. In F. D. Horowitz (Ed.) *Child development research,* vol. 4. Chicago: University of Chicago Press, 1975.

Scarr, S., & Weinberg, R. A. The influence of "family background" on intellectual attainment. *American Sociological Review,* 1978, *43,* 674–692.

Schaar, K. Crisis. *APA Monitor,* 1980, *11*(9, 10), 16.

Schacht, T., & Nathan, P. E. But is it good for the psychologists? Appraisal and status of DSM-III. *American Psychologist,* 1977, *32*(12), 1017–1025.

Schachter, S., & Latané, B. Crime, cognition and the autonomic nervous system. In D. Levine (Ed.) *Nebraska symposium on motivation,* vol. 12. Lincoln: University of Nebraska Press, 1964.

Schaefer, H. H., & Martin, P. L. *Behavioral therapy.* New York: McGraw-Hill, 1969.

Schaefer, J. M. Alcohol metabolism reactions among the Reddis of South India. *Alcoholism: Clinical and Experimental Research,* 1978, *2*(1), 61–69.

Schatzman, M. *Soul murder.* New York: Random House, 1973.

Scheff, T. J. *Being mentally ill: A sociological theory.* Chicago: Aldine, 1966.

Scheff, T. J. (Ed.) *Labelling madness.* Englewood Cliffs, N.J.: Prentice-Hall, 1975.

Scheftner, W. A. DSM-III and the schizophrenias. Presented at the symposium, The ABC's of DSM-III, Illinois Hospital Association, Illinois Psychiatric Society, and Illinois Medical Records Association, 1980.

Schein, E. H., Cooley, W. E., & Singer, M. T. A psychological follow-up of former POW's of the Chinese Communists: I. Results of interview study. M.I.T. Contract No. DA-49-007-MD-754, 1960.

Schendel, E., & Kourany, R. F. C. Cacodemonomania and exorcism in children. *Journal of Clinical Psychiatry,* 1980, *41*(4), 119–123.

Schizophrenia Bulletin, 1977, *3*(2), 180–181.

Schleifer, M., Weiss, G., Cohen, N., Elman, M.,

Evejic, H., & Kruger, E. Hyperactivity in preschoolers and the effect of methylphendate. *American Journal of Orthopsychiatry*, 1975, *45*(1), 38–50.

Schmauk, F. J. A study of the relationship between kinds of punishment, autonomic arousal, subjective anxiety and avoidance learning in the primary sociopath. Unpublished Doctoral Dissertation, Temple University, 1968.

Schmauk, F. J. Punishment, arousal and avoidance learning in sociopaths, *Journal of Abnormal Psychology*, 1970, *76*(3), 443–453.

Schmidt, C. W., Jr., Schaffer, J. W., Zlotowitz, H. I., & Fisher, R. S. Suicide by vehicular crash. *American Journal of Psychiatry*, 1977, *134*(2), 175–178.

Schneider, K. *Clinical psychopathology*. New York: Grune & Stratton, 1959.

Schneidman, E. S., & Farberow, N. L. A sociopsychological investigation of suicide. In E. S. Schneidman, N. L. Farberow, and R. E. Litman (Eds.) *The psychology of suicide*. New York: Science House, 1970.

Schooler, N. R., Levine, J., Severe, J. B., Brauzer, B., DiMascio, A., Klerman, G., & Tuason, V. B. Prevention of relapse in schizophrenia: An evaluation of fluphenazine decanoate. *Archives of General Psychiatry*, 1980, *37*(1), 16–24.

Schuckit, M. A., & Hoglund, R. M. J. An overview of the etiological theories on alcoholism. In N. J. Estes and M. E. Heinemann (Eds.) *Alcoholism: Development, consequences, and interventions*. St. Louis: Mosby, 1977.

Schulsinger, F. Psychopathy: Heredity and environment. *International Journal of Mental Health*, 1972, *1*, 190–206.

Schur, E. The addict and social problems. In S. C. Plog and R. B. Edgerton (Eds.) *Changing perspectives in mental illness*. New York: Holt, Rinehart and Winston, 1969.

Schwade, E. D., & Geiger, S. G. Abnormal electroencephalographic findings in severe behavior disorders. *Diseases of the Nervous System*, 1965, *17*, 307–317.

Schwartz, G. E. Biofeedback as therapy: Some theoretical and practical issues. *American Psychologist*, 1973, *28*(8), 666–673.

Schwartz, G. S. Devices to prevent masturbation. *Medical Aspects of Human Sexuality*, 1973, *7*(5), 141–193.

Schwartz, M. F., & Graham, J. R. Construct validity of the MacAndrew alcoholism scale. *Journal of Consulting and Clinical Psychology*, 1979, *47*(6), 1090–1095.

Schwartz-Place, E. J., & Gilmore, G. C. Perceptual organization in schizophrenia. *Journal of Abnormal Psychology*, 1980, *89*(3), 409–418.

Seffrin, J. R., & Seehafer, R. W. A survey of drug use beliefs, opinions and behaviors among junior and senior high school students. Part I: Group data. *Journal of School Health*, 1976, *46*(2), 263–268.

Selesnick, S. *The history of psychiatry*. New York: New American Library, 1968.

Seligman, M. E. P. Phobias and preparedness. *Behavior Therapy*, 1971, *2*, 307–320.

Seligman, M. E. P. Fall into helplessness. *Psychology Today*, June 1973.

Seligman, M. E. P. *Helplessness*. San Francisco: Freeman, 1975.

Seligman, M. E. P. Comment and integration. *Journal of Abnormal Psychology*, 1978, *87*(1), 165–179.

Selye, H. *Stress in health and disease*. Boston: Butterworths, 1976.

Serban, G. *Adjustment of schizophrenics in the community*. New York: Spectrum, 1980.

Shah, S. Dangerousness: Some definitional, conceptual, and public policy issues. In B. Sales (Ed.) *Perspectives in law and psychology*. New York: Plenum Press, 1977.

Shakow, D. Psychological deficit in schizophrenia. *Behavioral Science*, 1963, *8*, 275–305.

Shapiro, D., & Surwit, A. S. Learned control of physiological function and disease. In H. Leitenberg (Ed.) *Handbook of behavior modification and behavior therapy*. Englewood Cliffs, N.J.: Prentice-Hall, 1976.

Shatan, C. F. The grief of soldiers: Vietnam combat veterans' self-help movement. *American Journal of Orthopsychiatry*, 1973, *43*(4), 640–653.

Shatan, C. F. Stress disorders among Vietnam veterans: The emotional content of combat continues. In C. R. Figley (Ed.) *Stress disorders among Vietnam veterans: Theory, research and treatment*. New York: Brunner/Mazel, 1978.

Shevitz, S. A. Psychosurgery: Some current observations. *American Journal of Psychiatry*, 1976, *133*(3), 266–270.

Shoben, E. J. Towards a concept of the normal personality. *American Psychologist*, 1957, *12*, 183–189.

Showalter, C. V., & Thornton, W. E. Clinical pharmacology of phencyclidine toxicity. *American Journal of Psychiatry*, 1977, *34*, 1234–1237.

Siegel, R. A. Probability of punishment and suppression of behavior in psychopathic and nonpsychopathic offenders. *Journal of Abnormal Psychology*, 1978, *87*(5), 514–522.

Siegel, R. K., & Jarvik, M. E. Drug induced hallucinations in animals and man. In R. K. Siegel and L. J. West (Eds.) *Hallucinations: Behavior, experience, and theory*. New York: Wiley, 1975.

Siegel, R. K., & West, L. J. (Eds.) *Hallucinations: Behavior, experience, and theory*. New York: Wiley, 1975.

Siegelman, M. Parental background of male homosexuals and heterosexuals. *Archives of Sexual Behavior,* 1974, *3*(1), 3–18.

Siegl, E. Kindergarten is not compulsory. *Seattle's Child,* 1979, *1*(1), 6.

Sifneos, P. The prevalence of "alexithymic" characteristics in psychosomatic patients. *Psychotherapeutic Psychosomatics,* 1973, *22,* 225.

Silverman, L. Psychoanalytic theory: "The reports of my death are greatly exaggerated." *American Psychologist,* 1976, *31*(9), 621–637.

Singer, J., & Singer, I. Types of female orgasm. In J. LoPiccolo and L. LoPiccolo (Eds.) *Handbook of sex therapy.* New York: Plenum Press, 1978.

Sipe, N. P. Electroconvulsive therapy—No. *Illinois Issues,* November 1979, *12,* 12–15.

Skinner, B. F. *The behavior of organisms.* New York: Appleton-Century-Crofts, 1938.

Skinner, B. F. "Superstition" in the pigeon. *Journal of Experimental Psychology,* 1948, *38,* 168–172.

Skinner, B. F. *Science and human behavior.* New York: Macmillan, 1953.

Skinner, B. F. *About behaviorism.* New York: Knopf, 1974.

Skinner, H. A., & Jackson, D. N. A model of psychopathology based on an integration of MMPI actuarial systems. *Journal of Consulting and Clinical Psychology,* 1978, *46*(2), 231–238.

Slater, E. *Psychotic and neurotic illness in twins.* London: Her Majesty's Stationery Office, 1953.

Slater, E., & Cowie, V. A. *The genetics of mental disorder.* Oxford: Oxford University Press, 1971.

Slater, E., & Glithero, E. A. A follow-up of patients diagnosed as suffering from hysteria. *Journal of Psychosomatic Research,* 1965, *9,* 9–13.

Slater, E., & Shields, J. Genetic aspects of anxiety. In M. H. Lader (Ed.) *Studies of anxiety.* Ashford, England: Headley, 1969.

Sledge, W. H., Boydstein, J. A., & Rabe, A. J. Self-concept changes related to war captivity. *Archives of General Psychiatry,* 1980, *37*(4), 430–446.

Sloane, R. B., Staples, F. R., Cristol, A. H., Yorkston, N. J., & Whipple, K. *Short-term analytically oriented psychotherapy versus behavior therapy.* Cambridge, Mass.: Harvard University Press, 1975.

Sloane, R. B., Staples, F. R., Cristol, A. H., Yorkston, N. J., & Whipple, K. Patient characteristics and outcome in psychotherapy. *Journal of Consulting and Clinical Psychology,* 1976, *44,* 330–339.

Sloane, R. B., Staples, F. R., Whipple, K., & Cristol, A. H. Patients' attitudes toward behavior therapy and psychotherapy. *American Journal of Psychiatry,* 1977, *134*(1), 134–137.

Small, J. G., Small, I. F., & Moore, D. F. Experimental withdrawal of lithium in recovered manic depressive patients: A report of five cases. *American Journal of Psychiatry,* 1971, *127*(11), 1555–1558.

Smith, D. W., Jones, K. L., & Hanson, J. W. Perspectives on the cause and frequency of the fetal alcohol syndrome. *Annals of the New York Academy of Science,* 1976, *273*(1), 138–139.

Smith, D. W., & Wilson, A. A. *A child with Down's syndrome (Mongolism).* Philadelphia: Saunders, 1973.

Smith, E. V. Effect of the double-bind communication on the anxiety level of normals. *Journal of Abnormal Psychology,* 1976, *85*(4), 356–363.

Smith, J. Q. The life and death of a schizophrenic. *Psychotherapy: Theory, Research and Practice,* 1975, *12*(1), 2–7.

Smith, M. L., & Glass, G. V. Metaanalysis of psychotherapy outcome studies. *American Psychologist,* 1977, *32*(9), 752–760.

Smith, M. L., Glass, G. V., & Miller, T. I. *The benefits of psychotherapy.* Baltimore: Johns Hopkins University Press, 1980.

Smith, R. J. *The psychopath in society.* New York: Academic Press, 1978.

Snyder, S. H. *Use of marijuana.* New York: Oxford University Press, 1971.

Snyder, S. H. Catecholamines in the brain as mediators of amphetamine psychosis. *Archives of General Psychiatry,* 1972, *27*(2), 169–179.

Snyder, S. H. Amphetamine psychosis: A model schizophrenia mediated by catecholamines. *American Journal of Psychiatry,* 1973, *130*(1), 61–66.

Synder, S. H. *Madness and the brain.* New York: McGraw-Hill, 1974.

Snyder, S. H. The dopamine hypothesis of schizophrenia: Focus on the dopamine receptor. *American Journal of Psychiatry,* 1976, *133*(2), 197–202.

Snyder, S. H. The opiate receptor and morphine-like peptides in the brain. *American Journal of Psychiatry,* 1978, *135*(6), 645–652.

Sobel, D. E. Children of schizophrenic patients: Preliminary observations on early development. *American Journal of Psychiatry,* 1961, *118,* 512–517.

Sobell, M. B., & Sobell, L. C. *Behavioral treatment of alcohol problems: Individual therapy and controlled drinking.* New York: Plenum Press, 1978.

Sokolov, N. E. *Perception and the conditioned reflex.* New York: Pergamon Press, 1963.

Solomon, R. L. The opponent-process theory of acquired motivation: The costs of pleasure and the benefits of pain. *American Psychologist,* 1980, *35*(8), 691–712.

Solzhenitsyn, A. *One day in the life of Ivan Denisovich.* New York: Penguin, 1968.

Sperling, M. Conversion hysteria and conversion symptoms: A revision of classification and concepts. *Journal of the American Psychoanalytic Association*, 1973, *21*, 745–771.

Spitz, R. A. Hospitalism. *The Psychoanalytic Study of the Child*, 1945, *1*(1), 53–74.

Spitz, R. A. Anaclitic depression. *The Psychoanalytic Study of the Child*, 1946, *2*, 313–342.

Spitzer, R. L., Endicott, J., & Gibbon, M. Crossing the border into borderline personality and borderline schizophrenia. *Archives of General Psychiatry*, 1979, *36*(1), 17–24.

Spitzer, R. L., & Forman, J. B. W. DSM-III field trials: II. Initial experience with the multiaxial system. *American Journal of Psychiatry*, 1979, *136*(6), 818–820.

Spitzer, R. L., Forman, J. B. W., & Nee, J. DSM-III field trials: I. Initial interrater diagnostic reliability. *American Journal of Psychiatry*, 1979, *136*(6), 815–817.

Spitzer, R. L., Williams, J. B. W., & Skodol, A. E. DSM-III: The major achievements and an overview. *American Journal of Psychiatry*, 1980, *132*(2), 151–164.

Spohn, H. E., Lacoursiere, R. B., Thompson, K., & Coyne, L. Phenothiazine effects on psychological and psychophysiological dysfunction in chronic schizophrenics. *Archives of General Psychiatry*, 1977, *34*, 633–644.

Squire, L. R., Slater, P. C., & Miller, P. L. Retrograde amnesia and bilateral electroconvulsive therapy: A long term follow-up. *Archives of General Psychiatry*, 1981, *38*(1), 89–95.

Srole, L., & Fischer, A. K. The midtown Manhattan longitudinal study vs. "the mental paradise lost" doctrine: A controversy joined. *Archives of General Psychiatry*, 1980, *37*(2), 209–221.

Srole, L., Langner, T. S., Michael, S. T., Kirkpatrick, P., Opler, M. K., & Rennie, T. A. *Mental health in the metropolis: The midtown Manhattan study (rev. ed.)* New York: New York University Press, 1978.

Srole, L., Langer, T. S., Michael, S. T., Opler, M. K., & Rennie, T. A. *Mental health in the metropolis: The midtown Manhattan study*. New York: McGraw-Hill, 1962.

Stahl, W. L., & Swanson, P. D. Biochemical abnormalities in Huntington's chorea brains. *Neurology*, 1974, *24*, 813–819.

Stanovich, K. E., & Purcell, D. G. Comment on "Input capability and speed of processing in mental retardation" by Saccuzzo, Kerr, Marcus, and Brown. *Journal of Abnormal Psychology*, 1981, *90*(2), 168–171.

Staples, F. R., Sloane, R. B., Whipple, K., Cristol, A. H., & Yorkston, N. J. Differences between behavior therapists and psychotherapists. *Archives of General Psychiatry*, 1975, *32*(12), 1517–1522.

Steadman, H. J., & Cocozza, J. J. *Careers of the criminally insane.* Lexington, Mass.: Lexington Books, 1974.

Steer, R., & Schut, J. Types of psychopathology displayed by heroin addicts. *American Journal of Psychiatry*, 1979, *136*(11), 1463–1465.

Steinberg, E. P., & Schwartz, G. E. Biofeedback and electrodermal self-regulation in psychopathy. *Journal of Abnormal Psychology*, 1976, *85*(4), 408–415.

Steinmetz, S. A., & Strauss, M. A. (Eds.) *Violence in the family*. New York: Mead, 1974.

Stephens, B. Symposium: Developmental gains in the reasoning, moral judgements, and moral conduct of retarded and nonretarded persons. *American Journal of Mental Deficiency*, 1974, *79*(1), 113–115.

Stephens, B., Mahoney, D. J., & McLaughlin, J. A. Mental ages for achievement of Piagetian reasoning assessment. *Education and Training of the Mentally Retarded*, 1972, *7*(1), 124–128.

Stephens, J. H., & Kamp, M. On some aspects of hysteria: A clinical study. *Journal of Nervous and Mental Disease*, 1962, *134*(2), 305–315.

Stevens, C. B. *Special needs of long term patients*. Philadelphia: Lippincott, 1974.

Stevenson, I., & Wolpe, J. Recovery from sexual deviation through overcoming of non-sexual neurotic responses. *American Journal of Psychiatry*, 1960, *116*, 737–742.

Stoller, R. J. Transvestites' women. *American Journal of Psychiatry*, 1967, *124*(2), 333–339.

Stoller, R. J. *Sex and gender (vol. 1): The development of masculinity and femininity*. New York: Jason Aronson, 1974.

Stoller, R. J. Gender identity. In A. M. Freedman, H. I. Kaplan, and B. J. Sadock (Eds.) *Comprehensive textbook of psychiatry/II*, vol. 2 (2nd ed.). Baltimore: Williams & Wilkins, 1975.

Stoller, R. J. Sexual excitement. *Archives of General Psychiatry*, 1976, *33*(8), 899–909.

Storaska, F. *How to say no to a rapist and survive*. New York: Random House, 1975.

Stoyva, J. Self-regulation and stress-related disorders: A perspective on biofeedback. In D. I. Mostofsky (Ed.) *Behavior control and modification of physiological activity*. Englewood Cliffs, N.J.: Prentice-Hall, 1976.

Strahan, R. F. Comment: Six ways of looking at an elephant. *American Psychologist*, 1978, *33*(7), 693.

Strauss, J. S. Social and cultural influences on psychopathology. *Annual Review of Psychology*, 1979, *30*, 397–415.

Strauss, J. S., & Docherty, J. P. Subtypes of schizophrenia: Descriptive models. *Schizophrenia Bulletin*, 1979, *5*(3), 447–452.

Strauss, J. S., Kokes, R. F., Klorman, R., & Sacksteder, J. L. The concept of premorbid adjustment. *Schizophrenia Bulletin,* 1977, *3*(2), 182–185.

Strean, H. S. Psychotherapy with narcissistic character disorder. *Psychotherapy: Theory, Research and Practice,* 1972, *9*(3), 269–275.

Strub, R. L. Alzheimer's disease—Current perspectives. *Journal of Clinical Psychiatry,* 1980, *41*(4), 110–112.

Strupp, H. H. A psychodynamicist looks at modern behavior therapy. *Psychotherapy: Theory, Research and Practice,* 1979, *16*(2), 124–131.

Strupp, H. H., & Hadley, S. W. Specific versus nonspecific factors in psychotherapy: A controlled study of outcome. *Archives of General Psychiatry,* 1979, *36*(10), 1125–1136.

Strupp, H. H., Fox, R. E., & Lessler, K. *Patients view their psychotherapy.* Baltimore: Johns Hopkins University Press, 1969.

Sturgis, E. T., & Adams, H. E. The right to treatment: Issues in the treatment of homosexuality. *Journal of Consulting and Clinical Psychology,* 1978, *46*(1), 165–169.

Suicide Belt. *Time Magazine,* September 1, 1980, *116*(9), 56.

Suinn, R. M. *Fundamentals of behavior pathology* (2nd ed.). New York: Wiley, 1975.

Sullivan, H. S. *The interpersonal theory of psychiatry.* New York: Norton, 1953.

Summit, R. S., & Kryso, J. Sexual abuse of children: A clinical spectrum. *American Journal of Orthopsychiatry,* 1978, *48*(2), 237–251.

Surwit, R. S., Bradner, M. N., Fenton, C. H., & Pilon, R. N. Individual differences in response to the behavioral treatment of Raynaud's disease. *Journal of Consulting and Clinical Psychology,* 1979, *47*(2), 363–367.

Surwit, R. S., Shapiro, D., & Good, M. I. Comparison of cardiovascular biofeedback, neuromuscular biofeedback, and medication in the treatment of borderline essential hypertension. *Journal of Consulting and Clinical Psychology,* 1978, *40*(2), 252–263.

Sutker, P. B., & Archer, R. P. MMPI characteristics of opiate addicts, alcoholics and other addicts. In C. S. Newmark (Ed.) *MMPI: Current clinical and research trends.* New York: Praeger, 1979.

Swanson, D. W., Bohnert, P. J., & Smith, J. A. *The paranoid.* Boston: Little, Brown, 1970.

Szasz, T. *The myth of mental illness.* New York: Harper & Row, 1961.

Szasz, T. *The manufacture of madness.* New York: Harper & Row, 1970.

Szasz, T. From the slaughterhouse to the madhouse. *Psychotherapy,* 1971, *8*(1), 1–7.

Talbot, J. A. Care of the chronically mentally ill—Still a national disgrace. *American Journal of Psychiatry,* 1979, *136*(5), 688–689.

Talbot, J. A. *State mental hospitals: Problems and potentials.* New York: Human Services Press, 1980.

Talovic, S. A., Mednick, S. A., Schulsinger, F., & Fallon, I. R. H. Schizophrenia in high-risk subjects: Prognostic maternal characteristics. *Journal of Abnormal Psychology,* 1980, *89*(3), 501–504.

Tanna, V. L. Paranoid states: A selected review. *Comprehensive Psychiatry,* 1974, *15*(6), 453–490.

Tapp, J., & Levine, F. *Law, justice and the individual in society.* New York: Holt, Rinehart and Winston, 1977.

Tashkin, D. P., Shapiro, B. J., & Frank, I. M. Acute effects of smoked marihuana and oral delta-9—Tetrahydrocannabinal on specific airway conductance in asthmatic subjects. *American Review of Respiratory Diseases,* 1974, *109,* 420–428.

Tashkin, D. P., Shapiro, B. J., Lee, Y. E., & Harper, C. E. Subacute effects of heavy marihuana smoking on pulmonary functions. *New England Journal of Medicine,* 1976, *294*(1), 125–129.

Taube, C. A., & Redick, R. W. Provisional data on patient care episodes in mental health facilities, 1975. Statistical note 139, National Institute of Mental Health, Washington, D.C., 1977.

Taylor, C. B., Farquhar, J. W., Nelson, E., & Agras, S. Relaxation therapy and high blood pressure. *Archives of General Psychiatry,* 1977, *34*(3), 339–342.

Taylor, M. A., & Heiser, J. F. Phenomenology: An alternative approach to diagnosis of mental disease. *Comprehensive Psychiatry,* 1971, *12*(5), 480–486.

Taylor, P., & Fleminger, J. J. ECT for schizophrenia. *The Lancet,* June 28, 1980, pp. 1380–1383.

Taylor, V. The delivery of mental health services in the Xenia tornado. Unpublished doctoral dissertation, Ohio State University, 1976.

Telch, M. J. The present status of outcome studies. *Journal of Consulting and Clinical Psychology,* 1981, *49*(3), 472–475.

Templeman, T. L., & Wollersheim, J. P. A cognitive-behavioral approach to the treatment of psychopathy. *Psychotherapy: Theory, Research and Practice,* 1979, *16*(2), 132–139.

Terr, L. C. Psychic trauma in children: Observations following the Chowchilla school bus kidnapping. *American Journal of Psychiatry,* 1981, *138*(1), 14–19.

The curse of hyperactivity. *Newsweek Magazine,* June 23, 1980, 59–62.

Theodor, L. H., & Mandelcorn, M. S. Hysterical blindness: A case report and study using a modern psychophysiological technique. *Journal of Abnormal Psychology,* 1973, *82*(3), 552–553.

Thigpen, C. H., & Cleckley, H. *The three faces of Eve.* Kingsport, Tenn.: Kingsport Press, 1957.

Tienari, P. Schizophrenia and monozygotic twins. *Psychiatria Fennica,* 1971, pp. 97–104.

Tinklenberg, J. R., Roth, W. T., & Kopell, B. S. Marijuana and ethanol: Differential effects on time perception, heart rate, and subjective response. *Psychopharmacology, Berl.,* 1976, *49,* 275–279.

Titchener, J. L., Sheldon, M. B., & Ross, W. D. Changes in blood pressure of hypertensive patients with and without group psychotherapy. *Journal of Psychosomatic Research,* 1959, *4*(1), 10–12.

Titchener, J. L., & Kapp, F. T. Family and character change at Buffalo Creek. *American Journal of Psychiatry,* 1976, *133*(3), 295–299.

Tomlinson, B. E. The pathology of dementia. In C. E. Wells (Ed.) *Dementia* (2nd ed.). Philadelphia: Davis, 1977.

Torgersen, S. The nature and origin of common phobic fears. *British Journal of Psychiatry,* 1979, *134,* 343–351.

Tourney, G., Petrelli, A. J., & Hatfield, L. N. Hormonal relationships in homosexual men. *American Journal of Psychiatry,* 1975, *132*(3), 288–290.

Trice, H. M., & Beyer, J. M. A sociological property of drugs: Acceptance of users of alcohol and other drugs among university undergraduates. *Journal of Studies on Alcohol,* 1977, *38*(1), 58–74.

Tripp, C. A. *The homosexual matrix.* New York: McGraw-Hill, 1975.

Truax, C. B., & Carkhuff, N. C. *Toward effective counseling and psychotherapy.* Chicago: Aldine, 1967.

Tu, J. B. Survey of psychotropic medication in mental retardation facilities. *Journal of Clinical Psychiatry,* 1979, *40*(3), 125–128.

Tucker, J. A., Vuchivick, R. E., & Sobell, M. B. Differential discriminitive stimulus control of nonalcoholic beverage consumption in alcoholics and in normal drinkers. *Journal of Abnormal Psychology,* 1979, *88*(2), 145–152.

Tunis, M. M., & Wolff, H. G. Studies on headache: Cranial artery vasoconstriction and muscle contraction headache. *Archives of General Psychiatry,* 1954, *71,* 425–434.

Turk, D. C., Meichenbaum, D. H., & Berman, W. H. Application of biofeedback for the regulation of pain: A critical review. *Psychological Bulletin,* 1979, *86*(6), 1322–1338.

Turnbull, J. W. Asthma conceived as a learned response. *Journal of Psychosomatic Research,* 1962, *6*(1), 59–70.

Turner, R. J., & Wagonfeld, M. D. Occupational mobility and schizophrenia. *American Sociological Review,* 1967, *32*(1), 104–113.

Tyhurst, J. S. The role of transition states—Including disasters—In mental illness. *Symposium on social and preventive psychiatry.* Washington, D.C.: Walter Reed Army Institute of Research, 1957.

U.S. Department of Health, Education, and Welfare. *Alcohol and health.* Washington, D.C.: U.S. Government Printing Office, 1974.

Ullmann, L. P., & Krasner, L. *A psychological approach to abnormal behavior* (2nd ed.). Englewood Cliffs, N.J.: Prentice-Hall, 1975.

Usdin, E. Endorphins, dopamine, and schizophrenia: Two discussions. *Schizophrenia Bulletin,* 1979, *5*(2), 241–242.

Vaillant, G. E. Sociopathy as a human process: A viewpoint. *Archives of General Psychiatry,* 1975, *32*(2), 178–183.

Vaillant, G. E. *Adaptation to life.* Boston: Little, Brown, 1977.

Valenstein, E. S. *Brain control.* New York: Wiley, 1973.

Valins, S., & Nisbett, R. E. *Attribution process in the development and treatment of emotional disorders.* New York: General Learning Press, 1971.

Verville, E. *Behavior problems of children.* Philadelphia: Saunders, 1967.

Verwoerdt, A. *Clinical geropsychiatry.* Baltimore: Williams & Wilkins, 1976.

Vetter, A. J. *Psychology of abnormal behavior.* New York: Ronald Press, 1972.

Vogel-Sprott, M. Defining "light" and "heavy" social drinking: Research implications and hypothesis. *Quarterly Journal of Studies in Alcoholism,* 1974, *35,* 1388–1392.

Volavka, J., Davis, L. G., & Ehrlich, Y. H. Endorphins, dopamine and schizophrenia. *Schizophrenia Bulletin,* 1979, *5*(2), 227–239.

Wachtel, P. *Psychoanalysis and behavior therapy: Toward an integration.* New York: Basic Books, 1977.

Wadeson, H., & Carpenter, W. T. Impact of the seclusion room experience. *Journal of Nervous and Mental Disease,* 1976, *163*(5), 318–328.

Wagemaker, H., & Cade, R. The use of hemodialysis in chronic schizophrenia. *American Journal of Psychiatry,* 1977, *134,* 684–685.

Waggoner, R. Brain syndromes associated with intracranial neoplasm. In A. Freedman, H. I. Kaplan, and H. S. Kaplan (Eds.) *Comprehensive textbook of psychiatry.* Baltimore Williams & Wilkins, 1967.

Wahl, O. Six T.V. myths about mental illness. *TV Guide,* March 12, 1976, 4–8.

Waldron, S., Shrier, D. K., Stone, B., & Tobin, F. School phobia and other childhood neurosis: A systematic study of the children and their families. *American Journal of Psychiatry,* 1975, *132,* 802–808.

Wallen, V. Background characteristics, attitudes and self-concept of Air Force psychiatric casualties in Southeast Asia. In P. Bourne (Ed.) *The psychology and physiology of stress: With reference to special studies of the Vietnam War.* New York: Academic Press, 1969.

Wallick, M. M. Desensitization therapy with a fearful two-year-old. *American Journal of Psychiatry,* 1979, *136*(10), 1325–1326.

Waring, M., & Ricks, D. Family patterns of children who become adult schizophrenics. *Journal of Nervous and Mental Disease,* 1965, *140,* 351–364.

Warnes, H. Twenty years lines of advance in psychosomatic medicine. *The Psychiatric Journal of the University of Ottawa,* 1979, *4*(1), 85–92.

Warren, S. E., & O'Connor, D. T. Does a renal vasodilator system mediate racial differences in essential hypertension? *The American Journal of Medicine,* 1980, *69*(3), 425–429.

Watson, C. G., & Buranen, C. The frequencies of conversion reaction symptoms. *Journal of Abnormal Psychology,* 1979, *88*(2), 209–211.

Watson, J. B., & Rayner, R. Conditioned emotional reaction. *Journal of Experimental Psychology,* 1920, *3*(1), 1–14.

Watson, S. J., & Akil, H. Endorphins: Clinical issues. In R. Pickens and L. Heston (Eds.) *Psychiatric factors in drug abuse.* New York: Grune & Stratton, 1979.

Watson, S. J., & Akil, H. Endorphins, dopamine and schizophrenia: Two discussions. *Schizophrenia Bulletin,* 1979, *5*(2), 240–242.

Watson, S. J., Akil, H., Berger, P. A., & Barchas, J. D. Some observations on the opiate peptides and schizophrenia. *Archives of General Psychiatry,* 1979, *36*(1), 35–41.

Watt, J. A. G., Hall, D. J., & Olley, P. C. et al. Paranoid states of middle life: Familial occurrence and relationship to schizophrenia. *Acta Psychiatrica Scandinavia,* 1980, *61,* 413–426.

Wechsler, D. Intelligence: Definition, theory, and the I.Q. In R. Cancro (Ed.) *Intelligence: Genetic and environmental influences.* New York: Grune & Stratton, 1971.

Wechsler, D. Intelligence defined and undefined: A relativistic appraisal. *American Psychologist,* 1975, *30*(2), 135–139.

Weekes, C. Simple, effective treatment of agoraphobia. *American Journal of Psychotherapy,* 1978, *32*(3), 357–369.

Weiner, D. B. The apprenticeship of Philippe Pinel: A new document, "Observations of Citizen Pussin on the insane." *American Journal of Psychiatry,* 1979, *139*(9), 1128–1134.

Weiner, H. *Psychobiology and human disease.* New York: Elsevier-North Holland, 1977.

Weiner, H. T., Thaler, M., Reiser, M. F., & Mirsky, I. A. Etiology of duodenal ulcer: Relationship of specific psychological characteristics to rate of gastric secretion (serum pepsinogen). *Psychosomatic Medicine,* 1957, *19*(1), 1–11.

Weiner, R. D. The psychiatric use of electrically induced seizures. *American Journal of Psychiatry,* 1979, *136*(12), 1507–1517.

Weintraub, M. I. Hysteria: A clinical guide to diagnosis. *Clinical Symposia,* CIBA, 1977, *29*(6), 1–31.

Weiss, G., Hechtman, L., & Perlman, T. Hyperactives as young adults: School, employer, and self-rating scales obtained during ten-year follow-up evaluation. *American Journal of Orthopsychiatry,* 1978, *48*(3), 438–445.

Weiss, G., Kruger, E., Danielson, V., & Elman, M. Long term methylphenidate treatment of hyperkinetic children. *Psychopharmacology Bulletin,* 1974, *10*(1), 34–35.

Weiss, J. M. Effects of coping behavior in different warning signal conditions on stress pathology in rats. *Journal of Comparative and Physiological Psychology,* 1971, *77*(1), 22–30.

Weissman, M. M., Klerman, G. L., Prusoff, B. A., Sholomskas, D., & Padian, N. Depressed outpatients: Results one year after treatment with drugs and/or interpersonal psychotherapy. *Archives of General Psychiatry,* 1981, *38*(1), 51–55.

Weisz, J. R., & Zigler, E. Cognitive development in retarded and nonretarded persons. Piagetian tests of the similar sequence hypothesis. *Psychological Bulletin,* 1979, *86,* 831–851.

Weitkamp, L. R., Pardue, L. H., & Huntzinger, R. S. Genetic marker studies in a family with unipolar depression. *Archives of General Psychiatry,* 1980, *37*(10), 1187–1192.

Weitzel, W. D., Morgan, D. W., Guyden, T. E., & Robinson, J. A. Toward a more efficient mental status examination: Free form or operationally defined. *Archives of General Psychiatry,* 1973, *28*(2), 215–220.

Wells, C. E. Chronic brain disease: An overview. *American Journal of Psychiatry,* 1978, *135*(1), 1–12.

Welner, Z. Childhood depression: An overview. *Journal of Nervous and Mental Disease,* 1978, *166,* 588–593.

Wender, P. H., Rosenthal, D., Kety, S. S., Schulsinger, F., & Welver, J. Cross-fostering: A research strategy for clarifying the role of genetic and experiential factors in the etiology of schizophrenia. *Archives of General Psychiatry,* 1974, *30*(1), 121–128.

Wendkos, M. *Sudden death and psychiatric illness.* New York: Spectrum, 1979.

Werry, J. S. The childhood psychosis. In H. C. Quay and J. S. Werry (Eds.) *Psychopathological disorders of childhood.* New York: Wiley, 1979.

Wexler, L., Weissman, M. M., & Kasl, S. V. Suicide attempts 1970–75: Updating a United States study and comparisons with international trends. *British Journal of Psychiatry*, 1978, *132*(1), 180–185.

White, R. W. *The abnormal personality* (3rd ed.). New York: Ronald Press, 1964.

Wickramsera, I. Aversive behavior rehearsal for sexual exhibitionism. *Behavior Therapy*, 1976, *7*(2), 167–177.

Widom, C. S. A methodology for studying noninstitutionalized psychopathy. *Journal of Consulting and Clinical Psychology*, 1977, *45*(4), 674–683.

Wikler, A., Dixon, J. F., & Parker, J. B. Brain function in problem children and controls: Psychometric, neurological, and electroencephalographic comparisons. *American Journal of Psychiatry*, 1970, *127*(5), 634–645.

Wilder, J. The lure of magical thinking. *American Journal of Psychotherapy*, 1975, *29*(1), 37–55.

Willerman, L. Activity level and hyperactivity in twins. *Child Development*, 1973, *44*, 288–293.

Williams, M. *Brain damage, behavior and the mind.* New York: Wiley, 1979.

Williams, R. B., Jr. Headache. In R. B. Williams, Jr. and W. D. Gentry (Eds.) *Behavioral approaches to medical treatment.* Cambridge, Mass.: Ballinger, 1977.

Williams, T. Vietnam veterans. Unpublished paper presented at the University of Denver School of Professional Psychology. Denver, Col., April 1979.

Williams, T. *Post-traumatic stress disorders of the Vietnam veteran.* Cincinnati, Ohio: Disabled American Veterans, 1980.

Wilner, A., Reick, T., Robins, I., Fishman, R., & Van Doren, T. Obsessive-compulsive neurosis. *Comprehensive Psychiatry*, 1976, *17*, 527–539.

Wilson, G. T., & Lawson, D. M. Expectancies, alcohol, and sexual arousal in women. *Journal of Abnormal Psychology*, 1978, *87*(3), 358–367.

Wincze, J. P. Sexual deviance and dysfunction. In D. C. Rimm and J. W. Somerville (Eds.) *Abnormal psychology.* New York: Academic Press, 1977.

Winer, D. Anger and dissociation: A case study of multiple personality. *Journal of Abnormal Psychology*, 1978, *87*(3), 368–372.

Wing, J., Birley, J. L. T., Cooper, J. C., Graham, P., & Isaacs, A. D. Reliability of a procedure for measuring and classifying "present psychiatric state." *British Journal of Psychiatry*, 1967, *113*, 499–506.

Winick, M. Nutrition and mental development. *Mental Clinics of North America*, 1970, *54*, 1413–1428.

Winnik, H. Psychological problems after severe mental stress. *Excerpta Medica International Congress Series No. 150, Proceedings of the Fourth World Congress of Psychiatry*, Madrid, vol. II. September 1966, New York: Excerpta Medica Foundation, 1968.

Winoker, G. Genetic patterns as they affect psychiatric diagnosis. In V. M. Rakoff, H. C. Stancer, and H. B. Kedward (Eds.) *Psychiatric diagnosis.* New York: Brunner/Mazel, 1977.

Winoker, G. Unipolar depression: Is it divisible into autonomous subtypes? *Archives of General Psychiatry*, 1979, *36*(1), 47–52.

Wise, T. N. Personality profiles of impotent men. *Medical Aspects of Human Sexuality*, 1976, *10*(10), 144–160.

Witkin, H. A., Mednick, S. A., Schulsinger, F., Bakkestrom, E., Christiansen, K. O., Goodenough, D. R., Hirschorn, K., Lundsteen, C., Owen, D. R., Philip, J., Rubin, D. B., & Stocking, M. Criminality in XYY and XXY men. *Science*, 1976, *193*, 547–555.

Witkin, M. J. *Private psychiatric hospitals, 1974–1975.* Series A, No. 18, National Institute of Mental Health, 1977.

Witzig, J. S. The group treatment of male exhibitionists. *American Journal of Psychiatry*, 1968, *125*(1), 75–81.

Wolfe, B. The real life-death of Jim Morrison. *Esquire*, June 1971.

Wolff, H. G. The psychotherapeutic approach. In R. Hopkins and H. G. Wolff (Eds.) *Principles of treatments of psychosomatic disorders.* London: Pergamon Press, 1965.

Wolff, H. G. *Headache and other pain.* Revised by D. J. Dalessio. New York: Oxford University Press, 1972.

Wolkenstein, A. S. Evolution of a program for the management of child abuse. *Social Casework*, 1976, *52*(5), 309–316.

Wolpe, J. *Psychotherapy by reciprocal inhibition.* Stanford, Calif.: Stanford University Press, 1958.

Wolpe, J. Cognition and causation in human behavior and its therapy. *American Psychologist*, 1978, *33*(4), 437–446.

Wolpe, J. Behavior therapy versus psychoanalysis: Therapeutic and social implications. *American Psychologist*, 1981, *36*(2), 159–164.

Wolpe, J., & Rachman, S. Psychoanalytic "evidence": A critique based on Freud's case of little Hans. *Journal of Nervous and Mental Disease*, 1960, *130*(2), 135–148.

Wood, A. L. *Deviant behavior and control strategies.* Lexington, Mass.: Lexington Books, 1974.

Woodruff, R. A., Goodwin, D. W., & Guze, S. B. *Psychiatric diagnosis.* New York: Oxford University Press, 1974.

Wright, L. Conceptualizing and defining psychosomatic disorders. *American Psychologist*, 1977, *32*(8), 625–628.

Wright, M., & Hogan, T. P. Repeated LSD ingestion and performance on neuropsychological tests.

Journal of Nervous and Mental Disease, 1972, *154*(3), 432–438.

Wyatt, R. J., Potkin, S. G., Bridge, T. P., Phelps, B. H., & Wise, F. D. Monoamine oxidase in schizophrenia: An overview. *Schizophrenia Bulletin*, 1980, *6*(2), 199–207.

Yager, J. Post combat violent behavior in psychiatrically maladjusted soldiers. *Archives of General Psychiatry*, 1976, *33*(11), 1332–1335.

Yap, P. M. Koro—A culture-bound depersonalization syndrome. *The British Journal of Psychiatry*, 1965, *111*(1), 1–6.

Zax, M., & Stricker, G. *Patterns of psychopathology*. New York: Macmillan, 1963.

Zechnick, R. Exhibitionism: Genesis, dynamics and treatment. *Psychiatric Quarterly*, 1971, *45*(1), 70–75.

Zeichner, A., & Pihl, R. O. Effects of alcohol and behavior contingencies on human aggression. *Journal of Abnormal Psychology*, 1979, *88*(2), 153–160.

Zentner, M. The paranoid client. *Social Casework: The Journal of Contemporary Social Work*, 1980, *61*(3), 138–145.

Ziegler, F. J. Hysterical conversion reaction. *Postgraduate Medicine*, 1970, *47*, 174–179.

Zigler, E. Research in personality structure in the retardate. In N. R. Ellis (Ed.) *International review of research in mental retardation*, vol. 1. New York: Academic Press, 1966.

Zigler, E. Familial mental retardation: A continuing dilemma. *Science*, 1967, *153*, 292–298.

Zigler, E., & Phillips, L. Psychiatric diagnosis and symptomatology. *Journal of Abnormal and Social Psychology*, 1969, *63*(1), 69–75.

Zilbergeld, B., & Evans, M. The inadequacy of Masters and Johnson, *Psychology Today*, 1980, *14*, 28–43.

Zilboorge, G. *A history of medical psychology*. New York: Norton, 1941.

Zimering, S., & Calhoun, J. F. Is there an alcoholic personality? *Journal of Drug Education*, 1976, *6*(1), 97–103.

Zubin, J., & Spring, B. Vulnerability—A new view of schizophrenia. *Journal of Abnormal Psychology*, 1977, *86*(2), 103–126.

Zubin, J., & Steinhauer, S. How to break the log jam in schizophrenia: A look beyond genetics. *Journal of Nervous and Mental Disease*, 1981, *169*(8), 477–491.

Zuckerman, M., Eysenck, S., & Eysenck, H. J. Sensation seeking in England and America: Crosscultural, age, and sex comparisons. *Journal of Consulting and Clinical Psychology*, 1978, *46*(1), 139–149.

Chapter 4

page 95 American Psychiatric Association; *Diagnostic and Statistical Manual of Mental Disorders*, Third Edition, Washington, D.C., A.P.A., 1980. Reprinted by permission.

Chapter 5

page 107 Figure 5.1. Adapted with permission of the R. J. Brady Co., Bowie, Md. 20715, from their 1975 copyrighted work, *"Emergency Psychiatric Care: Management of Mental Health Crisis"*.

Chapter 6

page 126 *The American Journal of Psychiatry*, vol. 134:12, pp. 1426. Copyright, 1977, the American Psychiatric Association.

page 129 Table 6.2. Adapted from Table 8–1 "Sympathetic and Parasympathetic Functions of the Autonomic Nervous Systems" (p. 195) from *Essentials of Abnormal Psychology* by Benjamin Kleinmuntz. Copyright © 1974 by Benjamin Kleinmuntz. Reprinted by permission of Harper & Row, Publishers, Inc.

page 130 Figure 6.1. Adapted from Simulab 12 "The Autonomic Nervous System and the Organs It Innervates" (p. 501) from Krech, D., Crutchfield, R. S., Livson, N. and Krech, H. *Psychology: A Basic Course.* New York: A. A. Knopf, Inc., 1976. Courtesy of A. A. Knopf, Inc.

page 132 Table 6.3. Reprinted with permission from the *Journal of Psychosomatic Research*, 11 (2), T. H. Holmes and R. H. Rahe, "The Social Readjustment Rating Scale, Copyright 1967, Pergamon Press, Ltd.

page 133, 134 Rosen, E., Fox, R. E., and Gregory, I. *Abnormal Psychology*, 2nd Ed. Philadelphia: W. B. Saunders, 1972. By permission of current copyright holder, Holt, Rinehart and Winston, Inc.

page 136 Table 6.4. Reprinted with permission from the *Journal of Psychosomatic Research*, vol. 7, Rees, L., The Importance of Psychological, Allergic and Infective Factors in Childhood Asthma. Copyright 1964, Pergamon Press, Ltd.

page 137 Table 6.5. Reprinted with permission from the *Journal of Psychosomatic Research*, vol. 17, G. de Araujo, P. P. Van Arsdel, Jr., T. H. Holmes, and D. L. Dudley, Life Changes, Coping Ability and Chronic Intrinsic Asthma, Copyright 1973, Pergamon Press, Ltd.

page 139 Figure 6.3. Budzynski, T. H. Biofeedback Strategies in Headache Treatment. In J. V. Basmajian (Ed) *Biofeedback Principles and Practice for Clinicians*. Baltimore: Williams and Wilkins, 1979. By permission of the Williams and Wilkins Co., Baltimore.

page 139, 140 Vetter, A. J. *Psychology of Abnormal Behavior*. New York: Ronald Press Co., 1972. By permission of current copyright holder, John Wiley and Sons, Inc.

page 141 Table 6.6. Cobb, S. and Rose, A. M. Hypertension, Peptic Ulcer and Diabetes in Air Traffic Controllers. *Journal of the American Medical Association*, vol. 224, no. 4, pp. 489–492, copyright 1973, American Medical Association, reprinted by permission.

page 148 Reprinted, with permission, from the *American Journal of Orthopsychiatry*: copyright 1977 by the American Orthopsychiatric Association, Inc.

page 148, 149 *The American Journal of Psychiatry*, vol. 136:7, pp. 735–736, 1980. Copyright 1980, the American Psychiatric Association. Reprinted by permission.

Chapter 7

page 155 Figure 7.1. Prigatano, G. P. and Johnson, H. J. Autonomic Nervous System Changes Associated with a Spider Phobic Reaction. *Journal of Abnormal Psychology,* 83 (2), p. 174, 1974. Copyright 1974 by the American Psychological Association. Reprinted and adapted by permission of the author.

page 157 Table 7.1. Marks, I. and Lader, M. Anxiety States (anxiety neurosis): A Review. *Journal of Nervous and Mental Disease,* vol. 156, no. 1, pp. 3–18, 1973. Copyright 1973, the Williams and Wilkins Co. Baltimore. Reprinted and adapted by permission.

page 157, 158 Cameron, N. *The Psychology of Behavior Disorder.* Boston: Houghton Mifflin, Co., 1947. Courtesy of Houghton Mifflin Co. and David O. Hooke.

page 160 Figure 7.2. Geer, J. H., Davison, G. C. and Gatchel, R. I. Reduction of Stress in Humans Through Non-veridical Perceived Control of Aversive Stimulation. *Journal of Personality and Social Psychology.* Vol. 16, pp. 731–738, 1970. Copyright 1970 by the American Psychological Association. Reprinted and adapted by permission of the author.

page 162, 163 Henderson, D. K. and Gillespie, R. D. *Textbook of Psychiatry,* 10th Ed. New York: Oxford University Press, 1969. Reprinted by permission.

page 163 Figure 7.3. Agras, W. S., Sylvester, D. and Oliveau, D. C. The Epidemiology of Common Fears and Phobias. *Comprehensive Psychiatry,* vol. 10, p. 153, 1969. Reprinted by permission of Grune and Stratton, Inc. and the author.

page 167 Rachman, S. J. and Hodgson, R. J. *Obsessions and Compulsions,* © 1980, p. 59. Reprinted by permission of Prentice-Hall, Inc., Englewood Cliffs, N.J.

page 172 Figure 7.4. Foa, E. B., Steketee, G. and Milby, J. B. Differential Effects of Exposure and Response Prevention in Obsessive-compulsive Washers. *Journal of Consulting and Clinical Psychology,* vol. 48, no. 1, p. 73, 1980. Copyright 1980 by the American Psychological Association. Reprinted and adapted by permission of the author.

Chapter 8

page 177 Laughlin, H. P. *The Neurosis in Clinical Practice.* Philadelphia: W. B. Saunders, Co., 1956. Reprinted by permission of W. B. Saunders, Co.

page 178 Table 8.1. Watson, G. G. and Buranen, C. The Frequencies of Conversion Reaction Symptoms. *Journal of Abnormal Psychology,* vol. 88, no. 2, p. 210, 1979. Copyright 1979 by the American Psychological Association. Reprinted and adapted by permission of the author*.

page 179 Figure 8.1. From Lyle E. Bourne, Jr., and Bruce R. Ekstrand. Psychology: Its Principles and Meanings, 4th Ed., Copyright 1982, Holt, Rinehart and Winston, Inc.

page 179, 180 Cameron, N. *The Psychology of Behavior Disorder.* Boston: Houghton Mifflin, Co., 1947. Courtesy of Houghton Mifflin, Co. and David O. Hooke.

page 182 Figure 8.2. Hilgard, E. R., MacDonald, H., Morgan, A. H. and Johnson, L. S. The Reality of Hypnotic Analgesia: A Comparison of Highly Hypnotizable Simulators. *Journal of Abnormal Psychology,* vol. 87, no. 2, p. 243, 1978. Copyright 1978 by the American Psychological Association. Reprinted and adapted by permission of the author.

page 184, 185 Masserman, J. H. *Principles of Dynamic Psychiatry,* 2nd Ed. Philadelphia: W. B. Saunders, Co., 1961. Reprinted by permission of W. B. Saunders, Co.

page 189 Table 8.2. Bliss, E. L. Multiple personality: a report of 14 cases with implications for schizophrenia and hysteria. *Archives of General Psychiatry,* vol. 37, no. 12, p. 1392, 1980. Copyright 1980 by the American Medical Association. Reprinted by permission.

Chapter 9

page 206, 220 Ince, L. P. Behavior Modification of Sexual Disorders. *American Journal of Psychotherapy,* vol. 27, no. 3, pp. 447, 448–449, 1973. Reprinted by permission of the American Journal of Psychotherapy.

page 211 Hamilton J. W. Voyeurism: Some Clinical and Theoretical Considerations. *American Journal of Psychotherapy,* vol. 26, no. 2, pp. 277–284, 1972. Reprinted by permission of the American Journal of Psychotherapy.

page 211, 212 Cleckley, H. M. The Caricature of Love. New York: Ronald Press, 1957. Reprinted by permission of current copyright holder, John Wiley and Sons, Inc.

page 214 Krueger, D. W. Symptom Passing in a Transvestite Father and Three Sons. American Journal of Psychiatry, vol. 135, no. 6, pp. 739–742, 1978. Courtesy of the American Psychiatric Association.

Chapter 10

page 229 Figure 10.1. Kornetsky, C. *Pharmacology: Drugs Affecting Behavior.* New York: John Wiley and Sons, 1976. Reprinted by permission of John Wiley and Sons, Inc.

page 231 Table 10.2. Engs, R. C. Drinking Patterns and Drinking Problems of College Students. Reprinted by permission from *Journal of Studies on Alcohol,* vol. 38, pp. 2144–2156, 1977. Copyright by Journal of Studies on Alcohol, Inc. New Brunswick, N.J. 08903

page 235 Rosen, E., Fox, R. E. and Gregory, I. *Abnormal Psychology,* 2nd Ed. Philadelphia: W. B. Saunders, Co., 1972. By permission of current copyright holder, Holt, Rinehart and Winston, Inc.

page 240 Rosen, E., Fox, R. E. and Gregory, I. *Abnormal Psychology,* 2nd Ed. Philadelphia: W. B. Saunders, Co., 1972. By permission of current copyright holder, Holt, Rinehart and Winston, Inc.

page 243 Highlight 10.6. From *Narcotics–An American Plan* by Saul Jeffee. Paul S. Eriksson, Publisher. Reprinted by permission.

page 244, 245 Solomon, R. L. The Opponent-Process Theory of Acquired Motivation: The Costs of Pleasure and the Benefits of Pain. *American Psychologist,* vol. 35, no. 8, p. 696, 1980. Copyright 1980 by the American Psychological Association. Reprinted by permission of the author.

page 254 Figure 10.2. Miller, W. Behavioral Treatment of Problem Drinkers: A Comparative Outcome Study of Three Controlled Drinking Therapies. *Journal of Consulting and Clinical Psychology,* vol. 46, no. 1, p. 79, 1978. Copyright 1978 by the American Psychological Association. Reprinted and adapted by permission of the author.

Chapter 11

page 261, 262 Zentner, M. The Paranoid Client. *Social Casework: the Journal of Contemporary Social Work,* vol. 61, no. 3, p. 144, 1980. Reprinted by permission of the Family Service Association of America.

page 262, 263 Reprinted with permission of Macmillan Publishing Co., Inc. from *Patterns of Psychopathology* by M. Zax and G. Stricker. Copyright © 1963 by Macmillan Publishing Co., Inc.

page 264 Hopkins, W. R. and Fine, H. J. The End of Jim Morrison: A Schizoid Suicide–A Phenomenological Study in Object Relations. *Psychotherapy: Theory, Research and Practice,* vol. 4, no. 4, pp. 425, 426, 1977. Copyright 1977, the Division of Psychotherapy, American Psychological Association. Reprinted by permission.

page 266, 267 From McCall, R. J. *The Varieties of Abnormality,* 1975. Courtesy of Charles C. Thomas, Publisher, Springfield, Illinois.

page 271 McNeil Elton, B. *The Quiet Furies: Man and Disorder,* © 1967, pp. 83–90. Adapted by permission of Prentice-Hall, Inc., Englewood Cliffs, N.J.

page 272 Hare, R. D. *Psychopathy: Theory and Research.* Copyright © 1970 John Wiley and Sons, Inc. Reprinted by permission of John Wiley and Sons, Inc.

page 274 Figure 11.1. Hare, R. D. *Psychopathy: Theory and Research.* Copyright © 1970 John Wiley and Sons, Inc. Reprinted by permission of John Wiley and Sons, Inc.

page 276 Figure 11.2. Hare, R. D. *Psychopathy: Theory and Research.* Copyright © 1970 John Wiley & Sons, Inc. Reprinted by permission of John Wiley & Sons, Inc.

page 277 Figure 11.3. Schachter, S. and Latané, B. Crime, Cognition, and the Autonomic Nervous System. Reprinted from the 1964 *Nebraska Symposium on Motivation* edited by David Levine, by permission of University of Nebraska Press. Copyright © 1964 by the University of Nebraska Press.

page 278 Figure 11.4. Siegel, R. A. Probability of Punishment and Suppression of behavior in Psychopathic and Non-Psychopathic Offenders. *Journal of Abnormal Psychology,* vol. 87, no. 5, p. 518, 1978. Copyright 1978 by the American Psychological Association. Reprinted by permission of the author.

page 280, 281 Templeman, T. L. and Wollersheim, J. P. A Cognitive-Behavioral Approach to the Treatment of Psychopathy. *Psychotherapy: Theory, Research and Practice,* vol. 16, no. 2, p. 136, 1979. Copyright 1979, the Division of Psychotherapy, American Psychological Association. Reprinted by permission.

Chapter 12

page 289 Table 12.1 Reprinted by permission from Table 2, pages 196–197 in *Phenomenology and Treatment of Schizophrenia* by William E. Fann, Ismet Karacan, Alex D. Pokorny and Robert L. Williams (eds.) Copyright 1978, Spectrum Publications, Inc., New York City.

page 294 Highlight 12.2 Siegel, R. K. and Jarvik, M. Drug Induced Hallucinations in Animals and Man. In R. K. Siegel and L. G. West (Eds.) *Hallucinations: Behavior, Experience and Theory.* New York: John Wiley & Sons, 1975. Copyright © 1975 John Wiley & Sons, Inc. Reprinted by permission.

page 294 Highlight 12.2 Wadeson, H. and Carpenter, W. T. Impact of the Seclusion Room Experience. *Journal of Nervous and Mental Disease,* vol. 163, no. 5, p. 322, 1976. Copyright © 1976, the Williams & Wilkins Co., Baltimore. Reprinted by permission.

page 300 American Psychiatric Association; *Diagnostic and Statistical Manual of Mental Disorders,* Third Edition, Washington, D.C., A.P.A., 1980.

page 304 Table 12.4 Kantor, R. E., Wallner, J. M. and Windner, L. L. Process and Reactive Schizophrenia. *Journal of Consulting Psychology,* vol. 17, no. 1, pp. 157–163, 1953. Courtesy of the American Psychological Association.

page 306 Figure 12.2. Asarnow, R. F. and MacCrimmon, D. J. Residual performance deficits in clinically remitted schizophrenics: a marker for schizophrenia. *Journal of Abnormal Psychology,* vol. 87, no. 6, pp. 597–608, 1978. Copyright 1978 by the American Psychological Association. Reprinted by permission of the author.

page 307 Figure 12.3. Meiselman, K. C. Inducing Schizophrenic Associations in Normal Subjects. *Journal of Abnormal Psychology,* vol. 87, no. 3, p. 292, 1978. Copyright 1978 by the American Psychological Association. Reprinted by permission of the author.

page 308, 309 Betz, B. J. Curtain on Schizophrenia: A Twenty-five Year Clinical Follow-up. *American Journal of Psychotherapy,* vol. 34, no. 2, pp. 252–260, 1980. Reprinted by permission.

Chapter 13

page 315 Figure 13.1. Smith, E. K. Effect of double-bind communication on the anxiety levels of normals. *Journal of Abnormal Psychology,* vol. 85, no. 4, p. 361, 1978. Copyright 1978 by the American Psychological Association. Reprinted by permission of the author.

page 330 Figure 13.3. Zubin, J. and Steinhauer, S. How to break the log jam in schizophrenia: a look beyond genetics. *Journal of Nervous and Mental Disease,* vol. 169, no. 8, p. 481, 1981. Copyright © 1981 the Williams & Wilkins Co., Baltimore. Reprinted by permission.

page 332 Figure 13.4. Schooler, N. R., Levine, G., and Tuason, V. B. Prevention of relapse in schizophrenia: an evaluation of fluphenazine decanoate. *Archives of General Psychiatry,* vol. 37, no. 1, p. 19, 1980. Copyright 1980, American Medical Association. Reprinted by permission.

page 336 Figure 13.5. Matefy, R. E. Operant conditioning procedure to modify schizophrenic behavior: a case report. *Psychotherapy: Theory, Research and Practice,* vol. 9, no. 3, p. 228, 1972. Copyright 1972. Division of Psychotherapy, American Psychological Association. Reprinted by permission.

page 337 Table 13.4. Liberman, R. P. Behavior Therapy for Schizophrenia. In L. J. West and D. E. Flinn (Eds.) *Treatment of Schizophrenia: Progress and Prospects.* New York: Grune and Stratton, 1976. Reprinted by permission of Grune & Stratton, Inc. and the author.

Chapter 14

page 345, 346 Lemberg, R. W. Multi-sensory hallucinatory experiences: a diary account. *American Journal of Psychotherapy,* vol. 32, no. 3, pp. 461–464, 1978. Reprinted by permission.

page 346, 347 Suinn, R. M. *Fundamentals of Behavior Pathology* 2nd Ed., New York: John Wiley & Sons, 1975. Copyright 1975 John Wiley & Sons, Inc. Reprinted by permission.

page 347 Barnes, F. A Psychiatric unit serving an international community. *Hospital & Community Psychiatry,* vol. 31, no. 11, pp. 757–758, 1980. Reprinted by permission of Hospital & Community Psychiatry.

page 348 Figure 14.2. From *Soul Murder: Persecution in the Family* by Morton Schatzman. Courtesy of Random House, Inc.

page 351, 352 Swanson, D. W., Bohnert, P. J. and Smith, J. A. *The Paranoid.* Boston: Little, Brown and Co., 1970. Copyright 1970, Little, Brown and Co. Reprinted by permission.

page 352 Berger, K. and Zarit, S. Late life paranoid state: assessment and treatment. *American Journal of Orthopsychiatry,* vol. 48, no. 3, pp. 535–534, 1978. Reprinted with permission, from the American Journal of Orthopsychiatry: Copyright 1978 by the American Orthopsychiatric Association, Inc.

Chapter 15

page 363 Figure 15.1 Vetter, H. J. *Psychology of Abnormal Behavior* New York: Ronald Press Co., 1972. Reprinted by permission of current copyright holder, John Wiley & Sons, Inc.

page 364 Table 15.1 Beck, A. T. *Depression: Clinical, Experimental and Theoretical Aspects.* New York: Harper and Row, Publishers. Reprinted by permission of Lippencott/Harper & Row Publishers.

page 366 Table 15.2 Nelson, J. C. and Charney, D. S. The Symptoms of Major Depressive Illness. *American Journal of Psychiatry,* vol. 138, no. 1, p. 10, 1981. Copyright 1981, the American Psychiatric Association. Reprinted by permission.

page 367, 368 From Kolb, L. C.: *Noyes Modern Clinical Psychiatry,* Philadelphia: W. B. Saunders, 1968. Reprinted with permission.

page 368 Figure 15.2 Carlson, G. and Goodwin, F. K. The Stages of Mania: A Longitudinal Analysis of the Manic Episode. *Archives of General Psychiatry,* vol. 28, no. 2, pp. 221–228, 1973. Copyright 1973, American Medical Association. Reprinted by permission.

page 369 Norman Cameron and Ann Magaret: *Behavior Pathology,* p.332. Copyright © 1951 renewed 1979 by Houghton Mifflin Company. Reprinted by permission.

page 370 Akiskal, H. S., Djenderedjian, A. H., Rosenthal, R. H. and Khavi, M. K. Cyclothymic Disorder: Validation Criteria for Inclusion in the Bipolar Affective Group. *American Journal of Psychiatry,* vol. 134, no. 11, p. 1230, 1977. Courtesy of the American Psychiatric Association.

page 371 From Kolb, L. C.: *Noyes Modern Clinical Psychiatry.* Philadelphia: W. B. Saunders, 1968. Reprinted by permission.

page 372 Figure 15.4 Frederick, C. J. Current trends in suicidal behavior in the United States. *American Journal of Psychotherapy,* vol. 32, no. 2, pp. 117–200, 1978. Reprinted by permission of the American Journal of Psychotherapy.

page 372, 373 Litman, R. E. Suicide as acting out. In E. S. Schneidman, N. L. Farberow, and R. E. Litman (Eds.) *The Psychology of Suicide.* New York: Jason Aronson, Inc., 1970. Copyright © 1970, Jason Aronson, Inc. Reprinted by permission.

page 374, 375 Miller, J. Helping the suicidal client: some aspects of assessment and treatment. *Psychotherapy: Theory, Research and Practice,* vol. 17, no. 1, p. 100, 1980. Copyright 1980, the Division of Psychotherapy, American Psychological Association. Reprinted with permission.

Chapter 16

page 380 Figure 16.1 Lewinson, P. M., Mischel, W., Chaplin, W. and Barton, R. Social competence and depression: the role of illusory self-perceptions. *Journal of Abnormal Psychology,* vol. 89, no. 2, pp. 203–212, 1980. Copyright 1980 by the American Psychological Association. Reprinted by permission of the author.

page 382 Figure 16.2 Golin, S., Terrell, F., Weitz, J. and Drost, P. The illusion of control among depressed patients. *Journal of Abnormal Psychology,* vol. 88, no. 4, pp. 454–457, 1979. Copyright 1979 by the American Psychological Association. Reprinted by permission of the author.

page 389, 390 Arieti, S. Psychotherapy of Severe Depression. *American Journal of Psychiatry,* vol. 134, no. 8, pp. 864–868, 1977. Copyright 1977, the American Psychiatric Association.

page 391, 392 Kovacs, M. and Beck, A. T. Maladaptive cognitive structures in depression. *American Journal of Psychiatry,* vol. 135, no. 5, pp. 525–533, 1978. Copyright 1978, the American Psychiatric Association.

page 392 Figure 16.3 Kovacs, M., Rush, A. J. and Hollon, S. Depressed outpatients treated with cognitive therapy or pharmacotherapy. *Archives of General Psychiatry,* vol. 38, no. 1, pp. 33–39, 1981. Copyright 1981, American Medical Association. Reprinted by permission.

Chapter 17

page 401 Table 17.1. Earls, F. The prevalence of behavior problems in three year old children. *Archives of General Psychiatry,* vol. 37, no. 10, pp. 1153–1157, 1980. Copyright 1980, American Medical Association. Reprinted by permission.

page 402 Highlight 17.1. American Psychiatric Association, *Diagnostic and Statistical Manual of Mental Disorders,* Third Edition, Washington, D.C. Reprinted by permission.

page 407 Copyright 1980, by Newsweek, Inc. All Rights Reserved. Reprinted by permission.

page 414 Figure 17.1 Copyright 1980, by *Newsweek*, Inc. All Rights Reserved. Reprinted by permission.

page 415, 416 Hersen, M. The behavioral treatment of school phobia: current techniques. *Journal of Nervous and Mental Disease*, vol. 153, no. 2, pp. 99–106, 1971. Copyright 1971, the Williams & Wilkins Co., Baltimore. Reprinted by permission.

page 417 Figure 17.2 Azrin, N. H. and Thienes, P. M. Rapid Elimination of Enuresis by Intensive Learning without a Conditioning Apparatus. *Behavior Therapy*, vol. 9, pp. 342–354, 1978. Reprinted by permission of the Association for Advancement of Behavior Therapy.

page 417 Figure 17.3 Reprinted with permission from *Behavior Research and Therapy*, vol. 3, pp. 101–111, Azrin, N. H., Gottlieb, L., Hughart, L., Wesolowski, M. D. and Rahn, T. Eliminating self-injurious behavior by educative procedures. Copyright 1975, Pergamon Press, Ltd. Reprinted by permission.

Chapter 18

page 424 Bogdan, R. and Taylor, S. The Judged, Not the Judges: An Insiders View of Mental Retardation. *American Psychologist*, vol. 31, no. 1, pp. 47–52, 1976. Copyright 1976 by the American Psychological Association. Reprinted by permission of the publisher and author.

page 432 Figure 18.4 Birch, H. G., Richardson, S. A., Baird, D., Harobin, G. and Illsley, R. *Mental subnormality in the community: a clinical and epidemological study*. Baltimore: Williams and Wilkins, Co., 1970. Copyright © 1970, the Williams & Wilkins, Co., Baltimore. Reprinted by permission.

page 437 Table 18.2 Adapted from Reed, E. W. and Reed S. C. *Mental Retardation: a Family Study*. Philadelphia: W. B. Saunders, 1965.

page 441 Figure 18.5 Bigelow, G. and Griffiths, T. An Intensive Teaching Unit for Severely and Profoundly Retarded Women. From *Behaviior Modification of the Mentally Retarded*, Second Edition, edited by Travis Thompson and John Grabowski. Copyright © 1971, 1977 by Oxford University Press, Inc. Reprinted by permission.

Chapter 19

page 458 Figure 19.2 Gibbs, F. A., Gibbs, E. L. and Lennox, W. G. Influence of the Blood Sugar Level on the Wave Formation in Petit Mal Epilepsy. *Archives of Neurology and Psychiatry*, vol. 41, no. 6, pp. 1111–1116, 1939. Copyright 1939, American Medical Association. Reprinted by permission.

Chapter 20

page 470 Table 20.2 Karasu, T. B. Psychotherapies: an overview. *American Journal of Psychiatry*, vol. 134, no. 8, p. 853, 1977. Copyright 1977, the American Psychiatric Association. Reprinted by permission.

page 472 Figure 20.1 From Freeman, W. and Watts, T. W. *Psychosurgery in the treatment of mental disorder and intractable pain*. 2nd edition, 1950. Courtesy of Charles C. Thomas, Publisher, Springfield, Illinois.

page 480 Figure 20.2 Sloane, R. B., Staples, F. R., Cristol, A. H., Yorkston, N. J., and Whipple, K. Patients' Characteristics and Outcome in Psychotherapy. *Journal of Consulting and Clinical Psychology*, vol. 44, pp. 330–339, 1976. Copyright 1976 by the American Psychological Association. Reprinted by permission of the author.

page 489 Table 20.4 Meichenbaum, D. *Cognitive-Behavior Modification: An Integrated Approach*. New York: Plenum Publishing Co., 1977. Reprinted by permission.

Chapter 21

page 503 Figure 21.1 Paul, G. and Lentz, R. *Psychosocial Treatment of Chronic Mental Patients: Milieu vs Social Learning Program*. Cambridge, Mass: Harvard University Press, 1977. Copyright 1977 by Harvard University Press, Inc. Reprinted by permission.

PHOTO CREDITS

Chapter 1: pp. 3 & 6, Joel Gordon; p. 9, George Holton/Photo Researchers; p. 11 (left & right), United Press International.

Chapter 2: pp. 21 & 30 (bottom left), Bettmann Archive; p. 27 (top left) Forhistoriske Museum, Aarhus, Denmark; p. 27 (top right, bottom left & bottom right), Bettmann Archive; p. 30 (top left), The New York Public Library Picture Collection; p. 30 (top & bottom right), Bettmann Archive; p. 37 (left), National Library of Medicine; p. 37 (right), Magnum Photos; p. 39 (far left), United Press International; p. 39 (middle left & right), Wide World Photos; p. 39 (far right), National Library of Medicine.

Chapter 3: pp. 44 & 69 (bottom left) Bob Combs/Photo Researchers; p. 51, Charles Gatewood; p. 55, Bettmann Archive; p. 62 (left) Paul Seder/Taurus Photos; p. 62 (right), Erika Stone/Peter Arnold, Inc.; p. 69 (top left), Bill Stanton/Magnum Photos; p. 69 (right) Wide World Photos.

Chapter 4: pp. 74 & 81, Doug Tomsha; p. 79 (left), Doug Tomsha; p. 79 (right), Joel Gordon; p. 82, Doug Tomsha; p. 83, Harvard University Press; p. 84, Doug Tomsha.

Chapter 5: pp. 103 & 113, Martin Gershen/Photo Researchers; p. 104, Wide World Photos; p. 111, Murray Sill/*Miami Herald;* p. 115, United Press International; p. 117, United Press International; p. 118, Arthur Tress/Photo Researchers.

Chapter 6: pp. 125 & 138, Arthur Grace/Stock, Boston; p. 127, Odette Menneson-Rigaud/Photo Researchers; p. 134, Martin M. Rotker/Taurus Photos; p. 136, Robert Goldstein/Photo Researchers; p. 141, American Airlines; p. 148, Peter Menzel/Stock, Boston; p. 150, J. V. Basmajian, M.D./Chedoke Rehabilitation Center.

Chapter 7: pp. 153 & 158, Susan Rosenberg/Photo Researchers; p. 161, Jim Harrison/Stock, Boston; p. 162, HRW photo files; p. 171, Van Bucher/Photot Researchers.

Chapter 8: pp. 175 & 191, Gerald Martineau, The Washington Post; p. 181, Doug Tomsha; p. 186, Michael Weisbrot.

Chapter 9: p. 197, Wide World Photos; p. 202, Bob Levin/Black Star; p. 209, Sepp Seitz/Woodfin Camp & Associates; p. 216, Wide World Photos; p. 218 (top), Charles Gatewood; p. 218 (bottom), United Press International; p. 222, United Press International.

Chapter 10: pp. 227 & 246, Michael Weisbrot; p. 228, Ken Karp; p. 234, Erik Kroll/Taurus Photos; p. 237, United Press International; p. 241, Bettmann Archive; p. 244, Charles Marden Fitch/Taurus Photos; p. 250, Culver Pictures; p. 255 (left), Alcoholics Anonymous World Services, Inc.; p. 255 (right), United Press International.

Chapter 11: pp. 285 & 279, Michael Evans/Nancy Palmer Photo Agency; p. 261, Ed Lettau/Photo Researchers; p. 264, Wide World Photos; p. 269, United Press International; p. 271, United Press International.

Chapter 12: pp. 287 & 295, Elinor S. Reckwith/Taurus Photos; p. 290, Doug Tomsha; p. 292, Doug Tomsha; p. 297, National Library of Medicine; p. 301, Benyas-Kaufman/Black Star.

Chapter 13: p. 312, Bill Stanton/Magnum Photos; p. 314, Burk Uzzle/Magnum Photos; p. 316, James Gelvin/Magnum Photos; p. 324, Christopher S. Johnson/McLean Hospital; p. 327, Diane Walder/TIME Pix Syndication; p. 331, Ken Karp; p. 334, Doug Tomsha; p. 335, Doug Tomsha.

Chapter 14: p. 341, Ellen Pines Sheffield/Woodfin Camp & Associates; p. 346, Doug Tomsha; p. 351, Bill Stanton/Magnum Photos; p. 354, Ken Karp.

Chapter 15: pp. 361 & 363, United Press International; p. 367, Doug Tomsha; p. 372, United Press International; p. 375, Arthur Shay/TIME Pix Syndication.

Chapter 16: p. 377, Doug Tomsha; p. 379, Sylvia Johnson/Woodfin Camp & Associates; p. 382, Leo Choplin/Black Star; p. 383, Ellen Pines Sheffield/Woodfin Camp & Associates; p. 390, Owen Franker/Stock, Boston.

Chapter 17: pp. 399 & 406, Al Lowry/Photo Researchers; p. 415, Burt Glinn/Magnum Photos; p. 416, Linda Ferrer/Woodfin Camp & Associates; p. 418 (left), Michael Weisbrot; p. 418 (top & bottom right), Allan Grant.

Chapter 18: pp. 420 & 433 (left), Bruce Roberts/Photo Researchers; p. 433 (right), Photo Researchers; p. 436, W. Eugene Smith/Center for Creative Photography; p. 438, United Press International.

Chapter 19: p. 443, Armed Forces Institute of Pathology Photograph, Neg. Nos. 284425–01091 and 284425–01091; p. 445, Warren D. Jorgensen/Photo Researchers; p. 454, Woody Guthrie Publications, Inc.; p. 457, Culver Pictures.

Chapter 20: pp. 467 & 474, Doug Tomsha; p. 481, Paul Fusco/Magnum Photos; p. 485, Doug Tomsha; p. 486 (left & right) & 487 (left & right), Susan Rosenberg/Photo Researchers.

Chapter 21: pp. 495 & 511, Joel Gordon; p. 501, Jerry Cooke/Photo Researchers; p. 506, Wide World Photos; p. 508, United Press International; p. 509, Paul Fusco/Magnum Photos.

Name Index

Subject Index